The Handbook of
Forensic Rorschach Assessment

The LEA Series in Personality and Clinical Psychology
Irving B. Weiner, Editor

The Handbook of
Forensic Rorschach Assessment

Edited by
Carl B. Gacono · F. Barton Evans
with Nancy Kaser-Boyd · Lynne A. Gacono

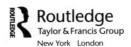
Routledge
Taylor & Francis Group
New York London

Cover design by Kathryn Houghtaling.

Lawrence Erlbaum Associates
Taylor & Francis Group
270 Madison Avenue
New York, NY 10016

Lawrence Erlbaum Associates
Taylor & Francis Group
2 Park Square
Milton Park, Abingdon
Oxon OX14 4RN

© 2008 by Taylor & Francis Group, LLC
Lawrence Erlbaum Associates is an imprint of Taylor & Francis Group, an Informa business

Printed in the United States of America on acid-free paper
10 9 8 7 6 5 4 3 2 1

International Standard Book Number-13: 978-0-8058-5823-5 (Hardcover)

Visit the Taylor & Francis Web site at
http://www.taylorandfrancis.com

This book is dedicated to
Paul Lerner and John Exner, Jr.

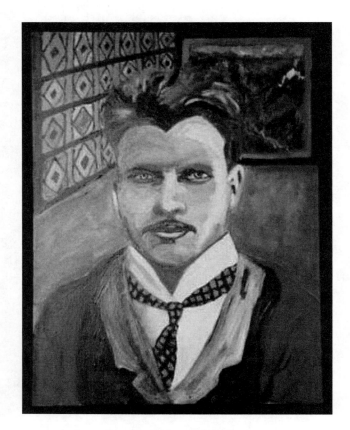

**Portrait of Hermann Rorschach
by Carl B. Gacono, PhD**

Contents

PREFACE

Carl B. Gacono
Private Practice, Austin, TX

Barton Evans
Private Practice, Bozeman, MT

The Rorschach Inkblot Method (RIM) has a long and noble tradition within the field of personality assessment. The number of RIM research studies and scholarly citations, second only to the MMPI/MMPI–2, speak to the amount of interest in the test's usage. The development of the Comprehensive System (Exner, 1997, 2003) has anchored the RIM within the mainstream of empirical personality assessment instruments, making it acceptable to use in forensic assessment (Gacono, Evans, & Vigilone, 2002).

The RIM provides an open-structured, performance-based cognitive perceptual problem-solving task that is quite different from self-report measures. As research has demonstrated (Ganellen, 1994, 1996), it is difficult to manipulate by conscious effort to underreport or overreport psychological difficulties. It is this unique element, which adds to the RIM's value in forensic assessment (Gacono, Evans, & Viglione, 2002; Ganellen, 1994, 1996; Ganellen, Wasyliw, Haywood, & Grossman, 1996; Grossman, Wasyliw, Benn, & Gyoerkoe, 2002). The refinement of a variety of relevant forensic groups (Gacono & Meloy, 1994; see chaps. 16–21, this vol.) has increased its usefulness as a forensic assessment tool.

Concurrent to these psychometric advances for the Rorschach,[1] psychology has witnessed a disturbing increase in psychological journals offering "pseudo-debates" concerning the relevance of various assessment methods or psychological tests to clinical and forensic practice (Gacono, Loving, & Bodholdt, 2001; Meyer, 1999, 2000; Weiner, 2001). We use the word "disturbing" because unqualified individuals, often academics who do not practice psychological assessment, have elevated themselves to a seemingly

---

[1]The position paper of the Board of the Society for Personality Assessment (2005), also known as the Rorschach White Paper, in which they carefully reviewed the scientific literature on the Rorschach, concluded, "This statement affirms that the Rorschach possesses reliability and validity similar to that of the generally accepted personality assessment instruments and it's responsible use in personality assessment is appropriate and justified."

expert role through their association in the literature with legitimate experts in psychological assessment. As Weiner (2001, p. 7) stated, "We've got some people who have come along and are raising criticisms ... who have never published any Rorschach research of their own and know very little about how to use the Rorschach in practice. They seem to be on some kind of crusade to bad-mouth the instrument."

Dedicated researchers and practitioners have responded by producing a substantial body of new validating research, as well as bringing a wealth of clinical/forensic experience about the inestimable value of the RIM in delivering mental health and forensic services as diagnostic consultants (Gacono, Evans, Jumes, & Loving, 2002; Meyer, 2000; Wiener, 2001). Persistent detractors have seldom demonstrated the same level of scientific rigor by weighing all available evidence, discriminating between compelling and questionable research findings, and drawing conclusions on the basis of a balanced and open-minded determination of where the facts lie (Gacono & Evans, 2004; Wiener, 2001). Rather, their rhetoric and tactics have been likened to advocacy. "An irony in this situation is the fact that contemporary Rorschach critics, while waving the banner of scientific legitimacy, are pursuing slash-and-burn tactics that have far more in common with advocacy than with science" (Weiner, 2001, p. 7). The result is that these "pseudo-debates" have an "armchair" quality about them (Hare, 1998, p.188)[2] that does little to further scientific exploration (Meyer, 2000).

The lack of applied knowledge on the part of assessment detractors, who are often not qualified as clinical or forensic experts, has resulted in a distorted picture of the issues. Their flawed or superficial understanding of essential applied theoretical and methodological issues directly impacts the manner in which the "debated" issues are presented (Gacono & Evans, 2004). More akin to politics than science, the authors demonstrate a very selective inattention to the literature, ignoring the well-designed studies demonstrating scientific robustness of the Rorschach, while emphasizing and summarizing any study they can find that seems to suggest something negative about the instrument (Meyer, 2000; Wiener, 2001). Although their "straw man" arguments sound reasonable to the naive reader (including well meaning academics who depend on peer-reviewed journals), the erroneous conclusions actually provide little useful information to either the practitioner who struggles with the ethical application of assessment measures or researchers facing the daunting work of Rorschach research. Additionally, these attacks on psychological assessment and psychological testing weaken rather than strengthen the public's view of applied psychology.

Like it or not, these "pseudo-debates," and the associated literature containing articles that do not meet the rigors of good science, eventually find their way into the court room and provide another source of distraction in an already difficult work arena. Forensic psychologists find themselves in the embarrassing and awkward position of having to ed-

---

[2]Concerning the "arm chair" quality Gacono and Bodholdt (2001) noted, "We would extend by drawing attention to the occasional recourse to rhetorical devices, including the straw man, and selective abstraction of a backwater of supposed conclusions, which on careful reading, run counter to the prevailing tone, substance or conclusion of the source-proper" (p. 66).

ucate the courts about inaccuracies on the part of these so-called experts.[3] Even psychologists very well qualified to educate the court and defend psychological assessment methods against these pseudo-debates often find themselves in lengthy and tedious cross-examinations designed to diminish the impact of their findings, sometimes by numbing juries and judges with highly technical "scientific" debate and thus losing the point of the forensic evaluation.

The aforementioned issues require active intervention by the forensic practitioner (Gacono et al., 2001). Forensic psychologists must educate their peers and others concerning what we do and how it works. Biased and scientifically unsupported attacks on one assessment instrument detract from the practice of forensic psychology as well as the practice of psychological assessment in general. It is in this spirit that we offer *The Handbook of Forensic Rorschach Assessment*. While focusing primarily on presenting guidelines for using the Rorschach in forensic practice, these chapters will assist evaluators, more broadly, in critically evaluating the advantages and disadvantages of psychological testing within the context of the forensic examination.

FORENSIC PSYCHOLOGICAL ASSESSMENT

A sophisticated and applied knowledge of psychological assessment and psychological testing, an understanding of psycholegal issues and the rules of evidence, and experience with forensic populations are essential to understanding the role of the Rorschach in forensic practice, including offering informed commentary on its efficacy. In order to evaluate the utility of the RIM in forensic assessment, one must understand what psychological assessment is and is not. First, psychological assessment does not equal psychological testing! Viewing the two as synonymous demonstrates a lack of understanding of the much broader scope of forensic work (Gacono et al., 2001; Gacono & Bodholdt, 2001). Such a misconception detracts from forensic psychologists' unique contribution to assessment, and encourages a de-emphasis of well-balanced and in-depth clinical training in graduate psychology programs. Psychological assessment is more broadly defined as a process that "integrate[s] the results of several carefully selected tests with relevant history, information and observation ... enabl[ing] the sophisticated clinician to form an accurate, in-depth understanding of the patient; formulate the most appropriate and cost-effective treatment plan; and later, monitor the course of intervention." (Meyer et al., 1998).

Alternately:

> Assessment is a *process* of deduction, selective inquiry, and also inference ... rooted in a knowledge of developmental psychology, personality and individual differences, statistics and measurement, with knowledge of limits (e.g. in prediction), in cognitive science, ethics, abnormal

---

[3]Some thoughts on how psychologists can handle challenges: Voir dire should be utilized to challenge the qualifications of these people related to their licensing status, their actual practice of psychological assessment (do they see and assess people), their knowledge of forensic practice and guidelines, their advanced standing in any recognized professional personality assessment group (i.e., fellow status in the Society for Personality Assessment), and so forth, before considering the testimony.

psychology including dynamics and defenses ... Assessment forms the cornerstone of the "forensic mind-set"—one that is data based, utilizing test data, observation, interviewing, and multi-sources of substantiated historical information in *forming, testing, and modifying hypotheses* ... Assessment is a multifaceted, ongoing, interactive process ... . (Gacono, 2000, pp. 194–195)

Forensic psychologists are always aware that psychological testing is only one component of psychological assessment, that no single data source can accurately assess the complexity inherent in forensic assessment, and that personality tests are not designed to directly assess psycholegal issues (see Otto, 2001).[4]

Having clarified the psycholegal issue and clearly understanding the limitations of any one method of obtaining information, the forensic examiner will find Monahan and Steadman's (1994) risk assessment model useful as a guide for directing specific assessment methods (Gacono, 2002a, 2000b, 2000c). Monahan et al. (2001) emphasized the need for gathering data using multiple methods from multiple domains:

1. Dispositional factors (including anger, impulsivity, psychopathy, and personality disorders).
2. Clinical or psychopathological factors (including diagnosis of mental disorder, alcohol or substance abuse, and the presence of delusions, hallucinations, or violent fantasies).
3. Historical or case history variables (including previous violence, arrest history, treatment history, history of self-harm, as well as social, work, and family history).
4. Contextual factors (including perceived stress, social support, and means for violence).

After the psychologist's role in assessing the relevant psycholegal issue is clearly defined, the forensic psychologist must determine which, if any, of the previous domains provide information needed to address the referral questions (psycholegal issue). Next, the forensic psychologist chooses reliable and valid methods and instruments for obtaining and organizing the data from the relevant domains.[5] Finally, valid results from the assessment methods are integrated into opinions that aid the trial of fact in addressing the psycholegal issue. This four-step process can be summarized as:

---

[4]Paradoxically, psychological assessment and psychological testing have been de-emphasized during a time when their usefulness has been clearly articulated (Meyer et al., 1998). In clinical settings, the de-emphasis of assessment has been rationalized as (a) too "costly" without a balanced accounting of the costs involved when it is ignored; and/or (b) "too time intensive" (actually it is the skill level of the clinician that prolongs the administration, scoring, and interpretation of the data—not inherent qualities of the test). There is also the practice of utilizing easily administered paper-and-pencil tests, which require minimal contact with the patient, with little consideration for the actual purpose of the evaluation (little if any relationship between the test and referral question). Of no surprise, these poorly conceived "window dressing" assessment protocols result in findings of little value; a finding that is subsequently used to justify the de-emphasis of formal assessment.

[5]The usefulness of psychological tests depends on the individual assessment context. For example, when assessing competency to stand trial, routine cases require semistructured interview questions to ascertain the individuals' understanding of their current legal situation, their ability to cooperate with counsel, and so forth; in a given case, personality testing may not be necessary. However, in the case of an identified psychopath (PCL–R ≥ 30) suspected of malingering Schizophrenia, the evaluation of malingering may necessitate administration of the SIRS (Rogers, 1986), observation of ward behavior, and assessment of thought disorder with the Rorschach. The same logic can be applied to other forensic issues including the assessment (not diagnosis) of psychopathy.

1. Establish referral questions/psycholegal issue.
2. Determine domains of information relevant to 1.
3. Choose assessment methods for addressing domains identified in 2.
4. Valid data is integrated into forensic opinions.

In the process of choosing assessment methods for forensic evaluations, we emphasize the need for using multiple assessment methods, such as review of collateral materials and records, clinical and semistructured interviewing, standardized psychological testing and so forth. For example, some methods, such as the PCL–R (Hare, 2003) and other semistructured interviews, are useful for collecting and quantifying certain dispositional and historical variables, whereas other methods such as the RIM and MMPI–2 add to understanding certain clinical and dispositional variables.

Although psycholegal issues suggest the relevant domains needed to be assessed, with the chosen domains guiding the psychologist's selection of assessment methods, the Federal Rules of Evidence and other legal standards guide the admissibility of psychological testimony. These standards require that expert testimony be relevant to the psycholegal issue, be of assistance to the fact finder, provide information beyond the understanding of a layperson, and not be overly prejudicial (Otto, 2001). Admissibility standards require that assessment methods, including psychological tests, must have *relevance* to the forensic issue and, as such, determine what constitutes a sound assessment strategy (McCann, 1998).

FORENSIC ASSESSMENT: ASSESSING HISTORICAL, DISPOSITIONAL, CLINICAL, AND CONTEXTUAL FACTORS

To better illustrate sound forensic assessment strategy, we use the following approach for assessing violence risk as an illustrative example. A first step in risk assessment involves a thorough review of historical and collateral information, including documentation relating to history of violence (including sexual assault), previous offenses, weapon use, and other factors relevant to specific risk concerns. This data provides historical and contextual information essential to forming an opinion. Next, the forensic psychologist assesses clinical and dispositional factors, including contemporary data on critical mental status markers, acute paranoid ideation, and delusions that require third-party corroboration from a review of treatment records, staff interviews, and other pertinent sources. Also, the evaluator reviews specific antecedents and consequents surrounding previous violent acts (contextual and dispositional) as well as the mode or type of violence (affective versus predatory). The evaluee's violence history is further clarified through interviewing concerning cognitive, affective, and behavioral patterns prior to, during, and consequent to violent episodes, as well as any current situational or dynamic factors that could be influenced by immediate intervention.[6] In addition to relevant historical, dispositional, clinical, and contextual factors, victim characteristics should also be assessed, such as age, gender, and the circumstances under which predation occurred.

---

[6]Record review and clinical interview allow identification of specific person-context factors (e.g., medication noncompliance, alcohol or drug use, level of supervision or custody) expected to mitigate or amplify more immediate risk of re-offense, including violent re-offense.

Subsequent to assessing history and mental status through a review of records and other documentation, and conducting forensic and collateral interviews, the forensic psychologist's opinions can be further enhanced by using an established actuarial risk assessment instrument such as the Violence Risk Appraisal Guide (VRAG), the Sex Offender Risk Appraisal Guide (SORAG; Quinsey, Harris, Rice, & Cormier, 1998), and/or, the HCR–20 (Webster, Douglas, Eaves, & Hart, 1997). Historical, clinical, dispositional, and contextual variables are quantified through the completion of such assessment procedures. For example, the VRAG and SORAG (Quinsey et al., 1998) are two protocols that produce a violence prediction probability estimate based on an empirically derived algorithm utilizing demographic, historical, and clinical variables, with a significant contribution made by the patient's psychopathy level assessed by the PCL–R (Hare, 1991, 2003). Although this actuarial data establishes an essential basis for forming opinions, the forensic psychologist must consider the limitations of primarily static, unchangeable data that are acquired through these methods (see Zamble & Quinsey, 1997, concerning the problems of "tombstone" predictors).

Forensic evaluation using the previous assessment domains provides a sound basis for case conceptualization. In addition, personality testing refines our understanding of dispositional or clinical factors such as impulsivity, levels of anger and hostility, presence of thought disorder, problems with affect regulation, and methods of coping with emotions (Gacono et al., 2001; Gacono & Meloy, 1994, 2002). Standardized psychological testing adds to understanding important similarities and differences among individuals to an extent not possible using only risk assessment guides and PCL–R scores that provide primarily nomothetic comparisons (Gacono, 1998). Combining historical information, risk assessment guide scores, PCL–R scores, and personality testing data allow the forensic psychologist to provide opinions emphasizing specific, individualized context-person dynamics—that is, under what circumstances a given patient is more likely to perpetrate a certain type of violence toward a particular type of victim. Such specificity allows the rigor of scientific knowledge to blend with the art of clinical insight to provide a uniquely comprehensive and human view of the individual being assessed. The forensic psychologist operates from the assumption that assessment is a multifaceted, ongoing, interactive process involving a continuous process of forming, testing, and modifying hypotheses.

CONCLUSIONS

In many jurisdictions, psychologists are called on to articulate how conclusions were derived (see *Daubert v. Merrell Dow Pharmaceuticals*, 1993). Under *Daubert* guidelines, the trier of fact evaluates the probative value of the forensic assessment using four criteria: the underlying theory or technique can and has been tested, the methodology employed has been subjected to scrutiny via peer review and publication, rates of error and classification obtained when using the technique are known and acceptable, and the degree to which the technique is accepted within the scientific community. Whereas these criteria are particularly relevant to specific methods of gathering data (individual tests), the use of the Monahan and Steadman (1994) domains for organizing global assessment strategies offers an especially comprehensive model for articulating the overall assessment process.

Additionally, it is of critical importance that forensic psychologists are cognizant of the nature and limitations of their data. For example, some data are static, whereas others are dynamic (changeable). Test scores should be considered in terms of error rates (i.e., within the context of a range of scores) and compared to corresponding normative data. Group comparisons (nomothetic data) may be only inferentially relevant to an individual case. In this manner, nomothetic data provides a starting point for interpretation; however, individual differences, teased out through multimethods and multilevels of assessment (collecting assessment data from multiple domains), are necessary to forming sound opinions.

Furthermore, the forensic psychologist has a special duty to understand how psychological tests work. This knowledge is essential for interpreting and reconciling "apparent" discrepancies among tests. Particularly relevant to the forensic context is the fact that results from self-report measures such as the MMPI–2 and MCMI–III may measure how people accurately see themselves or alternatively how they would like to appear others (McCann, 2001). As such, a given profile may be heavily influenced by the forensic context and not yield an accurate measure of the existing psychopathology. In this regard, forensic psychologists must consider the potential impact of the response style to the assessment process (Bannatyne, Gacono, & Greene, 1999). This critical issue is best assessed through a battery of tests that access different aspects of personality. In this manner, the Rorschach contributes uniquely to forensic practice (Gacono et al., 2001) in its demonstrated resistance to response style influence (Ganellen, 1994, 1996; Ganellen et al., 1996; Grossman et al., 2002).

All the chapters in this text purposely include at least one author who is a full or part-time licensed practicing forensic psychologist. The authors bring their practical expertise, guided by a systematic approach to personality assessment and knowledge of the good science, to their presentation of the Rorschach use in specific forensic contexts. In Part I (chaps. 1–6), the reader is provided with essential information related to the scientific and legal basis of the Rorschach. These chapters provide essential elements for preparing for informed court testimony. In Part II, models are presented for using the Rorschach in typical forensic evaluations (chaps. 7–15) involving both criminal (competency, insanity, risk assessment) and civil (custody, personal injury, fitness for duty). Part III contains updated references samples for various forensic populations, which are to be used as part of the ever-growing Comprehensive System database (chaps. 16–21).

In Part IV, the psychologist will find useful models for the Rorschach use in specialized areas of forensic practice (chaps. 22–25), such as with battered women, immigration court assessment, assessing impaired professionals, and working within the field of police psychology. Additionally, chapter 27 discusses how Rorschach findings are integrated with other assessment methods. It is our hope (Gacono, Evans, Kaser-Boyd, & Gacono) that this text will provide psychologists with a comprehensive resource to guide their forensic practice. It is within this context that we dedicate this text to John E. Exner and Paul Lerner, who passed away during the past year.

ACKNOWLEDGMENTS

A version of this chapter, "Introduction to a Special Series: Forensic Psychodiagnostic Testing," was previously published in *Journal of Forensic Psychology Practice, 2*(3), 1–10, 2002.

REFERENCES

Bannatyne, L., Gacono, C., & Greene, R. (1999). Differential patterns of responding among three groups of chronic, psychotic, forensic outpatients. Journal of Clinical Psychology, 55(12), 1553–1565.

Daubert v. Merrell Dow Pharmaceuticals, 516 US 869 (1995).

Exner, J. E. (1997, 2003). The Rorschach: A Comprehensive System: Basic foundations and principles of interpretation (4th ed.). Hoboken, NJ: Wiley.

Gacono, C. (1998). The use of the Psychopathy Checklist–Revised (PCL–R) and Rorschach in treatment planning with Antisocial Personality Disordered patients. *International Journal of Offender Therapy and Comparative Criminology, 42*(1), 49–64.

Gacono, C. (2000). Suggestions for the implementation and use of the Psychopathy Checklists in forensic and clinical practice. In C. B. Gacono (Ed.), *The clinical and forensic assessment of psychopathy: A practitioner's guide* (pp. 175–202). Mahwah, NJ: Lawrence Erlbaum Associates.

Gacono, C. B. (2002a). Guest editorial: Why there is a need for the personality assessment of offenders. *International Journal of Offender Therapy and Comparative Criminology, 46*, 271–273.

Gacono, C. B. (2002b). Introduction to a special series: Psychological testing in forensic settings. *International Journal of Offender Therapy and Comparative Criminology, 46*, 274–280.

Gacono, C. B. (2002c). Introduction to a special series: Forensic psychodiagnostic testing. *Journal of Forensic Psychology Practice, 2*, 1–10.

Gacono, C., & Bodholdt, R. (2001). The Role of the Psychopathy Checklist–Revised (PCL–R) in violence risk and threat assessment. *Journal of Threat Assessment, 1*(4), 65–79.

Gacono, C., & Evans, B. (2004). Entertaining reading but not science: Book review of What's wrong with the Rorschach. *International Journal of Offender Therapy & Comparative Criminology, 48*(2), 253–257.

Gacono, C., Evans, B., & Viglione, D. (2002). The Rorschach in forensic practice. *Journal of Forensic Psychology Practice, 2*(3), 33–53.

Gacono, C., Evans, B., Jumes, M., & Loving, J. (2002). The Psychopathy Checklist in forensic practice: PCL–R testimony. *Journal of Forensic Psychology Practice, 2*(3), 11–32.

Gacono, C., Loving, J., & Bodholdt, R. (2001). The Rorschach and psychopathy: Toward a more accurate understanding of the research findings. *Journal of Personality Assessment, 77*(1), 16–38.

Gacono, C., & Meloy, R. (1994). *The Rorschach assessment of aggressive and psychopathic personalities*. Hillsdale, NJ: Lawrence Erlbaum Associates.

Gacono, C., & Meloy, R. (2002). Assessing antisocial and psychopathic personalities. In J. Butcher (Ed.), *Clinical foundations of personality assessment* (2nd ed., pp. 361–375). New York: Oxford University Press.

Ganellan, R. J. (1994). Attempting to conceal psychological disturbance: MMPI defensive response sets and the Rorschach. *Journal of Personality Assessment, 63*, 423–437.

Ganellan, R. J. (1996). Exploring MMPI–Rorschach relationships. *Journal of Personality Assessment, 67*, 529–542.

Ganellen, R. J., Wasyliw, O. E., Haywood, T. W., & Grossman, L. S. (1996) Can psychosis be malingered on the Rorschach: An empirical study. *Journal of Personality Assessment, 66*, 65–80.

Grossman, L. S., Wasyliw, O. E., Benn, A. F., & Gyoerkoe, K. L. (2002). Can sex offenders who mini-mize on the MMPI conceal psychopathology on the Rorschach. *Journal of Personality Assessment, 78,* 484–501.

Hare, R. (1998). The Hare PCL–R: Some issues concerning its use and misuse. *Legal and Criminal Psychology, 3,* 99–119.

Hare, R. (1991). *Hare Psychopathy Checklist Revised (PCL–R) technical manual.* North Tonawanda, NY: Mutli-Health Systems.

Hare, R. (2003). Hare Psychopathy Checklist Revised (PCL–R) technical manual (2nd ed.). North Tonawanda, NY: Mutli-Health Systems.

McCann, J. T. (1998). Defending the Rorschach in court: An analysis of admissibility using legal and professional standards. *Journal of Personality Assessment, 70*(1), 125–144.

McCann, J. (2001). Guidelines for the forensic application of the MCMI–III. *Journal of Forensic Psychology Practice, 2.*

Meloy, R., & Gacono, C. (2000). Assessing psychopathy: psychological testing and report writing. In C. B. Gacono (Ed.), *The clinical and forensic assessment of psychopathy: A practitioner's guide* (pp. 231–250). Mahwah, NJ: Lawrence Erlbaum Associates.

Meyer, G. (1999). Introduction to the special series on the utility of the Rorschach for clinical assess-ment. *Psychological Assessment, 11*(3), 235–239.

Meyer, G. (2000). On the science of Rorschach research. *Journal of Personality Assessment, 75(1),* 46–81.

Meyer, G., Finn, S., Eyde, L., Kay, G., Kubiszyn, R., Moreland, K., Eisman, E., & Dies, R. (1998). *Ben-efits and costs of psychological assessment in healthcare delivery: Report of the Board of Profes-sional Affairs Psychological Assessment Work Group, Part I.* Washington, DC: American Psychological Association Practice Directorate.

Monahan, J., & Steadman, H. (1994). Toward a rejuvenation of risk assessment research. In J. Monahan & H. Steadman (Eds.), *Violence and mental disorder: Developments in risk assessment* (pp. 1–17). Chicago: University of Chicago Press.

Monahan, J., Steadman, H., Silver, E., Appelbaum, P., Robbins, P., Mulvey, E., Roth, L., Grisso, T., & Banks, S. (2001*). Rethinking risk assessment: The MacArthur study of mental disorder and vio-lence.* New York: Oxford.

Otto, R. (2001). Use of the MMPI–2 in forensic settings. *Journal of Forensic Psychology Practice,* 2.

Quinsey, V., Harris, G., Rice, M., & Cormier, C. (1998). *Violent offenders: Appraising and managing risk.* Washington, DC: American Psychological Association.

Webster, C. D., Douglas, K. S., Eaves, D., & Hart, S. D. (1997). *HCR–20 assessing risk for violence version 2.* Burnaby, British Columbia Mental Health Law and Policy Institute, Simon Fraser Uni-versity.

Weiner, I. (2001). Assessment advocacy—report of the SPA coordinator. *SPA Exchange, 12*(1), 7.

Zamble, E., & Quinsey, V. (1997). *The criminal recidivism process.* New York: Cambridge University Press.

ACKNOWLEDGMENTS

I would like to acknowledge, and thank, the individual authors for contributing their areas of Rorschach expertise to this volume. Their particular virtuosity and insight is evident in the exceptional quality of the text. A special acknowledgment is reserved for my wife, Lynne Gacono, for not only her emotional support and patience, but also for her tireless focus in reviewing and editing manuscripts. If not for her, this text would not have been finished.

I wish to thank Steve Rutter and Nicole Buchmann, production editors at Lawrence Erlbaum Publishers, for their patience in keeping me on track and offering encouragement throughout this project. Also, a special thanks to friends at LEA, Michele McEvoy and Lawrence (Larry) Erlbaum. Larry, as always, provided valued guidance and perspective unique among publishers.

It is with much affection that this book is dedicated to Paul M. Lerner and John Exner, Jr. They have not only severed as significant role models, but have been two of my most valued friends, colleagues, and mentors.

—*CBG*

The contributors to this book have each offered an important piece of the overall mosaic of the forensic use of the Rorschach. Far from being outside the mainstream, these authors together demonstrate in very real and practical ways that the Rorschach is alive, well, and making valuable contributions to the practice of forensic psychology.

My special appreciations are many. Endlessly energetic, relentlessly honest, creative, and brilliant, Carl Gacono is simply the very best collaborator with whom I have ever written. Deepest thanks go to dear friend Benjamin Schutz, who introduced me to the practice of forensic psychology, who has been my major forensic guide, and in many ways who is the inspiration for this book. Particular thanks also go Bruce Copeland, a long-time friend, colleague, and source of support on all things forensic and fly fishing. Sincere appreciation goes to our responsive and vastly competent editors Steve Rutter and Nicole Buchmann at LEA for their support, help, and encouragement. Words cannot begin to describe my gratitude to Larry Erlbaum, a man wise beyond his many years, who proves over and again that good relationships are the heart of good business.

On a more personal note, were it not for the sudden and devastating losses of two friends and lions of the Rorschach, Paul Lerner and John Exner, I would have dedicated this book to the following three people. I personally dedicate this book, along with my deepest love and appreciation, to my daughter Rebecca Evans and my son Samuel Evans, whose caring and honesty over the years have taught me more than they could possible imagine, and to Judy Maris, whose unwavering devotion to putting the head and the heart together inspires me like no other.

—FBE

CONTRIBUTORS

Marvin W. Acklin, Private Practice, Honolulu, HI

George I. Athey, Jr., PhD, Heritage Mental Health Clinic, Topeka, KS

Matthew R. Baity, PhD, Massachusetts General Hospital, Boston, MA

Michael Bridges, PhD, Temple University, Philadelphia, PA

Ted B. Cunliffe, PhD, California Department of Corrections and Rehabilitation, Susanville, CA

Philip S. Erdberg, PhD, Private Practice, Corte Madera, CA

F. Barton Evans, PhD, Private Practice, Bozeman, MT

Carl B. Gacono, PhD, ABAP, Clinical and Forensic Psychology, Austin, TX

Lynne A. Gacono, PhD, Austin State Hospital, Austin, TX

Ronald J. Ganellen, Northwestern University Medical School, Chicago, IL

James F. Gormally, PhD, Private Practice, Silver Spring, MD

Peter Graham, PhD, Acumen Assessments, Inc., Lawrence, KS

B. Thomas Gray, PhD, ABPP, North Texas State Hospital, Vernon, TX

Carl F. Hoppe, PhD, Private Practice, Beverly Hills, CA

Michael T. Jumes, PhD, North Texas State Hospital, Vernon, TX

Jerrald Justice, Private Practice, Walnut Creek, CA

Nancy Kaser-Boyd, PhD, Geffen School of Medicine, UCLA, Los Angeles, CA

Margaret Lee, PhD, Private Practice, Greenbrae, CA

Hale Martin, PhD, Denver University, Denver, CO

Joseph McCann, PsyD, JD, UHS Hospitals, Binghamton, NY

J. Reid Meloy, PhD, ABPP, University of California, San Diego, CA

Greg J. Meyer, PhD, University of Toledo, Toledo, OH

Nancy W. Olesen, PhD, Private Practice, San Rafael, CA

Benjamin M. Schutz, PhD, Private Practice, Springfield, VA

Jacqueline Singer, PhD, Private Practice, Sonoma, CA

Bruce L. Smith, PhD, University of California, Berkley, CA

Scott C. Stacy, PsyD, Acumen Assessments, Inc., Lawrence, KS

Donald J. Viglione, Alliant International University, San Diego, CA

Marjorie G. Walters, PhD, Private Practice, San Rafael, CA

Irving B. Weiner, PhD, ABPP, ABAP, University of South Florida, Tampa, FL

Peter A. Weiss, PhD, Interfaith Medical Center, Brooklyn, NY

William U. Weiss, PhD, University of Evansville, IN
Myla H. Young, Private Practice, Walnut Creek, CA

About the Editors

Carl B. Gacono, PhD, is a licensed psychologist who maintains a clinical and forensic private practice in Austin, Texas. Formerly the Assessment Center Director at Atascadero State Hospital and, later, the Chief Psychologist at the Federal Correctional Institution, Bastrop, Texas, he has over 20 years of correctional and institutional experience. Dr. Gacono is the author of *The Clinical and Forensic Interview Schedule for the Hare Psychopathy Checklist: Revised* and *Screening Version*, senior author of *The Rorschach Assessment of Aggressive and Psychopathic Personalities*, coeditor of *Contemporary Rorschach Interpretation*, editor of *The Clinical and Forensic Assessment of Psychopathy: A Practitioner's Guide*, and has authored or coauthored over 80 scientific articles and book chapters. He is the 1994 recipient of the Samuel J. And Anne G. Beck Award for excellence in early career research, the 2000 Walter G. Klopfer Award, a member of the American Board of Assessment Psychology, and a Fellow of the Society for Personality Assessment. Dr. Gacono is sought as an expert in the area of criminal behavior, psychopathy, treatment of conduct and antisocial personality disorders, and clinical, forensic, and research applications of the Rorschach and Psychopathy Checklists.

F. Barton Evans, PhD, is a licensed psychologist who maintains a clinical and forensic private practice in Bozeman, MT. He has practiced psychology for 30 years in wide variety of settings, including Yale University School of Medicine and Georgetown University. Dr. Evans is Clinical Professor of Psychiatry and Behavior Science at George Washington University Medical School. He is the author of a book, *Harry Stack Sullivan: Interpersonal Theory and Psychotherapy*, and has authored or coauthored over 20 scientific articles and book chapters. He is a Fellow of the Society for Personality Assessment, an officer of its Board of Trustees, and chaired its ad hoc committee responsible for the development of "The Status of the Rorschach in Clinical and Forensic Practice," also known as the Rorschach White Paper. Dr. Evans is sought as an expert in the areas of psychological issues in immigration matters, parenting plan evaluations, psychological trauma, and forensic applications of the Rorschach.

Nancy Kaser-Boyd, PhD, is a licensed psychologist who has maintained a clinical and forensic practice in Los Angeles for 25 years. She is Associate Clinical Professor in the Department of Psychiatry and Biobehavioral Sciences at UCLA Medical School, where she teaches the use of psychological tests to evaluate difficult clinical cases (e.g., factitious disorders, complicated mood disorders, effects of trauma, personality disorders) and forensic issues (e.g., dangerousness, insanity, malingering). Dr. Kaser-Boyd is coauthor of *Essentials of Rorschach Assessment*, and numerous book chapters and journal articles on evaluating trauma and forensic topics. Dr. Kaser-Boyd completed a postdoctoral fellowship at the University of Southern California Institute of Psychiatry and Law. She is member of the American Board of Assessment Psychology, and a Fellow in the Society for Personality Assessment. A member of two Los Angeles County Superior Court Panels (Criminal and Dependency), her expertise is sought in cases of severe child neglect and abuse, in family homicide, and in psychological assessments of forensic issues where she has used the Rorschach to illustrate critical mental states.

Lynne A. Gacono, PhD, is a licensed psychologist in both private and public practice. Dr. Gacono is the chairperson for the Manifest Dangerousness Committee at Austin State Hospital. She is also a member of the Texas State Forensic Committee. Her research interests and publications have involved the use of the Rorschach and MMPI–2 in assessing forensic psychiatric patients. Dr. Gacono maintains a private clinical and forensic practice in Austin, Texas, where she works with women's issues, eating disorders, addictions, chronic pain, and physical conditions.

THE HANDBOOK OF FORENSIC
RORSCHACH ASSESSMENT

I

SCIENTIFIC AND LEGAL FOUNDATIONS

1

ESSENTIAL ISSUES IN THE FORENSIC USE OF THE RORSCHACH

Carl B. Gacono
Private Practice, Austin, TX

F. Barton Evans III
Private Practice, Bozeman, MT

Donald J. Viglione
Alliant International University

The Rorschach is one of the most widely used, openly accepted, and frequently requested tests in forensic psychology practice (Meloy, 1991; Piotrowski, 1996; Weiner, Exner, & Sciara, 1996). It consistently meets the rigors of forensic scrutiny (Weiner et al., 1996). Weiner et al. (1996) found that in 7,934 recent federal and state court cases, in which psychologists presented Rorschach data, 6 cases were challenged and in just one the testimony was excluded. Uniformly, where challenges are sustained, it has not been the Rorschach's psychometric properties (Viglione & Meyer, chap. 2, this vol.) that have been impeached, but rather the psychologist's interpretations (Meloy, chap. 4, this vol.; Meloy, Hanson, & Weiner, 1997). Discredited interpretations were either too broad (used to prove a crime was committed), too narrow (aiding in diagnosis formulation without linking them to the forensic issue), or irrelevant to the legal issue before the court. Accordingly, these three caveats suggest potential pitfalls in Rorschach testimony.

Despite its favorable status and a substantial body of literature attesting to its reliability and validity (Viglione & Meyer, chap. 2, this vol.; Weiner, 1996), the Rorschach has been targeted for attack by a small group of psychologists. In fact, as with Neuropsychological assessment, it is this very acclaim and acceptance that has induced method critics to attack the test (Board of Professional Affairs, 1998; Wood & Lilienfeld, 1999). Under the guise of "good" science, the rhetoric and tactics of these detractors has been likened instead to "advocacy" or politics (Weiner, 2001a, p. 7). Weiner noted that, instead of a neutral, dispassionate, and thorough review of the literature, these critics ignored methodologically sound studies, while citing studies that emphasized negative aspects of the Rorschach (Meyer, 2000; Weiner, 2001a).[1] Such a practice ignores the very dictates of good science.

These attacks on the Rorschach are largely polemical and editorial. As Atkinson (1986) suggested, upon completing a meta-analysis with favorable results for the Rorschach, the "deprecation of the Rorschach is a sociocultural, rather than scientific, phenomenon" (p. 244). These attacks rest on a misunderstanding of clinical and forensic practice and a misrepresentation of the empirical literature.

The most vexing problem about these attacks is the manner in which ethical and moralistic language is used as a vehicle for conveying polarized positions as moral imperatives. Historically, this moralistic point of view about the Rorschach and performance based testing occurred episodically since the 1920s and these modern-day biased Rorschach criticisms are the latest incarnation of a longer tradition (Exner, 2003; Viglione & Rivera, 2003). These moral pretensions make claims about the righteousness of science and its empirical foundations, but offer no new empirical data and eschew comprehensive and balanced syntheses of the empirical based Rorschach literature. Under careful examination, the misleading tactics of these detractors becomes evident (Gacono & Evans, 2004; Martin, 2003). As stated by Gacono and Bodholdt (2001, p. 66), "We would extend by drawing attention to the occasional recourse to rhetorical devices, including the straw man, and selective abstraction of a backwater of supposed conclusions, which on careful reading, run counter to the prevailing tone, substance or conclusion of the source-proper."

Beyond any intentional biases, the conclusions of these detractors suggest that they do not understand how the Rorschach actually works (Gacono & Evans, 2004; Martin, 2003; see appendix B).[2] As noted by Weiner (1995, p. 73), "Those who currently believed the Rorschach is an unscientific or unsound test with limited utility have not read the relevant literature of the last 20 years; or, having read it, they have not grasped its meaning."

Well-trained psychologists with a sophisticated understanding of psychological constructs use the Rorschach to derive information beyond what is available from diagnosis, self-report tests, and interview. From a broader perspective, the Rorschach plays a valuable role in the description of the complex interaction among psychological, biological, environmental, and behavioral domains (Viglione & Perry, 1991), and therefore is frequently relied on in forensic evaluations (Ackerman & Ackerman, 1996, 1997).

---

[1]Summaries and meta-analyses of Rorschach research (Atkinson, Quarrington, Alp, & Cyr, 1986; Bornstein, 1996, 1999; Gacono, Loving, & Bodholdt, 2001; Meyer & Archer, in press; Hiller, Rosenthal, Bornstein, Berry, & Brunell Neuleib, 1999; Parker, Hanson, & Hunley, 1988; Viglione, 1999) reveal that Rorschach variables are associated with many criteria relevant to forensic contexts and incremental validity beyond interview, diagnosis, self-report test, and ability tests. Also, respondents' efforts to minimize problems and to present themselves in a positive light do not greatly influence Rorschach and projective test variables in contrast to self-report tests (Brems & Johnson, 1991; Bornstein, Rossner, Hill, & Stepnian, 1994; Ganellen, 1994; Harder, 1984; Shedler, Erdberg, & Haroian, 1993).

[2]Voire dire can be utilized to challenge the qualifications of these individuals regarding their licensing status, their practice of psychological assessment (do they see and assess people), their advanced standing in any recognized professional personality group (i.e., fellow staus in the Society for Personality Assessment), and so forth. In some cases, testimony might be encouraged in order to expose their lack of competence and discredit their ethical violations (i.e., practicing in areas beyond their expertise, training, and competence).

Weiner (1996) observed that critics had ignored 20 years of empirical support for the Rorschach. Taking up this challenge, Viglione (1999) reviewed 20 years of empirical investigations of the Rorschach in five major journals and found that the available data supported its validity and utility in a variety of areas. An excellent example of Weiner's observation of critics' ignoring the empirical data can be found in Grove and Barden's (1999) work advocating for the inadmissibility of the Rorschach under *Daubert/Kumho*. Ostensibly offering a "scientific" review of the evidence on reliability and validity of the instrument, these authors systematically ignored the numerous positive reliability and validity studies. Given the persistent bias against "Projective tests,"[3] Masling (1997) questioned whether data supporting the Rorschach would change the mind of the critics. He attributes some of this rigidity, politicization, and bias to the fact that former students, emboldened by their teachers, have become critics of Projective tests. This bias against the Rorschach has existed since the 1920s among American academic psychology departments and, despite the research in support of the Rorschach, a reading of the recent criticisms suggests that Masling's speculations are true.

Like it or not, these biased and unscientific opinions find their way into the courtroom through published articles and even books. Although they do little to promote scientific study (Meyer, 2000) or provide useful information to the trier of fact, such biased criticisms present an avenue for opposing attorneys to challenge when they search for possible weaknesses in psychological testimony. Forensic psychologists using the Rorschach need to prepare for this additional challenge (see chaps. 1–6 this vol.). This chapter summarizes key issues from several essential articles that will aid the examiner in preparing for forensic testimony.

ESSENTIAL ARTICLES

One positive outcome of these pseudo-debates[4] has been the publication of a plethora of excellent, scientific articles that serve as a guide for forensic Rorschach usage. The following summarizes four articles that provide a starting point for anchoring the contents of this handbook. We recommend that forensic psychologists thoroughly review the original sources.

Rorschach Testimony

Meloy (1991) provides an excellent overview for using the Rorschach in court. He emphasized six major points:
    1. The training of the examiner.

---

[3]The correct term for describing the Rorschach is a "performance-based test." It has been demonstrated that the Rorschach is a cognitive perceptual task that involves only limited amounts of "projection."

[4]We use the term "pseudo-debate" as, for the most part, Rorschach detractors have presented "legal briefs" rather than scientific reviews (Weiner, 2001b). Legal briefs are designed to present convincing arguments and evidence to support these arguments (presenting alternative evidence is the responsibility of the opposing party). A scientific review, on the other hand, is expected to present an unbiased account of the literature and to report contradictory evidence when it exists" (Barrett & Morris, 1993, pp. 201–202). Inviting individuals with little working knowledge of the test to debate has been counterproductive. By nature of the resultant publications, it has elevated unqualified professionals to the role of "Rorschach expert" and given them a voice that offers little to Rorschach science.

2. Ensuring accurate scoring and administration.
3. Having a thorough knowledge of the validity data.
4. Not overinterpreting the data.
5. Avoiding the use of psychological jargon.
6. Use of the Rorschach data in court.

Training, Scoring, and Administration.   Unlike most self-report measures, the Rorschach requires extensive course work and supervised practice to become proficient with its basic administration and scoring. In addition to course work in graduate school, achieving scoring proficiency requires advanced training with the Exner Comprehensive System (CS),[5] as well as supervision on administration and scoring. Because of the higher standards of expertise required in Forensic assessment, psychologists holding themselves out as experts on the Rorschach CS should have experience scoring 50 to 100 protocols at a minimum. Rorschach users understand that proficient scoring alone does not equal Rorschach mastery, including skillful interpretation (Gacono, DeCato, Brabender, & Goertzel, 1997).

We cannot emphasize enough the importance of proper administration. Whereas reliable scoring is seldom an issue—research has found most Rorschach variables achieve an acceptable level of agreement—inadequate inquiry can be. Specifically, because scoring is based on recorded verbalizations that are directly linked to inquiry, high levels of scoring agreement can be achieved without "proper" inquiry. For example, CBG consulted on a case where the defense hypothesized that their client committed an act of affective, rather than predatory, violence. Although the floating MMPI–2 protocol was consistent with this hypothesis, Rorschach results yielding +3 *D* and +3 *AdjD* and a *RIAP* stating that "this person has a sturdier tolerance for stress than most people and he is unlikely to experience problems with controls ..." were not. Whereas a careful examination of the protocol revealed only two nonsignificant content scoring errors, close inspection of the responses recorded during administration indicated that the examiner failed to inquire whenever the presence of shading or inanimate movement was suggested. The absence of inquiry concerning these key variables, which contribute significantly to the *D* and *AdjD*, occurred in over 12 responses. When the Structural Summary was recalculated including these "missed" *shading and inanimate movement* responses, the resultant –3 *D* and –1 *AdjD* was more consistent with both the MMPI–2 findings and the defense attorney's hypothesis. This underscores a critical point, namely, scoring reliability should only be examined after it has been determined that the test was properly administered and inquired.

Validity.   Whereas we discuss Rorschach validity at greater length in the next section, we concur with Meloy (1991) concerning the need for the forensic Rorschach examiner to not only be familiar with the validity research related to specific CS variables, but also be conversant with relevant forensic comparative data and the implications for forensic practice. These forensic reference groups (also see chaps. 16–21) have included

---

[5]Due to the extensive research and normative data, the Exner Comprehensive System has been consistently endorsed by forensic psychologists as the only system that can meet the standards of forensic scrutiny (McCann, 1998).

specific data available for: forensic psychiatric patients (Bannatyne, Gacono, & Greene, 1999; Gacono & Meloy, 1994; Gacono & Gacono, chap. 20, this vol.; Nieberding et al., 2003; Young, Justice, Erdberg, & Gacono, 2000), sex offenders (Bridges, Wilson, & Gacono, 1998; Cohan, 1998; Gacono & Meloy, 1994; Gacono, Meloy, & Bridges, 2000; Gacono, Meloy, & Bridges, chap. 18, this vol.), conduct disordered children and adolescents (Gacono, Gacono, & Evans, chap. 16, this vol.; Gacono & Meloy, 1994; Loving & Russell, 2000; Smith, Gacono, & Kaufman, 1995; Weber, Meloy, & Gacono, 1992), and antisocial and psychopathic males and females (Cunliffe, 2002; Cunliffe & Gacono, 2005; Cunliffe & Gacono, chap. 17, this vol.; Gacono & Meloy, 1994; Gacono, Meloy, & Berg, 1992; Gacono et al., 2000; Gacono, Gacono, & Evans, chap. 16, this vol.).

Interpretations, Psychological Jargon, and Rorschach Data in Court.   Psychologists' interpretations should be firmly anchored in validity research. Equally important is the manner in which Rorschach information is presented (Weiner, chap. 6, this vol.). A common trap for forensic psychologists is for attorneys on cross-examination to elicit responses to questions about reliability and validity that mimic dissertation defenses or presentations at scientific meetings. Although extraordinary technical detail about statistics, methodology, and research are important survival tactics in such settings, this kind of response in court will often bore the judge or jury to tears. This reaction is exactly what the attorney intends. Paradoxically, by going down the Alice in Wonderland rabbit hole of detailed, technical exposition of kappa, chance corrected reliabilities, and base rate sensitivities, vivid and cogent Rorschach findings can be lost and the credibility of the Forensic examiner to the trier of fact can be seriously eroded. It is incumbent on forensic psychologists to prepare counsel calling them to testify for such challenges, to use plain language in the courtroom, and to prepare short, precise, confidently stated, and understandable explanations of complex topics suitable to the average lay person.

Recent research lends support for this position. Krause and Sales (2001) found that clinical expert opinion was more persuasive than actuarial expert opinion in mock jurors' ratings about dangerousness determination and that adversarial procedures such as cross-examination or competing expert testimony had less impact on clinical expert opinion. Additionally, in a large national survey of state court judges, Gatowski et al. (2001) found that, although judges strongly endorse (91%) the utility of *Daubert/Kumho* guidelines, their clear understanding particularly behind the scientific concepts of falsifiablity (5%) and error rate (4%) was quite low. Together these studies suggest that scientific expert opinion is likely to be most persuasive when it is rich with clinical examples and where it does not overwhelm the trier of fact with arcane scientific exegesis.

As with all psychological tests, Meloy (1991) reaffirmed the ethical requirement of protecting the security of psychological tests and measures, as essential to forensic Rorschach use. Examiners should avoid photocopying copy written materials, such as location charts, and/or taking the actual Rorschach cards to court. Forensic lore includes the story of the examiner who takes the Rorschach cards to court, only to have them taken away while testifying and passed among the judge and jury. Subsequently, a rendition of the examinee's verbatim responses is used to discredit the test.

Rorschach Validity

As noted by Weiner (1996), addressing the current attacks on the Rorschach requires an understanding of the validity of psychological tests. Tests are inferential measures, and as such, their correlation with other tests provides only limited information concerning their validity. Several tests may correlate with each other, but not with observable behavior (Weiner, 1996). Correlations with observed thoughts, feelings, and actions provide more powerful information than correlations with other assessment instruments. Furthermore, the validity of any test can only be addressed by specifying the purposes for which they are more or less valid, that is, valid for what? (Weiner, 1996).

Key meta-analytic studies have confirmed that conceptual, theory-based studies demonstrate substantially higher validity coefficients for Rorschach variables than research undertaken without a theoretical or empirical rationale (Viglione & Hilsenroth, 2001; Weiner, 2001a). Conceptual validation studies of the Rorschach indicate adequate validity values equivalent to those found for the MMPI: "The MMPI and Rorschach are valid, stable, and reliable under certain circumstances. When either test is used in the manner for which it was designed and validated, its psychometric properties are likely to be adequate for either clinical or research purposes" (Parker, Hanson, & Hunsley, 1988, p. 373). Furthermore, there are at least six well-designed, original meta-analyses addressing Rorschach validity, which all find empirical support for the validity of the test (Atkinson et al., 1986; Bornstein, 1996, 1999; Hiller et al., 1999; Meyer & Archer, 2001; Parker et al., 1988).

As Weiner et al. (1996) and Meloy et al. (1997) found, validity of the Rorschach was most often questioned when interpretations were too broad, too narrow, or irrelevant to the legal issue before the court. All of these challenges fall squarely into concerns about test validity. The question for personality assessors is not whether the Rorschach is valid, rather to answer the question, "What can the Rorschach do for you?" (i.e., What is it valid for?; Weiner, 1999). These general cautions suggest an approach to Rorschach interpretation based on the specific psycholegal questions asked for the forensic assessment. Whereas Exner's (2000) interpretative search strategy is the most sophisticated method available for mining the rich data yield available in the Rorschach CS for clinical interpretation, not all CS variables are relevant to the psycholegal questions to be assessed or are empirically sturdy enough to draw definitive conclusions. It is incumbent on the Forensic psychologist to understand the construct validity research behind the CS variables and sets of variables relevant to the legal questions.

On a related note, a test must be reliable in order to be valid. Careful reading of the Rorschach literature is essential to defending the test's reliability and for revealing when a critic is only using studies that support their biases or to reveal inconsistencies and misinterpretation of existing data (Viglione & Meyer, chap. 2, this vol.). For example, in commentaries on the research, the only empirical data cited (Garb et al., 2001; Wood & Lilienfeld, 1999) to support claims of unreliability in Rorschach scoring are 8 reliability coefficients (2%) selected from 403 reported by Acklin, McDowell, Verschell, and Chan

(2000). Three of these 8 intraclass correlation coefficients (ICC) were less than .60, and mistakenly described as "low" (Garb et al., 2001, p. 436).[6]

In another criticism of Rorschach's reliability, the critics failed to include 16 studies that produced findings counter to their arguments (see Meyer, 1997a, 1997b).[7] Rorschach reliability coefficients compare quite favorably to those for other tests (Acklin et al., 2000; Exner, 1993; McDowell & Acklin, 1996; Meyer, 1997a; Meyer et al., 2002; Viglione, 1999; Viglione & Hilsenroth, 2001). Well-trained raters can score both high and low base rate CS variables with good (Kappa and ICC > .60) to excellent (> .75–. 80) reliability (Garb, 1998; Shrout & Fliess, 1979). The majority of the CS variables that are central to the interpretive variables are also reliable (Exner, 1993). Those variables without test–retest data are, for the most part, not central to interpretation or contained in other variables for which we have test–retest coefficients (Viglione & Hilsenroth, 2001).

The most glaring example related to interrater reliability is the manner in which Wood, Nezworski, Lilienfeld, and Garb (2003) misrepresent how it is computed. As noted by Gacono and Evans (2004, p. 234):

> The straw person rhetoric is no more evident than in the authors' discussion of interrater reliability (pp. 227–228). The authors provide a method for computing interrater reliability and then indicate why it is faulty. Although their presentation sounds and is plausible, it is based on a disquietingly inaccurate portrayal of how percentage agreement is computed ... which is methodologically completely and unequivocally erroneous. From a scientific perspective, what is disturbing about this example is that, even when presented with information to the contrary, the authors have stuck with their inaccurate beliefs and continue to use them as a basis for supporting their arguments.

Finally, studies reporting less than acceptable temporal consistency reliability for the CS have serious methodological flaws. These flawed studies include research with a nonstandard form of administration (Schwartz, Mebane, & Malony, 1990); a dissertation involving only 17 older adults with an unspecified test–retest interval (Erstad, 1996); and a sample of Schizophrenic patients with various illness courses, medications, hospitalizations, psychotherapies and test–retest intervals ranging from 1 to 18 years (averaging 6.4 years; Adair & Wagner, 1992).

The great majority of individual CS variables are coded with good or excellent interrater reliability (e.g., 95% in Acklin et al., 2000). Only a few very low base rate variables, typically of little interpretive significance (e.g., *MQ none*) occasionally produce poor re-

---

[6]In previous research conducted by Garb (1998), he, in agreement with experts in the psychometric literature (Cicchetti, 1981; Landis & Koch, 1977; Shrout & Fliess, 1979), defined coefficients greater than .60 as indicating "good" reliability. Additionally, among the 403 coefficients in Acklin et al. (2000), a range of over and underestimates of the true reliability would be expected due to standard errors of measurement. Standard error of measurement are especially large with low base rate variables in small samples as those included in Acklin et al. (2000).

[7]Meyer (1997a) conducted a meta-analysis of these studies and found a mean estimated Kappa of .86 and a mean percent agreement of 92% for the variables.

liability coefficients, but they have not yet been analyzed with sufficiently large samples given their minuscule base rates (Viglione & Meyer, chap. 2, this vol.).

Admissibility

McCann (1998) analyzed the admissibility of the Rorschach in court using both legal and professional standards (McCann, 1998). He systematically evaluated the Rorschach using two major sources of admissibility: expert evidence and psychometric evidence. First, McCann outlines the three most important legal tests for admissibility: the *Federal Rules of Evidence* (1992), the *Frye* test (*United States v. Frye,* 1923), and the *Daubert* standard (*Daubert v. Merrell Dow Pharmaceuticals, Inc.* 1993). Secondly, he summarizes the standards for forensic use of psychological tests set forth by two important professional articles: Heilbrun (1992) and Marlowe (1995).

Using both legal tests and professional standards, McCann ambitiously derives nine standards, including publication and peer review, standard administration and norms, reliability, validity, rate of error, general acceptance, relevance and helpfulness, falsifiability, and response style interpretation. McCann's standards go beyond legal standards, offering a more stringent test for acceptability of psychological tests in forensic settings. Using these higher standards, McCann analyzes the admissibility of the Rorschach in legal and forensic settings. In summary, McCann (1998) concludes:

> An analysis of the current clinical and research status of the Rorschach reveals that it meets professional and legal standards for admissibility of psychometric evidence and expert testimony. This conclusion rests on the foundation of a large body of literature that exists for the Exner Comprehensive System because this method of administration and scoring is standardized, has documented psychometric characteristics, and has been the primary subject of Rorschach research over the past 20 years. … Legal admissibility does not require that all scientific issues be completely resolved to the satisfaction of all members of the professional community. Expert testimony must rest on methodology that is generally accepted, testable, standardized, relevant, and helpful. In all of these respects, the Rorschach is an appropriate methodology to utilize in forensic evaluation. (pp. 140–141)

Addressing the Critics

Gacono, Loving, and Bodholdt (2001) provide an alternate format for reviewing the Rorschach's status, improving Rorschach research, and addressing biased criticisms. Rather than encouraging pseudodebates that do little to contribute to assessment improvements, Gacono et al. (2001) offer guidelines for evaluating Rorschach research related to Antisocial Personality and Psychopathy, and recommend that other experts do the same in their conceptual areas. They provided five areas of conceptual understanding that are essential to responsible criticisms of the psychopathy/ Rorschach literature:

1. Antisocial Personality Disorder (ASPD; American Psychiatric Association, 1994) and Psychopathy are related but distinct constructs, differing from each other along important historical, theoretical, and definitional lines.

2. Psychopathy may be conceptualized both in dimensional terms (i.e., along a continuum of severity) and in categorical terms (i.e., as a taxon or discrete syndrome), and that applying one of these approaches versus the other to PCL–R scores affects research findings;

3. Psychopathy may manifest in varying forms across various populations, for example across gender or throughout development from youth into adulthood.

4. Personality testing is only one facet of both psychological assessment and diagnosis. It contributes to the assessment of the dimensional aspects of Psychopathy. Research findings must be adapted for clinical application.

5. While methodological limitations inherent to certain Rorschach/Psychopathy studies may limit our ability to generalize these particular findings to other settings, they in no way invalidate the compendium of well-designed studies as certain rather persistent Rorschach detractors would have us believe. (p. 17)

Seemingly plausible sounding arguments have been presented by critics that are actually quite biased and hold little weight. For example, critics may present ASPD and Psychopathy as synonymous, lower cut-off scores for designating Psychopathy as a category, equate diagnosis with assessment, and so on (Gacono, Bodholdt, & Loving, 2001; Gacono & Evans, 2004; Gacono & Gacono, 2006). When a study includes these errors, either the critic is being naive or they are consciously promoting their own biases. In either case, ignoring any of the previous five principles provides a foothold for impeaching Rorschach critics.

In addition to outlining five key conceptual issues, Gacono et al. (2001) offered four essential criteria for reviewing the methodology of individual Psychopathy/Rorschach studies:

1. CD and ASPD are comprised of heterogeneous groups of individuals. Studies that treat Psychopathy as a taxon must validate groups with an appropriate measure (e.g. the [Psychopathology Checklist–Revised] PCL–R with adults, the PCL:YV for adolescents [or a PCL:YV prepublication—modified version of the PCL–R]) and use the accepted cut-off scores (PCL–R $\geq$ 30).

2. Studies need to account for (control or delineate) the limitations imposed by factors such as gender, sexual deviance, concurrent Axis I psychosis, age, IQ, testing setting, and legal status. These factors can influence the production of certain Rorschach variables.

3. R (number of responses) must be considered. Increased R is found in certain sex offender groups (Bridges, et al., 1998; Gacono et al., 2000), whereas low R is typical among many criminal groups (Viglione, 1999). Thus, R can act as a moderator influencing the relationship between Rorschach variables and criterion variables. Research should investigate this hypothesis by controlling R and examining the relationship between Rorschach variables and criterion constructs at different levels of R (e.g., $R = 14–17$, etc.).

4. Response style must be considered (Bannatyne et al., 1999). Variables and styles such as R, *Lambda*, *Extratensiveness,* and *Introversiveness* can impact the production of

certain Rorschach variables (Exner, 1995), contributing to seemingly discrepant findings among studies.

When a reader understands these five conceptual and four methodological criteria, they know "what to look for" in sorting pseudodebates from legitimate scientific debate. It is essential to avoid being seduced by the plausible sound of conclusions based on studies that fail to consider these issues (e.g., Brody & Rosenfeld, 2000). These conclusions are easily impeached with closer scrutiny.

For example, two recent articles addressing forensic issues (Dawes, 1999; Grove & Barden, 1999) presented a biased and unbalanced picture of the Rorschach with obvious glaring deficiencies in the authors' claims. Both of these publications fail to incorporate large bodies of empirical evidence from refereed journals demonstrating the validity of the Rorschach. (e.g., Blais, Hilsenroth, Castlebury, Fowler, & Baity, 2001; Meyer, 1997a, 1997b; 2000; Meyer & Archer, 2001; Shedler, Mayman, & Manis, 1993; Viglione, 1999; Viglione & Hilsenroth, 2001). Dawes (1999, p. 301) referred to the "deficiency" of the Rorschach in relation to the criterion of reasonable certainty employed in forensic applications. His argument is based on some elusive and illogical juxtaposition of incremental validity statistical analysis with the forensic notion that expert testimony should be "incremental" in the forensic sense of aiding the trier of facts. In making his sweeping conclusions, Dawes ignores much of the available information and research support from incremental and criterion validity for the Rorschach. In the worst case, Dawes misunderstands the Rorschach itself. For example, the requirement that the Ego Impairment Index show incremental validity over its own subcomponent in a small sample, reveals a lack of awareness of the structure of the test. Such lack of expertise is more vividly demonstrated by a description in a previous attack on the Rorschach: "Six of the Rorschach cards are black or various shades of gray, and the remaining four are colored" (Dawes, 1994, p. 146). Anyone who is familiar with the test would know that five cards are all black and gray, two are black and gray with shades of red, and three are chromatically colored without prominent black and grey features.

These unscientific and prejudiced attacks on the Rorschach obfuscate forensic issues and mislead jurists and practitioners. Most useful to the forensic psychologist would be additional Rorschach articles that, following the lead of Gacono et al. (2001), offer conceptual and methodological guidelines for evaluating other relevant bodies of literature central to Rorschach usage.

THE RORSCHACH'S ROLE IN FORENSIC ASSESSMENT

Criticisms of the Rorschach have observed that reliability and validity in the research lab is different from what might be called "field" reliability and validity (i.e., whether the test is reliable and valid as used by practitioners; e.g., Hunsley & Bailey, 1999). Following this lead, Weiner (1999) demonstrated that field incremental validity only actually manifests within a single case when it adds some unique information to an assessment. The Rorschach does this. In addition to its scores and ratios, the Rorschach provides an additional opportunity to observe the client's behavior in response to novel and complex stimuli (their performance). Observing the clients "performance" provides an added dimension to more traditional face-to-face interviewing, both essential components of most forensic evaluations.

The Rorschach also adds incrementally to the information obtained by self-report measures such as the MMPI–2. It is well-established that Rorschach scores are minimally, if at all, correlated with self-report scores in any direct or one-dimensional fashion (Archer & Krishnamurthy, 1993a, 1993b). Ironically, this difference supports the utility of the test. By measuring different aspects of personality functioning and/or measuring personality in a different way, the Rorschach's incremental validity is ensured.

Additionally, a benefit of the Rorschach rests in its ability to partially bypass an individual's volitional controls. Research supports the view that the Rorschach is most useful in contexts in which the respondent may be unwilling or unable to engage in the examination fully. Such opportunities for the Rorschach would include employment, criminal forensic, and custody evaluations that involve adversarial relationship components.

Under these adversarial conditions, response manipulation can skew or even invalidate reliable findings from self-report (Bannatyne et al., 1999). As a result, self-report data may provide little usable information in forensic contexts, beyond acknowledging distorted response style. For example, research supports the practitioners' decision to embrace the Rorschach in custody evaluations in the context of the limitations of self-report instruments. Bathurst, A. W. Gottfried, and A. E. Gottfried (1997) found that 508 custody litigation participants produced defensive MMPI–2s. Mean L, F, and K elevations were 56, 45, and 59, with 20% producing profiles with $L \geq 65$ and 25% with $K \geq 65$. Bagby, Nicholson, Buis, Radovanovic, and Fidler (1999) reported similar results, with MMPI–2 means for 115 custody litigants of 62, 48, and 58. They noted that 52% of their subjects produced either L or $K \geq 65$, and that Wiggins Social Desirability Scale and the Superlative Scale identified 74% as underreporting. Consistently, these data demonstrate that the MMPI–2 produce a limited yield in custody evaluations with 40% to 75% of litigants' results providing indeterminate and noncontributory findings. Bathurst et al. (1997) conclude, "It was not possible to determine from the MMPI–2 per se whether this approach is an overestimate of mental health in a psychologically healthy population or an attempt by psychologically disturbed individuals to conceal symptomatology"(p. 209). Bagby et al. commented that the answer to the Bathurst question "necessitates the collection of extra test data" (p. 28).

Additionally, Haywood, Grossman, Kravitz, and Wasyliw (1994) found that alleged child molesters produced even more defensive findings, with 75% of their subjects minimizing pathology according to a standard MMPI criterion. Haywood et al. also found that sexual cognitive distortions on a specific self-report instrument (Cognition Scale; Abel, Becker, & Cunningham-Rather, 1984) were similarly confounded by defensive responding. Defensiveness and constriction are consistent with findings with Antisocial offenders (Gacono & Meloy, 1994) and other forensic populations (Bannatyne et al., 1999; Nieberding et al., 2003), which further indicated the limited usefulness for self-reported tests in many, if not most, forensic settings (Gacono & Meloy, 2002). The utility of self-report scales is limited in that they do not distinguish between healthy and defensive functioning (Shedler et al., 1993) and emphasize characteristics mediated by social convention and role behavior rather than implicit motives and tacit traits (McClelland, Koestner, & Weinberger, 1989).

"What the Rorschach can do for you?" is most relevant in custody evaluations. Defensive response styles on the MMPI–2 (see Baer & Miller, 2002; Bagby et al., 1999; Bathhurst et al., 1997; Medhoff 1999; Posthuma & Harper 1998) and the MCMI (Lampel, 1999; Halon, 2001) are common in these contexts. Participants in custody battles understandably may not be willing or able to portray themselves accurately with self-report measures, making the Rorschach more valuable. This may be the reason that psychologists conducting custody evaluations often use the Rorschach for both for adults and children (Ackerman & Ackerman, 1997).

Whereas the Rorschach is often used in conjunction with other assessment methods in addressing a variety of forensic issues, it is least likely to be requested for determinations of competency to stand trial, and most likely to be sought in answering questions of sanity at the time of the crime, treatability, or dangerousness (Rogers & Cavanaugh, 1983). These trends do not eliminate its usefulness to any given forensic evaluation (see Acklin, chap. 8, this vol.; Gacono & Evans, 2004, introduction, this vol.; Gray & Acklin, 2007). For example, in the case of an identified psychopath (PCL–R $\geq$ 30) suspected of malingering Schizophrenia, the evaluation of competency to stand trial would be aided by a strategy that incorporates the Rorschach, the SIRS (Structured Interview of Reported Symptoms), the PCL–R, and collateral data. Whereas the assessment of malingering may necessitate administration of the SIRS (Rogers, Bagby, & Dickens, 1986), an observation of ward behavior, the assessment of thought disorder (with the Rorschach), and an evaluation of Psychopathy level would add weight to the examiner's conclusions. First and foremost, the context of the evaluation suggests high motivation for feigning a mental illness. Second, ward observations might reveal inconsistencies in the patient's presentation, such as interacting in a normal manner when the patient doesn't realize staff is observing. Next, the Rorschach's unusual thinking, perceptual accuracy, and reality testing indices may be inconsistent for psychosis, but consistent with character disordered or nonpatient samples. Finally, the elevated PCL–R total score along with a substantiated history of lying and conning and manipulation (PCL–R items 4 & 5 = 2s) add additional data to the hypothesis that this patient is malingering. Knowing the research and literature as suggested earlier in this chapter would lead one to know that information is also available about malingering Schizophrenia on the Rorschach (Netter & Viglione, 1994). Thus, within multiple assessment methods, the Rorschach also has multiple impacts on the evaluation outcomes. The same logic can be applied to other forensic and clinical issues.

It is important for the forensic examiner to develop a systematic strategy for inclusion of Rorschach variables in a forensic assessment. Suggested guidelines for assessing the validity of CS variables are outlined next. These guidelines are ordered from most to least relevant in terms of cogency for the forensic evaluation:

1. Are there Rorschach variables directly relevant to the legal issue before the court?
2. Where Rorschach variables are directly relevant, are there norms and construct validity research on the target forensic population?

3. Where Rorschach variables are not directly relevant to the legal issue before the court, are there CS variables with sufficient validity to be informative about pertinent personality attributes and behavioral propensities?

First, are there Rorschach variables directly relevant to the legal issue before the court? Clearly, the Rorschach is not going to directly answer the question of whether someone is competent to stand trial such as measures like Grisso's (1988) Competency Assessment Procedure. On the other hand, although not a direct measure of a legal or forensic issue, the Rorschach can quite nicely lend important data when the individual's mental health is at issue before the court (Acklin, chap. 8, this vol.; Gray & Acklin, chap. 7, this vol.). For example, the Rorschach can provide important information about whether or not an individual's thinking and perception is indicative of an underlying psychotic process.

Second, where Rorschach variables are directly relevant, are there norms and construct validity research on the target forensic population? Clearly, Exner's (2003) nonforensic, patient and nonpatient samples, and Gacono and Meloy's (1994) Forensic samples provide essential populations for comparison. Part III of this volume adds to these Forensic samples (Cunliffe & Gacono, chap. 17, this vol.; Gacono, Gacono, & Evans, chap. 16, this vol.; Gacono & Gacono, chap. 20, this vol.; Singer et al., chap. 21, this vol.).

Third, where Rorschach variables are not directly relevant to the legal issue before the court, are there CS variables with sufficient validity to be informative about pertinent personality attributes and behavioral propensities? For example, in a custody case in which one parent is alleged to have chronic difficulties with anger management, CS variables involving affect modulation, anger, and aggression, and their durability over time (such as Exner's, 1993, Test–retest studies) are likely to be relevant. Lastly, are there CS variables that due to their singular nature or to the problems of response style on other psychological tests or clinical interview shed some light on the question at hand? These variables may not have the strongest validity research (e.g., *Sx* Content variable) or may be in an experimental stage, namely, acceptance in the Comprehensive System (e.g., Armstrong's Trauma Content Index, Armstrong & Lowenstein 1990; Gacono & Meloy, 1994, Aggressive Content Scales; Gacono, Gacono, Meloy, & Baity, 2005; chap. 26, this vol.). Clearly, the Forensic psychologist will rely incrementally less on those interpretations, which either have little bearing on the specific legal question or, alternatively, lack strong validity research for a given *CS* variable.

Forensic psychologists are always cognizant of the fact that the Rorschach should be part of a multimethod approach to assessment utilizing such methods as self-report measures, clinical and structured interviews, and collateral information. All of these sources of data are needed to assess the historical, clinical, dispositional, and contextual variables required in a Forensic Psychological Assessment (Gacono, 2002; Preston & Liebert, 1990). When properly administered, scored, and interpreted, however, the Rorschach is an invaluable tool that adds incrementally to the practitioner's armament. Despite the recent re-emergence of attacks on the Rorschach, the solid research of the past

20 years, including an analysis of the test's acceptance in the courtroom, suggests that the Rorschach will continue to be widely used in clinical and forensic work for years to come.

ACKNOWLEDGMENT

This chapter is a modified version of "Introduction to a Special Series: Forensic Psychodiagnostic Testing," published in the *Journal of Forensic Psychology Practice, 2*(3), 1–10, (2002).

REFERENCES

Abel, G. G., Becker, J. V., & Cunningham-Rathner, J. (1984). Complications, consent, and cognitions in sex between children and adults. *International Journal of Law and Psychiatry, 7,* 89–103.

Ackerman, M. J., & Ackerman, M. C. (1996). Child custody practices: A 1996 survey of psychologists. Family Law Quarterly, 30, 565–586.

Ackerman, M. J., & Ackerman, M. C. (1997). Child custody evaluation practices: A survey of experienced professionals (revisited). *Professional psychology: Research and Practice, 28,* 137–145.

Acklin, M. W., McDowell II, C. J., Verschell, M. S., & Chan, D. (2000). Inter-observer agreement, intra-observer reliability, and the Rorschach comprehensive system. *Journal of Personality Assessment, 74,* 15–47

Adair, H. E., & Wagner, E. E. (1992). Stability of unusual verbalizations on the Rorschach for outpatients with schizophrenia. *Journal of Clinical Psychology, 48*(2), 250–256.

American Psychiatric Association (1994). Diagnostic and statistical manual of mental disorders (4th ed.). Washington, DC: Author.

Armstrong, J., & Lowenstein, R. (1990). Characteristics of patients with multiple personality and dissociative disorders on psychological testing. *Journal of Nervous and Mental Disease, 174,* 448–454.

Atkinson, L. (1986). The comparative validities of the Rorschach and MMPI: A meta-analysis. Canadian Psychology/Psychologie Canadienn, 27(3), 238–247.

Atkinson, L., Quarrington, B., Alp, I. E., & Cyr, J. J. (1986). Rorschach validity: An empirical approach to the literature. *Journal of Clinical Psychology, 42,* 360–362.

Archer, R. P., & Krishnamurthy, R. (1993a). Combining the Rorschach and the MMPI in the assessment of adolescents. *Journal of Personality Assessment, 60,* 132–140.

Archer, R. P., & Krishnamurthy, R. (1993b). A review of MMPI and Rorschach interrelationships in adult samples. *Journal of Personality Assessment, 61,* 277–293.

Baer, R., & Miller, J. (2002) Underreporting of psychopathology on the MMPI–2: A meta-analytic review. *Psychological Assessment, 14,* 16–26.

Bagby, R. M., Nicholson, R. A., Buis, T., & Radovanovic, H. (1999). Defensive responding on the MMPI–2 in family custody and access evaluations. *Psychological Assessment, 11,* 24–28.

Bannatyne, L. A., Gacono, C. B., & Greene, R. (1999). Differential patterns of responding among three groups of chronic psychotic forensic outpatients. *Journal of Clinical Psychology, 55*(12), 1553–1565.

Barrett, G., & Morris, S. (1993). The American Psychological Associations' amicus curiae brief in *Price Waterhaouse v. Hopkins*: The values of science versus the values of the law. *Law and Human Behavior, 17,* 201–216.

Bathurst, K., Gottfried, A. W., & Gottfried, A. E. (1997). Normative data for the MMPI–2 in child custody litigation. *Psychological Assessment, 7,* 419–423.

Blais, M. A., Hilsenroth, M. J., Castlebury, F., Fowler, J. C., & Baity, M. R. (2001). Predicting DSM–IV Cluster B personality disorder criteria from MMPI–2 and Rorschach data: A test of incremental validity. *Journal of Personality Assessment, 76,* 150–168.

Board of Professional Affairs (1998). Awards for distinguished professional contributions: John Exner. *American Psychologist, 53,* 391–392.

Bornstein, R. F. (1996). Construct validity of the Rorschach Oral Dependency scale: 1967–1995. *Psychological Assessment, 8,* 200–205.

Bornstein, R. F. (1999). Criterion validity of objective and projective dependency tests: A meta-analytic assessment of behavioral prediction. *Psychological Assessment, 11*(1), 48–57.

Bornstein, R. F., Rossner, S. C., Hill, E. L., & Stepanian, M. L. (1994). Face validity and fakability of objective and projective measures of dependency. *Journal of Personality Assessment, 63,* 363–386.

Brems, C., & Johnson, M. E. (1991). Subtle–Obvious scales of the MMPI: Indicators of profile validity in a psychiatric population. *Journal of Personality Assessment, 56*(3), 536–544.

Bridges, M., Wilson, J., & Gacono, C. B. (1998). A Rorschach investigation of defensiveness, self-perception, interpersonal relations, and affective states in incarcerated pedophiles. *Journal of Personality Assessment, 70,* 365–385.

Brody, & Rosenfeld, (2002). Object Relations in Criminal Psychopaths. *International Journal of Offender Therapy and Comparative Criminology, 46,* 4.

Cicchetti, D. V. (1994). Guidelines, criteria, and rules of thumb for evaluating normed and standardized assessment instruments in psychology. *Psychological Assessment, 6,* 284–290.

Cohan, R. (1998). *A comparison of sex offenders against minors and rapists of adults on selected Rorschach variables.* Unpublished doctoral dissertation, Wright Institute, Berkeley, CA.

Cunliffe, T. (2002). *A Rorschach investigation of incarcerated female psychopaths.* Unpublished doctoral dissertation, Pacific Graduate School of Psychology, Palo Alto, CA.

Cunliffe, T., & Gacono, C. (2005). A Rorschach investigation of incarcerated female offenders with antisocial personality disorder. *International Journal of Offender Therapy and Comparative Criminology, 49*(5), 530–546.

Daubert v. Merrell Dow Pharmaceuticals, Inc. 113 S. Ct. 2786 (1993).

Dawes, R. M. (1994). *House of cards: Psychology and psychotherapy built on myth.* New York: The Free Press.

Dawes, R. M. (1999). Two methods for studying incremental validity of a Rorschach variable. *Psychological Assessment, 11,* 297–302.

Erstad, D. (1996). *An investigation of older adults' less frequent human movement and color responses on the Rorschach.* Unpublished doctoral dissertation, Marquette University.

Exner, J. E. (1993). *The Rorschach: A Comprehensive System: Vol. 1. Basic foundations* (3rd ed.). New York: Wiley.

Exner, J. E. (1995). *A Rorschach workbook for the Comprehensive System* (5th ed.). Ashville, NC: Rorschach Workshops.

Exner. J. E. (2000). *A primer for Rorschach interpretation.* Asheville, NC: Rorschach Workshops.

Exner, J. E. (2003). *The Rorschach: A Comprehensive System: Vol. 1. Basic foundations* (4th ed.). New York: Wiley.

Federal rules of evidence. (1992). Boston: Little, Brown

Gacono, C. B. (2002). Introduction to a special series: Forensic psychodiagnostic testing. *Journal of Forensic Psychology Practice, 2*(3), 1–10.

Gacono, C., & Bodholdt, R. (2001). The role of the Psychopathy Checklist–Revised (PCL–R) in violence risk and threat assessment. *Journal of Threat Assessment, 1*(4), 65–79.

Gacono, C., DeCato, C., Brabender, V., & Goertzel, T. (1997). Vitamin C or pure C: The Rorschach of Linus Pauling. In J. R. Meloy, M. W. Acklin, C. B. Gacono, J. R. Murray, & C. A. Peterson (Eds.), *Contemporary Rorschach interpretation* (pp. 421–451). Hillsdale, NJ: Lawrence Erlbaum Associates.

Gacono, C. B., & Evans, B. (2004). Entertaining reading but not science: Book review of What's wrong with the Rorschach. *International Journal of Offender Therapy and Comparative Criminology, 48*(2), 253–257.

Gacono, C. B., & Gacono, L. A. (2006, April). Some caveats for evaluating the research on psychopathy. *The Correctional Psychologist, 38*(2), 7–9.

Gacono, C. B., Gacono, L. A., Meloy, J. R., & Baity, M. (2005). The Rorschach Extended Aggression Scores. *Rorschachiana, 27*, 164–190.

Gacono, C. B., Loving, J., & Bodholdt, R. (2001). The Rorschach and psychopathy: Toward a more accurate understanding of the research findings. *Journal of Personality Assessment, 77*(1), 16–38.

Gacono, C. B., & Meloy, J. R. (1994). *The Rorschach assessment of aggressive and psychopathic personalities*. Hillsdale, NJ: Lawrence Erlbaum Associates.

Gacono, C. B., & Meloy, J. R. (2002). Assessing antisocial and psychopathic personalities. In J. Butcher (Ed.), *Foundations of clinical personality assessment* (2nd ed.). Oxford, England: Oxford University Press.

Gacono, C., Meloy, J., & Berg, J. (1992). Object relations, defensive operations, and affective states in narcissistic, borderline, and antisocial personality. *Journal of Personality Assessment, 59*, 32–49.

Gacono, C. B., Meloy, J. R., & Bridges, M. (2000). A Rorschach study of psychopaths, sexual homicide perpetrators, and nonviolent pedophiles: Where Angels fear to tread. *Journal of Clinical Psychology, 55*(6), 1–21.

Ganellen, R. J. (1994). Attempting to conceal psychological disturbance: MMPI defensive sets and the Rorschach. *Journal or Personality Assessment, 6*, 423–437.

Garb, H. N. (1998). *Studying the clinician: Judgment research and psychological assessment*. Washington, DC: American Psychological Association.

Garb, H. N., Wood, J. M., Nezworski, M. T., Grove, W. M., & Stejskal, W. J. (2001). Towards a resolution of the Rorschach controversy. *Psychological Assessment, 13*, 433–448.

Gatowski, S. I., Dobbin, S. A., Richardson, J. T., Ginsberg, G. P., Merlino, M. I., & Dahir, V. (2001). Asking the gatekeepers: A national survey of judges in judging expert evidence in a *post-Daubert world*. *Law and Human Behavior, 25*(5), 433–458.

Grisso, T. (1988). *Competency to stand trial evaluations: A manual for practice*. Sarasota, FL: Professional Resource Exchange.

Grove, W. M., & Barden, R. C. (1999). Protecting the integrity of the legal system: The admissibility of testimony from mental health experts under *Daubert/Kumho* analyses. *Psychology, Public Policy, and Law, 5*(1), 224–242.

Halon, R. (2001). The Millon Clinical Multiaxial Inventory–III: The normal quartet in child custody cases. *American Journal of Forensic Psychology, 19*, 57–75.

Harder, D. W. (1984). Character style of the defensively high self-esteem man. *Journal of Clinical Psychology, 40*(1), 26–35.

Haywood, T. W., Kravitz, H. M., Grossman, L. S., & Wasyliw, O. E. (1994). Profiling psychological distortion in alleged child molesters. *Psychological Reports, 75*, 915–927.

Heilbrun, K. (1992). The role of psychological testing in forensic assessment. *Law and Human Behavior, 16*, 257–272.

Hiller, J. B., Rosenthal, R., Bornstein, R. F., Berry, D. T. R., & Brunell Neuleib, S. (1999). A comparative meta-analysis of Rorschach and MMPI validity. *Psychological Assessment, 11*(3), 278–296.

Hunsley, J., & Bailey, J. M. (1999). The clinical utility of the Rorschach: Unfulfilled promises and an uncertain future. *Psychological Assessment, 11*, 266–277.

Krause, D. A., & Sales, B. D. (2001). The effects of clinical and scientific expert testimony on juror decision making in capital sentencing. *Psychology, Public Policy, and Law, 7*(2), 276–310.

Landis, J. R., & Koch, G. G. (1977). The measurement of observer agreement for categorical data. *Biometrics, 33*, 159–174.

Lampel, A. (1999) Use of the Millon Clinical Multiaxial Inventory–III in evaluating child custody litigants. *American Journal of Forensic Psychology, 17*, 19–31.

Loving, J., & Russell, W. (2000). Selected Rorschach variables of psychopathic juvenile offenders. *Journal of Personality Assessment, 75*, 126–142.

Marlowe, D. B. (1995) A hybrid decision framework for evaluating psychometric evidence. *Behavioral Sciences and the Law, 13*, 207–228.

Martin, H. (2003). Scientific critique or confirmation bias? *The National Psychologist, 121*(5), 19.

Masling, J. M. (1997). On the nature and utility of projective tests and objective tests. *Journal of Personality Assessment, 69,* 257–270.

McCann, J. (1998). Defending the Rorschach in court: An analysis of admissibility using legal and professional standards. *Journal of Personality Assessment, 70*(1), 125–144.

McClelland, D. C., Koestner, R., & Weinberger, J. (1989). How do self-attributed and implicit motives differ? *Psychological Review, 96,* 690–702

McDowell, C., & Acklin, M. W. (1996). Standardizing procedures for calculating Rorschach interrater reliability: Conceptual and empirical foundations. *Journal of Personality Assessment, 66*(2), 308–320.

Medhoff, D. (1999). MMPI–2 validity scales in child custody evaluations: Clinical versus statistical significance. *Behavioral Sciences and the Law, 17,* 409–411.

Meloy, J. R. (1991, Fall/Winter). Rorschach testimony. *Journal of Psychiatry and the Law,* 221–235.

Meloy, R., Hansen, T., & Weiner, I. (1997). Authority of the Rorschach: Legal citations during the past 50 years. *Journal of Personality Assessment, 69,* 53–62.

Meyer, G. J. (1997a). Assessing reliability: Critical corrections for a critical examination of the Rorschach Comprehensive System. *Psychological Assessment, 9*(4), 480–489.

Meyer, G. J. (1997b). Thinking clearly about reliability: More critical correlations regarding the Rorschach Comprehensive system. *Psychological Assessment, 9,* 495–498.

Meyer, G. J. (2000). On the science of Rorschach research. *Journal of Personality Assessment, 75*(1), 46–81.

Meyer, G. J., & Archer, R. P. (2001). The hard science of Rorschach research: What do we know and where do we go? *Psychological Assessment, 13,* 486–502.

Meyer, G. J., Baxter, D., Exner, J. E., Jr., Fowler, C. J., Hilsenroth, M. J., Piers, C. C., & Resnick, J. (2002). An examination of interrater reliability for scoring the Rorschach Comprehensive System in eight data sets. *Journal of Personality Assessment, 78,* 219–274.

Netter, B., & Viglione, D. J. (1994). An empirical study of malingering schizophrenia on the Rorschach. *Journal of Personality Assessment, 62,* 45–57.

Nieberding, R., Gacono, C., Pirie, M., Bannatyne, L., Viglione, D., Cooper, B., Bodholdt, R., & Frackowiak, M. (2003). MMPI–2 based classification of forensic psychiatric outpatients: An exploratory cluster analytic study. *Journal of Clinical Psychology, 59*(9), 907–920.

Parker, K. C., Hanson, R. K., & Hunsley, J. (1988). MMPI, Rorschach, and WAIS: A meta-analytic comparison of reliability, stability, and validity. *Psychological Bulletin, 103*(3), 367–373.

Piotrowski, C. (1996). Use of the Rorschach in forensic practice. *Perceptual and Motor Skills, 82,* 254.

Posthuma, A, & Harper, J. (1998). Comparison of MMPI–2 responses of child custody and personal injury litigants. *Professional Psychology: Research and Practice, 2,* 437–443.

Preston, J., & Liebert, D. (1990). Defending the Rorschach in forensic cases. *American Journal of Forensic Psychology, 8*(1), 59–66.

Rogers, R., Bagby, R. M., &Dickens, S. E. (1986). *Structured Interview of Reported Symptoms manual.* Lutz, FL: PAR.

Rogers, R., & Cavanaugh, J. (1983). Usefulness of the Rorschach: A survey of forensic psychiatrists. *Journal of Psychiatry and the Law, 11,* 55–67.

Schwartz, N. S., Mebane, D. L., & Malony, H. N. (1990). Effects of alternate modes of administration on Rorschach performance of deaf adults. *Journal of Personality Assessment, 54*(3–4), 671–683.

Shaffer, T., Erdberg, P., & Haroian, J. (1999). Current nonpatient data for the Rorschach, WAIS–R, and MMPI–2. *Journal of Personality Assessment, 73,* 305–316.

Shedler, J., Mayman, M., & Manis, M. (1993). The illusion of mental health. *American Psychologist, 48,* 1117–1131.

Shrout, P. E., & Fliess, J. L. (1979). Intraclass correlations: Uses in assessing rater reliability. *Psychological Bulletin, 86,* 420–428.

Smith, A. M., Gacono, C. B., & Kaufman, L. (1997). A Rorschach comparison of psychopathic and non-psychopathic conduct disordered adolescents. *Journal of Clinical Psychology, 53*(4), 239–300.

United States v. Frye 293F. 1013 (D. C. Cir. 1923).

Viglione, D. J. (1999). A review of recent research addressing the utility of the Rorschach. *Psychological Assessment, 11*, 251–265.

Viglione, D. J., & Hilsenroth, M. (2001). The Rorschach: Facts, fictions, and future. *Psychological Assessment, 13*, 452–471.

Viglione, D. J., & Perry, W. (1991). A general model for psychological assessment and psychopathology applied to depression. *British Journal of Projective Psychology, 36*, 1–16.

Viglione, D. J., & Rivera, B. (2003). Assessing personality and psychopathology with projective tests. In J. R. Graham & J. A. Naglieri & I. B. Weiner (Eds.), *Comprehensive handbook of psychology: Assessment psychology* (Vol. 10, pp. 531–553). New York: Wiley.

Weber, C., Meloy, J., & Gacono, C. (1992). A Rorschach study of attachment and anxiety in inpatient conduct-disordered and dysthymic adolescents. *Journal of Personality Assessment, 58*, 435–438.

Weiner, I. (1995). Variable selection in Rorschach research. In J. Exner, Jr. (Ed.), *Issues and methods in Rorschach research* (pp. 73–98). Mahwah, NJ: Lawrence Erlbaum Associates.

Weiner, I. (1996). Some observations on the validity of the Rorschach Inkblot Method. *Psychological Assessment, 8*(2), 206–213.

Weiner, I. (2001a). Considerations in collecting Rorschach reference data. *Journal of Personality Assessment, 77*(1), 122–127.

Weiner, I. (2001b). Assessment advocacy—report of the SPA coordinator. *SPA Exchange, 12*, 7.

Weiner, I., Exner, J., & Sciara, A. (1996). Is the Rorschach welcome in the courtroom? *Journal of Personality Assessment, 67*(2), 422–424.

Weiner, I. B. (1999). What the Rorschach can do for you: Incremental validity in clinical applications. *Assessment, 6*, 327–339.

Wood, J. M., & Lilienfeld, S. O. (1999). The Rorschach Inkblot Test: A case of overstatement? *Assessment, 6*, 341–349.

Wood, J. M., Nezworski, M. T., Lilienfeld, S. O., & Garb, H. N. (2003). *What's wrong with the Rorschach?* San Francisco: Wiley.

Young, M. H., Justice, J. V., Erdberg, P. S., & Gacono, C. B. (2000). The incarcerated psychopath in psychiatric treatment: Management or treatment? In C. B. Gacono (Ed.), *The clinical and forensic assessment of psychopathy: A practitioner's guide* (pp. 313–331). Mahwah, NJ: Lawrence Erlbaum Associates.

2

AN OVERVIEW OF RORSCHACH PSYCHOMETRICS FOR FORENSIC PRACTICE

Donald J. Viglione
Alliant International University

Gregory J. Meyer
University of Toledo

This chapter addresses current evidence concerning the Rorschach Inkblot Test relevant to forensic practice. We present a selective overview of research findings and some new data to help explicate the scientific and empirical foundations of the test. The focus is primarily on psychometric issues of reliability, validity, normative reference values, and utility. Even when limiting ourselves to these topics, we are selective because it is not possible to address them comprehensively within a single chapter. We focus on topics of most interest in the forensic arena and that have attracted the most research and controversy lately.[1] There is no attempt to select research that supports or does not support the test, but rather a bias for selecting recent versus older and well-known and established evidence.

This review emphasizes Rorschach variables from the Comprehensive System (CS; Exner, 2003), but non-CS variables are included where relevant. In response to pressing concerns of most forensic psychologists when using the Rorschach, we address the recent criticisms of the Rorschach by synthesizing research findings. In doing so, we identify legitimate and spurious criticisms and describe and illuminate related limitations of the Rorschach. This entails our using the existing research literature and theory about the Rorschach to recommend certain alterations to interpretive practices and to identify important research needs.

CRITICISMS OF THE RORSCHACH FROM A HISTORICAL PERSPECTIVE

Before addressing psychometric issues, we present a brief historical perspective. Exner (1974) published the first edition of the Comprehensive System (CS), which was eventually recognized as being largely successful in meeting historical psychometric chal-

---

[1] For coverage of issues not included in the chapter, see Meyer and Archer (2001) and Viglione and Hilsenroth (2001).

lenges of reliability and validity. In the 1980s into the 1990s, the CS became the dominant system in teaching and practice (Hilsenroth & Handler, 1995; Mihura & Weinle, 2002) and it has become to be used extensively on an international basis (e.g., in Argentina, Belgium, Brazil, Denmark, Finland, France, Holland, Japan, Israel, Italy, Peru, Portugal, Sweden, and Spain). Exner's works are contained in three volumes with eight editions and in five editions of his workbook.

Since 1995, the Rorschach has once again been subjected to a series of repetitive critical reviews from a group of coauthors (e.g., Garb, 1999; Grove, Barden, Garb, & Lilienfeld, 2002; Hunsley & Bailey, 1999, 2001; Lilienfeld, Wood, & Garb, 2000; Nezworski & Wood, 1995; Wood & Lilienfeld, 1999; Wood, Nezworski, Garb, & Lilienfeld, 2001a; Wood, Nezworski, Garb, & Lilienfeld, 2001b; Wood, Nezworski, & Stejskal, 1996), although controversy has existed since its origin (e.g., Hirt, 1962; Murstein, 1965; Rabin, 1981; Viglione & Rivera, 2003). Some of these criticisms are written to challenge the Rorschach in court (e.g., Dawes, 1999; Grove & Barden, 1999; Grove et al, 2002; Lilienfeld et al., 2000; Wood et al., 1996). Criticisms and controversies have waxed and waned in the literature. A regular tension has emerged between practitioners using the Rorschach, many of whom find the Rorschach to be indispensable in their applied work, and some academic researchers who consider the Rorschach and its evidentiary foundation to be fundamentally flawed.

Atkinson, Quarrington, Alp, and Cyr (1986), after presenting results from one of the earliest meta-analytic reviews on Rorschach validity, questioned why its validity is continuously challenged despite the evidence. They asserted bluntly, "The oft-cited explanation is that deprecation of the Rorschach is a sociocultural, rather than scientific, phenomenon" (p. 244). Others have asked whether the debate about the utility of the Rorschach is more philosophical and political, rather than academic and scientific (Viglione & Rivera, 2003).

To a degree, these recent challenges of the Rorschach and the CS prompted the current book on forensic issues. Although the controversy is part political and philosophical debate and part scientific and rational debate, one goal is to focus on the latter. Nevertheless, because it is probably impossible to step outside of the former, we note that we consider ourselves political centrists when it comes to the Rorschach. That is, we believe the evidence supports its use in clinical practice, but we also believe that, like all tests, it has its limitations. Continued research is needed to specify the applications and limitation for many interpretive postulates. Like all tests, it needs to be used cautiously and conscientiously.

RELIABILITY: DO WE MEASURE CONSISTENTLY?

Reliability can be globally defined as the extent to which a construct is assessed consistently. Once we are measuring something consistently, it is necessary to establish that what is being measured is actually what we want to measure (validity) and that the measured information is helpful in some applied manner (utility). We focus on reliability first.

There are four main types of reliability—internal consistency, stability, alternate forms, and interrater. *Internal consistency reliability* refers to the consistency or homogeneity of content over items, that is, whether the items of a scale or test measure the same construct. In the Rorschach, the notion of an item would have two meanings. First, responses or cards could be considered items. This form of internal consistency reliability entails an assumption that each card or response provides an equal opportunity to measure the same construct (Exner, Armbruster, & Viglione, 1978). However, it is readily recognized that each card does not allow an equal opportunity for all scores (e.g., cards vary greatly in their pull for color or texture determinants), so that internal consistency reliability is infrequently evaluated or reported and it is considered largely inapplicable to the test.

In terms of internal consistency reliability, an item also translates to the individual subcomponents or criteria of composite indices (e.g., the subcomponents of the *DEPI* or Ego Impairment Index, *EII*). As an example of this version of internal consistency research, Hilsenroth, Fowler, and Padawer (1998) and Stokes, Pogge, Grosso, and Zaccario (2001) examined the internal consistency of the six criteria forming the Schizophrenia Index (*SCZI*), whereas Dao and Prevatt (2006) examined the five criteria of its successor, the Perceptual Thinking Index (*PTI*). Although they found evidence for a reasonable degree of homogeneity (*KR—20* = .79, .70, and .75, respectively), these analyses are difficult to interpret because the six *SCZI* and five *PTI* criteria draw on just two types of scores, form quality and the cognitive special scores. As such, there should be a certain degree of artificial correlation among the criteria, although the precise magnitude would be hard to determine.

More substantively, the *SCZI* or *PTI* and all the other CS Constellation Indices were created as composites that draw on the full range of information available in a protocol to maximize validity; they were not developed as scales designed to measure a single homogeneous construct. As Streiner (2003) has pointed out, internal consistency reliability is important for scales assessing a homogenous construct but immaterial for a composite index. Indeed, efficiency in measurement is achieved through low rather than high intercorrelations among subcomponents or items. Accordingly, weak internal consistency reliability can accompany strong validity and utility.

Another type of reliability that has been largely considered inapplicable to the Rorschach is *alternate forms reliability*, which assesses the consistency of scores across parallel versions of an instrument. Although Holtzman specifically developed his set of inkblots to have two parallel forms and Behn-Eschenberg made an early effort at developing a set of inkblots to parallel Rorschach's inkblots (see, e.g., Exner, 2003, p. 12), at present a good parallel set of the 10 standard Rorschach inkblots does not exist.

Stability reliability, also known as temporal consistency or test–retest reliability, is essentially the consistency of scores over time. It has been applied to the Rorschach and the results generally have been acceptable to good (Grønnerød, 2003; Meyer & Archer, 2001; Viglione & Hilsenroth, 2001). Comprehensive System scores thought to measure traitlike aspects of personality have produced relatively high retest coefficients, even over extended time periods. Also, scores thought to reflect statelike emotional process have produced relatively low retest coefficients even over short time intervals.

However, the most recent large-scale and well-designed study of CS stability found lower than anticipated consistency over a 3-month retest period (Sultan, Andronikof, Réveilòre, & Lemmel, 2006). For instance, stability coefficients for *R* and *Lambda*, which index the overall richness or complexity of a protocol, were .75 and .72, respectively. Because these scores are related to the frequency of other scores in the protocol, when they are unstable most other scores will be unstable as well. Indeed, in this study the median level of stability reliability across a core set of 47 scores was .53 and the median across 87 ratios, percentages, and derivations in the lower portion of the Structural Summary was .55. Number of responses (R) and *Lambda*, as markers of task engagement, moderated stability. Stability reliability was greater among those individuals whose R and *Lambda* did not change much over time, as compared to the stability among those individuals whose R and *Lambda* differed at the two testings.

Conducted in France, the Sultan et al. study was a carefully executed investigation with a sound methodology and adequate controls. It also used the most sophisticated statistical analyses to date to examine potential moderators of stability, and several were identified that would increase stability if they were controlled (e.g., engagement with the Rorschach task, situational distress/emotional status). Variation over time due to situational distress or emotional status is not related to the true stability reliability of the test, so that test–retest statistics underestimate the Rorschach's true reliability. Nevertheless, even taking this situational variation into consideration, the stability for the majority of the Rorschach CS variables in this study was limited.

More investigation of Rorschach stability reliability is needed (Meyer & Archer, 2001; Viglione & Hilsenroth, 2001), and Sultan et al.'s (2006) findings should be replicated. However, given the care that went into designing and executing this study, forensic examiners should be aware of the challenges to the CS that might emerge in the courtroom from these data. The Sultan data indicate that nonpatient volunteers for a study can provide notably different protocols when tested by one reasonably trained examiner and again 3 months later by a different reasonably trained examiner. This finding will remain even if it is subsequently discovered that certain methodological factors account for the lower than expected stability or if the majority of future studies find superior stability.

Putting these results in context might be illuminating. Forensic examiners should recognize that the global stability of Rorschach scores might, under some circumstances, be more similar to the stability of memory tests than the stability of intelligence tests. For instance, although the manual for the third edition of the Wechsler Memory scale (WMS; Psychological Corporation, 1997) does not report data for all subscales, the 1-month stability for 13 of its subscores is .71 ($N = 297$). Over a 7 ½-month retest interval, the average stability coefficient for 5 of its subscores was .66 (Dikmen, Heaton, Grant, & Temkin, 1999) and over a 9-month interval the average stability for 10 scores was .68 (Martin et al., 2002). Although these coefficients are higher than those observed in Sultan et al., more similar stability values are found for tests like the California Verbal Learning Test (CVLT) and the Hopkins Verbal Learning Test (HVLT). Over a retest interval of 1 to 2 months, the average stability of HVLT scores was about .50 (Barr, 2003; Benedict, Schretlen, Groninger, & Brandt, 1998). Average stability for CVLT scores also has been about .50 over a 1-year retest interval (Paolo, Tröster, & Ryan, 1997). Finally, as another example, the average stability of scores on the Extended Complex Figure Test was .46 over the course of a 1-week interval ($N = 55$; Woodrome & Fastenau, 2005). It should be pointed out that memory ability is thought to be a stable trait similar to many personality and information-processing variables accessed by the Rorschach and, as such, should possess stability reliability.

Forensic examiners addressing work-related issues might also note that the Sultan et al. (2006) findings are similar to the stability of job performance measures. In a recent meta-analysis, Sturman, Cheramie, and Cashen (2005) found that over a 6-month retest interval, the temporal consistency of objective job performance measures was .45. For both objective and subjective measures of job performance, consistency was .56.

In a summary of the research data available at the time, Viglione and Hilsenroth (2001) reported that CS stability was adequate or better in all respects, especially in the context of comparing Rorschach findings to other personality tests. Revisiting the data about other tests leads to the conclusion that the level of stability reported by Sultan is similar to that reported for the MMPI in a meta-analysis over a 1-year period (Mauger, 1972; Stone, 1965; Sines, Silver, & Lucero, 1961; all as cited in Dahlstrom, Welsh, & Dahlstrom, 1975; Milott, Lira, & Miller, 1977; Ryan, Dunn, & Paolo, 1995). The Sultan stability reliability coefficients are also similar to those reported in a comprehensive meta-analysis of self-report, observer, and performance tests of personality (Roberts & Del Vecchio, 2000), but less than that reported in a more limited and less definitive meta-analysis of eight self-report tests over a 1-year period (Schuerger, Zarrella, & Holtz, 1989). At this point, forensic examiners should be alert to the possibility, based on this one study, that CS scores can be more changeable and responsive to statelike influences than previously thought. In forensic cases, when making dispositional attributions, examiners might consider repeating a Rorschach and other personality assessment measures to more definitively differentiate state and trait influences.

The type of reliability that has received the most attention recently—and one that may be most relevant to forensic practice—is *interrater reliability,* or the consistency of judgments across raters. For the Rorschach, this type of reliability concerns coding (scoring) reliability as well as the reliability of interpretation across test users. We address research in coding reliability because it has received most of the recent research attention. For issues involving interpretive reliability, we refer to Meyer, Mihura, and Smith (2005).

Exner (2003) has primarily presented percentage agreement (%A) between coders as a means of addressing interrater reliability and coding accuracy. Percentage agreement is the proportion of responses in which two raters agree on a code, that is, code a given response parameter the same way. He had required that any code have a %A of 80% to be included in the CS. Weiner (1991) also required that studies submitted to the *Journal of Personality Assessment* meet this %A benchmark for 20 records. For example, for *Human Movement (M)*, if two raters independently code 50 responses and agree 45 times on the presence or absence of M, then %A = 90%. However, M only occurs in about one fifth of responses from adults, so that two raters are expected to agree, by chance, about 70% of the time. This high incidence of chance agreement occurs largely because raters with knowledge of base rates could agree that M is absent even if they randomly scored M. Accordingly, %A does not consider base rates and chance agreement, and it overestimates reliability for single scores, so that it has been subjected to criticism (Wood et al., 1996).

Although true in some respects, criticism of %A has been greatly overextended to all types of coding and response combinations. It is not nearly as problematic for response segments that have multiple choices for codes. The term *response segment* refers to a coding category, for example, determinants or content. To achieve agreement for determinants, one would have to agree on all determinants in a given response (e.g., *FT.CF* and *FT.CF* represents an agreement, whereas *FT.CF* and *FT.FC* do not.) Obviously, chance agreement for response segments (e.g., determinants or content) is much lower than it is for individual codes. For determinants and content chance %A is about 20%; for all special scores chance %A is about 40%; for location, *DQ*, and *FQ* chance %A is about 30%–50% (Meyer, 1997a, 1997c). Thus, it is mathematically impossible to discount 80% agreement for response segments among 20 records as being due to chance.

Nevertheless, there are preferred statistics that do take base rate into consideration, namely, kappa for response level data and the intraclass correlation (ICC) for protocol level data. Kappa is appropriate for nominal or categorical variables, as represented by individual Rorschach scores or codes. Accordingly, if one wanted to evaluate how reliably two raters or two teams of raters scored *Texture* (*T*) on a response by response basis, one could use kappa. This statistic could, for example, estimate reliability for the presence or absence of any form of *T*. Alternatively, it could detect whether or not raters reliably distinguished between *FT, TF, T* and no Texture.

Whereas kappa is applied to response-level variables, the ICC is applied to dimensional variables at the protocol level. In other words, if one wanted to evaluate the reliability of the sum of all *T* responses, *X* – %, or the Suicide Constellation across records, ICC is ideal. Score levels and interpretation of ICC are equivalent to kappa, and it is an excellent statistic for Rorschach summary scores (i.e., those types of scores that are found on the CS Structural Summary). Given that the preponderance of interpretive inferences emerges from the Structural Summary, the ICC is more related to the foundation of interpretation and how the test is used in practice. Kappa, however, may be more useful in training raters and evaluating the ease to which a new score can be coded.

Janson (Janson & Olsson, 2001, 2004) has introduced a new statistic called iota. As a more general statistic, it can be used instead of kappa or ICC. It is a multivariable extension of kappa and can be applied to response level variables (e.g., individual codes), response segments (e.g., determinants or contents in a given response), or even all the codes of a response or protocol in its entirety. Like the ICC, it also can also be applied to dimensional or protocol level variables. Accordingly, it has considerable flexibility and is recommended for research and training. For training or forensic applications, one could measure the reliability or agreement of two raters for a single record across all scores.

Given that kappa, ICC, and iota are more demanding types of reliability statistics, the benchmarks for interpreting their magnitude differ from those associated with Pearson *r* and %A. Kappa, ICC, and iota at .75 or above is considered excellent, .60 and above good, and .40 and above fair (Cicchetti, 1994; Shrout & Fliess, 1979).

There are four meta-analyses addressing Rorschach interrater reliability. Two related studies address CS reliability (Meyer, 1997a, 1997c; Meyer et al., 2002) and the others address two non-CS scales, the Rorschach Prognostic Rating scale and the Rorschach Oral Dependency scale (see Meyer, 2004). Meyer (2004) compared these interrater reliability data to all the other meta-analyses of interrater reliability available at the time. Comparisons with these other types of judgments allow forensic psychologists—or indeed an attorney, judge, or jury—to derive a "gut feel" sense of how the reliability of the Rorschach fares.

These interrater reliability comparisons are presented in Table 2–1.[2] Reliabilities are presented separately for scale-level judgments and item-level judgments. With each type of judgment, the average reliability coefficient is listed along with the number of pairs of ratings summarized. For the Rorschach, scale data corresponds to protocol level summary scores, whereas item data corresponds to coding determinations made on individual responses. A consistent pattern is that scale reliabilities exceed item reliabilities because random errors tend to cancel each other out when items are aggregated to form scales. The overall reliability of the Rorschach CS and Rorschach Oral Dependent scale are excellent with summary score coefficients about .90 and response-level judgments in the range between .80 and .85. The Rorschach Prognostic Rating scale reliability is not as high, with $r = .84$ for summary scores, but still more than adequate.

Thus, one must conclude that the Rorschach interrater reliability is good to excellent and compares favorably to a wide range of determinations made in psychology and medicine. Attorneys, judges, or juries may be very interested to know that the Rorschach raters agree much more than do superiors' evaluations of job performance, surgeons/nurses' diagnoses of breast abnormalities, and physicians' estimations of the quality of medical care from record review, all of which are subject to considerable disagreement and inconsistency across raters. Rorschach CS and Oral Dependent scale coding determinations have the same degree of agreement or reliability as do simple, physical measurements in medicine. For example, Rorschach coding is as reliable as estimating the size of the spinal canal and spinal cord from MRI, CT, or x-ray scans, or counts of decayed, filled, or missing teeth in early childhood. These comparisons are consistent with the conclusion that Rorschach coding for the trained examiner is typically a relatively straightforward process, one in which consistency and agreement are attainable across raters.

Clearly, the answer to the question, "Do we code reliably?" is yes, as well-trained and motivated raters code reliably. However, there are limitations. Several studies reported that standard errors of reliabilities of low base rate variables are large so that their reliability estimates are erratic (Acklin, 1999; Acklin, McDowell, & Verschell, 2000; Meyer, 1997a, 1997c; Meyer et al., 2002; Viglione & Taylor, 2001). Low base rate variables, for example, sex, reflections, color projection, or refined variables[3] can be loosely defined as occurring on the average once or less often per record. This is a

---

[2]Meyer (2004) compared types of statistics, contrasting r with kappa or the ICC. Across 16 topics that provided both types of statistics, the mean kappa/ICC was .70 and the mean r was .74. Because these differences are not large, the findings for those 16 topics were combined in our version of the table. Our table also differs slightly from Meyer's (2004) in that it presents two coefficients for job selection interviews (one for joint interviews and one for separately conducted interviews), rather than just a single undifferentiated coefficient.

[3]Weiner (2001) described refined variables as coding combinations that encompass multiple categories, so that $M-$, $WS+$, or M^a with *Pure H* are refined variables. In contrast, M, W, and H are unrefined variables. He stated that refined variables are more likely to demonstrate validity in research. There is not a great deal of research with refined variables, presumably because large samples are needed.

TABLE 2–1

Meta-Analyses of Interrater Reliability in the Psychological and Medical Literature

Target reliability construct	n(k–1) = independent pairs of judgments		Reliability r/κ/ICC	
	Scale	Item	Scale	Item
1. Measured bladder volume by real-time ultrasound		360		.92[b]
2. Measured size of spinal canal and spinal cord on MRI, CT, or X-ray	200	86	.90[a]	.88[a]
3. Count of decayed, filled, or missing teeth (or surfaces) in young children	113	237	.97[a]	.79[c]
4. Rorschach Oral Dependency Scale scoring	974	6,430	.91[b]	.84[c]
5. Scoring the Rorschach Comprehensive System: Summary scores	784		.91[b]	
Response segments		11,518		.86[c]
Scores per response		11,572		.83[c]
6. Neuropsychologists' test-based judgments of cognitive impairment		901		.80[c]
7. Hamilton Depression Rating Scale scoring from joint interviews[d]	3,847	495	.86[b]	.71[b]
8. Level of drug sedation by ICU physicians or nurses	1,116	165	.86[b]	.71[c]
9. Functional independence measure scoring (joint and separate interviews)	1,365	1,345	.91[c]	.62[c]
10. TAT Personal Problem-Solving Scale scoring	385		.85[b]	
11. Rorschach Prognostic Rating Scale scoring	472		.84[a]	
12. TAT Social Cognition and Object Relations Scale scoring	934		.82[b]	
13. TAT Defense Mechanism Manual scoring	743		.80[b]	
14. Hamilton Anxiety Rating Scale scoring from joint interviews[d]	752	214	.80[b]	.72[c]
15. Borderline personality disorder (joint and separate interviews) Diagnosis	402		.82[c]	
Specific symptoms		198		.64[c]
16. Signs and symptoms of temporomandibular disorder (separate exams)	192	562	.86[c]	.56[c]
17. Hamilton Depression Rating Scale scoring from separate interviews	1,012	597	.82[b]	.52[b]
18. Therapist or observer ratings of therapeutic alliance in treatment	(S = 31)		.78[a]	
19. Job selection ratings by joint interviews	9,364		.77[a]	
20. Hamilton Anxiety Rating Scale scoring from separate interviews	268	208	.76[b]	.58[c]
21. Axis I psychiatric diagnosis by SCID in joint interviews	216		.75[c]	
22. Type A behavior pattern by structured interview	(S = 3)		.74[a]	
23. Axis II psychiatric diagnosis by semistructured joint interviews	740		.73[c]	
24. Personality or temperament of mammals (variable observations)	151	637	.71[a]	.49[a]

		$n(k-1)$ = independent pairs of judgments		Reliability $r/\kappa/ICC$	
Target reliability construct		Scale	Item	Scale	Item
25. Visual analysis of plotted behavior change in single-case research			1,277		.57[b]
26. Editors' ratings of the quality of manuscript reviews or reviewers			3,721		.54[b]
27. Presence of clubbing in fingers or toes[e]			630		.52[c]
28. Stroke classification by neurologists			1,362		.51[c]
29. Child or adolescent problems:	Teacher ratings	2,100		.64[a]	
	Parent ratings	4,666		.59[a]	
	Externalizing	7,710		.60[a]	
	Internalizing	5,178		.54[a]	
	Direct observers	231		.57[a]	
	Clinicians	729		.54[a]	
30. Job performance ratings by supervisors		1,603	10,119	.57[a]	.48[a]
31. Axis I psychiatric diagnosis by SCID in separate interviews		693		.56[c]	
32. Job selection ratings by separate interviews		3,185		.53[a]	
33. Axis II Psychiatric diagnosis by semistructured separate interviews		358		.52[c]	
34. Self and partner ratings of conflict:	Men's aggression	616		.55[a]	
	Women's aggression	616		.51[a]	
35. Determination of systolic heart murmur by cardiologists			500		.45[c]
36. Abnormalities on clinical breast examination by surgeons or nurses			1,720		.42[c]
37. Mean quality scores from two grant panels:	Dimensional ratings		2,467		.43[b]
	Yes/No decision		398		.39[c]
38. Job performance ratings by peers		1,215	6,049	.43[a]	.37[a]
39. Number of factors in a correlation matrix by scree plots[f]			2,300		.35[c]
40. Medical quality of care as determined by physician peers			9,841		.31[c]
41. Job performance ratings by subordinates		533	4,500	.29[a]	.31[a]
42. Definitions of invasive fungal infection in the research literature			21,653		.25[c]
43. Research quality by peer-reviewers:	Dimensional ratings		31,068	.25[b]	
	Yes/No decision		4,807		.21[c]

Note. Adapted from Meyer (2004), which provides a complete description of the meta-analytic data sources contributing to this table. ICC = intraclass correlation, ICU = intensive care unit, S = number of studies contributing data, SCID = Structured Clinical Interview for the *Diagnostic and Statistical Manual of Mental Disorders* (DSM), and TAT = Thematic Apperception Test.

[a]Pearson's *r*. [b]Combination of *r* and κ or agreement ICC. [c]κ or agreement ICC. [d]Category includes videotaped interviews and instances when the patient's report fully determined both sets of ratings (e.g., identical questions in written and oral format). [e]One study produced outlier results (κ = .90) relative to the others (κ range from .36–.45) so the results should be considered tentative. [f]Finding should be treated cautiously because agreement varied widely across studies, with values below .10 in several samples but above .70 in several others.

statistical issue and one would need large samples to accurately estimate reliability for low base rate variables.

In addition, there are some codes for which reliabilities are lower so that they are presumably more of a challenge to code accurately. Table 2–2 identifies these CS codes associated with lower reliabilities in multiple research reports. Forensic examiners should pay special care to code these variables accurately, consistent with CS principles. Some examiners have protocols in high-stakes cases blindly rescored by a colleague. Viglione wrote *Rorschach Coding Solutions* (2002) to address these and other coding challenges. Along with the workbook (Exner et al., 2001) and volume I text (Exner, 2003), it is a good resource to consult to eliminate rater drift from CS standards. Indeed, interrater reliability is not a fixed property of the score or instrument. In forensic practice, this means that what counts is the reliability of the person who coded the protocol, not the general reliability found in the literature. As such, it would behoove forensic examiners to document that they have achieved good interrater reliability with another expert rater.

In the forensic arena, the single most problematic implication of the data on variables with lower reliabilities might be the possibility of over coding *ALOG*, *DR*, and *FQ–* so as to overestimate pathology, thought disorder, and the likelihood of a psychotic or schizo-

TABLE 2–2

CS Codes Decisions with Lower Reliabilities in Some Studies

Developmental Quality

   DQv and *DQv/+*

Form Dominance

   FC vs. *CF* vs. *C*

   Form Shading vs. *Shading Form* vs. *Shading*

Shading Subtypes

   Y vs. *T* vs. *C'* vs. *V*

Form Quality

   Occasionally *FQ* subcategories, especially *FQu*

   Failure to code or neglect of *FQ+*

Contents

   Art, Ay, Sc, Bt vs. *Na* vs. *Ls, Id*

Special Scores

   DV vs. *INC*

   ALOG vs. no special score, coding too many *ALOG*s

   CONTAM vs. *INC*

   PER or *DR* vs. task comment, coding too many *DR*s

   Level 1 vs. *Level 2*

phrenic diagnosis. In forensic assessment, such an error might translate to underestimates of, for example, sanity, capacity, culpability, or parenting ability. Some comfort can be drawn by the fact that the research indicates that the summary scores for cognitive special scores, *WSum6* and *Sum6*, generally demonstrate better reliability than do the individual scores (e.g., *DV2* or *ALOG* individually). This superior reliability is important because interpretation is primarily based on these summary scores rather than on individual cognitive special score codes.

Research reports from around the world (Erdberg, 2005; Viglione, 1999; Viglione & Hilsenroth, 2001) also reveal that the CS is transportable to other languages and cultures and that coding reliability is very similar to the results from the meta-analyses. For the most part, those codes that achieve lower or more variable reliabilities in U.S. samples are the same as codes that are more variable in the international samples (Exner et al., 1999).

Another issue or complication is that most reliability research studies generally use raters who work or train in the same setting. If local guidelines develop to contend with scoring ambiguity, agreement among those who work or train together may be greater than agreement across different sites or workgroups. Thus, existing reliability research may then give an overly optimistic view of reliability across sites or across forensic examiners working independently.

In a preliminary presentation, Meyer, Viglione, Erdberg, Exner, and Shaffer (2004) examined this across site interreliability issue by having 40 randomly selected protocols from Exner's new CS nonpatient reference group sample and 40 protocols from Shaffer, Erdberg, and Haroian's (1999) from a California (CA) sample recoded by a third group of trained raters. This third group, advanced graduate students supervised in Viglione's lab, were blind to the original coding, the origin of the samples, and the nature and purpose of the study. The coding assigned by the original sites was compared to the coding assigned by this single additional site and yielded an across site median ICC of .72, an acceptable level of reliability in the good range.

These across site results can be contrasted with within site data sets, that is, samples coded by raters working in the same setting. We have three such relevant within site research reports available to us: (a) the meta-analysis data in Table 2–1, (b) a large international sample (Erdberg, 2005), and (c) a smaller sample from Viglione's lab. All report greater reliabilities than our across site median ICC of .72. As noted earlier, the Table 2–1 meta-analysis yields a reliability estimate for summary scores of .91. Erdberg (2005) compiled 467 protocols from 17 internationally collected nonpatient reference samples. The initial median within site ICC from the international sample was .82, a reliability estimate in the excellent range. Although the pool of protocols was collected from many different countries, all the scoring for each protocol took place locally by examiners who trained together. Thus, these data provide a reasonable sample of within site scoring reliability across the world and attest to the cultural adaptability of the test and its administration procedures. The third within site reliability estimate is pertinent because it is from the same lab that provided the across site coding. Viglione and Taylor (2001) reported a median within site reliability of .92 for 84 protocols.

Although the across site reliability estimates are preliminary, these findings suggest that there are complexities in the coding process that are not fully clarified in the standard

CS training materials (Exner 2003; Exner et al., 2001). As a result, training sites (e.g., specific graduate programs) may develop guidelines for coding that help resolve these residual complexities but they may not generalize well to other training sites. Forensic examiners may find it helpful to consult an advanced coding text (Viglione, 2003) or to practice coding with colleagues trained in a different setting.

NORMATIVE DATA: HOW ADEQUATE ARE CS NORMS?

Rorschach normative reference group data have been criticized for pathologizing examinees. Wood et al. (2001b) compared CS reference values on 14 selected variables to the values reported in 8 to 19 comparison samples from the literature. They reported small to very large differences (Cohen's d from .18 to 1.67)[4] for the 13 variables where mean differences could be computed.[5] All differences were in the more pathological or problematic direction for the comparison samples. There were nine variables for which these differences were at least medium size: (a) lower values for $X+\%$, Afr, FC, P, $WSumC$, and $Pure H$; and (b) higher values for reflections, $X-\%$ and Y. Variability of these scores (i.e., the SD) was greater than in the original CS sample—a worrisome finding because it might suggest that current confidence intervals and normative interpretive ranges are too narrow.

The samples in the Wood et al. report were portrayed as nonpatient or normative reference samples but had serious problems and were not fully representative of nonpatients (Meyer, 2001). From a total pool of 32 studies, 22 samples (69%) did not have a procedure to exclude patients or low functioning or disturbed individuals; 16 (50%) samples were college students or the elderly; one had a mean R of 15, whereas another had a mean R of 39, suggesting atypical administration; respondents in one sample were held motionless with electrodes on their head; and just two samples had data for all 14 scores. Obviously, these samples are not representative of nonpatients and are not a good source for comparisons. Nevertheless, it is hard to dismiss these findings totally, as others (Viglione & Hilsenroth, 2001) have examined similar data and found that the distributions for form quality and R appeared to diverge to some degree from CS expectations.

To investigate these normative issues with a better comparison sample, Meyer (2001) contrasted Exner et al.'s (1993) original CS adult normative reference sample to a composite of 2,125 protocols from nine adult samples presented in Erdberg and Shaffer's (1999) symposium on international CS reference data. These samples (which include the Shaffer et al., 1999, sample from the United States) provided data on all CS variables and encompassed great variability and thus generalizability across subject selection procedures, examiner training, examination context, language, culture, and national boundaries. Across 69 composite scores from the lower portion of the Structural Summary, distributions for 49 variables were similar in the original CS sample and international

---

[4]Cohen's d is an effect size measure for comparing two groups. It basically is the difference between the means of the groups in standard deviation units, i.e. the z-score for the differences. For example, a difference of 10 IQ points should result in a Cohen's d of 0.67.

[5]The 14th variable was EB style, a categorical variable for which means could not be computed.

data, a finding consistent with the conclusion that the original CS norms are generally adequate. These data, in addition to the similarities between U.S. and international findings for interrater reliability, again indicate considerable cultural and international adaptability of the Rorschach. One can adapt it to different cultures, languages, and regions, and the test behaves largely as it does in the United States.

Nevertheless, some differences between the CS sample and the composite of international samples persist, so that we need to adjust our normative expectations. International samples have higher scores for *Dd, S, FQu, FQ–, Hd, (Hd)*, and *Sum6*, and lower scores for *WSumC, EA, FQo, P, COP, AG*, and *Afr*. In all cases, the CS norms come across as "healthier." In other words comparison to the CS norms would lead to more pathological interpretations than would comparisons to the international norms. Accordingly, normative expectations for these and for variables that subsume them (e.g., *X–%* for *FQ–*) need to be adjusted. More specific recommendations are given here.

A reasonable question becomes, "Why do the original CS norms look healthier than other normative approximation samples?" The CS respondents were recruited largely through work, unions, or social organizations. Compensation was in the altruistic form of contributions to charity in name of the place of business or organizations, so that respondents were not paid themselves as volunteers. Thus, differences could be due to situational differences or examination context. The CS respondents may feel that their responses matter more than do volunteers in other studies, so that they may "tidy-up" their answers a bit more through filtering in the response process (Exner, 2003). One might speculate that making the examination matter to the respondent is a better approximation of the use of the test in the real world, and thus a better contrast sample. Alternatively, these recruiting practices involving employment and social involvement might lead to a selection bias in terms of attracting healthier and better adapted individuals to volunteer. Indeed, the literature indicates that the garden variety volunteers tend to possess problematic characteristics and are less well-adapted (Berman, Fallon, & Coccaro, 1998; Rosenthal & Rosnow, 1975).

Other explanations of the observed health in the CS norms include differences in administration or coding. There are considerable differences between the initial CS form quality tables first published in 1974 (Exner, 1974) and the current version (Exner et al., 2001), with most of these differences resulting in more *FQ–* and fewer *FQo* responses (Meyer & Richardson, 2001; Viglione, 1989). In addition, criteria and examples for other coding distinctions have changed or been elaborated on over time in ways that alter the benchmarks for assigning a score (Meyer, 2001). Another explanation is simple aging of the norms and increasing mental health difficulties over time.

To address these normative issues, Exner started collecting a new adult normative reference group in 1999 (Exner, 2002; Exner & Erdberg, 2005). This new sample, which is now approaching 500 respondents, was collected largely in the same way as the original CS sample, but there are some differences. The new sample involves the workplace or organizations less formally, so that individuals may feel that they represent themselves instead of an organization. For example, charity donations are made in a respondent's name rather than the organization's name. In the original CS sample, a manager acted as the liaison between examiners and data collection sites and actually solicited respondents. In the new sample, examiners recruit participants on their own. Respondents are now excluded due to "prolonged or significant history" of psychotropic medications or illegal drug use.

Exner and Erdberg (2005) provided data for 450 of the individuals in this sample. The more important differences in terms of mean differences and interpretive cutoffs between the two groups are summarized in Table 2–3. The selected frequencies differ by 5% in the two samples. As can be seen, form quality is less optimal in the new reference sample. There are fewer *Populars*, more special scores, and more of the serious *Level 2 Cognitive Special Scores*. There is less color overall and more color-dominated relative to form-dominated color responses. The *Afr* is lower, there is a notable increase in space responses, and there is a lower frequency of both cooperative and aggressive movement scores. In addition, it is more common for passive movement to exceed active and for the *Depression Index (DEPI)* to be elevated. Although the frequencies remain low, it is worth pointing out that the *SCON* did not exceed 7 in any of the old 600 records, but it does for 11 of the current 450 records. These changes incorporate many of the same variables discussed earlier as divergences between the old CS samples and the international composite pool of references samples collected by other researchers.

Another notable finding is that the standard deviation for *R* is 5.68, as compared to 4.40 in the original CS sample of 600. This change may be problematic because this increased variability of *R* should be associated with more variability for all other scores. Indeed, the great majority of *SD*s is larger in the new sample as compared to the original. This greater variability means that interpretive postulates need to have wider confidence intervals (i.e., the range of expected scores is broader).

Although the new CS reference sample reduces some of the differences with the composite of international reference samples, it does not eliminate them. For example, the new CS sample still has means for *Dd* and *X–%* that are lower and means for *X+%* and *EA* that are higher than other reference samples.

The study that initiated the concerns about the original CS normative reference sample is mentioned in the previous reliability discussion and was published by Shaffer, Erdberg, and Haroian (1999). Its respondents had MMPI–2 *T* score means at approximately 50 and WAIS–R IQs of about 100, thus at normative values. Most Rorschach values were consistent with the original CS normative reference group, but values for the variables already identified as diverging from normative expectations also demonstrated such divergence in this sample. The Shaffer et al. California (CA) sample also differed from both the original and new CS samples in terms of overall complexity. The mean for *R* in the Shaffer et al. sample is only 20.8 versus 23.36 for the new CS sample, and the *Lambda* is 1.22 (median = .75) versus .58 (median = .47) in the new CS sample, with 41% of the Shaffer et al. sample having a *Lambda* greater than .99 versus 14% in the new CS sample. These findings indicate that the Shaffer et al. sample was not very productive and they produced relatively simplistic records in comparison to the CS and other samples included in the international group.

Along with our interrater reliability investigations with these samples (Meyer et al., 2004), we have conducted some initial investigations into the differences between the CA normative reference sample and the new CS reference sample. In this research, we ex-

TABLE 2–3

Illustrative Changes in the New Target Reliability Construct Versus Original CS Normative Reference Samples

Domain/Score	Original 600	New 450
Quality of Perception and Thinking		
X+%	.77	.68
Xu%	.15	.20
X–%	.07	.11
X+% < .55	2%	12%
X% > .20	22%	45%
X–% > .20	3%	10%
XA% > .89	74%	45%
WDA% < .85	5%	16%
P > 7	31%	18%
Sum6	1.91	2.54
WSum6	4.48	7.12
Lvl2 SS > 0	6%	13%
Color		
FC > CF +C + 2	25%	15%
FC > CF +C + 1	41%	26%
CF + C > FC + 1	12%	26%
CF + C > FC + 2	4%	14%
Extratensive	38%	31%
Miscellaneous		
S > 2	14%	38%
DQv > 2	12%	2%
T > 1	11%	17%
Ego < .33	13%	20%
Ego > .44	23%	30%
Afr < .40	3%	9%
Afr < .50	11%	24%
Zd < 3.0	7%	14%
Intell > 5	2%	8%
COP = 0	17%	11%
AG = 0	37%	44%
Hd	.84	1.14
(Hd)	.21	.62
DEPI > 4	5%	14%
p > a + 1	2%	10%
Mp > Ma	14%	23%

amined whether coding conventions might contribute to the differences between the data sets. More specifically, we wondered if CS–CA differences would be reduced when records from both samples were recoded at a third site. If the Shaffer et al. records were coded according to somewhat different benchmarks than Exner's protocols, the differences between the two samples would be reduced if records from both samples were coded by a third group.

To address this question and as described earlier, we obtained 80 protocols from both the CA and CS samples. These 80 protocols were then recoded by a new group of examiners who were trained together in one setting. We then computed two sets of difference scores, using Cohen's d as the effect size index. The first difference score compared mean scores for the CS and CA samples using the original coding from the two sites. The second difference score compared the means for the CS and CA samples based on the new coding. Because the new coding was done by raters who trained together within one site, it eliminates the potential influence of site-specific differences in coding conventions. We anticipated that the initial differences would decrease with the revised coding; that is, the second set of differences from single site scores would be smaller than the first set of differences generated from separate sites.

Initially, with the original CS and CA scoring, across 129 structural summary variables the differences for 36 scores (28%) were moderate to large, with d values greater than .40 or less than −.40. Thus, the normative expectations differed for 36 of the 129 variables in our randomly selected protocols from both samples. However, with the new single site coding, there were only three means (2%) that remained different at this magnitude. Thus, almost all the seemingly important differences between the new CS sample and the CA sample disappeared when the protocols were rescored by a different group. In general, for most variables, our new coding split the difference between the CS sample and Shaffer et al. sample. By and large, the groups now were much more similar: Relative to the original scores, with the new coding, the CS sample looked less healthy than before and the Shaffer et al. sample looked healthier than before.

However, there were instances when the new scores were more similar to one of the reference samples than the other. For complexity variables (*Lambda*, *DQ+*, *Blends*, etc.) and for *Dd*, the values from the rescored protocols more closely resembled the CS reference sample than the CA sample. Furthermore, with the possible exception of *Dd*, the CS reference sample is more similar than the CA sample to the internationally collected reference samples for these particular complexity scores. In contrast, form quality values from the rescored protocols were more in line with the Shaffer et al. CA sample than the CS sample. Equally important, the CA reference sample is more similar than Exner's CS sample to the form quality values observed in other U.S. and international reference samples.

The overall findings suggest that site-specific coding practices may contribute in important and previously unappreciated ways to some of the seeming differences across normative approximation samples. In addition, these initial data suggest a convergence between the CS and CA sample, with the international normative sample. These suggestions are hypotheses that need to be tested with additional samples and coding sites.

There is less research into the suitability of the CS normative reference samples for children. In a study similar to the Shaffer et al. (1999) study and from the same group of researchers, Hamel, Shaffer, and Erdberg (2000) reported on 100 6- to 12-year-old children. This research has also attracted a lot of attention. To establish this group as a normative reference sample, their parents identified them as average to psychologically healthy on a commonly used multidimensional rating scale. However, once again, the Rorschach data diverged from the CS normative reference groups in some respects. In many ways, the differences are similar to those found in the adult normative reference samples. Like the adult samples, Hamel et al. found more distorted form quality values, less color, more use of unusual blot locations, elevated rates of dysfunction on the constellation indices, and less complexity. However, unlike the adult CA versus CS sample differences, the reference values observed by Hamel et al. tended to be more extreme. For instance, the average *Dd* was 8.3, the average *X–%* was .41, 62% of the sample had an elevated *SCZI* (value of 4 or more), and the median *Lambda* value was 1.14 (mean = 1.91).[6]

Although Hamel et al. (2000) took a careful and conscientious approach to their study, several characteristics of the sample suggest it is idiosyncratic and challenge its trustworthiness as a contemporary CS reference sample for children. First, all administration and coding was done by a single examiner, so that generalizability may be limited. Second, for interrater reliability, *%A* was reported in an unusual way.[7] This method would lead to the undetected possibility of coding inaccuracies for determinants, contents, and special scores. Also, in comparison to most research reports, *%A* was low for location and form quality. Third, the authors strongly emphasized the necessity for precision in documenting blot areas on the location sheet that appear to drift from CS standards:

> Students should be clearly taught to very carefully and accurately encircle the precise portion of the blot utilized by the examinee … to enable any other clinician to precisely replicate the coding for location. The precision of location cannot be overemphasized; not only does the location code clearly depend upon an accurate location sheet, but so do other segments of the coding. Form quality and Popular are heavily dependent upon location. A Form Quality of ordinary can easily be altered to unusual or minus on the basis of location alone. (Hamel et al., 2000, p. 291)

If carried through in administration, this emphasis on precision may distort the interaction between the examiner and respondent in the inquiry and also influence the documentation of response areas on the location sheet. Moreover, along with the slack in interrater reliability, it may be related to the extraordinary *Dd* elevation. Excessive *Dd* locations, in turn, could negatively affect form quality codes and *Popular* responses, as well as *SCZI* scores. Accordingly, we do not recommend using the Hamel et al. (2000) sample as a normative approximation sample.

Nevertheless, other samples suggest clinicians should be cautious about using the existing CS reference values for children. Besides Hamel et al. (2000), other child and ado-

---

[6]Because of the skew inherent with *Lambda*, we recommend that median *Lambda* values be reported and that *Pure F%* (*Pure F/R*) be used (Meyer, Viglione, & Exner, 2001).

[7]It should be pointed out that the Hamel reliability data was derived using an across site coding procedure where the comparison scoring was done by a person trained in the same lab that did the rescoring for the Meyer et al. (2004) across site reliability study.

lescent reference samples have been collected in the United States and abroad (Erdberg, 2005; Erdberg & Shaffer, 1999), including France, Italy, Japan, and Portugal. These samples show some notable variability, particularly for *Dd*, *Lambda*, and form quality scores. It is too early to determine whether these differences reflect genuine cultural differences in personality and/or childrearing practices or if they are artifacts due to differences in administration, inquiry, or scoring conventions. However, the composite of data suggest that the adjustments offered earlier for adults should be made for children. In addition, for children, forensic examiners need to factor in developmental trends. The available international data suggest trends consistent with those for Exner's CS reference data (Wenar & Curtis, 1991) across the ages from 5 to 16. These include developmental increases in complexity markers like *DQ+*, *Blends*, and *Zf*, as well as increases in *M* and *P*. In addition, there is a decrease in *WSum6* and to a lesser extent in *DQv*. Unlike Exner's CS reference samples, the composite of alternative reference samples suggests clinicians should anticipate a decrease in *Lambda* as children age and an improvement in form quality scores. Ultimately, the same reasons that instigated the collection of a new adult CS normative reference group also apply to children, so that a new carefully collected age-stratified children's sample is desirable.

Based on the available evidence from the new CS adult reference sample and the other reference samples collected in the United States and internationally, we offer the following recommendations regarding normative expectations and use of nonpatient reference samples with the CS. For adults, we recommend that examiners use the new CS sample as their primary benchmark, but adjust for those variables that have consistently looked different in normative approximation and international samples. Examiners should consider the Shaffer et al. sample as an outer boundary for what might be expected from reasonably functioning nonpatients, because it shows what can be observed for nonpatients within the limits of current administration, inquiry, and scoring guidelines. Table 2–4 summarizes our current recommendations for modifications in normative expectations for crucial variables that have consistently diverged from CS norms. These include adjustments to form quality, color, texture, and human representations.

For children, we would recommend using the available age norms and make similar recommendations or adjustments to the same variables. Although we would not recommend the Hamel et al. sample as an outer boundary for what could be expected for younger U.S. children, its data illustrate how ambiguity or flexibility in current administration and scoring guidelines can result in obtaining some unhealthy looking data from apparently normal functioning children.

POTENTIAL MODERATORS FOR NORMATIVE EXPECTATIONS

Recent CS texts (Exner, 2003; Exner & Erdberg, 2005; Exner et al., 2001) have presented normative reference sample data broken out by *Lambda* and *EB* style. There are three *EB* styles formed by the ratio of *M* to *WSumC*: *Ambitent* ($M \approx WSumC$), *Extratensive* ($M < WSumC$), and *Introversive* ($M > WSumC$), all with *Lambda* less than 1. The fourth style is the *Avoidant* type, with *Lambda* greater than or equal to 1. Thus, the CS position is that style acts as a moderator variable. In other words, the association between a given Rorschach variable and an outcome or construct differs according to style. For example, one might interpret an Affective Ratio of .40 differently according to *EB/Lambda* style, that is, for a person with an *Ambitent* style versus an *Avoidant* style. If the *EB* and *Lambda* styles were such a moderator, then one would need to use different normative tables for each of the four styles, as recommended by the CS.

However, research support for *Lambda/EB* style as a moderator is lacking. The only such published empirical support known to us is greater validity for an old version of the *DEPI* among extratensives (Viglione, Brager, & Haller, 1988). Subsequently, in a study with adolescents, Krishnamurthy and Archer (2001) failed to find support for *EB* as a moderator for the current *DEPI*. Most of the support in CS texts for these four styles (Exner, 2003) relies solely on the fact that the norms differ for the four groups. For the most part, the differences in mean values across groups are redundant with *EB* and *Lambda*. For example, Extratensives produce a higher *Affective Ratio* and more *Blood* responses. These responses involve color or color cards, so that they are redundant with the Extratensive style, because they are concomitant to the *WSumC* elevation, $M < WSumC$.

There is considerable research support for *EB* as a measure of coping characteristics and for *Lambda* with simplification and coping limitations. There is no systematic or comprehensive data demonstrating incremental validity for other variables when taking *EB/Lambda* style into consideration. Or, put another way, there is no body of evidence to suggest that interpretation of other variables routinely varies by *EB/Lambda* style. Accordingly, we recommend that the forensic psychologists not rely on the normative reference group tables broken out by *EB/Lambda* style. Instead, as already recommended, use the tables that encompass all *EB/Lambda* styles, the $N = 450$ sample found in the new volume II (Exner & Erdberg, 2005), along with the interpretive adjustments recommended in Table 2–4.

This recommendation does not mean that there are no variables that might act as moderators for the interpretation of other variables. The most likely candidate is *R*, the number of responses. The relationship between *R* and other variables, as well as whether *R* is a moderator that should be controlled, has been argued in the Rorschach literature for a long time (Cronbach, 1949; Exner, 1974, 1992; Fiske & Baughman, 1953; Holtzman, 1958; Kinder, 1992; Lipgar, 1992; Meyer, 1992a). Research findings suggest that just about every score is associated with *R* and every other score when *R* is not controlled (Exner, Viglione, & Gillespie, 1984). Number of responses is closely related to the first factor on the Rorschach, characterized by Meyer (1992b) as "task engagement." This factor accounts for approximately 25% of Rorschach variance. Number of responses is already often controlled to some extent in percentages and ratios. The percentages ($X+\%$, *Affective Ratio, Egocentricity Index*) are the variables with the most normal distributions, a desirable quality for applying psychometrics to refine interpretations and for efficiently evaluating validity through research.

Exner (1974) originally decided to let *R* vary and to use the less directive Klopfer (Klopfer & Kelley, 1942) response phase administration. This decision was partially based on the idea that the variation of *R* in the initial normative reference sample was considerably less compared to other research (e.g., Fiske & Baughman, 1953). However, as noted earlier, the new CS normative reference group sample ($SD = 5.68$; Exner &

TABLE 2–4

Recommendations for Adjustments to CS Adult Normative Expectations

Variable	Research Adjustments to Expectations	vs. New CS Sample[a]
Location + Form Quality		
Dd	3–4	1
X–%	.15–.25	.09–.14
X+%	.50–.60	.65–.70
XA%/WDA%	.70–.85	.80–.95
Human Representations		
Pure H	2 or 3	3 or 4
H : Non Pure H	H + 1 = Non Pure H	H > Non Pure H
COP	1	2
Ratio of GHR to PHR (HRV)	Between 3:2 and 1:1	2 to 1 ratio
AG	1 in 2 records	1 every record
Color + Related Variables		
FC: CF + C	FC = or < CF + C	FC > CF + C + 1
WSumC	2.5–3.5	4.5
Afr	.45–.55	.55–.65
Extratensive	1 in 5 records	1 in 3 records
EA	6–7	9
Texture		
T = 0	1 in 3 records	1 in 6
T = 1	1 in 3	2 in 3
T = 2	1 in 3	1 in 6
Miscellaneous		
Ambitent	1 in 2 or 3 records	1 in 5 records

[a]Exner & Erdberg, 2005, $N = 450$

Erdberg, 2005) is more variable than the previous normative reference group ($SD = 4.40$; Exner, 2001). Given that other scores are associated with R, this increased variation makes most other scores more variable. Thus, CS interpretive bands may be too narrow or may need to be modified by R. Eventually, research will need to supply the specifics: which variables and which criteria or interpretations are most affected by levels of R. We already know that the variables in the percentages, especially the *FQ* percentage scores, remain valid when R levels are considered. Also, the *Ego Impairment Index* contains an R correction that apparently contributes to interpretive accuracy.

Overall, the CS variables' association with R suggests that R should be at least considered in interpretation. To provide some data about which variables are most sensitive to levels of R, Table 2–5 classifies the correlations between CS variables and R by their magnitude. For those variables in the categories of very strong ($r > .6$) and strong ($r > .5$), and to some extent moderate ($r > .4$), it is probably advisable and perspicacious to take R into consideration when interpreting a protocol. A number of these variables, particularly the FQ variables and pairs (2), already have corrections for R in the form of percentages of R calculations. Correlations are quite abstract, so it is difficult to get a gut feel for the score differences that correspond to these correlations. Table 2–6 is provided to give the forensic examiners a feel for the various levels of correlations in Table 2–5. It is very clear that normative expectations for short and long records diverge considerably for variables that have moderate to strong correlations with R.

Looking at individual variables, the FQ percentage variables, for example X–% or XA%, and the *Egocentricity Index*, are typically relatively unaffected by R, except in very long records. Interpreting these variables in ratios to other variables partially corrects for R, although not completely. For other variables, notably the HVI and OBS, longer records are expected given the overproductive and detail-oriented coping styles exhibited by hypervigilant and obsessive individuals.

For the remaining variables, it is probably wise to consider R. These would include Dd and D locations; individual Developmental Quality and Z-*scores*; FM, m, shading, es,

TABLE 2–5

Score Correlations with R in a Mixed Patient, Offender, and Nonpatient sample ($N = 1,342$)

Correlation with R	Location, DQ and Z	Determinants	FQ	Contents	Special Scores	Actuarial
Very strong (> .6)	D, Dd, DQo	F	FQo, FQu, FQ–	All A, Hd+(Hd)+Ad +(Ad)		
Strong (> .5)	ZF	(2), es		A, All H, Non Pure H	PHR	
Moderate (> .4)	S, DQ+, ZSum	FM + m, SumSh, EA		Hd, Ad		HVI-tot, OBS-tot
Weak (> .3)		M, FM, m, C', Y, a, p, Blends, WSumC, D-Score[a]		An + Xy, Cg, Sc	GHR, Lvl 2	
Minimal (> .15)	W, DQv, DQv/+, Afr	FC, CF+C, T, V, FD, Mp, Ma, MQ–, C-Sh-Blend	X–%, X+%, Xu%, WDA%, F + %	H, (H), (Hd), (A), (Ad), Art, Bt, Fd, Ge, Ls, Na, Sx, Iso/R, P	MOR, PER, HRV[a], Individual Cog. SS, Sum6, WSum6	DEPI, SCZI-tot,
Virtually none (≈ .0)	W:D+Dd, Zd, W:M		FQ+, XA%, S–%,	H:Non pure H	AG, COP, CP	PTI, SCZI-pos, CDI, SCON, HVI-pos, EII

[a]The correlations between R and both D-Score and HRV are negative.

TABLE 2–6

Examples of Changes in Mean Scores for Selected Variables Corresponding to Levels of Correlation With R in a Mixed Patient, Offender, and Nonpatient Sample (N = 1,342)

Correlation With R	Example Variable	Low R n = 493	Optimal R n = 619	High R n = 230
		R = 14–17 Mean R = 15.4	R = 18–27 Mean R = 21.7	R > 27 Mean R = 35.1
Very strong (> .6)	Dd	1.6	2.8	7.1
Strong (> .5)	es	6.1	8.9	14.5
Moderate (> .4)	S	1.7	2.7	4.7
Weak (> .3)	Y	1.1	1.6	2.7
Minimal (> .15)	HRV	0.6	0.4	−1.3
Virtually none (≈ .0)	CDI	3.2	2.9	2.8

and to a lesser degree *EA*; all summary scores encompassing multiple human and animal contents and *A*, and to a lesser degree *Hd* and *Ad*; and *PHR*. For these variables within records containing less than 18 responses, the CS reference tables probably overestimate their expected frequency.

On the other hand, CS tables probably underestimate frequencies for long records with 28 responses or more. When possible, these "*R*-sensitive" variables should be interpreted with ratios or other arrays. For example, interpreting the pattern and interrelationships of the four *DQ* scores, or *HRV* rather than *PHR* or *GHR* individually, will reduce distortions due to *R*.

For records with 18 to 27 responses, the normative reference group tables probably provide excellent estimates of normative expectations, when modified by our recommendations in Table 2–4. Most likely, the Rorschach has the most validity for records of this length. For records outside of that range, interpretations might be more tentative and interpretations based on incorporating *R* adjustments should be considered.

VALIDITY: DOES THE RORSCHACH MEASURE WHAT WE THINK IT MEASURES?

We focus on construct validity, whether or not the test scale is measuring what we intend it to measure. Do the Rorschach variables, as a whole, show a pattern of convergent and discriminant validity? In other words, what is the evidence that given Rorschach variables are associated with appropriate and relevant criteria and not correlated with irrelevant or conceptually independent criteria? Oftentimes, distinctions in construct validity are made in terms of timing: An empirical association demonstrated at the same time the test is administered is referred to as concurrent validity, whereas an association with a criterion collected sometime in the future is referred to as predictive validity. Incremental validity concerns whether we are deriving information that is not attainable elsewhere, a type of validity that we consider under utility, which concerns the usefulness of the test.

Of course, validity is ultimately demonstrated between a specific Rorschach variable and a specific construct or criterion relevant to that particular variable. However, organizing the vast literature by all the variables is a nearly insurmountable task, so that we address the global validity of the test. Does the evidence suggest that the Rorschach as a test produces valid measures of appropriated and relevant outcomes and constructs?

There have been thousands of studies addressing Rorschach validity from around the world (e.g., see summaries in Exner & Erdberg, 2005; Viglione, 1999), demonstrating considerable support for its validity and cultural adaptability. Based on these studies, Meyer and Archer (2001; also see Meyer, 2004) summarized the available evidence from Rorschach meta-analyses, including those that examined the global validity of the test and those that examined the validity of specific scales in relation to particular criteria. The scales included CS and non-CS variables. They then considered the evidence for the Rorschach in the context of evidence from meta-analyses on other psychological and medical tests (Meyer, Finn et al., 2001).

A number of factors make it challenging to compare findings across meta-analyses. Coefficients were not corrected for unreliability, range restriction, or the imperfect construct validity of criterion measures. Moreover, results emerged from different types of research designs and types of validation tasks. These differences cause effect sizes to fluctuate and make definitive comparisons of effect sizes difficult.

Nonetheless, the results of these meta-analyses indicate that psychological and medical tests have varying degrees of validity, ranging from tests that were essentially unrelated to a criterion, to tests that were strongly associated with relevant criteria. Contrary to some opinions, it was difficult to distinguish between medical tests and psychological tests in terms of their effects size patterns. At the same time, it was clear that test validity was a function of the criteria used to evaluate the instrument: Validity for a particular test was greater with some criteria and weaker with others. Within these findings, validity for the Rorschach was much the same as it was for other instruments. Thus, Meyer and Archer concluded that the systematically collected data showed the Rorschach produced validity coefficients that were on par with other personality tests, with meta-analytic effect sizes that supported its overall validity and usefulness. More specifically, they concluded that the results demonstrated that "across journal outlets, decades of research, aggregation procedures, predictor scales, criterion measures, and types of participants, reasonable hypotheses for the vast array of Rorschach ... scales that have been empirically tested produce convincing evidence for their construct validity" (Meyer & Archer, 2001, p. 491).

Consistent with Atkinson et al.'s 1986 comment that criticism of the Rorschach might be as much political as it is scientific, Meyer and Archer also express some puzzlement as to why the Rorschach might be singled out for intense scrutiny and criticism when its broadband validity is equal to other psychological tests.

Some individual meta-analyses have identified moderators of Rorschach validity, that is, factors or conditions that influence the validity of the test. Bornstein (1999) found considerable support for the validity of the Rorschach Oral Dependency scale as a predictor of observed dependent behavior. Although his moderator analyses examined inkblot data combined with Thematic Apperception Test (TAT) data, he found that validity was consistent across criteria derived from lab, field, or classroom settings. It is true that in the single study from a hospital-clinic setting validity was nonsignificant. Bornstein also found that validity was consistent across ratings made by researchers or other observers and regardless of whether behavior was classified dichotomously or measured dimensionally. Thus, on the whole, the findings were generalizable across settings and methodology.

Hiller and Rosenthal and their coworkers (Hiller, Rosenthal, Bornstein, Berry, & Brunell-Neuleib, 1999) produced a comparative meta-analysis of Rorschach and MMPI research. They found that the Rorschach demonstrated greater association with what they called "objective" criteria. In contrast, the MMPI was more closely associated with psychiatric diagnostic classification and other self-reported measurements. A wide variety of events or outcomes was encompassed under the objective modifier. These criteria were largely behavioral events, medical conditions, behavioral interactions with the environment, or classifications that required minimal to no judgment from others, for example, dropping out of treatment, history of abuse or not, number of driving accidents, history of criminal offenses, medical disorder versus control, cognitive test performance, behavioral test of ability to delay gratification, or response to medication. Such characteristics and events were also identified as valid Rorschach criteria in a descriptive review of the same literature (Viglione, 1999). Many are behavioral events and life outcomes involving interactions between the individual and the environment that emerge over time. From a concrete perspective, these criteria for which the Rorschach is most valid might also be identified by an exclusionary definition as not self-report and not diagnostic classification. On the other hand, the data are clear that the Rorschach does identify psychotic diagnoses and measure psychotic symptoms well (Meyer & Archer, 2001; Perry, Minassian, Cadenhead, & Braff, 2003; Viglione, 1999, Viglione & Hilsenroth, 2001). Unlike many other disorders, these diagnoses are often based more on patients' observed behavior than on their self-reported presenting complaints.

In a recent meta-analysis, Grønnerød (2004) reviewed the literature examining the extent to which Rorschach variables changed as a function of psychological treatment. The Rorschach produced a level of validity that was equivalent to alternative instruments, so that it was as sensitive and able to measure change as self-report and clinician rating scales. Like Bornstein (1999) and Hiller et al. (1999), Grønnerød examined moderators to Rorschach validity. He found that Rorschach scores changed more with longer treatment, presumably because of more personality change over time. He also addressed some methodological issues. Suggesting some potential bias, when coders were blind to whether the protocol was obtained before or after treatment, there was less change. Another methodological note was that those studies that paid more attention to coding reliability, and how coding was accomplished, yielded greater validity coefficients. This is one of the few demonstrations of reliability constraining validity with real-world assessment applications.

Overall, the meta-analytic evidence supports the general validity of the Rorschach. Globally, the test appears to function as well as other assessment instruments. To date, only a few meta-analyses have systematically examined the validity literature for specific scales in relation to particular criteria. The evidence has been positive and supportive for the *ROD*, *RPRS*, and *SCZI/PTI*, although not for the *DEPI* when used as a diagnostic indicator. As is true for other commonly used tests, such as the MMPI–2, PAI, MCMI, or Wechsler scales, additional focused meta-analytic reviews that systematically catalog the validity of particular Rorschach variables relative to specific types of criteria will continue to refine and enhance clinical and forensic practice.

UTILITY: IS THE RORSCHACH USEFUL?

Utility of an assessment instrument can be globally defined as the practical value of the information it provides. It may be further specified as a function of the beneficial influence of a test on information, decisions, and outcomes relative to its costs (Viglione, 1999). Taking into consideration cost–benefit issues and the time necessary for examination and interpretation, the Rorschach "should provide information that is not routinely available through less time-consuming self-report, interview, or observational methods" (Viglione, 1999, p. 251). As an example, Viglione and Hilsenroth's (2001) review of the research on the CS Suicide Constellation revealed that it provided information about self-harm risk that was not easily attainable from the client through interview or from direct observation. This cost–benefit approach is typically translated statistically, even if it oversimplifies the issue, into an evaluation of incremental validity. In other words, the Rorschach and a more readily available or less time-intensive method are compared statistically. The requirement for incremental validity then would be the Rorschach accounts for variance in the outcome beyond that accounted for by the simpler method. Such a finding demonstrates statistically that the Rorschach provides unique information. Equating utility with statistical demonstrations of incremental validity is certainly reductionistic and research reports frequently lack adequate sample sizes to test it sufficiently. Nevertheless, much of the literature referring to utility uses this statistical method.

In addition to incremental validity, utility involves the prediction of real-world behavior and life outcomes, as demonstrated by the Hiller et al. (1999) meta-analysis. Research demonstrating validity within clinical or forensic practice, referred to as ecological validity, is especially important because it demonstrates the usefulness of the test in that applied context (i.e., utility). Having information about what is going to happen in the future and about patterns over time also provides great benefit. In this way, predictive validity, as contrasted to concurrent validity, also supports utility.

The empirical literature demonstrates that the Rorschach possesses utility in all of these forms. Research reviews (Viglione, 1999; Viglione & Hilsenroth, 2001; Weiner, 2001) contain empirical data consistent with the conclusion that Rorschach variables possess incremental validity over other tests, including self-report scales, intelligence test scores, demographic data, and other types of information. Meta-analyses (Hiller et al., 1999; Meyer, 2000a; Meyer & Archer, 2001) have reached the same conclusion. Moreover, these reviews and meta-analyses have demonstrated that the test is especially relevant for real-world behaviors, characteristics manifested over time, and life outcomes.

It is beyond the scope of this chapter to review individual studies, but a sampling of recent utility findings, many of them quite impressive, are presented here. This Rorschach research has continued to support the validity of the test through demonstrations of incremental validity with real-life outcome criteria. Thus, this sampling of studies from the United States and Europe continue to support the conclusion that the Rorschach yields important information that is not attainable through simpler, less time-consuming methods. Among the outcomes included in these studies are future success in naval special forces training in Norway (Hartmann, Sunde, Kristensen, & Martinussen, 2003), future adolescent and adult delinquency from clinician ratings of ego strength from Rorschach protocols taken at ages 4 to 8 in Sweden (Janson & Stattin, 2003), future psychiatric relapse among previously hospitalized children (Stokes et al., 2003), previous glucose stability levels among diabetic children in France (Sultan, Jebrane, & Heurtier-Hartemann, 2002), and future emergency medical transfers and drug overdoses in inpatients during a 60-day posttest period (Fowler, Hilsenroth, & Piers, 2001). In these studies, the Rorschach has demonstrated incremental validity over, for example, various self-report scales, collateral reports, *DSM* diagnoses, and intelligence tests.

Other studies demonstrate utility by using real-life behavioral and life outcome criteria. Several different research projects conducted in Sweden illustrate this nicely, using criteria such as eating behavior in an experimental setting, eventual weight loss, and positive response to obesity medication in an obesity treatment program (Elfhag, Barkeling, Carlsson, Lindgren, & Rossner, 2004; Elfhag, Barkeling, Carlsson, & Rossner, 2003; Elfhag, Carlsson, & Rossner, 2003; Elfhag, Rossner, & Carlsson, 2004); agreement between therapist's planned goals for treatment and what they actually focused on (Bihlar, 2001; Bihlar & Carlsson, 2001); and selection for intensive, long-term psychoanalytic therapy (Nygren, 2004a, 2004b). Many of these studies demonstrated predictive validity, which is another way of demonstrating utility because such information is not easily attainable.

This summary of recent utility studies is limited in a number of ways. Largely, the studies support the overall or broadband utility of the Rorschach. In other words, they support the test as a useful instrument. This summary does not address the utility of specific variables for specific applications. Most importantly, the findings for specific variables need to be replicated. Also, a strength shared by all of these studies was that the researchers articulated thoughtful hypothesized associations for specific Rorschach variables. Although the results were largely supportive, there also were negative findings, where results did not support the hypothesized variables. For instance, Elfhag et al. did not find support for the *ROD* in relation to eating behavior and Nygren did not find support for *m*, *X–%*, or *FD* as predictors of who would be selected for intensive psychotherapy.

As with reliability and validity research reports, most of these utility studies have used CS variables, but considerable incremental validity utility has also been demonstrated for some non-CS scales (Garb, 1999). These include the Rorschach Prognostic Rating scale (Meyer, 2000a; Meyer & Handler, 1997), the Rorschach Oral Dependency scale (Bornstein & O'Neill, 1997), and the *Ego Impairment Index* (Perry & Viglione, 1991; Viglione, Perry, & Meyer, 2003). The *Ego Impairment Index* is derived from standard CS variables, including *HRV*, *FQ–*, *WSum6*, *M–*, and certain critical contents—*An, Bl, Ex,*

Fd, Fi, Sex, X-Ray, MOR, and *AG,* in addition to *R* as a control variable. It has a great deal of empirical validity and utility support in the literature (Dawes, 1999; Perry & Viglione, 1991; Perry et al., 2003; Stokes et al., 2003, Viglione, Perry, & Meyer, 2003).

It has been demonstrated and reported many times in the literature that like-named Rorschach and self-report scales that purportedly measure similar constructs are weakly associated with one another, if at all (see, e.g., Archer & Krishnamurthy, 1993a, 1993b, 1997; Krishnamurthy, Archer, & House, 1996; Meyer, 1996, 1999; Meyer & Archer, 2001; Meyer, Riethmiller, Brooks, Benoit, & Handler, 2000; Viglione, 1996). Most of this work has used the MMPI as the self-report measure. These data suggest that the Rorschach should display incremental validity over self-report scales. From a logical and mathematical point of view, if both the Rorschach and a given self-report test are related with a given real-life outcome, and the Rorschach and self-report measure are not related to each other, both should be uniquely related to that outcome and both should provide incremental validity over the other. Nevertheless, the lack of association between the two methods and by implication the amount of method variance involved in assessment techniques, forces the forensic psychologist to employ a multimethod strategy (see Erdberg, chap. 27, this volume). Findings suggest that CS and self-reports are more highly correlated when patients take similar open/ guarded approach to both tests, and may be negatively correlated when they adopt opposing styles (Meyer, 1997b, 1999). Research also indicates that self-report is more easily manipulated (e.g., Meyer & Archer, 2001; Viglione, 1999). Accordingly, the Rorschach may be more useful in forensic assessment contexts when the respondent is motivated to exaggerate or minimize certain features. However, it has been demonstrated that many individuals—but not all—can influence obvious or dramatic Rorschach content and, to lesser extent, actuarial indices (Exner & Erdberg, 2005; Ganellen, chap. 5, this vol.; Meisner, 1988; Morgan & Viglione, 1992; Netter, 1991; Perry & Kinder, 1990).

CONCLUSIONS

Overall, the empirical evidence is consistent with the conclusion that the Rorschach can be reliably scored, is valid, and provides unique information. Generalizability of administrative procedures and global reliability, validity, and utility findings has been demonstrated in many countries internationally so that applicability to domestic subcultural groups is not problematic. However, there is much more to learn and document. The Rorschach is a complex instrument and, like any complex assessment tool, it poses challenges for reliable and accurate administration, scoring, and interpretation. We have highlighted some of the issues that we think are most important for forensic examiners to consider and have offered guidelines for revised interpretation based on the literature. The test will continue to be challenged in forensic practice because it is considered controversial by some and a symbol of problems with clinical practice and judgment by others. However, because it provides utility in the form of information that cannot necessarily be obtained easily from other sources, it will continue to be used in forensic contexts. We hope what we provided here assists forensic practitioners in accurately describing litigants and clients in an empirically defensible fashion, while being cognizant of the strengths and limitations of the test so that the legal system is served well.

REFERENCES

Acklin, M. W. (1999). Behavioral science foundations of the Rorschach test: Research and clinical applications. *Assessment, 6,* 319–324.

Acklin, M. W., McDowell, C. J., & Verschell, M. S. (2000). Interobserver agreement, intraobserver reliability, and the Rorschach Comprehensive System. *Journal of Personality Assessment, 74,* 15–47.

Archer, R. P., & Krishnamurthy, R. (1993a). Combining the Rorschach and the MMPI in the assessment of adolescents. *Journal of Personality Assessment, 60*(1), 132–140.

Archer, R. P., & Krishnamurthy, R. (1993b). A review of MMPI and Rorschach interrelationships in adult samples. *Journal of Personality Assessment, 61*(2), 277–293.

Archer, R. P., & Krishnamurthy, R. (1997). MMPI–A and Rorschach indices related to depression and conduct disorder: An evaluation of the incremental validity hypothesis. *Journal of Personality Assessment, 69(3),* 517–533.

Atkinson, L., Quarrington, B., Alp, I. E., & Cyr, J. J. (1986). Rorschach validity: An empirical approach to the literature. *Journal of Clinical Psychology, 42,* 360–362.

Barr, W. B. (2003). Neuropsychological testing of high school athletes: Preliminary norms and test–retest indices. *Archives of Clinical Neuropsychology, 18,* 91–101.

Benedict, R. H. B., Schretlen, D., Groninger, L., & Brandt, J. (1998). Hopkins Verbal Learning Test–Revised: Normative data and analysis of inter-form and test–retest reliability. *The Clinical Neuropsychologist, 12,* 43–55.

Berman, M. E., Fallon, A., & Coccaro, E. F. (1998). The relationship between personality psychopathology and aggressive behavior in research volunteers. *Journal of Abnormal Psychology, 107,* 651–658.

Bihlar, B., & Carlsson, A. M. (2000). An exploratory study of agreement between therapists' goals and patients' problems revealed by the Rorschach. *Psychotherapy Research, 10*(2), 196–214.

bihlar, B., & Carlsson, A. M. (2001). Planned and actual goals in psychodynamic psychotherapies; Do patients' personality characteristics relate to agreement? *Psychotherapy Research, 11*(4), 383–400.

Bornstein, R. F. (1999). Criterion validity of objective and projective dependency tests: A meta-analytic assessment of behavioral prediction. *Psychological Assessment, 11,* 48–57.

Bornstein, R. F., & O'Neill, R. M. (1997). Construct validity of the Rorschach Oral Dependency (ROD) scale: Relationship of ROD scores to WAIS–R scores in a psychiatric inpatient sample. *Journal of Clinical Psychology, 53*(2), 99–105.

Cicchetti, D. V. (1994). Guidelines, criteria, and rules of thumb for evaluating normed and standardized assessment instruments in psychology. *Psychological Assessment, 6,* 284–290.

Cronbach, L. J. (1949). Statistical methods applied to Rorschach scores: A review. *Psychological Bulletin, 46,* 393–429.

Dahlstrom, W. G., Welsh, G. S., & Dahlstrom, L. E. (1972). *A MMPI handbook: Vol. 1: Clinical interpretation.* Minneapolis: University of Minnesota Press.

Dao, T. K., & Prevatt F. (2006). A psychometric evaluation of the Rorschach Comprehensive System's Perceptual Thinking Index. *Journal of Personality Assessment, 86,* 180–189.

Dawes, R. M. (1999). Two methods for studying the incremental validity of a Rorschach variable. *Psychological Assessment, 11*(3), 297–302.

Dikmen, S. S., Heaton, R. K., Grant, I., & Temkin, N. R. (1999). Test–retest reliability and practice effects of Expanded Halstead–Reitan Neuropsychological Test Battery. *Journal of the International Neuropsychological Society, 5,* 346–356.

Elfhag, K., Barkeling, B., Carlsson, A. M., Lindgren, T., & Rossner, S. (2004). Food intake with an antiobesity drug (sibutramine) versus placebo and Rorschach data: A crossover within-subjects study. *Journal of Personality Assessment, 82*(2), 158–168.

Elfhag, K., Barkeling, B., Carlsson, A. M., & Rossner, S. (2003). Microstructure of eating behavior associated with Rorschach characteristics in obesity. *Journal of Personality Assessment, 81*(1), 40–50.

Elfhag, K., Carlsson, A. M., & Rossner, S. (2003). Subgrouping in obesity based on Rorschach person-ality characteristics. *Scandinavian Journal of Psychology, 44*(5), 399–407.

Elfhag, K., Rossner, S., & Carlsson, A. M. (2004). Degree of body weight in obesity and Rorschach per-sonality aspects of mental distress. *Eating & Weight Disorders, 9*(1), 35–43.

Erdberg, P. (2005, July). *Intercoder agreement as a measure of ambiguity of coding guidelines* Paper presented at the 18th International Congress of Rorschach and Projective Methods, Barcelona.

Erdberg, P., & Schaffer, T. W. (1999, July). *International symposium on Rorschach nonpatient data: Findings from around the world.* Paper presented at the International Congress of Rorschach and Projective Methods, Amsterdam, The Netherlands.

Exner, J. E. (1974). *The Rorschach: A Comprehensive System.* Oxford, England: Wiley.

Exner, J. E. (1992). R in Rorschach research: A ghost revisited. *Journal of Personality Assessment, 58,* 245–251.

Exner, J. E. (2002). A new nonpatient sample for the Rorschach Comprehensive System: A progress report. *Journal of Personality Assessment, 78,* 391–404.

Exner, J. E. (2003). *The Rorschach: A Comprehensive System* (4th ed.). New York: Wiley.

Exner, J. E., Armbruster, G. L., & Viglione, D. (1978). The temporal stability of some Rorschach fea-tures. *Journal of Personality Assessment, 42*(5), 474–482.

Exner, J. E., Colligan, S. C., Hillman, L. B., Metts, A. S., Ritzler, B., Rogers, K. T., Sciara, A., D., & Viglione, D. J. (2001). *A Rorschach workbook for the Comprehensive System* (5th ed.). Asheville, NC: Rorschach Workshops.

Exner, J. E., & Erdberg, P. (2005). *The Rorschach: A Comprehensive System: Vol. 2. Interpretation* (3rd ed.). Oxford, England: Wiley.

Exner, J. E., Meyer, G. J., Renteria, L., Mattlar, C.-E., Tuset, A. M., Gonzalez, Y., Nakamura, N., & Nihashi, N. (1999, July). *A cross-national review of Rorschach interscorer reliability.* Paper presented at the 16th congress of the International Rorschach Society, Amsterdam, The Netherlands.

Exner, J. E., Viglione, D. J., & Gillespie, R. (1984). Relationships between Rorschach variables as rele-vant to the interpretation of structural data. *Journal of Personality Assessment, 48*(1), 65–70.

Fiske, D. W., & Baughman, E. E. (1953). Relationships between Rorschach scoring categories and the total number of responses. *Journal of Abnormal and Social Psychology, 48,* 25–32.

Fowler, J. C., Hilsenroth, M. J., & Piers, C. (2001). An empirical study of seriously disturbed suicidal patients. *Journal of the American Psychoanalytic Association, 49*(1), 161–186.

Garb, H. N. (1999). Call for a moratorium on the use of the Rorschach inkblot test in clinical and foren-sic settings. *Assessment, 6*(4), 313–317.

Grønnerød, C. (2003). Temporal stability in the Rorschach method: A meta-analytic review. *Journal of Personality Assessment, 80*(3), 272–293.

Grønnerød, C. (2004). Rorschach assessment of changes following psychotherapy: A meta-analytic review. *Journal of Personality Assessment, 83,* 256–276.

Grove, W. M., & Barden, R. C. (1999). Protecting the integrity of the legal system: The admissibility of testimony from mental health experts under *Daubert/Kumho* analyses. *Psychology, Public Policy, & Law, 5*(1), 224–242.

Grove, W. M., Barden, R. C., Garb, H. N., & Lilienfeld, S. O. (2002). Failure of Rorschach-comprehen-sive-system-based testimony to be admissible under the Daubert–Joiner–Kumho standard. *Psychol-ogy, Public Policy, & Law, 8*(2), 216–234.

Hamel, M., Shaffer, T. W., & Erdberg, P. (2000). A study of nonpatient preadolescent Rorschach proto-cols. *Journal of Personality Assessment, 75,* 280–294.

Hartmann, E., Sunde, T., Kristensen, W., & Martinussen, M. (2003). Psychological measures as predic-tors of military training performance. *Journal of Personality Assessment, 80,* 87–98.

Hiller, J. B., Rosenthal, R., Bornstein, R. F., Berry, D. T. R., & Brunell-Neuleib, S. (1999). A compara-tive meta-analysis of Rorschach and MMPI validity. *Psychological Assessment, 11*(3), 278–296.

Hilsenroth, M. J., Fowler, J. C., & Padawer, J. R. (1998). The Rorschach Schizophrenia Index (SCZI): An examination of reliability, validity, and diagnostic efficiency. *Journal of Personality Assessment, 10*, 514–534.

Hilsenroth, M. J., & Handler, L. (1995). A survey of graduate students' experiences, interests, and attitudes about learning the Rorschach. *Journal of Personality Assessment, 64*, 243–257.

Hirt, M. E. (1962). *Rorschach science: Readings in theory and method.* Oxford, England: Free Press Glencoe.

Holtzman, W. H. (1958). *Holtzman inkblot technique.* San Antonio, TX: Psychological Corporation.

Hunsley, J., & Bailey, J. M. (1999). The clinical utility of the Rorschach: Unfulfilled promises and an uncertain future. *Psychological Assessment, 11*(3), 266–277.

Hunsley, J., & Bailey, J. M. (2001). Whither the Rorschach? An analysis of the evidence. *Psychological Assessment, 13*(4), 472–485.

Janson, H., & Olsson, U. (2001). A measure of agreement for interval or nominal multivariate observations. *Educational and Psychological Measurement, 61*, 277–289.

Janson, H., & Olsson, U. (2004). A measure of agreement for interval or nominal multivariate observations by different sets of judges. *Educational and Psychological Measurement, 64*, 62–70.

Janson, H., & Stattin, H. (2003). Prediction of adolescent and adult antisociality from childhood Rorschach ratings. *Journal of Personality Assessment, 81*, 51–63.

Kinder, B. N. (1992). The problems of *R* in clinical settings and in research: Suggestions for the future. *Journal of Personality Assessment, 58*, 252–259.

Klopfer, B., & Kelley, D. M. (1942). *The Rorschach technique.* Oxford, England: World Book.

Krishnamurthy, R., & Archer, R. P. (2001). An evaluation of the effects of Rorschach *eb* style on the diagnostic utility of the depression index. *Assessment, 8*(1), 105–109.

Krishnamurthy, R., Archer, R. P., & House, J. J. (1996). The MMPI–A and Rorschach: A failure to establish convergent validity. *Assessment, 3*(2), 179–191.

Lilienfeld, S. O., Wood, J. M., & Garb, H. N. (2000). The scientific status of projective techniques. *Psychological Science in the Public Interest, 1*(2), 27–66.

Lipgar, R. M. (1992). The problem of *R* in the Rorschach: The value of varying responses. *Journal of Personality Assessment, 58*, 223–230.

Martin, R., Sawrie, S., Gilliam, F., Mackey, M., Faught, E., Knowlton, R., & Kuzniekcy, R. (2002). Determining reliable cognitive change after epilepsy surgery: Development of reliable change indices and standardized regression-based change norms for the WMS–III and WAIS–III. *Epilepsia, 43*, 1551–1558.

Mauger, P. A. (1972). *The test–retest reliability of persons: An empirical investigation utilizing the MMPI and the Personality Research Form.* Unpublished doctoral dissertation, University of Minnesota.

Meisner, S. (1988). Susceptibility of Rorschach distress correlates to malingering. *Journal of Personality Assessment, 52*(3), 564–571.

Meyer, G. J. (1992a). Response frequency problems in the Rorschach: Clinical and research implications with suggestions for the future. *Journal of Personality Assessment, 58*(2), 231–244.

Meyer, G. J. (1992b). The Rorschach's factor structure: A contemporary investigation and historical review. *Journal of Personality Assessment, 59*(1), 117–136.

Meyer, G. J. (1996). The Rorschach and MMPI: Toward a more scientifically differentiated understanding of cross-method assessment. *Journal of Personality Assessment, 67*, 558–578.

Meyer, G. J. (1999). The convergent validity of MMPI and Rorschach scales: An extension using profile scores to define response/character styles on both methods and a re-examination of simple Rorschach response frequency. *Journal of Personality Assessment, 72*, 1–35.

Meyer, G. J. (1997a). Assessing reliability: Critical corrections for a critical examination of the Rorschach Comprehensive System. *Psychological Assessment, 9*(4), 480–489.

Meyer, G. J. (1997b). On the integration of personality assessment methods: The Rorschach and MMPI. *Journal of Personality Assessment, 68*(2), 297–330.

Meyer, G. J. (1997c). Thinking clearly about reliability: More critical corrections regarding the Rorschach Comprehensive System. *Psychological Assessment, 9*(4), 495–498.

Meyer, G. J. (2000a). Incremental validity of the Rorschach Prognostic Rating scale over the MMPI
Ego Strength scale and IQ. *Journal of Personality Assessment, 74*(3), 356–370.

Meyer, G. J. (2000b). On the science of Rorschach research. *Journal of Personality Assessment, 75*(1),
46–81.

Meyer, G. J. (2001). Evidence to correct misperceptions about Rorschach norms. *Clinical Psychology:
Science & Practice, 8*(3), 389–396.

Meyer, G. J. (2004). The reliability and validity of the Rorschach and TAT compared to other psychological and medical procedures: An analysis of systematically gathered evidence. In M. Hilsenroth
& D. Segal (Eds.), *Personality assessment: Vol. 2. Comprehensive handbook of psychological
assessment* (pp. 315–342). Hoboken, NJ: Wiley.

Meyer, G. J., & Archer, R. P. (2001). The hard science of Rorschach research: What do we know and
where do we go? *Psychological Assessment, 13*, 486–502.

Meyer, G. J., Finn, S. E., Eyde, L., Kay, G. G., Moreland, K. L., Dies, R. R., Eisman, E. J., Kubiszyn, T.
W., & Reed, G. M. (2001). Psychological testing and psychological assessment: A review of evidence and issues. *American Psychologist, 56*, 128–165.

Meyer, G. J., & Handler, L. (1997). The ability of the Rorschach to predict subsequent outcome: A meta-
analysis of the Rorschach prognostic rating scale. *Journal of Personality Assessment, 69*(1), 1–38.

Meyer, G. J., Hilsenroth, M. J., Baxter, D., Exner, J. E., Jr., Fowler, J. C., Piers, C. C., et al. (2002). An
examination of interrater reliability for scoring the Rorschach Comprehensive System in eight data
sets. *Journal of Personality Assessment, 78*(2), 219–274.

Meyer, G. J., Mihura, J. L., & Smith, B. L. (2005). The interclinician reliability of Rorschach interpretation in four data sets. *Journal of Personality Assessment, 84*(3), 296–314.

Meyer, G. J., & Richardson, C. (2001, March). *An examination of changes in form quality codes in the
Rorschach Comprehensive System from 1974 to 1995.* Paper presented at the annual meeting of the
Society for Personality Assessment, Philadelphia, PA.

Meyer, G. J., Riethmiller, R. J., Brooks, R. D., Benoit, W. A., & Handler, L. (2000). A replication of
Rorschach and MMPI–2 convergent validity. *Journal of Personality Assessment, 74*(2), 175–215.

Meyer, G. J., Viglione, D. J., Erdberg, P., Exner, J. E., Jr., & Shaffer, T. (2004, March). *CS scoring differences in the Rorschach Workshop and Fresno nonpatient samples.* Paper presented at the annual
meeting of the Society for Personality Assessment, Miami, FL.

Meyer G. J, Viglione, D. J., & Exner, J. E., Jr. (2001). Superiority of *Form %* over *Lambda* for research
on the Rorschach. *Journal of Personality Assessment, 76*, 68–75.

Mihura, J. L., & Weinle, C. A. (2002). Rorschach training: Doctoral students' experiences and prefer-
ences. *Journal of Personality Assessment, 79*, 39–52.

Milott, S. R., Lira, F. T., & Miller, W. C. (1977). Psychological assessment of the burned patient. *Journal of Clinical Psychology, 33*, 425–430.

Morgan, L., & Viglione, D. J. (1992). Sexual disturbances, Rorschach sexual responses, and mediating
factors. *Psychological Assessment, 4*(4), 530–536.

Murstein, B. I. E. (1965). *Handbook of projective techniques.* Oxford, England: Basic Books.

Netter, B. C., & Viglione, D. J., Jr. (1994). An empirical study of malingering schizophrenia on the Rorschach. *Journal of Personality Assessment, 62*(1), 45–57.

Nezworski, M. T., & Wood, J. M. (1995). Narcissism in the Comprehensive System for the Rorschach.
Clinical Psychology: Science & Practice, 2(2), 179–199.

Nygren, M. (2004a). Differences in Comprehensive System Rorschach variables between groups differing in therapy suitability. In A. Andronikof (Ed.), *Rorschachiana xxvi: Yearbook of the International Rorschach Society* (pp. 110–146). Ashland, OH, US: Hogrefe & Huber.

Nygren, M. (2004b). Rorschach Comprehensive System variables in relation to assessing dynamic
capacity and ego strength for psychodynamic psychotherapy. *Journal of Personality Assessment,
83(3)*, 277–292.

Paolo, A. M., Tröster, A. I., & Ryan, J. J. (1997). Test–retest stability of the California Verbal Learning Test in older persons. *Neuropsychology, 11*, 613–613.

Perry, G. G., & Kinder, B. N. (1990). The susceptibility of the Rorschach to malingering: A critical review. Journal of Personality Assessment, 54(1–2), 47–57.

Perry, W., Minassian, A., Cadenhead, K., Sprock, J., & Braff, D. (2003). The use of the Ego Impairment Index across the schizophrenia spectrum. *Journal of Personality Assessment, 80*(1), 50–57.

Perry, W., & Viglione, D. J. (1991). The Ego Impairment Index as a predictor of outcome in melancholic depressed patients treated with tricyclic antidepressants. *Journal of Personality Assessment, 56(3)*, 487–501.

The Psychological Corporation. (1997). *WAIS–III—WMS–III technical manual*. San Antonio: Author.

Rabin, A. I. (1981). *Assessment with projective techniques: A concise introduction*. New York: Springer.

Roberts, B. W., & DelVecchio, W. F. (2000). The rank-order consistency of personality traits from childhood to old Age: A quantitative review of longitudinal studies. *Psychological Bulletin, 126*, 3–25.

Rosenthal, R., & Rosnow, R. L. (1975). *The volunteer subject*. New York: Wiley.

Ryan, J. J., Dunn, G. E., & Paolo, A. M. (1995). Temporal stability of the MMPI–2 in a substance abuse sample. *Psychotherapy in Private Practice, 14*, 33–41.

Schuerger, J. M., Zarrella, K. L., & Holtz, A. S. (1989). Factors that influence the temporal stability of personality by questionnaire. *Journal of Personality and Social Psychology, 56*, 777–783.

Shaffer, T. W., Erdberg, P., & Haroian, J. (1999). Current nonpatient data for the Rorschach, WAIS–R, and MMPI–2. *Journal of Personality Assessment, 73*(2), 305–316.

Shrout, P. E., & Fliess, J. L. (1979). Intraclass correlations: Uses in assessing rater reliability. *Psychological Bulletin, 86*, 420–428.

Sines, L. K., Silver, R. J., & Lucero, R. J. (1961). The effect of therapeutic intervention by untrained "therapists." *Journal of Clinical Psychology, 17*, 394–396.

Stokes, J. M., Pogge, D. L., Grosso, C., & Zaccario, M. (2001). The relationship of the Rorschach Schizophrenia Index to psychotic features in a child psychiatric sample. *Journal of Personality Assessment, 76*, 209–228

Stokes, J. M., Pogge, D. L., Powell-Lunder, J., Ward, A. W., Bilginer, L., & DeLuca, V. A. (2003). The Rorschach Ego Impairment Index: Prediction of treatment outcome in a child psychiatric population. *Journal of Personality Assessment, 81*, 11–19.

Stone, L. A. (1965). Test–retest stability of the MMPI scales. *Psychological Reports, 16*, 619–620.

Streiner, D. L. (2003). Being inconsistent about consistency: When coefficient alpha does and doesn't matter. *Journal of Personality Assessment, 80*, 217–222.

Sturman, M. C., Cheramie, R. A., & Cashen, L. H. (2005). The impact of job complexity and performance measurement on the temporal consistency, stability, and test–retest reliability of employee job performance ratings. *Journal of Applied Psychology, 90*, 269–283.

Sultan, S., Andronikof, A., Réveilère, C., & Lemmel, G. (2006). A Rorschach stability study in a non-patient adult sample. *Journal of Personality Assessment, 87*, 330–348.

Sultan, S., Jebrane, A., & Heurtier-Hartemann, A. (2002). Rorschach variables related to blood glucose control in insulin-dependent diabetes patients. *Journal of Personality Assessment, 79*(1), 122–141.

Viglione, D. J. (1989). Rorschach science and art. *Journal of Personality Assessment, 53*, 195–197.

Viglione, D. J. (1996). Data and issues to consider in reconciling self report and the Rorschach. *Journal of Personality Assessment, 67*, 579–587.

Viglione, D. J. (1999). A review of recent research addressing the utility of the Rorschach. *Psychological Assessment, 11*(3), 251–265.

Viglione, D. J. (2003). *Rorschach coding solutions: A reference guide for the Comprehensive System*. San Diego: Author.

Viglione, D. J., & Hilsenroth, M. J. (2001). The Rorschach: Facts, fictions, and future. *Psychological Assessment, 13*(4), 452–471.

Viglione, D. J., & Rivera, B. (2003). Assessing personality and psychopathology with projective methods. In J. R. Graham & J. A. Naglieri (Eds.), *Handbook of psychology: Assessment psychology* (Vol. 10, pp. 531–552). New York: Wiley.

Viglione, D. J., & Taylor, N. (2003). Empirical support for interrater reliability of the Rorschach Comprehensive System coding. *Journal of Clinical Psychology, 59*(1), 111–121.

Viglione, D. J., Brager, R. C., & Haller, N. (1988). Usefulness of structural Rorschach data in identifying inpatients with depressive symptoms: A preliminary study. *Journal of Personality Assessment, 52*(3), 524–529.

Viglione, D. J., Perry, W., & Meyer, G. (2003). Refinements in the Rorschach Ego Impairment Index incorporating the Human Representational Variable. *Journal of Personality Assessment, 81*(2), 149–156.

Wenar & Curtis (1991). The validity of the Rorschach for assessing cognitive and affective changes, *Journal of Personality Assessment, 57*, 291–308.

Weiner, I. B. (1991). Editor's note: Interscorer agreement in Rorschach research. *Journal of Personality Assessment, 56*, 1.

Weiner, I. B. (2001). Advancing the science of psychological assessment: The Rorschach inkblot method as exemplar. *Psychological Assessment, 13*, 423–434

Wood, J. M., & Lilienfeld, S. O. (1999). The Rorschach Inkblot Test: A case of overstatement? *Assessment, 6*(4), 341–351.

Wood, J. M., Nezworski, M. T., Garb, H. N., & Lilienfeld, S. O. (2001a). The misperception of psychopathology: Problems with norms of the Comprehensive System for the Rorschach. *Clinical Psychology: Science & Practice, 8*(3), 350–373.

Wood, J. M., Nezworski, M. T., Garb, H. N., & Lilienfeld, S. O. (2001b). Problems with the norms of the Comprehensive System for the Rorschach: Methodological and conceptual considerations. *Clinical Psychology: Science & Practice, 8*(3), 397–402.

Wood, J. M., Nezworski, M. T., & Stejskal, W. J. (1996). The Comprehensive System for the Rorschach: A critical examination. *Psychological Science, 7*(1), 3–10.

Wood, J. M., Nezworski, M. T., Stejskal, W. J., & McKinzey, R. K. (2001). Problems of the Comprehensive System for the Rorschach in forensic settings: Recent developments. *Journal of Forensic Psychology Practice, 1*(3), 89–103.

Woodrome, S. E. & Fastenau, P. S. (2005). Test–retest reliability of the Extended Complex Figure Test–Motor Independent administration (ECFT–MI). *Archives of Clinical Neuropsychology, 20*, 291–299.

3

ADMISSIBILITY OF THE RORSCHACH

Joseph T. McCann
UHS Hospital, Binghamton, NY

F. Barton Evans
Private Practice, Bozeman, MT

Defending the Rorschach in Court: An Analysis of Admissibility Using Legal and Pofessional Standards

Joseph T. McCann

There are a number of legal and professional standards that guide admissibility of expert testimony and psychometric evidence. The most important legal tests for admissibility include the *Federal Rules of Evidence* (1992), the *Frye* test (*United States v. Frye,* 1923), and the *Daubert* standard (*Daubert v. Merrell Dow Pharmaceuticals, Inc.,* 1993). Within the profession, Heilbrun (1992) and Marlowe (1995) have outlined criteria for the selection of psychological tests in forensic settings. Using these legal and professional standards, the Rorschach is analyzed according to individual criteria. Although several issues require additional research, it is concluded that the status of the Rorschach Inkblot Method is such that it satisfies legal tests of admissibility and professional criteria that have been suggested. In those cases where the Rorschach is apt to be deemed inadmissible, it is likely due to how data from the instrument are utilized, rather than characteristics of the instrument itself.

Professional sentiments about use of the Rorschach Inkblot Method in forensic settings have ranged widely. There are those who suggest that the Rorschach is an instrument that has absolutely no validity and should not be used in any clinical or forensic settings. The strongest proponent of this position is Dawes (1994), who contended that the Rorschach is a "shoddy" instrument and "is not a valid test of anything" (p. vii). He went so far as to recommend to everyone that if they ever undergo a psychological evaluation and someone takes out the Rorschach, that the person should leave the room. There are, of course, others who contend that the Rorschach is a valid and reliable instrument that can yield

Joseph T. McCann's article originally appeared in the *Journal of Personality Assessment* (1998). It is reprinted here with permission.

F. Barton Evans is the sole author of the update regarding McCann's article.

very useful information when used properly. The clearest position on this approach has been outlined by Weiner (1996), who stated that those who are critical of the Rorschach have "not read the relevant literature of the last 20 years; or, having read it, they have not grasped its meaning" (p. 206). Given the need for empirically based methods when conducting forensic evaluations, the issues raised in this debate over use of the Rorschach Inkblot Method are of extreme importance to those who use the instrument in settings where their findings may be presented and challenged in court.

The Rorschach continues to hold a prominent place in training and practice settings. In surveys of training programs, teaching of the Rorschach Inkblot Method continues at a very high level, with 94% of programs accredited by the American Psychological Association teaching the instrument in 1974, 93% teaching it in 1984, and 85% teaching it in 1993 (Piotrowski & Zalewski, 1993; Ritzler & Alter, 1986). In addition, clinical use of the Rorschach has not diminished in the last several decades. Surveys of professional test usage document that the Rorschach is among the most widely used psychological assessment instruments in the United States. It has been shown consistently that the Rorschach is used by more than 80% of agencies or practitioners who engage in psychological assessment (Lubin, Larsen, & Matarazzo, 1984; Lubin, Wallis, & Paine, 1971; Piotrowski & Keller, 1989; Sundberg, 1961; Watkins, Campbell, Nieberding, & Hallmark, 1995).

Despite the favorable status that the Rorschach apparently has within the profession, there are still strong critics who state that the instrument lacks validity and reliability and should not be viewed as a measure of anything (Dawes, 1994; Ziskin & Faust, 1988). Moreover, as managed care and other economic pressures have impacted on the professional practice of psychology, mental health practitioners are finding themselves searching for alternative avenues of professional practice. Mental health professionals are engaging in forensic work with greater frequency, and this area of practice is often where comprehensive personality assessment, involving broad-based approaches to testing that include the Rorschach, has been relatively untouched by economic concerns (Acklin, 1996).

Given the increased frequency with which mental health professionals have become involved in evaluating individuals in legal settings, there has been a concomitant increase in commentary in the literature on the appropriate use of various psychological testing instruments in forensic practice. In particular, there are guides for using the MMPI (Pope, Butcher, & Seelen, 1993) and Millon inventories (McCann & Dyer, 1996) in forensic settings. However, there is limited literature on use of the Rorschach in forensic settings.

Some exceptions to this state of affairs are articles that document the psychometric characteristics of the Rorschach (Weiner, 1996, 1997) and the experiences of a large sample of professionals who use the Rorschach in forensic settings; who find that the instrument does not encounter significant challenge in the courtroom (Weiner, Exner, & Sciara, 1996). Meloy, Hansen, and Weiner (1997) also found that the Rorschach has been given legal weight by appellate courts throughout the United States. These articles document useful information on the reliability, validity, and clinical utility of the Rorschach as an instrument for describing personality, assisting in differential diagnosis, and identifying important psychological variables in forensic settings.

The purpose of this article is to reformulate the issues in this debate by analyzing its psychometric properties and its current scientific and clinical status within the context of established standards for admissibility of expert testimony. Legal standards established through case law and formal rules of evidence, and proposed guidelines found in the professional literature, constitute the two major sources from which criteria are drawn to analyze the appropriateness of using the Rorschach in forensic settings. Note that legal rules on admissibility of expert testimony vary across jurisdictions, and in many instances it is within the presiding judge's discretion whether proffered testimony and the methodology on which it is based are ultimately admitted into court. The following analysis does not constitute legal or professional advice but is offered as a guideline that can be used in establishing the admissibility of one's reliance on the Rorschach when answering psycholegal questions and performing psychological evaluations in forensic matters.

LEGAL STANDARDS FOR EXPERT TESTIMONY

It is the job of the trier of fact (i.e., judge or jury) in legal settings to decide ultimate issues such as the determination of guilt or innocence, appropriate monetary damages, and other matters critical to the outcome of a case. This process is done by weighing and evaluating evidence offered before a court. Mental health professionals frequently appear as expert witnesses to assist the trier of fact by providing information that is deemed important for deciding the legal issues. Because expert witnesses offer opinions that are based on knowledge that is assumed to be outside the range of familiarity for the typical juror, expert opinions typically serve to make information available to jurors that will assist their decision making.

Legal standards in the form of evidentiary rules serve to guide judges in deciding whether proffered expert testimony will be admissible. Evidentiary rules vary across jurisdictions, with Federal courts relying on the *Federal Rules of Evidence (FRE;* 1992) and state courts relying either on codified rules of evidence or extensive case law. Some state courts model their rules of evidence after the *FRE;* other state courts (e.g., New York) have a large body of case law governing the admissibility of evidence. Regardless of the specific jurisdiction in which an expert might testify, one of three major legal standards is likely to guide admissibility of testimony; these standards are the *FRE,* the *Frye* test *(United States v. Frye,* 1923), and the *Daubert* standard *(Daubert v. Merrell Dow Pharmaceuticals, Inc.,* 1993).

FRE

According to the *FRE,* evidence is admissible if it is "relevant" (Rule 401); more specifically, the evidence must make the existence of any fact that is of consequence to the outcome of the case more or less probable. However, not all relevant evidence is admissible, and Rules 402 and 403 of the *FRE* outline exceptions to the admissibility of relevant evidence, such as evidence that is not permitted by the U.S. Constitution (e.g., if a criminal defendant's testimony violates the Fifth Amendment right against self-incrimination) or evidence that is prejudicial, confusing, or a waste of time.

Article VII of the *FRE* outlines the parameters for opinion and expert testimony. In particular, Rule 702 governs the testimony of experts:

> If scientific, technical, or other specialized knowledge will assist the trier of fact to understand the evidence or to determine a fact in issue, a witness qualified as an expert by knowledge, skill experience, training, or education, may testify thereto in the form of an opinion or otherwise.

A careful reading of this rule suggests that the standard for admissibility of expert testimony under the *FRE* is *helpfulness*—testimony must merely be helpful to the trier of fact in making his or her decision.

Under Rule 703 of the *FRE,* the bases of opinion testimony by experts are guided by the following:

> The facts or data in the particular case on which as expert bases an opinion or inference may be those perceived by or made known to the expert at or before the hearing. If of a type reasonably relied upon by experts in the particular field in forming opinions or inferences upon the participant, the facts or data need not be admissible in evidence.

This rule suggests that any method on which an expert relies may be admissible if it is of a type that is reasonably relied on by others in one's professional community.

With respect to the use of the Rorschach, therefore, the issue under the *FRE* becomes whether reliance on this method is reasonable in light of what others in the professional community rely on and whether opinions derived, in part from Rorschach results, will be helpful to the jury. The *FRE* were designed to be fairly liberal in that they were intended to give judges latitude in deciding on the admissibility of evidence.

The *Frye* Standard

A second major legal standard governing admissibility of expert testimony is the *Frye* test that has been outlined in the original court decision in *United States v. Frye* (1923). Although this case represents a Federal opinion, it has been adopted by many state courts as the appropriate standard for determining admissibility of expert testimony. According to the *Frye* test, expert testimony is admissible if it is based on a methodology that has been sufficiently established to have gained *general acceptance* in the field to which it belongs. Therefore, the *Frye* test examines whether a particular theory, technique, or methodology is generally accepted in the field when determining if expert testimony is admissible.

Again with respect to the Rorschach, an important consideration will be whether the instrument is generally accepted in the field of clinical psychology and forensic assessment. This issue will be examined more carefully later in light of recent findings on use of the Rorschach in both clinical and forensic psychological evaluations.

The *Daubert* Standard

A third major legal standard for examining the admissibility of expert testimony is the U.S. Supreme Court decision in *Daubert v. Merrell Dow Pharmaceuticals, Inc.* (1993).

Although the case dealt with a civil action brought against the manufacturer of an anti-nausea drug for damages related to resultant birth, defects, the *Daubert* decision addressed a critical issue on the admissibility of expert testimony in federal courts. Prior to the decision, federal courts had been essentially divided on whether the *FRE* or *Frye* test was the appropriate test for admissibility of proposed expert testimony. In a detailed decision, the *Daubert* court held that the appropriate standard of admissibility in federal courts was the *FRE* and that the general acceptance test under *Frye* was no longer appropriate as the sole determinative factor. In essence, the court stated that the *FRE* "assign to the trial judge the task of ensuring that an expert's testimony both rests on a reliable foundation and is relevant to the task at hand" (p. 2799).

However, the *Daubert* decision outlined a variety of factors that judges might consider when making a determination as to whether expert testimony is admissible. The four major factors outlined in the decision include the following: (a) The theory or technique is scientific knowledge that can or has been tested, (b) the theory or technique has been subjected to peer review, (c) there is a known or potential rate of error, and (d) general acceptance in the field. These four factors were offered by the *Daubert* court as a guide for judges when deciding what expert testimony should be admitted.

The first of the four criteria suggests that courts give consideration to whether a specific technique or theory has been tested. In particular, it is important to determine the extent to which the methodology is falsifiable and capable of empirical testing. Although mental health professionals are not generally oriented toward the concept of falsifiability, this concept refers to the extent to which hypotheses have been generated about a theory or methodology and tested to determine their validity. The second of the four factors recommends that courts evaluate the extent to which the methodology has been subjected to peer review and publication. This factor is "relevant, but not dispositive" (p. 2797) in evaluating the extent to which flaws in the technique or methodology have been uncovered by the scientific community. The third factor refers not only to "known or potential" error rates, but also to the "existence and maintenance of standards controlling the technique's operation" (p. 2797). Here the court appears to recommend that courts consider whether standards have been developed for using the methodology and for drawing conclusions from the data. Finally, the fourth criterion outlined in the *Daubert* decision is general acceptance, as it has been outlined earlier in the *Frye* opinion. That is, acceptance of the methodology is important reformation that should be considered when evaluating admissibility, but it is not the sole controlling factor as it is under the *Frye* test.

The *Daubert* opinion has generated a considerable amount of academic discussion and there is no consensus about implications of the opinion. There are some who have argued that the *Daubert* opinion will result in more liberal acceptance of expert testimony because of the FRE's liberal "helpfulness" approach, whereas others argue that the *Daubert* criteria will result in more critical judicial analysis of proposed testimony and thus greater restrictions on expert opinion (Goodman-Delahunty, 1997). Despite this interesting issue, the major implication of the *Daubert* opinion is that judges continue to have broad discretion in deciding what expert testimony will be permitted in Federal courts.

Another important point to consider is that the *Daubert* decision does not spell the end of the *Frye* standard. Some states (e.g. Arizona, California, Florida, Nebraska, & New York) have explicitly rejected the "gatekeeping" role of the court outlined by *Daubert* and have instead retained the *Frye* general acceptance test. Therefore, the *Frye* standard will still apply in those state courts where the test remains in effect, whereas *Daubert* will control admissibility in all federal courts, or in those state courts that explicitly adopt that particular standard. Thus, regardless of the specific jurisdiction in which an expert testifies, the standard for admissibility will be either the FRE—*Daubert* or the *Frye* standard.

PROFESSIONAL STANDARDS FOR FORENSIC PSYCHOLOGICAL USAGE

Although rules of evidence provide the framework within which the ultimate determination of admissibility of expert testimony is made, there have been guidelines offered in the professional literature in recent years to provide direction on the selection of psychological assessment instruments in forensic settings. It is important to recognize that these guidelines do not represent formal standards adopted by any particular professional organization or credential-issuing body. Nevertheless, they provide assistance to forensic mental health professionals who use psychological instruments to help answer psycholegal questions. The two major presentations on this issue are those by Heilbrun (1992) and Marlowe (1995).

Heilbrun's Guidelines

According to Heilbrun (1992), the selection of a psychological assessment instrument for use in forensic evaluation must be guided by the relevance of the instrument to the legal standard that provides the framework for the forensic issues being evaluated. In particular, the relevance of any psychometric instrument can take one of two forms. The first type of relevancy pertains to those instruments that are direct measures of a legal construct that lie at the heart of a particular forensic assessment. Examples of such instruments include specific interviews and measures for assessing competency to stand trial. (Grisso, 1988), the Gudjonsson Suggestibility Scales as measures of interrogative suggestibility (Gudjonsson, 1997), and the Rogers Criminal Responsibility Assessment Scales (Rogers, 1984). A second form of relevancy described by Heilbrun is when a psychological assessment instrument measures a psychological construct (e.g., reality testing, impulsivity, etc.) that is a critical part of some issue (e.g., mental disease or defect) that must be addressed when answering a psycholegal question. In these situations, the relation between the psychological assessment instrument and forensic issues must be outlined in the professional's written report or testimony.

The Rorschach is not a direct measure of any legal or forensic issue and instead falls in the second form of relevancy just described. That is, forensic use of the Rorschach typically involves the assessment of some personality variable that is a part of some underlying legal standard, and the clinician must make the connection between Rorschach results and the forensic issue being addressed clear in the report or through testimony. In more direct terms, the Rorschach is a personality assessment instrument and is likely to have some relevance when any forensic issue can be connected in some way to the participant's personality.

Although admissibility of expert testimony based in part on results from psychological testing is determined by legal rules of evidence, Heilbrun stated that mental health professionals should also formulate their own standards. Toward this end, he proposed seven guidelines that can serve as a framework for selecting psychological tests in forensic assessments. These seven guidelines fall under the three general categories of test selection, administration, and interpretation. The standards proposed by Heilbrun include the following:

1. The test should be commercially available and adequately documented in a manual and should be peer reviewed.
2. Reliability should be established, with a coefficient of .80 advisable or explicit justification for lower coefficients.
3. The test should be relevant to the legal issue or some psychological construct underlying the legal issue with available validation research.
4. The test should have a standard method of administration.
5. The test should be applicable to the population and purpose for which it is used.
6. Objective tests and actuarial data applications are preferred.
7. There should be some method for interpreting test results within the context of the individual's response style.

These guidelines serve as a useful outline to assess the suitability of a particular psychological testing instrument for forensic assessment. Although they do not represent adopted standards by any format credential-issuing or professional organization, they do represent a useful outline to follow.

Marlowe's Hybrid Model

In an attempt to operationalize an approach to evaluating admissibility of psychometric evidence, Marlowe (1995) developed a hybrid model (i.e., a blend of scientific and legal principles) for examining psychometric evidence. This model is comprised of a flowchart that formulates seven basic questions that are addressed in sequential order. According to Marlowe, the first question that must be addressed is whether the witness is recognized as an expert possessing scientific, technical, or specialized knowledge that will assist the trier of fact; this question is similar to the standard outlined in *FRE* Rule 702. The second question addresses whether the theory underlying the data collection is recognized, time tested, falsifiable, and committed to refinement. Once this question has been addressed, the third step in Marlowe's model is to determine whether the psychometric instrument is recognized. In particular, the concern is that an instrument have adequate reliability, standardized norms, professional standards governing appropriate use, and that constructs measured by the instrument have some relevance to the forensic issue at hand. The fourth step in Marlowe's hybrid model is that the instrument have appropriate data collection, reduction, and analysis procedures. The specific concerns at this stage of analysis are that the instrument have justified norms, standardized administration procedures, and accepted methods for analyzing and scoring data.

The last three steps in Marlowe's hybrid model are concerned less with the psychometric properties of the test and more with the manner in which the instrument and the data it yields are utilized. The fifth question addresses whether the data are irrelevant, prejudicial, or duplicative. These issues are more legally based and do not have particular scientific counterparts; they deal mainly with assuring that admissibility of psychometric data will not impede expediency in the judicial process. At the sixth stage in Marlowe's model is whether the psychometric data should be excluded because they run afoul of prevailing social policies. The concern here is that the data do not contribute to the violation of constitutional or statutory rights, such as discrimination, racial bias, and the like.

The seventh step in Marlowe's hybrid model is the most complex because it refers to the issue of validity of the expert's reasoning when relying on particular psychometric data. The issue becomes whether the expert has developed a proper psycholegal formulation into which the data fit, the extent to which there are explicit empirical foundations (e.g. error rates, test validity, etc.) for using the test in a particular manner, and using sound reasoning and an acceptable level of expressed certainty in one's opinion. In short, the seventh stage in this hybrid model constitutes a large portion of what would be covered during direct testimony and cross-examination.

ADMISSIBILITY OF THE RORSCHACH: AN ANALYSIS

A review of each legal and professional standard just presented will quickly reveal that there are many areas of overlap and several common themes run across the various standards. For instance, the *Daubert* opinion, Heilbrun's guidelines, and Marlowe's hybrid model are all concerned with the extent to which a particular psychometric instrument has been subjected to peer review. Likewise, general acceptance is the major consideration under *Frye* and is also one of many factors that the *Daubert* standard cites as a factor that judges should consider when deciding on the admissibility of expert testimony. Moreover, the extent to which there is an adequate scientific foundation on which an expert can rest his or her opinion is a major theme in each of the legal tests or professional guidelines presented.

One could go through each of the frameworks presented and analyze admissibility of the Rorschach; however, there would be considerable repetition in such an approach because of overlap that exists across the various approaches. Instead, major factors or issues presented across the various models are presented next and the Rorschach is examined in terms of how well it satisfies those major concerns.

Publication and Peer Review

One major standard for evaluating admissibility of expert testimony is whether the methodology has been published and subjected to peer review. This issue is explicitly stated in the *Daubert* opinion and is also a standard in Heilbrun's guidelines and Marlowe's hybrid model. Therefore, the operational criteria become whether the test is commercially available, has an adequate technical manual, and has research that has been published in peer-reviewed journals.

The Rorschach meets this criterion in several respects. In particular, the Rorschach plates are commercially available from most test publishers and they have been standardized perceptual stimuli for almost 80 years. Moreover, publication of the Comprehensive System method for scoring the Rorschach (Exner. 1974, 1978, 1986, 1991, 1993; Exner & Weiner, 1982, 1994) has become the clinical and forensic standard. Moreover, a considerable amount of methodologically sound research has been generated in the last 20 years on the Rorschach and published in peer-reviewed journals. According to Butcher and Rouse (1996), an average of 95.8 articles are published on the Rorschach each year, and this rate has held fairly constant over the past 20 years.

Some concerns about the Comprehensive System were raised by Wood, Nezworski, and Stejskal (1996a, 1996b) in that a large portion of the research on which Exner's Comprehensive System is based consists of unpublished data that have not undergone peer review. However, Exner (1996) noted in response that many of these unpublished studies were integrated into several of his publications that have appeared in peer-reviewed journals. Moreover, the frequency of Rorschach-based research articles cited by Butcher and Rouse (1996) indicate that several independent researchers have investigated the instrument and published findings in a peer-reviewed journal. For example, Gacono and Meloy's (1994) detailed research on antisocial disorders and the Rorschach produced over a dozen scientific studies, which appeared in four different peer-reviewed psychological and psychiatric journals.

None of the legal or professional standards make any specifications as to what constitutes adequate peer review. Moreover, the *Daubert* court seemed to be concerned more with the fact that the instrument be submitted to "the scrutiny of the scientific community...because it increases the likelihood that substantive flaws in methodology will be detected" (p. 2797). Perhaps no other psychological assessment instrument has been subjected to such intense scrutiny as the Rorschach, and major flaws that were uncovered in its scoring methodology were the impetus behind development of the Comprehensive System.

Standard Administration and Norms

The presence of a standard method for administering, scoring, and interpreting data from a psychometric instrument is one of the main criteria that has been set forth in professional guidelines for forensic use of psychological tests (Heilbrun, 1992; Marlowe, 1995); this criteria has not explicitly appeared in any of the legal tests for admissibility, but there are a number of scoring systems that have been developed for the Rorschach. The most widely used system is Exner's Comprehensive System (Piotrowski, Sherry, & Keller, 1985). This system depends on a specific method of administration and scoring that is outlined in detail by Exner (1995). Moreover, there are clinical norms available for a variety of diagnostic groups as well as nonpatient adults, adolescents, and children (Exner, 1993, 1995). Based on the extensive normative data available for the Comprehensive System, and the fact that most recent research is based on this particular scoring method, it can be concluded that forensic applications of the Rorschach satisfy the criterion of standardized administration and extensive normative data when the Comprehensive System is utilized (Meloy, 1991; Weiner, 1997). The use of an alternative system of scoring may not satisfy this particular professional guideline.

Reliability

The reliability of a psychometric instrument is explicitly identified by Heilbrun and Marlowe as a vital criterion to consider when selecting an instrument for use in forensic assessments. Moreover, the *Daubert* standard indirectly points to reliability as an important criterion for admissibility of expert testimony. With respect to Rorschach data. it is important to identify the type of reliability coefficients that can be calculated. McCann and Dyer (1996) outlined reasons why internal consistency is a preferred measure of reliability because it reflects the precision of measurement, whereas test—retest reliability is often affected by changes in the construct being assessed. However, internal consistency is a reliability measure that is well suited for multi-item psychometric scales, but it is not applicable to Rorschach data, which rely on discrete determinants and ratios. Instead, interrater and test—retest reliability are most applicable to Rorschach data.

Exner (1993) reported on the test-retest reliability of various determinants, ratios, and percentages from the Comprehensive System for both adults and children. The magnitude of the correlations for the ratios and percentages generally equal or exceed .80 and show good stability for both children and adults. One exception is *es*. which is composed of the sum of nonhuman movement and shading determinants. Data provided by Exner (1993) reveal that the test—retest reliability of inanimate movement (*m*) and diffuse shading (*Y*) are the lowest among all determinants at .26 and .31, respectively, over a 1-year period. These two determinants are used to compute *es* and account for the low stability. These variables are measures of situational stress and represent state affect; therefore, stability is expected to be low because of changes in state affect. These low reliability coefficients could instead be viewed as indicative of the validity of these measures.

Nearly all of the stability coefficients cited by Exner (1993) meet or exceed the criterion of .80 cited by Heilbrun, who stated that "the use of tests with a reliability coefficient of less than .80 is not advisable. The use of less reliable tests would require an explicit justification by the psychologist" (p. 265). A survey of Exner's (1993) data reveals that those determinants that are reflective of trait aspects of personality have reliability coefficients that meet or exceed this criterion, whereas those Rorschach data with coefficients below this level represent state aspects of personality. Therefore, the explicit justification that could be offered for relying on Rorschach measures with lower reliability is that because they measure state versus trait aspects of personality, the lower stability is expected and supports the interpretive significance attributed to these data.

Another issue that is worthy of note concerning Rorschach reliability is the concern raised by Wood and his colleagues (Wood et al., 1996a, 1996b) that interrater reliability of the Rorschach is unknown because the percentage of agreement figures cited by Exner (1993) are not reliability coefficients, for the reason that they do not take into consideration chance levels of agreement between raters as would a coefficient such as kappa. However, the stability coefficients cited by Exner (1993), which in fact are reliability measures, could not be achieved without adequate interrater reliability. If interrater reliability of the Rorschach were low, then there would be too much error variance and the high levels of test—retest reliability could not be achieved. Therefore, the most critical form of reliability for Rorschach data (i.e., test—retest reliability) offers a reliable measure that satisfies the criterion outlined in professional and legal standards for forensic psychological test use.

Validity

The validity of the Rorschach has been extensively discussed by a number of authors, and this topic is beyond the scope of this article. However, it is important to note that validity of a psychometric instrument is an explicit criterion outlined by Heilbrun and Marlowe. It is also mentioned in the *Daubert* standard. Despite unresolved issues about what is specifically being measured by a few Rorschach measures (cf. Exner, 1996; Wood et al., 1996a, 1996b), there are several articles documenting the validity of the Rorschach.

Weiner (1996, 1997) outlined how the Rorschach is capable of differentiating state and trait personality variables, measuring developmental change in children and adolescents, monitoring treatment improvement, and identifying distress in individuals with posttraumatic stress disorder. Other reviews have documented validity of the Rorschach for a variety of clinical symptoms and with various populations such as children and adolescents (Atkinson, 1986; Meyer, 1993; Ornberg & Zalewski, 1994; Parker, Hanson, & Hunsley, 1988). The validity of the Rorschach can therefore be supported by citing the research noted in these various reviews.

Rate of Error

The *Daubert* opinion states that when judges evaluate the admissibility of proffered expert testimony that the known or potential rate of error should be considered. However, the opinion does not explicitly state how rate of error should be defined. With respect to this criterion, the Rorschach data that have a rate of error established are those indexes that are utilized to assign a diagnostic classification to a particular participant. Although the Rorschach data have uses that extend beyond the assignment of a diagnostic classification (e.g., description of personality dynamics, assessment of personality structure, etc.), when use of the instrument is extended into the realm of diagnosis, the rate of error becomes an important consideration.

Several studies have examined the rate of error associated with use of the constellation scores from the Comprehensive System, such as the Schizophrenia Index (SCZI), Depression Index (DEPI), Coping Deficit Index, Hypervigilance Index, Suicide Constellation, and Obsessive Style Index. For example, Ganellen (1996) cited findings showing that the SCZI has an overall correct classification rate of 92% and 86% for psychotic disorders and that the DEPI has correct classification rates of 79% and 88% for identifying depression. Meyer (1993) demonstrated that response frequency is a mediating factor that impacts on the ability of the Rorschach indexes to discriminate between various diagnostic groups, and when response frequency is average or high, the diagnostic validity of Rorschach indexes is better than in brief records.

Wood et al. (1996a, 1996b) pointed out that the DEPI has shown rather poor diagnostic power in cross-validation studies and falls prone to what is termed *shrinkage* during cross-validation. The results of independent studies have shown that the DEPI does not have a strong relation with self-report measures of depression (Bail, Archer, Gordon, & French, 1991; Meyer, 1993). Moreover, the Rorschach indexes need to be investigated further in independent research. However, the *Daubert* opinion does not require that a particular rate of error be zero; it is only necessary that expert opinion be based on a foundation where the potential rate of error can be established. In this respect, the Rorschach indexes have rates of error established, and the statistical power of the Rorschach as a research instrument, although relatively low in some respects, is similar to that found in other areas of behavioral science (Acklin, McDowell, & Ornduff, 1992). Therefore, the Rorschach's rate of error for certain decisions can be determined and cited when using Rorschach data in forensic evaluations.

General Acceptance

Under the *Frye* test, general acceptance of a particular method or technique is the central factor that determines whether expert testimony is admissible. Under the *Daubert* standard, general acceptance is a major but not primary consideration. Therefore, whether a psychometric instrument has achieved wide acceptance is a major consideration when selecting psychological tests for forensic application.

The best measure of general, acceptance is the pattern and frequency of psychological test use by practicing professionals. As noted earlier, the Rorschach has achieved wide acceptance as defined by frequency of its use. Surveys have consistently shown that the Rorschach is utilized by over 80% of mental health agencies (Lubin et al., 1971, 1984; Piotrowski & Keller, 1989). In a recent survey, the Rorschach was cited as the third most widely used psychological assessment instrument; it was utilized by 82% of a sample of 412 practicing clinical psychologists engaged in psychological assessment services (Watkins, Campbell, Nieberding, & Hallmark, 1995).

In a study of psychological test use in criminal forensic examinations, Borum and Grisso (1995) found that the Rorschach was used in 32% of criminal responsibility evaluations and 30% of evaluations of competency to stand trial. Another study by Ackerman and Ackerman (1997) on child custody evaluation practices showed that the Rorschach was the second most widely used instrument with adults (used by 48% of respondents) and the sixth most commonly used instrument for children (used by 27% of respondents). Although the relevance of Rorschach data to competency to stand trial and child custody evaluations is not as clear as it is for criminal responsibility evaluations, the data cited in surveys demonstrate that the Rorschach is a widely used instrument. Its general acceptance among those who use psychological tests can be demonstrated.

Relevance and Helpfulness

The *FRE* and the *Daubert* standard require that any proposed expert testimony be both relevant and helpful to the trier of fact. In addition, the criteria outlined by Heilbrun and Marlowe emphasize the need for psychometric evidence to be relevant in some way to the psycholegal issue being addressed by the expert witness. With respect to Rorschach testimony, admissibility under this standard will be determined not by any psychometric properties of the instrument, but rather by the manner in which it is used by the mental health professional. In other words, the forensic professional who relies on the Rorschach must demonstrate, through written reports or oral testimony, how Rorschach results are used in a particular case.

Rorschach results are likely to have some direct relation to the legal issues at hand when the test participant's personality structure is directly relevant. For example, reality testing, the capacity to handle stress, and how one handles emotions may all be directly related to issues such as mental state at the time of offense or risk of violence to others. In other cases, the. connection between Rorschach data may be less clear, and the relevancy will need to be more clearly stated. For instance, Rorschach data in child custody cases do not address directly parenting capacity or the quality of the parent-child relationship; however, the instrument can provide useful data on issues that have an impact on these factors, such as personality characteristics of the parents. Again, it is up to the mental health professional to establish the relevance of the Rorschach data to the issue being litigated.

Overall, admissibility or inadmissibility of Rorschach-based testimony, where relevance and helpfulness are primary issues, appears to be determined by how the test data are utilized, rather than by any specific characteristics of the instrument itself. This is supported by a survey of legal decisions on the Rorschach that documents when Rorschach testimony is deemed inadmissible, it is primarily due to invalid references being made by the expert witness (Meloy et al., 1997).

Falsifiability

The *Daubert* opinion cites falsifiability as a criterion to point out that expert testimony must be capable of being empirically testable for it to be admissible. In other words, the statements constituting a scientific explanation must be capable of being subjected to empirical test. In fact, the debate over the validity of the Rorschach is itself a reflection of the testability and falsifiability of the instrument; there are those who have for many years been trying to "falsify" the instrument.

The use of Rorschach data for explaining and describing personality is particularly germane because some of the explanations derived from the instrument are fully capable of being tested as the research cited herein suggests. Problems arise when Rorschach data are utilized to provide explanations about unconscious processes and psychoanalytic hypotheses that are more difficult to subject to empirical testing. Of course, there are exceptions to these limitations, such as the work of Bornstein (1996) on oral dependency. The mental health professional who utilizes the Rorschach in forensic settings can establish the testability, or falsifiability, of the method by using data that have been subjected to emperical analysis. Therefore, reliance on the Structural Summary from the Comprehensive System or other empirically established indexes will keep the expert's utilization of the Rorschach within the permissible bounds of testability or falsifiability.

Response Style Interpretation

Although none of the legal tests for admissibility require an instrument to have some method for evaluating the individual's response style to be deemed admissible. Heilbrun recommended that this be a criterion for test selection in forensic evaluations. Objective instruments such as the MMPI–2, MCMI-III, and PAI all have scales that measure response style, and one specialized measure, the Structured Interview of Reported Symptoms (Rogers, Bagby, & Dickens, 1992) has shown particularly good capacity for identifying malingering and dissimulation.

The Rorschach was once thought to be impervious to faking, malingering, and other forms of response bias (Stermac, 1988); however, the capacity of the instrument to identify various forms of biased responding has been studied. Participants who have been instructed to portray an impression of psychological health have been shown to provide significantly more popular responses (*P*), fewer stress related determinants (*es*), fewer inappropriate combinations (*FABCOM, INCOM*), and fewer dramatic or sensational contents (Seamons, Howell, Carlisle, & Roe, 1981). Exner (1991) reported on research that has shown individuals undergoing child custody evaluations, where the motivation to deny psychopathology is high, provide a high number of personalized (*PER*) and popular (*P*) responses and show high levels of intellectualization.

Malingering has also been examined on the Rorschach by a number of investigators. Essentially, the results suggest that there are trends in Rorschach data that may be indicative of malingering, but no definitive patterns emerge. For instance, informed malingerers could not be distinguished from patients with genuine psychosis (Albert, Fox, & Kahn, 1980), and a specific Rorschach index designed to detect malingering has not shown sensitivity (Basch & Alpert, 1980). Other studies have supported the finding that Rorschach protocols characterized by good form quality that include bizarre or inappropriate combinations are suggestive, but not conclusive, of malingering (Seamons et al., 1981). A restricted number of responses has also been a consistent finding among studies in which some form of dissimulation (i.e., denial, malingering, etc.) is suspected (Perry & Kinder, 1990).

In general, the studies conducted on dissimulation and the Rorschach have established trends in structural summary data that are suggestive of biased responding. However, no clear diagnostic cutoffs or operating characteristics have been established. Therefore, it is important to integrate other data sources when arriving at conclusions related to the possibility that a particular participant is dissimulating. Nevertheless, the Rorschach data can be reviewed for possible signs of biased responding because there are methods to evaluate the validity of the Rorschach data for a particular participant (e.g. number of responses, relative number of form-only responses, etc.).

CONCLUSIONS

An analysis of the current clinical and research status of the Rorschach reveals that it meets professional and legal standards for admissibility of psychometric evidence and expert testimony. This conclusion rests on the foundation of a large body of literature that exists for the Exner Comprehensive System because this method of administration and scoring is standardized, has documented psychometric characteristics, and has been the primary subject of Rorschach research over the past 20 years. Other Rorschach systems have not been as well documented and it is therefore recommended that any forensic application of the Rorschach rely primarily on the Comprehensive System. Moreover, primary use of structural summary data, as opposed to sequence and nonstandardized content analysis, is recommended because of the availability of research to support reliability and validity.

There are those who may continue to argue that the Rorschach is not an appropriate psychometric instrument for any use and that it should be banned not only from forensic but also clinical settings. However, as surveys of test usage continue to demonstrate, the Rorschach has maintained a very high level of acceptance and use. Moreover, debates such as the one between Wood et al. (1996a, 1996b) and Exner (1996) are fruitful because they contribute to refinements of the instrument's use and also constitute "'good science' in part because it increases the likelihood that substantive flaws in methodology will be detected" (*Daubert,* 1993, p. 2797). One should also consider the fact that no legal or professional standard requires that a psychometric instrument be a perfect measure of psychological constructs. Moreover, legal admissibility does not require that all scientific issues be completely resolved to the satisfaction of all members of the professional community. Expert testimony must rest on methodology that is generally accepted, testable, standardized, relevant, and helpful. In all of these respects, the Rorschach is an appropriate methodology to utilize in forensic evaluation. However, satisfaction of these criteria does not guarantee that one's testimony or reliance on the Rorschach will be admissible or given weight in any particular court of law.

As both Heilbrun and Marlowe noted, a major governing factor in use of psychometric instruments is the burden placed on the forensic professional to provide clear reasoning concerning how psychometric data relates to the specific psycholegal issue being evaluated. Meloy et al. (1997) found that although the Rorschach is cited favorably by courts; in those few instances where Rorschach testimony was limited or excluded it was due to invalid inferences being made by the psychologist, rather than the individual properties or characteristics of the instrument. Therefore, it is incumbent on the professional using the Rorschach in forensic settings to make clear inferences that have relevance to the issues being addressed. In some forensic evaluations, such as fitness to proceed or child custody evaluations, the connection may not be clear at first and the expert may need to provide more explicit reasoning that ties the data to a given issue. In other forensic evaluations, such as risk of violence or mental state at the time of offense, the connection may be more evident.

The Rorschach appears to be a useful instrument for addressing various diagnostic issues in forensic assessment. However, one must be aware of the various legal and professional standards guiding use of psychometric tests in this area. Although not all Rorschach issues have been resolved, this does not preclude its use in forensic settings. As noted in the *Daubert* opinion, "vigorous cross-examination, presentation of contrary evidence, and careful instruction on the burden of proof" (p. 2798) are the most appropriate methods for attacking evidence. Disagreement among professionals does not constitute adequate grounds for the preclusion of evidence in legal settings; it is rules of evidence and case law that guide admissibility. The Rorschach can be defended in court adequately if the professional has a sound grasp of the professional literature and familiarity with legal standards for admissibility of expert testimony. The professional must also be prepared to articulate clearly his or her reasoning surrounding Rorschach data and its relevance to a particular psycholegal issue, and to know the research to address any attacks raised on cross-examination.

ACKNOWLEDGMENT

I thank J. Reid Meloy for his assistance during the completion of this article and two anonymous reviewers for their helpful comments and suggestions.

REFERENCES

Ackerman, M. J., & Ackerman, M. C. (1997). Custody evaluation practice: A survey of experienced professionals (revisited). *Professional Psychology: Research & Practice, 28,* 137–145.

Acklin, M. W. (1996). Personality assessment and managed care. *Journal of Personality Assessment, 66,* 194–201.

Acklin, M. W., McDowell, C J., & Ornduff, S. (1992). Statistical power and the Rorschach: 1975–1991. *Journal of Personality Assessment, 59,* 366–379.

Albert, S., Fox, H. M., & Kahn, M. W. (1980). Faking psychosis on the Rorschach: Can expert judges detect malingering? *Journal of Personality Assessment, 44,* 115–119.

Atkinson, L. (1986). The comparative validities of the Rorschach and the MMPI: A meta-analysis. *Canadian Psychology, 27,* 238–247.

Ball, J. D., Archer, R. P., Gordon, R. A., & French, J. (1991). Rorschach depression indices with children and adolescents: Concurrent validity findings. *Journal of Personality Assessment, 57,* 465–476.

Bash, I. Y., & Alpert, M. (1980). The determination of malingering. *Annals of the New York Academy of Sciences, 347,* 86–99.

Bornstein, R. R. (1996). Construct validity of the Rorschach oral dependency scale: 1967–1995. *Psychological Assessment, 8,* 200–205.

Borum, R., & Grisso, T. (1995). Psychological test use in criminal forensic evaluations. *Professional Psychology: Research & Practice, 26,* 465–473.

Butcher, J. N., & Rouse, S. V. (1996). Personality: Individual differences and clinical assessment. *Annual Review of Psychology, 47,* 87–111.

Dawes, R. M. (1994). *House of cards: Psychology and psychotherapy built on myth.* New York: Free Press.

Daubert v. Merrell Dow Pharmaceuticals, Inc., 113 S.Ct. 2786 (1993).

Exner, J. E. (1974). *The Rorschach: A comprehensive system: Vol. 1.* New York: Wiley.

Exner, J. E. (1978). *The Rorschach: A comprehensive system: Vol. 2.* New York: Wiley.

Exner, J. E. (1986). *The Rorschach: A comprehensive system: Vol. 1. Basic foundations* (2nd ed.). New York: Wiley.

Exner, J. E. (1991). *The Rorschach: A comprehensive system: Vol. 2. Interpretation* (2nd ed.). New York: Wiley.

Exner, J. E. (1993). *The Rorschach: A comprehensive system: Vol. 1. Basic foundations* (3rd ed.). New York: Wiley.

Exner, J. E. (1995). *A Rorschach workbook for the comprehensive system* (4th ed.) Asheville, NC: Rorschach Workshops.

Exner, J. E. (1996). A comment on the comprehensive system for the Roschach: A critical examination *Psychological Science, 7,* 11–13.

Exner, J. E., & Weiner, I. B (1982). *The Rorschach: A comprehensive system: Vol. 3. Assessment of children and adolescents.* New York: Wiley.

Exner, J. E., & Weiner, I. B. (1994). *The Rorschach: A comprehensive system: Vol 3: Assessment of children and adolescents* (2nd ed.). New York: Wiley.

Federal rules of evidence. (1992). Boston: Little, Brown.

Gacono, C., & Meloy, J. R. (1994). *Rorschach assessment of aggressive and psychopathic personalities.* Hillsdale, NJ: Lawrence Erlbaum Associates, Inc.

Ganellen, R. J. (1996). Comparing the diagnostic efficiency of the MMPI, MCMI-II, and Rorschach: A review. *Journal of Personality Assessment, 67,* 219–243.

Goodman-Delahunty, J. (1997). Forensic psychological expertise in the wake of *Daubert, Law and Human Behavior, 21,* 121–140.

Grisso, T. (1988). *Competency to stand trial evaluations: A manual for practice.* Sarasota, FL Professional Resource Exchange.

Gudjonsson, G. (1997). *The Gudjonsson Suggestibility Scales manual.* East Sussex, England: Psychology Press.

Heilbrun, K. (1992). The role of psychological testing in forensic assessment. *Law and Human Behavior, 16,* 257–272.

Lubin, B., Larsen, R. M., & Matarazzo, J. (1984). Patterns of psychological test usage in the United States: 1935–1982. *American Psychologist, 39,* 451–454.

Lubin, B., Wallis, R. R., & Paine, C. (1971). Patterns of psychological test usage in the United States. *Professional Psychology, 2,* 70–74.

Marlowe, D. B. (1995). A hybrid decision framework for evaluating psychometric evidence. *Behavioral Sciences & the Law, 13,* 207–228.

McCann, J. T., & Dyer, F. J. (1996). *Forensic assessment with the Million inventories.* New York: Guilford.

Meloy, J. R. (1991). Rorschach testimony. *Journal of Psychiatry & Law, 8,* 221–235.

Meloy, J. R., Hansen, T. L., & Weiner, I. B. (1997). The authority of the Rorschach: Legal citations during the past 50 years. *Journal of Personality Assessment, 69,* 53–62.

Meyer, G. J. (1993). The impact of response frequency on the Rorschach constellation indices and on their validity with diagnostic and MMPI–2 criteria. *Journal of Personality Assessment, 60,* 153–180.

Ornberg, B., & Zalewski, C. (1994). Assessment of adolescents with the Rorschach: A critical review. *Assessment, 1,* 209–217.

Parker, K. C. H., Hanson, R. K., & Hunsley, J (1988). MMPI, rorschach, and WAIS: A meta-analytic comparison of reliability, stability, and validity. *Psychological Bulletin, 103,* 367–373.

Perry, G. G., & Kinder, B. N. (1990). The susceptibility of the Rorschach to malingering. A critical review. *Journal of Personality Assessment, 54,* 47–57.

Piotrowski, C., & Keller, J. W. (1989). Psychological testing in outpatient mental health facilities: A national study *Professional Psychology, 20,* 423–425.

Piotrowski, C., Sherry, D., & Keller, J. W. (1985). Psychodiagnostic test usage: A survey of the Society for Personality Assessment. *Journal of Personality Assessment, 49,* 115–119.

Piotrowski, C., & Zalewski, C. (1993). Training in psychodiagnostic testing in APA-approved PsyD and PhD clinical psychology programs. *Journal of Personality Assessment, 61,* 394–405.

Pope, K. S., Butcher, J.N., & Seelen, J. (1993). *The MMPI, MMPI–2, & MMPI—A in court.* Washington, DC: American Psychological Association.

Ritzier, B., & Alter, B. (1986). Rorschach teaching in APA-approved clinical graduate programs: Ten years later. *Journal of Personality Assessment, 50,* 44–49.

Rogers, R. (1984). *Rogers criminal responsibility assessment scales.* Odessa, FL: Psychological Assessment Resources.

Seamons, D. T., Howell, R. J., Carlisle, A. L., & Roe, A. L. (1981). Rorschach simulation of mental illness and normality. *Journal of Personality Assessment, 45,* 130–135.

Stermac, L. (1988). Projective testing and dissimulation. In R. Rogers (Ed.), *Clinical assessment of malingering and deception* (pp. 159–168). New York: Guilford.

Sundberg, N.D. (1961). The practice of psychological testing in clinical services in the United States *American Psychologist, 16,* 79–83.

United States v. Frye, 293 F. 1013 (DC Cir. 1923).

Watkins, C. E., Campbell, V. L., Nieberding, R., & Hallmark, R. (1995). Contemporary practice of psychological assessment by clinical psychologists. *Professional Psychology, 26,* 54–60.

Weiner, I. B. (1996). Some observations on the validity of the Rorschach inkblot method. *Psychological Assessment, 8,* 206–213.

Weiner, I. B. (1997). Current status of the Rorschach inkblot method. *Journal of Personality Assessment, 68,* 5–19.

Weiner, I. B., Exner, J. E., & Sciara, A. (1996). Is the Rorschach welcome in the courtroom? *Journal of Personality Assessment, 67,* 422–424.

Wood, J. M., Nezworski, M. T., & Stejskal, W. J. (1996a). The comprehensive system for the Rorschach: A critical examination. *Psychological Science, 7,* 3–10.

Wood, J. M., Nezworski, M. T., & Stejskal, W. J. (1996b). Thinking critically about the comprehensive system for the Rorschach: A reply to Exner. *Psychological Science, 7,* 14–17.

Ziskin, J., & Faust, D. (1988). *Coping with psychiatric and psychological testimony* (4th ed.). Los Angeles: Law and Psychology Press.

An Update of McCann's "Defending the Rorschach in Court"

F. Barton Evans

McCann's (1998) article on the admissibility of the Rorschach stands out in the literature on both the Rorschach and forensic psychological testing in general as an exemplary model for assessing the soundness of psychometric evidence for court and the expert testimony that flows from it. Because McCann's overall structure and clarity of analysis remains fresh today, his original article is included in this book as an essential resource for forensic psychologists using the Rorschach. He reviewed the legal tests for admissibility, as well as professional standards for deciding what psychological tests to use in forensic settings. McCann noted that the Rorschach fared well in these analyses and that, when the Rorschach was deemed inadmissible, the judicial judgment arose from misuse of the data, rather than characteristics of Rorschach itself. The purpose of this section is to provide the reader with a brief update of relevant literature since McCann's article.

McCann (1998) noted a growing difference of professional opinion about the Rorschach and its use in forensic settings. Although the Rorschach has met with controversy since its beginning (see Viglione & Rivera, 2003), a series of criticisms began to surface claiming that the Rorschach lacked scientific reliability and validity (Dawes, 1994; Wood, Nezworski, & Stejskal, 1996) and the suggestion was made that it should not be used in court (Wood et al., 1996). Indeed, Garb (1999) made an unprecedented call for a moratorium on use of the Rorschach, and Grove and Barden (1999) argued for the inadmissibility of the Rorschach in court under *Daubert/Kumho*. This small, but vocal, faction of authors spawned a series of repetitious articles critical of the Rorschach (e.g., Grove, Barden, Garb, & Lilienfeld, 2002; Hunsley & Bailey, 1999, 2001; Lilienfeld, Wood, & Garb, 2000; Nezworski & Wood, 1995; Wood & Lilienfeld, 1999; Wood, Nezworski, Garb, & Lilienfeld, 2001a, 2001b; Wood, Nezworski, & Stejskal, 1996; Wood, Nezworski, Stejskal, & McKinzey, 2001), as well as those in support of excluding Rorschach testimony in the court room (Dawes, 1999; Grove & Barden, 1999; Grove et al., 2002; Lilienfeld et al., 2000). Forensic psychologists using the Rorschach are strongly encouraged to read these papers and be prepared to address the points raised in them.

Rorschach researchers have responded in strength and numbers to these critiques. For example, Weiner (1996) stated that those who are critical of the Rorschach have "not read the relevant literature of the past 20 years, or, having read it, have not grasped its meaning" (p. 206). Since Weiner's article, well-designed meta-analyses (see Gronnerod, 2006, 2003; Hiller, Rosenthal, Bornstein, Berry, & Brunell-Neuleib, 1999; Rosenthal, Hiller, Bornstein, Berry, & Brunell-Neuleib, 2001) and other research have demonstrated that, when properly used, the Rorschach is a valid and reliable instrument that can yield valuable information. Rather than list the voluminous research support for the Rorschach, the reader is referred to Viglione and Meyer (chap. 2, this vol.) as a primary contemporaneous resource providing a thorough review of the scientific status of the Rorschach. In response to the growing discrepancy between the mounting evidence of scientific robustness of the Rorschach and the public's perception of the Rorschach as "junk science" (fueled by the small faction disparaging the Rorschach in the media), the Board of Trustees of the Society for Personality Assessment (2005) published "The Status of the Rorschach in Clinical and Forensic Practice: An Official Statement by the Board of Trustees of the Society for Personality Assessment," also known as the Rorschach White Paper (copy of this article can be found on the Web site of the Society for Personality Assessment at www.personality.org). The statement is written in a language suitable for judges, attorneys, administrators, and the public and also includes a substantial compilation of research references and tables to support its claims. Based on a careful review of the science underlying the test, the Rorschach White Paper concludes that "the Rorschach possesses documented reliability and validity similar to other generally accepted test instruments used in the assessment of personality and psychopathology and that its responsible use in personality assessment is appropriate and justified" (p. 221).

Furthermore, since McCann (1998), there are several important articles challenging the claims that the Rorschach is inadmissible as a scientifically valid instrument in court. Gacono, Evans, and Viglione (2002; chap. 1, this vol.) summarized the main issues for the forensic psychologist preparing for forensic testimony and contrasted the polemical debate of Rorschach detractors with a review of the substantial literature supporting the use of the Rorschach in court. In an article on the Rorschach as exemplar of dealing with challenges to psychological assessment instruments in forensic settings, Hilsenroth and Striker (2004) provided essential reference materials and offered guidelines for proceeding with challenges to the Rorschach in court. They emphasized that debate or the lack of unanimous agreement among the scientific community about a psychological instrument does not automatically translate into inadmissibility. They also pointed out that forensic expertise resides primarily in how the psychological instrument is used, rather than the Rorschach itself. In addition, Hilsenroth and Striker (2004) cogently informed the reader that legal debate does not require the same neutrality or objectivity as scientific debate and the critiques of Rorschach detractors often fall into the category of legal debate. Next, Ritzler, Erard, and Pettigrew (2002a, 2002b) specifically challenged Grove and Barden's (1999) and Grove et al.'s (2002) contentions for the inadmissibility of the Rorschach in court. Ritzler et al. (2002a) leveled a strongly worded criticism of Grove and Barden, stating that they "overlooked or minimized a substantial body of empirical data supporting the reliability and validity of the Rorschach Comprehensive System" and further "misinterpreted the language and intent of the Supreme Court decisions." The articles by Ritzler et al. contribute to the growing chorus of concern about the selective use of the scientific literature by Rorschach detractors to bolster their arguments (see also Gacono, Evans, & Viglione, 2002). Erard and Evans (2006) took the Rorschach detractors to task for failing to follow the very principles of good science that they claim as the basis of their critiques, specifically factual accuracy (acceptance of the value of empirical data and analysis), thoroughness (objective review of all existing literature, including research contrary to one's opinions), and humility (admission of potential limitations in conclusions). In conclusion, although there is debate about the use of the Rorschach in court, for the well-prepared Rorschach expert, little has changed substantively to contradict McCann's (1998) conclusions regarding its acceptability in court other than an abundance of new meta-analyses and research supporting the underlying science of the Rorschach.

Since McCann's article, the Rorschach has maintained an important role and wide acceptance in professional practice settings. More recent surveys of professional test usage document that the Rorschach remains a commonly used psychological assessment instrument in the United States. Camara, Nathan, and Puente's (2000) survey found that the Rorschach is the second most widely used personality assessment instrument among clinical psychologists and neuropsychologists. Archer and Newsome (2000) found it continued to be the second most widely used personality assessment instrument used in the assessment of adolescents. In forensic assessment, Quinnell and Bow (2001) and Boccaccini and Brodsky (1999) found that the Rorschach was the third most widely utilized personality assessment instrument used respectively in custody evaluations and personal injury evaluations. These surveys replicate the findings reported by McCann (1998), suggesting a noteworthy history of stable use of the Rorschach.

Despite the weight of evidence supporting the clinical and forensic use of the Rorschach, Lillienfeld et al. (2000) claimed that the Rorschach is "highly controversial" and not widely accepted in the relevant scientific community, citing "sustained and often withering criticisms directed at projective testing during the past several decades" (p. 27). Schutz and Evans (chap.12, this vol.) criticize Lilienfeld et al. for failing to mention or reference research in refereed journals contrary to their opinion and for essentially misinterpreting and misrepresenting the meaning of research by Piotrowski, Belter, and Keller (1998) on the impact of managed care on the decreased use of projective techniques. Lally's survey (2003) of diplomates in forensic psychology assessed these experts' opinion on the use of specific psychological tests in six areas: mental state at the time of offense, risk for future violence, risk for future sexual violence, competency to stand trial, competency to waive *Miranda* rights, and malingering. He categorized experts' ratings of the Rorschach as equivocal-unacceptable for mental state at the time of offense and unacceptable to risk of violence assessment (53%), risk for future sexual violence (52%), competency to stand trial (60%), and to waive *Miranda* rights (63%), and malingering (55%). Whereas clearly this study suggests the possibility of a limited, if any, role for the Rorschach in these criminal matters, the survey leaves open the question of the basis for these judgments, especially background and training of the experts and their knowledge of the psychological literature on the use of the Rorschach in criminal matters. In light of the substantial research on the Rorschach with criminal populations beginning with Gacono and Meloy (1994) and of applications amply demonstrated in this book (chaps. 7–11, 16–20, 22, and parts of 23), the results of the Lally (2003) survey could be substantially misleading in the court room, if accepted uncritically.

McCann (1998) expressed his concern that there was an appearance of limited literature on use of the Rorschach in forensic settings. Unlike books for using the MMPI (Pope, Butcher, & Seelen, 2006) and the Millon inventories (McCann & Dyer, 1996) in forensic settings, Rorschach experts heretofore had no central resource for the Rorschach, but were limited to scouring the psychological literature for guidance in its use in court. The publication of *The Handbook of Forensic Rorschach Assessment* addresses McCann's concern and demonstrates the broad use of the Rorschach in a variety of forensic settings.

Lastly, McCann noted that the Rorschach fared well in both in published legal decisions both in the courts in general (Weiner, Exner, & Sciara, 1996) and in appellate courts (Meloy, Hansen, & Weiner 1997). Updating the 10 years since Meloy, Hansen, and Weiner's study, Meloy (chap. 4, this vol.) reported on the authority of the Rorschach in court, reviewing 150 published appellate citations from federal, state, and military courts between 1996 and 2005. He reported an average yearly citation rate nearly three times the rate of the previous study and found that, most frequently, the Rorschach did not receive special attention, but was discussed as one of a battery of psychological tests. Meloy found that, when the Rorschach was singled out, such legal cases could be classified in four categories: "the definitions and functions of the test in the court's eyes; inappropriate use of the test; qualified use of the test; and d) criticism of the test" (p. 80). He noted that none of these cases included a *Daubert* challenge to the scientific adequacy of the test and that "There was not one case in which the Rorschach was ridiculed or disparaged by opposing counsel" (p. 85). Meloy concluded "it is clear that the test continues to have authority, or weight, in higher courts of appeal throughout the United States" (p. 86).

Additionally, Evans and Schutz (chap. 12, this vol.) conducted a Lexis Nexus search using "Rorschach and Child Custody" for legal citations from the last 50 years

(1956–2005), which yielded 43 hits. They found only five cases that touched on the admissibility or scientific status of the Rorschach, which fell into three of Meloy's (2007) categories: the inappropriate use of the Rorschach, qualified use of the Rorschach, and criticism of the Rorschach. These legal cases showed that the court understood bad practice when they saw it, it recognized potential problems with the Rorschach were not sufficient grounds for appeal, and in the two cases, the court was split on whether or not the Rorschach was useful or unreliable. In the one case where the court found the Rorschach unreliable, a published dissent from one of the state appellate judges noted that the Rorschach had been admitted two previous times in that state, suggesting a further split in the opinion about the Rorschach.

In conclusion, McCann's (1998) opinions about the legal admissibility of the Rorschach continue to be supported and confirmed. The Rorschach continues to demonstrate impressive scientific sturdiness that meets applicable guidelines for legal admissibility. It persists in its wide acceptance in both clinical and forensic professional practice settings and its legal authority within the courtroom has been affirmed. With the publication of *The Handbook of Forensic Rorschach Assessment*, the use of the Rorschach in a broad variety of forensic settings is now clearly established

ACKNOWLEDGMENT

I wish to express my gratitude to Judy Maris for her support and invaluable editing help.

REFERENCES

Archer, R. P., & Newsome, C. R. (2000). Psychological test usage with adolescent clients: Survey update. *Assessment, 7,* 227–235.

Belter, R. W., & Piotrowski, C. (2001). Current status of doctoral-level training in psychological testing. *Journal of Clinical Psychology, 57,* 717–726.

Boccaccini, M. T., & Brodsky, S. L. (1999). Diagnostic test usage by forensic psychologists in emotional injury cases. *Professional Psychology: Research and Practice, 30,* 253–259.

Board of Trustees of the Society for Personality Assessment. (2005). The status of the Rorschach in clinical and forensic practice: An official statement by the Board of Trustees of the Society for Personality Assessment. *Journal of Personality Assessment, 85,* 219–237.

Camara, W. J., Nathan, J. S., & Puente, A. E. (2000). Psychological test usage: Implications in professional psychology. *Professional Psychology: Research and Practice, 31,* 141–154.

Dawes, R. M. (1999). Two methods for studying the incremental validity of a Rorschach variable. *Psychological Assessment, 11*(3), 297–302.

Dawes, R. M. (1994). *House of cards: Psychology and psychotherapy built on myth.* New York: The Free Press.

Erard, R. E., & Evans, F. B. (2006). Rorschach: Not what cracks and potshots claim it is. *The National Psychologist, 15(4),* 13.

Gacono, C. B., Evans, F. B., III, & Viglione, D. J. (2002). The Rorschach in forensic practice. *Journal of Forensic Psychology Practice, 2,* 33–54.

Gacono, C. B., & Meloy, J. R. (1994). *The Rorschach assessment of aggressive and psychopathic personalities.* Hillsdale, NJ: Lawrence Erlbaum Associates.

Garb, H. N. (1999). Call for a moratorium on the use of the Rorschach Inkblot Test in clinical and forensic settings. *Assessment, 6,* 313–315.

Gronnerod, C. (2006). Reanalysis of the Gronnerod (2003) Rorschach temporal stability meta-analysis data set. *Journal of Personality Assessment, 86,* 222–225.

Gronnerod, C. (2003). Temporal stability in the Rorschach method: A meta-analytic review. *Journal of Personality Assessment, 80,* 272–293.

Grove, W. M., & Barden, R. C. (1999). Protecting the integrity of the legal system: The admissibility of testimony from mental health experts under *Daubert/Kumho* analyses. *Psychology, Public Policy, & Law, 5*(1), 224–242.

Grove, W. M., Barden, R. C., Garb, H. N., & Lilienfeld, S. O. (2002). Failure of Rorschach-comprehensive-system-based testimony to be admissible under the Daubert–Joiner–Kumho standard. *Psychology, Public Policy, & Law, 8*(2), 216–234.

Hiller, J. B., Rosenthal, R., Bornstein, R. F., Berry, D. T. R., & Brunell-Neuleib, S. (1999). A comparative meta-analysis of Rorschach and MMPI validity. *Psychological Assessment, 11,* 278–296.

Hilsenroth, M. J., & Stricker, G. (2004). A consideration of challenges to psychological assessment instruments used in forensic settings: Rorschach as exemplar. *Journal of Personality Assessment, 83,* 141–152.

Hunsley, J., & Bailey, J. M. (1999). The clinical utility of the Rorschach: Unfulfilled promises and an uncertain future. *Psychological Assessment, 11*(3), 266–277.

Hunsley, J., & Bailey, J. M. (2001). Whither the Rorschach? An analysis of the evidence. *Psychological Assessment, 13*(4), 472–485.

Lally, S. J. (2003). What tests are acceptable for use in forensic evaluations? A survey of experts. *Professional Psychology: Research and Practice, 34,* 491–498.

Lilienfeld, S. O., Wood, J. M., & Garb, H. N. (2000). The scientific status of projective techniques. *Psychological Science in the Public Interest, 1*(2), 27–66.

McCann, J. T. (1998). Defending the Rorschach in court: An analysis of admissibility using legal and professional standards. *Journal of Personality Assessment, 70*(1), 125–144.

McCann, J. T., & Dyer, F. J. (1996). *Forensic assessment with the Millon inventories.* New York: Guilford.

Meloy, J. R., Hansen, T. L., & Weiner, I. B. (1997). Authority of the Rorschach: legal citations during the past 50 years. *Journal of Personality Assessment, 69,* 53–62.

Nezworski, M. T., & Wood, J. M. (1995). Narcissism in the Comprehensive System for the Rorschach. *Clinical Psychology: Science & Practice, 2*(2), 179–199.

Piotrowski, C., Belter, R. W., & Keller, J. W. (1998). The impact of "managed care" on the practice of psychological testing: Preliminary findings. *Journal of Personality Assessment, 70,* 441–447.

Pope, K. S., Butcher, J. N., & Seelen, J. (2006). *The MMPI, MMPI–2, & MMPI–A in court: A practical guide for expert witnesses and attorneys* (3rd ed.). Washington, DC: American Psychological Association.

Quinnell, F. A., & Bow, J. N. (2001). Psychological tests used in child custody evaluations. *Behavioral Sciences & the Law, 19,* 491–501.

Ritzler, B., Erard, R., & Pettigrew, G. (2002). A final reply to Grove and Barden: The relevance of the Rorschach Comprehensive System for expert testimony. *Psychology, Public Policy, and Law, 8,* 235–246.

Ritzler, B., Erard, R., & Pettigrew, G. (2002). Protecting the integrity of Rorschach expert witnesses: A reply to Grove and Barden (1999) re: The admissibility of testimony under *Daubert/Kumho* analyses. *Psychology, Public Policy, and Law, 8,* 201–215.

Rosenthal, R., Hiller, J. B., Bornstein, R. F., Berry, D. T. R., & Brunell-Neuleib, S. (2001). Meta-analytic methods, the Rorschach, and the MMPI. *Psychological Assessment, 13,* 449–451.

Viglione, D. J., & Rivera, B. (2003). Assessing personality and psychopathology with projective methods. In J. R. Graham & J. A. Naglieri (Eds.), *Handbook of psychology: Assessment psychology* (Vol. 10, pp. 531–552). New York: Wiley.

Weiner, I. B. (1996). Some observations on the validity of the Rorschach Inkblot Method. *Psychological Assessment, 8,* 206–213.

Weiner, I. B., Ixner, J. E., & Sciara, A. (1966). Is the Rorschach welcome in the courtroom? *Journal of Personality Assessment, 67,* 422–424.

Wood, J. M., & Lilienfeld, S. O. (1999). The Rorschach inkblot test: A case of overstatement? *Assessment, 6*(4), 341–351.

Wood, J. M., Nezworski, M. T., Garb, H. N., & Lilienfeld, S. O. (2001a). The misperception of psychopathology: Problems with norms of the Comprehensive System for the Rorschach. *Clinical Psychology: Science & Practice, 8*(3), 350–373.

Wood, J. M., Nezworski, M. T., Garb, H. N., & Lilienfeld, S. O. (2001b). Problems with the norms of the Comprehensive System for the Rorschach: Methodological and conceptual considerations. *Clinical Psychology: Science & Practice, 8*(3), 397–402.

Wood, J. M., Nezworski, M. T., & Stejskal, W. J. (1996). The Comprehensive System for the Rorschach: A critical examination. *Psychological Science, 7*(1), 3–10.

Wood, J. M., Nezworski, M. T., Stejskal, W. J., & McKinzey, R. K. (2001). Problems of the Comprehensive System for the Rorschach in forensic settings: Recent developments. *Journal of Forensic Psychology Practice, 1*(3), 89–103.

CHAPTER

4

THE AUTHORITY OF THE RORSCHACH: AN UPDATE

J. Reid Meloy
University of California, San Diego

It has been a decade since Meloy, Hansen, and Weiner (1997) reported on the authority of the Rorschach in court between 1945 and1995. In their study of a half century of legal citations that appeared in federal, state, and military courts of appeal concerning the Rorschach, the test was cited in 247 published cases, and issues concerning the scientific nature of the test arose in 10.5% of the citations. After studying these particular cases, they concluded that "despite occasional disparagement by prosecutors, the majority of the courts found the test findings to be both reliable and valid" (p. 53).

Much has transpired over the past decade concerning the Rorschach, including both scientific and *ad hominem* attacks against its use, particularly in forensic settings (Wood, Nezworski, Lilienfeld, & Garb, 2003). Research concerning the test has also continued unabated, and the third edition of the advanced interpretation of the Comprehensive System was published (Exner & Erdberg, 2005) just prior to the 2006 deaths of two Rorschach pioneers, John Exner, Jr. and Paul Lerner. A search of PsycInfo indicates that during 2005 there were over 100 different scientific papers, dissertations, book chapters, and books published on the Rorschach both in the United States and Europe.

The question of legal weight of the Rorschach, moreover, remains central to its use in forensic settings. Weight is the "influence, effectiveness, or power to influence judgment or conduct" (Black, 1979, p. 1429), and for our purposes, it is the consideration the Rorschach test is given by the trier of fact in its decision making. This is the authority of the Rorschach, and a new study was conducted to see if the past decade has witnessed a change in the court's perspective on the test.

METHOD

The measures selected for study were the quantity and content of legal citations between 1996 and 2005 that mentioned the word *Rorschach*. Legal citations in this study were all published and unpublished federal, state, and military case law opinions written by various courts of appeal throughout the United States. The reference word *Rorschach* was entered into the Lexis computer database at the University of San Diego School of Law, and all cases in which the word was mentioned were identified and printed in full text form. All cases were read to determine whether the reference word referred to the inkblot test or something else. Cases in which the test was utilized were studied for content and meaning, with a particular focus on whether or not the test's scientific status was accepted, challenged, or rejected.

RESULTS

There were 191 appellate cases between 1996 and 2005 in which the word *Rorschach* appeared. Twenty of these cases were unpublished (cannot be cited), and 21 additional cases did not refer to the test, but instead the word was used as a metaphor, adjective, or to name a person.[1] The Rorschach test was therefore cited in 150 appellate cases, averaging 15 times per year, *three times* the rate of citation during the previous half century (Meloy et al., 1997). The Rorschach test was utilized by forensic clinicians in a wide variety of civil and criminal case appeals, including death penalty, emotional disability, child custody, competency to stand trial, Miranda competency, workman's competency, termination of parental rights, habeas corpus petitions, conditional release and parole, alimony, sexually violent predator status, guardianship, family visitation, revocation of passport, SSI disability, child sexual abuse, and other criminal appeals. The test was most often cited in death penalty appeals. In the vast majority of all appeal cases, the test was mentioned by the court as one of several psychological tests utilized by examiners in their evaluation of the defendant, plaintiff, or subject of interest in the case. Other tests frequently mentioned included the Minnesota Multiphasic Personality Inventory–2 (MMPI–2), the Millon Clinical Multiaxial Inventory–III (MCMI–III), various measures of intelligence, and various measures of neuropsychological functioning. The Rorschach test was neither focused on, nor singled out, in these cases, but was treated, instead, as one test in a battery that provided useful psychological information to the court.

There were a minority of cases in which the Rorschach test received additional attention by the courts, and these cases fell into four categories: the definitions and functions of the test in the court's eyes, inappropriate use of the test, qualified use of the test, and criticism of the test.

Definitions and Functions of the Rorschach Test

The definitions and functions of the test were mentioned in 12 appellate cases. In *Hall v. State of Tennessee* (2005), the Court of Criminal Appeals defined the Rorschach as a "traditional inkblot test to test personality style and functioning" (p. 14). In *Rompilla v. Horn* (2004), the U.S. Court of Appeals, Third Circuit, drew on the definition of the test in *Stedman's Medical Dictionary* (27th ed.): "a projective psychological test in which the subject reveals his or her attitudes, emotions, and personality by reporting what is seen in each of 10 inkblot pictures" (p. 1808). In a death penalty appeal through the U.S. District

---

[1]Don J. Rorschach, the City Attorney of Irving, Texas, was mentioned by name in one case. In our first study, we contacted him and he told us that his father's great uncle was, indeed, Dr. Hermann Rorschach.

Court in Nebraska, Dr. Daniel Martell in *Ryan v. Clarke* (2003) explained that the method of scoring the Rorschach was standardized by Exner in the 1970s to validate the testing and eliminate the subjective results, and that absent such scoring, the test results are not reliable (p. 45). In *State v. Raiford* (2003), the Court of Appeals of Louisiana defined the Rorschach as "a projective personality test" (p. 11). In *Thompson v. Bell* (2001), another death penalty appeal, the Rorschach was defined as the "inkblot test" (p. 6). In a custody case in the Family Court of Delaware, the court in *Martin v. Martin* (2002) spelled out the function of the Rorschach: "This is a test that involves people's statements of reactions when looking at various ink blots. The responses are then compared to a large data base of the responses of others with various known characteristics" (p. 9). Likewise, the Supreme Court of California in a death penalty appeal noted that Dr. Don Viglione had used the test to determine whether the defendant's personality was more consistent with dependent traits or antisocial traits (*People v. Box*, 2000). That same year, the Court of Appeal in Louisiana in a termination of parental rights case found the Rorschach to be "an important diagnostic test" (p. 16) in *State of Louisiana in the Interest of Emma Hair* (2000). In Puerto Rico 3 years earlier, the U.S. District Court in *U.S. v. R.I.M.A.*, a juvenile transfer case to adult court, opined that the Rorschach's function was to "determine the individual's psychological profile and dynamics, that is, identify the decision making process and the meaning that an individual attributes to his surroundings" (p. 6).

Inappropriate Use of the Rorschach Test

Courts of appeal cited the inappropriate use of the test in four cases (2.6%). In *State v. Walker* (2005), the Court of Appeals of Ohio upheld a finding of a proper determination of a "sexual predator." However, a psychologist testified that solely on the basis of the Rorschach findings, the defendant had no sexual preoccupation, had no mental condition, excluding mental retardation, and was not a pedophile. The court noted that the psychologist did not use any other tests commonly geared toward addressing sexual issues, and he admitted under cross-examination that the Rorschach cannot yield diagnoses of sexual deviance.

In *Commonwealth v. DeBerardinis* (2004), the Superior Court of Massachusetts considered a motion to determine competency to stand trial. A psychologist administered the Rorschach using the Thought Disorder Index and also the vocabulary subtest of the Wechsler Adult Intelligence Scale–Revised (WAIS–R). She found moderately elevated formal thought disorder consistent with a chronic organic condition, presumably vascular dementia. She concluded that the defendant was psychotic. The court of appeal responded, "These conclusions are simply not supported by the factual evidence, and they appear to exaggerate the strength of her findings. Indeed, when asked to confirm her report's conclusion that DeBerardinis was psychotic, she amended her opinion by stating that he had the capacity to be psychotic or the propensity for psychotic thinking ... the court finds that the doctor's conclusions do not support a determination of incompetence to stand trial in this case" (p. 5).

In *State v. Parker* (2002), the Court of Appeals of Washington reviewed the trial court's exclusion of the testimony of a prominent neuropsychologist in a double sexual murder case. In the trial, the neuropsychologist determined that the defendant had "generally low average to borderline mental ability" but was not mentally retarded. In addition, she testified that the defendant's responses to the Rorschach did not suggest a violent predisposition because no sexual associations were given, nor any associations suggesting violent or destructive activity (Footnote 8). During an interview with the prosecution before trial, she stated that what she knew about the defendant from her testing and interview and the details of the crimes—she did not review any police reports, lab tests, autopsy reports, or other discovery—did not "mesh." "He doesn't seem like the kind of person, or have the kind of capacity for mental elaboration and mental imagery and complexity that performing these two murders in such a similar manner would suggest" (Footnote 11). She further stated that his Rorschach responses did not indicate sexual pathology, aggression, or anger, and that she doubted he committed the murders because he didn't come across as an angry person (Footnote 15). She admitted, however, that the Rorschach test is not an accepted method of evaluating the likelihood that someone committed a crime. The court requested a detailed explanation from the neuropsychologist as to how her tests indicated the defendant was incapable of performing the acts committed by the murderer. She subsequently submitted a certified letter stating that she was unable to reach any conclusions about whether the defendant committed the murders. The trial court found her testimony irrelevant and speculative. The Court of Appeals affirmed the decision and, on the basis of Federal Rules of Evidence 401 and 702, ruled that she had not provided an adequate evidentiary foundation for her opinions, and therefore the trial court had not abused its discretion in excluding her testimony.

In the Supreme Court of Texas (*S. V. v. R.V.*, 1996), the judges agreed to review a case in which an adult child intervened in her parents' divorce proceeding, alleging that her father was negligent by sexually abusing her until she was 17 years old. A forensic psychologist testified during the subsequent court proceeding that the daughter's MMPI test showed that she fit the classic "V profile" of someone who had been abused, and that several aspects of the father's Rorschach test were also consistent with what one would expect to see in a child abuser. The Supreme Court did not comment directly on this psychologist's testimony, but ruled that expert opinions regarding recovered memories of childhood sexual abuse could not be objectively verified to extend the discovery rule, and thus the action was barred due to the passage of time.

Qualified Use of the Rorschach Test

In the Court of Appeal of Louisiana, a customer brought a personal injury action against a discount department store for injuries she sustained when a shelving display stocked with crawfish platters allegedly fell on her (*Green v. K-Mart Corporation*, 2003). The examining psychologist eventually diagnosed her with psychotic depression, but testified that her Rorschach test results were invalid because she only responded to three cards.

In *U.S. v. Battle* (2003), the U.S. District Court in Atlanta heard a petition for postconviction relief following a murder conviction and death penalty. The 133-page opinion included, among other things, a lengthy analysis of the use of the Rorschach *WSum6* score and *SCZI* in the determination of schizophrenia, relying most heavily on the testimony of

Mark Hazelrigg, at the time a psychologist from the Federal Bureau of Prisons. The court noted that the Exner scoring system was "widely accepted," reviewed several studies concerning the validity of these indices, and reiterated that the psychologists on the case agreed that the Rorschach scores were only suggestive of the presence or absence of schizophrenia. On a more stylistic note, the court opined that another defense psychologist's testimony at trial was "lengthy, repetitious, and obscure" (p. 110). "The court could tell that some of the jurors were struggling to stay focused on his testimony ... occasionally, a juror or two closed her eyes, but only momentarily. In the case of one juror, the intervention of the Court Security Officer was required occasionally to make sure that the juror did not fall asleep" (p. 110). The defense psychologist's testimony, likely causing the sleepiness of the jurors, resulted in a petition filed by the defense attorneys that a hearing should be held to determine jury misconduct. The court denied their motion.

In the Court of Appeals of Michigan, two minors petitioned for the termination of their father's parental rights (*In re Hamlet*, 1997). A psychologist who examined the father determined on the basis of the Rorschach test that he had an antisocial personality disorder. This finding was challenged by the father's counsel on the basis that the Rorschach is not a reliable determiner of narcissism. The court opined that both sides agreed the father would need years of therapy before he could adequately parent his children, therefore the outcome would be the same whether or not the psychologist's test findings were accurate. The termination of the father's parental rights was affirmed.

Criticism of the Rorschach Test

The appellate courts criticized the test in three cases (2%). The U.S. District Court in Atlanta heard a death penalty appeal in 2001 in the case of Anthony Battle (*U.S. v. Battle*), an inmate who had killed a federal corrections officer with a hammer in 1994. This hearing was 2 years prior to the postconviction relief hearing noted previously before the same court. The judges wrote, "The Rorschach is a test frequently used in diagnosing schizophrenia, but it does not have an objective scoring system. Rather, the Rorschach is scored by using the Exner guideline system which allows some discretion to the scorer" (p. 8).

In another criminal juvenile transfer case to adult court (*State ex rel. H.H.*, 1999), two psychologists examined the adolescent charged with murder. The Superior Court of New Jersey, Atlantic County, wrote, "It should be noted Dr. Witt testified that the Rorschach and house-tree drawing tests administered by Dr. Bogacki are somewhat controversial and considered to be of questionable validity in the field of psychology. During cross-examination, Dr. Bogacki admitted that there is disagreement about the effectiveness of the house-tree drawing test, and that many psychologists do not believe much in the validity or effectiveness of the Rorschach test" (p. 12).

The U.S. District Court for the Northern District of Indiana reviewed a denial of an application for supplemental security income (*Jones v. Apfel*, 1997). The examining psychologist used the Rorschach and attempted to use the MMPI. The court wrote in a footnote, quoting from the *Attorney's Textbook of Medicine* by Roscoe Gray: "The Rorschach test is the most widely used objective personality test. However, there is no obvious socially desirable answer to these tests, results do not meet the requirements of standardization, reliability, or validity of clinical diagnostic tests, and interpretation thus is often controversial" (93–76.2).

A Rorschach by Any Other Name

The word *Rorschach* continues to be widely used as a metaphor and adjective in courts of appeal throughout the United States. In a family trust case in California, the inconsistency of the Probate Code became a "Rorschach test for the parties" (*Huscher v. Wells Fargo Bank*, 2004). In *Baker v. Welch* (2003), a U.S. District Court wrestled with an action brought by a parolee because his female parole officer viewed his penis while taking a urine test, thus violating his right to privacy. The court opined that much of the Bill of Rights is a Rorschach test, wherein "what the judge sees in it is the reflection of his or her own values, values shaped by personal experience and temperament as well as by historical reflection ..." (p. 23). In *Harris v. City of Chicago* (2002), the Picasso statue in Daley Plaza cast a "Rorschach shadow" in an action against the city to prevent the reading of a prayer at a commemoration ceremony. In a firearm conviction appeal, the U.S. Court of Appeals for the First Circuit wrote, "Engaging in any mode of analysis without first establishing a statutory definition would be like administering a Rorschach test without any inkblots" (*U.S. v. Nason*, 2001, p. 6).

Increasingly, the word *Rorschach* is used to describe a process by which a jurist projects his individualized notion of justice into a particular matter before the court (*Michigan United Conservation Clubs v. Secretary of State*, 2001; *Temps by Ann, Inc. v. City State Services*, 2000; *Pallisco v. Pallisco*, 1999; *U.S. v. Epps, 1997; Kevorkian v. Thompson*, 1997). In one case, Fourth Amendment search and seizure law was at risk of becoming "one immense Rorschach blot" (*State v. Smith*, 1997). By far the most common recent use of the word *Rorschach* as judicial metaphor is to describe the shape of redistricting to rearrange voter demographics, often to the advantage of one political party over another (*Luidens v. 63rd District Court*, 1996; *Johnson v. Miller*, 1996; *Johnson v. Mortham*, 1996; *King v. State Board of Elections*, 1996). One court even referred to the process of creating a congressional district as "racial Rorschach-ism" (*Ray Hays v. State of Louisiana*, 1996).

The most striking quote found in this study, however, concerned an attorney's challenge to a psychologist after he testified that the Rorschach could measure what was unconscious (*In the Interest of M.C.M. et al.*, 2001). The Court of Appeals of Texas transcript read as follows:

Opposing counsel: "Doctor, the unconscious that you previously say it measures, in part, the Rorschach Test, can you name one empirical study that has ever proven the unconscious to exist?"

Psychologist: "Not off the top of my head."

Opposing counsel: "So what you are telling the Court is that you use a test that measures something that doesn't exist to determine that?"

Psychologist: "I am sorry, what is your question?"

Court: "Before you finish that question, I don't know where we are going with what tests are proven what, but so it may help us on other examinations of this sort, this court is of the opinion that there is an unconscious whether it's been proven or not. I think it's empirically known that there is an unconscious state and I take judicial notice of the existence of such."

Opposing counsel: "The Court takes judicial notice of something that has never been proven to exist, Your Honor? Do I understand the Court to say that?"

Court: "However you are defining it. I am saying that the Court takes judicial notice of the fact that this Court believes there is an unconscious state." (pp. 7–8)

Another judge was appointed to hear this motion.

CONCLUSIONS

The Rorschach has been cited significantly more frequently (15 times compared to 5 times per year) and with significantly less criticism (2% vs. 10.5%) when this previous decade's appellate cases (1996–2005) are compared to the last half century's cases (1945–1995) (Meloy et al., 1997). There was not one case in which the Rorschach was ridiculed or disparaged by opposing counsel. More importantly, two earlier court decisions which completely devalued the Rorschach as a psychological test—in *Alto v. State* (1977) the Rorschach was labeled a technique, not a test; and, in *Usher v. Lakewood Engineering & Mfg. Co.* (1994), a protection order was issued against all psychological testing due to questionable validity—did not serve as precedent for any subsequent case opinions in the last decade. There has been no Daubert challenge to the scientific status of the Rorschach in any state, federal, or military court of appeal since the U.S. Supreme Court decision in 1993 set the federal standard for admissibility of scientific evidence (*Daubert v. Merrell Dow Pharmaceuticals, Inc.*, 1993). This does not preclude the existence of challenges at the trial court level, which quantitatively cannot be known, but it is reasonable to assume that such challenges, if they occurred, were not serious enough to rise to the level of an appeal.

These empirical findings invite two alternative explanations: first, the scientific criticism of the Rorschach, most notably the publications of Wood et al. (2003), which in turn stimulated a rigorous scientific debate and studies to measure and improve the reliability, validity, and norms for the test (Board of Trustees of the Society for Personality Assessment, 2005), have paradoxically resulted in a much firmer scientific footing for the Rorschach. Or, second, the swirling scientific debates in the academic journals have been a tempest in a teapot, and have largely gone unnoticed and unheralded by both forensic clinicians who regularly use the Rorschach and the appellate courts who consider the test one of several valid measures of personality and psychology. The word itself continues to be deeply embedded as a metaphor in the lexicon of the judiciary, rarely misused and often colorfully embellished.

When the test was mishandled by experts, the same pattern emerges as we found in our previous study. The psychologist's inferences and conclusions derived from the Rorschach went far beyond the data, and were considered unfounded and speculative by the court. It is frankly astonishing that an occasional psychologist will still attempt to determine whether or not a crime was committed by studying a defendant's Rorschach. Other inferential leaps, although there were few in these appellate cases, were characterized by an attempt to criminally profile or diagnose a subject solely on the basis of his Rorschach test.

The recommendations from Meloy et al. (1997) are still applicable given the last decade's findings, and bear repeating:

> Psychologists who use the Rorschach in court should pay particular attention to the inferences that they develop from the data. These inferences should be closely linked to one another, previously validated in published research, and consistent with other findings in the case derived from other sources of evidence. These other sources of evidence should typically include self-report of the examinee, historical and contemporaneous data independent of self-report, and other administered tests. The decision to use the Rorschach in a forensic case should also have some bearing on the psycholegal question that is to be addressed. (p. 61)

The empirical findings of this new study substantiate and extend the findings from our previous work. Although judges are not scientists, and it is the obligation of psychologists who use the Rorschach to know the scientific parameters of the instrument, it is clear that the test continues to have authority, or weight, in higher courts of appeal throughout the United States.

ACKNOWLEDGMENTS

I thank Grant Morris and Alessandria Driussi, without whom this study could not have been completed. This study was funded by a grant from Forensis, Inc. (www.forensis.org).

REFERENCES

Alto v. State, 565 P. 2d 492 (Sup. Ct. Alaska, 1977).

Baker v. Welch, WL 22901051 (2003).

Black, H. C. (1979). *Black's law dictionary* (5th ed.). St. Paul, MN: West.

Board of Trustees of the Society for Personality Assessment. (2005). The status of the Rorschach in clinical and forensic practice. *Journal of Personality Assessment, 85*, 219–237.

Commonwealth v. DeBerardinis, 17 Mass. L. Rptr. 641 (2004).

Daubert v. Merrell Dow Pharmaceuticals, Inc., 113 S. Ct. 2786 (1993).

Exner, J., & Erdberg, P. (2005). *The Rorschach: A comprehensive system. Vol. 2. Advanced Interpretation* (3rd ed.). New York: Wiley.

Green v. K-Mart Corp., 849 So. 2d 814 (2003).

Hall v. State, WL 22951 (2005).

Harris v. City of Chicago, 218 F. Supp. 2d 990 (2002).

Hays v. State of La., 936 F. Supp. 360 (1996).

Huscher v. Wells Fargo Bank, 121 Ca. App. 4th 956 (2004).

In re Hamlet, 225 Mich. 505 (1997).

In re M.C.M., 57 S.W. 3d 27 (2001).

Johnson v. Miller, 929 F. Supp. 1529 (1996).

Johnson v. Mortham, 926 F. Supp. 1460 (1996).

Jones v. Apfel, 997 F. Supp. 1085 (1997).

Kevorkian v. Thompson, 947 F. Supp. 1152 (1997).

King v. State Board of Elections, 979 F. Supp. 582 (1996).

Luidens v. 63rd Dist. Court, 219 Mich. App. 24 (1996).

Martin v. Martin, 820 A.2d 410 (2002).

Meloy, J. R., Hansen, T. L., & Weiner, I. B. (1997). Authority of the Rorschach: Legal citations during the past 50 years. *Journal of Personality Assessment, 69*, 53–62.

Michigan United Conservation Clubs v. Secretary of State, 464 Mich. 359 (2001).

Pallisco v. Pallisco, WL 33444279 (1999).

People v. Box, 23 Cal.4th 1153 (2000).

Rompilla v. Horn, 355 F.3d 233 (2004).

Ryan v. Clarke, 281 F.Supp.2d 1008 (2003).

State v. Parker, 114 Wash. App. 1070 (2002).

State v. Raiford, 846 So. 2d 913 (2003).

State v. Smith, 148 Or. App. 235 (1997).

State v. Walker, WL 1620491 (2005).

State ex rel. Hair, 757 So.2d 754 (2000).

State ex rel. H.H., 333 N.J. Super. 141 (1999).

S.V. v. R.V., 933 S.W. 2d 1 (1996).

Temps by Ann, Inc. v. City State Services, Inc., WL 33522104 (2000).

Thompson v. Bell, 315 F.3d 566 (2001).

U.S. v. Battle, 235 F. Supp. 2d 1301 (2001).

U.S. v. Battle, 264 F. Supp. 2d 1088 (2003).

U.S. v. Epps, 987 F. Supp. 22 (1997).

U.S. v. Nason, 269 F. 3d 10 (2001).

U.S. v. R.I.M.A., 963 F. Supp. 1264 (1997).

Usher v. Lakewood Engineering & Mfg. Co., 158 F.R.D. 411 (1994).

Wood, J., Nezworski, M., Lilienfeld, S., & Garb, H. (2003). *What's wrong with the Rorschach?* San Francisco: Jossey-Bass.

5

RORSCHACH ASSESSMENT OF MALINGERING AND DEFENSIVE RESPONSE SETS

Ronald J. Ganellen
Northwestern University Medical School

One critical issue that has to be systematically addressed during a forensic psychological evaluation involves determining whether the individuals being evaluated are truthfully reporting symptoms of any claimed psychological disorder and the extent to which their ability to function is affected by their psychological condition. Although determining the accuracy of responses is an important part of any psychological evaluation, there may be different reasons individuals distort their account of their psychological functioning during clinical as opposed to forensic evaluations. In clinical evaluations, individuals may be motivated to exaggerate problems as a "plea for help" if they doubt a clinician will take their problems seriously, or may want to downplay or conceal difficulties because of a desire to control how others see them (Greene, 2000; Paulhaus, 1986) or to protect their view of themselves (Huprich & Ganellen, 2005). In contrast, individuals evaluated in the context of a legal proceeding may be motivated to exaggerate problems to obtain a financial settlement in a civil case; avoid punishment by feigning incompetence to stand trial; claim insanity at the time of the crime; or receive a reduced sentence, such as avoiding the death penalty in a capital murder case.

The possibility an individual evaluated during legal proceedings may skew their report of psychological difficulties should not be underestimated. Investigations of the incidence of malingering suggest that malingering occurs with considerable frequency in both clinical and forensic settings. For instance, Rogers, Sewell, and Goldstein (1994) surveyed 320 forensic psychologists, who estimated that 15.7% of individuals evaluated in a forensic context and 7.4% of individuals evaluated in a clinical context were malingering.

The survey conducted by Rogers et al. (1994) investigated the base rate of malingering in forensic cases in general. It is possible that malingering may occur more frequently during certain types of legal proceedings (e.g., civil vs. criminal cases) than others. The base rates of malingering in different conditions was estimated by Mittenberg, Patton, Canyock, and Condit (2002) based on survey results provided by psychologists concerning a total of 33,531 cases. After taking into account multiple sources of information, including record review, self-report, observed behavior, scores on forced choice symptom tests, or implausible accounts of symptoms and history, Mittenberg et al. found that 29% of personal injury claimants, 30% of disability claimants, 19% of criminal defendants, and 39% of individuals with mild closed head injuries were identified as malingerers or as exaggerating their symptoms to some extent. Similarly, Rogers (1986) determined that 20.8% of defendants evaluated in the context of an insanity defense engaged in definite or suspected malingering.

Interestingly, some investigations of criminal offenders have found this population has relatively low rates of defensiveness (Rogers & McKee, 1995). In contrast, defensiveness has been found to occur quite frequently in populations who undergo psychological evaluations for other legal purposes. Defensiveness is considered by some investigators to be nearly normative for individuals evaluated during child custody proceedings (Bagby, Nicholson, Buis, Radanovic, & Fidler, 1999; Bathurst, Gottfried, & Gottfried, 1997; Medoff, 1999; Posthuma & Harper, 1998), for instance, and occurs quite frequently in other forensic settings, including individuals invested in returning to work seen during fitness to work evaluations (Gormally, chap. 15, this vol.; Greene, 2000), as well as in populations of alleged sex offenders (Haywood, Grossman, & Hardy, 1993).

The results of these studies should alert clinicians conducting psychological evaluations during any legal proceeding to the sobering fact that a substantial percentage of the individuals they evaluate will make a deliberate attempt to skew their account of their psychological condition in a manner favorable to their case. One issue that must be carefully, systematically, and objectively addressed during any psychological evaluation, therefore, is a determination of whether an individuals' report of their emotional state, the symptoms they claim to experience, the severity of behavioral problems, and the disability caused by their psychological condition should be considered valid and reliable. This chapter presents an overview of issues concerning distinctions among different types of self-favorable and self-unfavorable response sets, discusses the strengths and weaknesses of the Rorschach Comprehensive System (CS; Exner, 2003) for detecting attempts to skew findings, and suggests ways in which the CS and Minnesota Multiphasic Personality Inventory–2 (MMPI–2; Butcher, Dahlstrom, Graham, Tellegen, & Kaemmer, 1989) can be used conjointly to effectively identify exaggerating and minimizing approaches to forensic psychological evaluations.

DEFINITIONS OF MALINGERING

Some disagreement exists concerning the definition of malingering. The *DSM–IV* (APA, 1994) states that malingering is diagnosed when there is "intentional production of false or grossly exaggerated physical or psychological symptoms, motivated by external incentives such as avoiding military service, avoiding work, obtaining financial compensation, evading criminal prosecution, or obtaining drugs" (p. 297). Furthermore, the *DSM–IV* states the index of suspicion for malingering should be high if any combination of the following are present: an individual is seen in a medicolegal or psycholegal context, there is a marked discrepancy between claimed symptoms or disability and objective findings, there is evidence of a lack of cooperation during the evaluation process, or an individual has an Antisocial Personality Disorder.

Some writers have criticized *DSM–IV* criteria developed to identify malingering because of concerns that these criteria spread too broad a net, which increases the risk of high rates of false positive classification of malingering. For instance, according to the *DSM–IV* criteria, the index of suspicion of malingering should be considered to be elevated for any individual evaluated in the context of medicolegal or psycholegal proceedings. However, based on the surveys reported previously, whereas 29% of personal injury claimants exaggerate symptoms and reports of disability, 71% report problems accurately (Mittenberg et al., 2002). Examination of the base rate of malingering in samples of personal injury litigants suggests that the *DSM–IV* criteria may inaccurately identify high rates of honest individuals pursuing a personal injury action as malingering. A similar point was made by Rogers (1990), who examined rates of classification of forensic patients as responding honestly or malingering. Rogers found that two thirds of malingerers in his sample were correctly classified using the *DSM–IV* criteria. However, a large percentage of bona fide patients were miscategorized on the basis of *DSM–IV* criteria as malingering. Based on these findings, Rogers concluded that among patients evaluated in a forensic context *DSM–IV* criteria alone do not effectively discriminate between honest and feigned mental disorders.

In a sophisticated discussion of the dilemmas clinicians face in diagnosing malingering, Slick, Sherman, and Iverson (1999) emphasized that two elements are critical in differentiating malingering from honest responding and from other clinical conditions characterized by symptoms that are difficult to explain, such as a Conversion Disorder or Factitious Disorder. These two elements are a determination that individuals consciously overreported problems and that the individuals deliberately gave a false account of their psychological status in order to obtain an external incentive. They point out that these two elements are clinically useful as some patients with a Conversion Disorder may present with symptoms that appear extreme, unbelievable, fabricated, or out of proportion to objective findings. However, the motivation for an individual with a Conversion Disorder is psychological or unconscious in nature, whereas an individual who is malingering is motivated by a tangible external incentive.

Another issue to consider in identifying malingering concerns whether malingering is conceptualized as a dichotomous or continuous variable. Traditional discussions of malingering have given the impression that individuals evaluated during some legal proceedings either report psychological problems accurately and honestly or produce false, inaccurate, feigned accounts of their condition. Other writers have observed that there may be gradations in individuals' accounts of symptoms and disability.

This distinction has the following important implication. If one accepts the dichotomous view of malingering, one might conclude that an individual found to deliberately exaggerate certain emotional and behavioral difficulties should be viewed as having no psychological problems. However, it is certainly possible that individuals who meet *DSM–IV* criteria for a specific diagnosis (e.g., Major Depression) may attempt to convince others they have a different disorder (e.g., Schizophrenia) when they do not. It is also possible that one individual who meets *DSM–IV* criteria for a specific disorder (e.g., Major Depression) may describe the severity of symptoms and limitations in functioning caused by that disorder in a mildly exaggerated manner, whereas another individual may falsely claim severe symptoms and limitation in functioning. In other words, differing degrees of exaggeration may be observed in different patients or when one patient is evaluated at different points in time.

Furthermore, during an evaluation, individuals may report some parts of their history and clinical symptoms honestly, but give an inaccurate, exaggerated account when describing other circumstances and problems. As pointed out by Sweet (1999) in a discussion of malingered neuropsychological deficits, "valid performances on some measures do not rule out malingering, and, conversely, malingered performances on some measures do not rule out valid performance on others. In fact, in a minority of cases, both conditions may be present simultaneously" (p. 258). In contrast to a dichotomous perspective, conceptualizing malingering phenomena as potentially involving a continuum of degrees and types of feigning psychological disorders permits the clinician the opportunity to make these important distinctions.

Resnick (1997) recommended that several terms may be useful in describing the range of malingering phenomena. He suggested the term *pure malingering* be used if a particular patient feigns having symptoms of a specific disorder when in actuality that patient does not have those symptoms. In contrast, Resnick suggested that the term *partial malingering* be applied when an individual exaggerates the nature or severity symptoms or problems that actually exist. Resnick also recommended that partial malingering be used if an individual falsely claims that symptoms that genuinely existed at some time in the past but then resolved are still present at the time the individual is evaluated for the purposes of a legal proceeding.

I encountered an instance of partial malingering when I evaluated a man embroiled in divorce proceedings concerning his financial responsibilities to his soon-to-be ex-wife and children. This man claimed he was unable to continue working as the president and CEO of the business he had taken over from his ex-wife's family when his father-in-law retired because of symptoms of a Bipolar Disorder and therefore should not be obligated to make child custody payments. The results of the evaluation and review of collateral information indicated that although this man had relinquished control of the family business and explained that he was no longer working because of his psychiatric condition, in actuality he was being followed by a psychiatrist, was stable on appropriate medication, and had laid the foundation to purchase a company in the same industry from a colleague with the understanding that the deal would be consummated once the divorce proceedings were resolved. This information demonstrated that this man was not fabricating symptoms of a Bipolar Disorder, but was making exaggerated claims of the extent to which he was impaired as a result of this condition.

Another useful term relating to determinations of malingering is *false imputation*. This refers to a specific type of malingering in which an individual attributes causality for actual emotional problems or psychosocial difficulties to an event or situation that the individual consciously knows has no causal relationship to their symptoms. For example, one individual I evaluated in the context of a personal injury lawsuit claimed that he began having problems with alcohol and drugs as a result of the traumatic incident that was the basis for the lawsuit. This explanation had been accepted by the psychiatrist and psychologist who treated this man following the industrial accident. Records produced by the treating mental health professionals indicated they conceptualized this man's history of abuse of alcohol and drug abuse as a reaction to the trauma and efforts to "self-medicate and dampen the emotional distress" caused by the accident. In contrast to this account of events, treatment records obtained from other sources revealed the plaintiff had a history of drug and alcohol abuse for many years before the traumatic incident and had been in at least one substance abuse treatment program in the past. These records made it clear that the plaintiff had neglected to disclose to his psychiatrist and psychologist relevant information and instead presented an account of his problems that seemed designed to lead others to conclude that he was damaged by the industrial accident.

An observation I have made over the years is that treating clinicians are vulnerable to being misled when patients engage in false imputation and attribute all of their psychological problems to a specific traumatic event, such as the claim made by the plaintiff in the brief case example discussed earlier. Often, such explanations are plausible and are easy to accept, particularly by a mental health professional functioning in the role of a treating clinician who attempts to understand and empathize with a patient's situation, rather than carefully examining and weighing the veracity of the claims made by particular individual. The fact of the matter is that it is often difficult, if not impossible, to determine whether the patients' account of the onset of psychological problems, such as substance abuse or depression, is accurate without obtaining collateral information. This underscores the importance of obtaining not only a thorough, detailed history from an individual involved in legal proceedings during a clinical interview and by review of records, but also of corroborating this account by administering standardized, objective assessment measures, such as the MMPI–2 or Rorschach. The use of objective assessment instruments is essential not only to provide evidence that substantiates or refutes claims of specific troubling symptoms, behaviors, and disability, but also of identifying response sets that may bias or skew findings from a psychological evaluation.

ASSESSMENT PROCEDURES

Evaluation of the specific symptoms needed to diagnose an individual with a mental or psychological disorder depends to a large extent on the patient's self-report of subjective symptoms. Determining that a Delusional Disorder with persecutory features exists, for instance, requires evidence that individuals believe other people are following or trying to harm them, whereas determining whether or not individuals have Posttraumatic Stress Disorder involves evidence that they experience flashbacks or recurrent, intrusive distressing thoughts or images of the traumatic event, as well as other symptoms. It is quite conceivable that a resourceful individual can learn enough about a particular condition to present a convincing portrayal of that condition using information accessible to the public at many public libraries or easily obtained by conducting an Internet search.

Considerable evidence exists that clinical acumen alone does not reliably differentiate between genuine and feigned accounts of psychological disorders (Bourg, Connor, & Landis, 1995). For this reason, the use of standardized clinical assessment methods is highly recommended both to assess the validity of patients' self-report, as well as the nature and severity of the symptoms they experience. For instance, at the request of an attorney, I evaluated an individual who claimed to be disabled because of significant depression that developed during the course of a chronic pain disorder. This man earned a *T*-score of 52 on MMPI–2 Scale 2 and a *T*-score of 50 on the Depression Content scale, whereas his Rorschach Structural Summary contained the following values: *DEPI* = 0, *D score* = +1, *C′* = 1, *FD* and *FV* = 0. These findings provide no objective support for this man's claim that he was impaired because of severe depression.

One strength of the MMPI–2 is the validity scales, which have long played a role in the assessment of symptom exaggeration or minimization. A strong body of evidence exists demonstrating that the family of *F* scales (*F, FBack*, and *Fp*) are robust, objective indicators of overreporting and underreporting symptoms of psychological disturbance (Berry, Baer, & Harris, 1991; Greene, 2000; Rogers, Sewell, & Salekin, 1994). Substantial evidence also shows that other, supplementary MMPI–2 validity scales accurately discriminate between honest and malingered profiles. These include the Dissimulation scale (*DS*; Gough, 1954), the Fake Bad scale (*FBS*; Lees-Haley, English, & Glenn, 1991), and the Obvious–Subtle scales (*O–S*; Wiener, 1948), although some controversy exists about these measures (Greene, 2000).

The CS (Exner, 2003) does not include validity indices parallel to the MMPI–2 validity scales, which clinicians can rely on to identify fake bad or fake good response sets. Over the years, relatively little attention has been paid to the possibility that conscious efforts to exaggerate or to deny psychological difficulties could affect responses to the Rorschach because of a widely accepted belief that the Rorschach is impervious to response bias or faking. Historically, this belief was based on the general assumption that the Rorschach, a projective assessment instrument that uses ambiguous stimuli, taps into unconscious psychological processes that, by definition, are not consciously controlled and therefore cannot be intentionally manipulated.

The belief that the Rorschach could not be skewed by response sets was reinforced by early studies by Fosberg (1938, 1941, 1943). Fosberg investigated whether individuals could alter their responses to the Rorschach when given instructions concerning how to approach the test. In an initial study, Fosberg (1938) found no differences when the profiles of four groups administered the Rorschach under different instructional sets were compared. Based on the results of a second study in which the test–retest reliability of participants who took the Rorschach twice and who were given different instructions prior to one administration, Fosberg (1941) concluded that the Rorschach was impervious to conscious attempts to respond in ways that would make an individual look better or worse adjusted.

A different approach was taken by Rosenberg and Feldberg (1944), who examined the Rorschach protocols of 93 soldiers who on the basis of psychiatric interviews were identified as "known" or suspected malingerers. They identified 15 characteristics that occurred frequently in the Rorschachs of this group. These characteristics included a low number of responses, percepts with vague form, and a tendency to repeatedly ask the examiner questions about the nature of the test and testing procedures. One limitation of Rosenberg and Feldberg's (1944) study was the absence of a control group. Despite this, they concluded that 87% of the Rorschach protocols of known or suspected malingerers contained four of more of the 15 characteristics.

Similar findings were reported by other researchers who investigated the responses of known or suspected malingerers. Based primarily on clinical observations, rather than empirical studies, these researchers (Benton, 1945; Hunt, 1946; Wachspress, Berenberg, & Jacobson, 1953) characterized the Rorschach protocols of malingerers as involving a low number of responses; slow reaction times; frequent card rejections; a failure to produce an adequate number of *Popular* responses in some cases, or an elevated number of *Populars* in others; as well as a tendency to produce dramatic, deviant responses.

Several empirical studies provide support for these clinical observations. For instance, two studies (Easton & Feigenbaum, 1967; Feldman & Graley, 1954) used a within-subjects design. In these studies, the Rorschach was administered in two conditions, one in which the Rorschach was administered using standard instructions and the other in which participants were instructed to feign psychological disturbance. Consistent with findings from previous studies, faked protocols differed from standard protocols in terms of a lower number of responses and fewer *Popular* responses. In addition, Feldman and Graley (1954) found that faked protocols contained a higher level of what was termed "dramatic" content, responses involving fire, blood, explosions, smoke, and sexual anatomy responses. The findings from the studies summarized thus far suggest that, contrary to popularly held beliefs, responses to the Rorschach may be skewed by conscious response sets.

In addition to these early studies, contemporary approaches to the Rorschach also repudiate the early assumption that Rorschach responses cannot be consciously manipulated because of the projective nature of the test. Exner (2003), for instance, pointedly dismissed the premise that Rorschach stimuli are ambiguous, as well as the assumption that responses to the Rorschach are impervious to conscious response sets.

Reviews of older studies investigating whether Rorschach profiles can be affected by deliberate efforts to create a positive or negative impression have pointed out important methodological and statistical shortcomings of these studies (Exner, 1991; Perry & Kinder, 1990). For instance, some early studies used group rather than individual administration of the Rorschach (Feldman & Graley, 1954; Pettigrew, Tuma, Pickering, & Whelton, 1983). The extent to which results based on group Rorschach administration can be generalized to current clinical practice, which relies on individual administration of the Rorschach, is questionable. Furthermore, because studies conducted prior to 1974 did not use the Comprehensive System, the method of administration and scoring used in earlier studies differed from contemporary administration and scoring practices and specific variables and patterns of scores contained in the CS could not be investigated.

Other studies have investigated whether raters experienced in the use of the Rorschach could judge whether Rorschach protocols were valid or malingered (Albert, Fox, & Kahn, 1980; Mittman, 1983). These studies found that expert judges could not reliably differentiate between valid and malingered protocols. However, one important methodological limitation of these findings concerns the method by which judges determined whether or not a protocol was valid. Judges were not required to use any formal scoring method and may have relied on the content of responses. The researchers did not provide judges with any specific guidelines to use to differentiate between valid and malingered protocols and, as discussed earlier, the Rorschach itself does not contain specific validity scales. Thus, it should not be surprising that judges did not accurate identify valid and malingered protocols if no clearly defined criteria exist by which malingering on the Rorschach can be identified. Rather than showing that the Rorschach contributes little to the assessment of malingering, these studies may simply show that judgments based on content analysis using nonstandardized, subjective decision rules are not effective in distinguishing between valid and malingered Rorschach protocols.

MALINGERING PSYCHOTIC DISORDERS: EMPIRICAL STUDIES

Simulation Studies

Albert et al. (1980) investigated how easy it would be for individuals to fake schizophrenia when administered the Rorschach. They administered the Rorschach to six nonpatients, the control group, six patients diagnosed with paranoid schizophrenia, and two groups of nonpatients instructed to feign schizophrenia. One group of simulators, an "uninformed" group of malingerers, was instructed to simulate schizophrenia during administration of the Rorschach, whereas the other group of simulators, the "informed" malingerers, was instructed to respond as a paranoid schizophrenic would and was also informed about the clinical characteristics of this disorder before the test was administered. The protocols from these participants were rated by judges on dimensions, including the presence or absence of a psychotic disorder and whether or not the protocol was faked. Judges were also asked to assign a psychiatric diagnosis to each participant. Albert et al. (1980) found that judges could not reliably identify participants as psychotic or nonpsychotic and could not reliably distinguish between genuine and faked protocols.

As discussed earlier, there are several methodological limitations in this study. These include the absence of specific guidelines to be used to identify malingering on the Rorschach. In addition, judges were not required to use any formal scoring system. Exner (1991) also pointed out that all protocols were administered by Albert who may not have been blind to participants' group assignment. This could result in inadvertent examiner influence on participants' responses.

Kahn, Fox, and Rhode (1988) attempted to correct for some of the limitation in the Albert et al. (1980) study, specifically the absence of formal scoring and interpretation guidelines. Kahn et al. used a subset of Rorschach protocols from each of the four groups in the Albert et al. (1980) study, protocols obtained from the control group, from inpatients with paranoid schizophrenia, from college students instructed to malinger paranoid schizophrenia after being coached about characteristics of schizophrenia, and from college students instructed to malinger schizophrenia without any coaching. Rorschach protocols were scored according to CS guidelines and scores were input into a computer interpretation program developed by Exner (1991).

Kahn et al. (1988) reported that the computer program did not accurately classify protocols produced by the malingering groups as invalid. The only protocol identified by the computer program as invalid was, in fact, produced by a schizophrenic patient. It should be noted, however, that the interpretation program was not developed to identify malingering, but did classify protocols as being valid or invalid based on the total number of responses (e.g., whether R was less than or greater than 14). In a comment on this study, Cohen (1990) pointed out that one should not equate profile invalidity with malingering. In other words, these results showed that simulators did not differ from the control and patient groups in terms of the number of responses they produced, but did not address whether there were meaningful differences on other Rorschach variables.

Mittman (1983) collected Rorschach protocols under standard administration procedures from 6 nonpatient adults, 6 psychiatric inpatients diagnosed with schizophrenia, and 6 psychiatric inpatients diagnosed with depression. In addition the Rorschach was administered to six nonpatients asked to simulate schizophrenia without any coaching and six nonpatients instructed to simulate schizophrenia who were given information about this disorder. The protocols were scored according to the Comprehensive System and Structural Summaries were calculated. It should be noted that the *SCZI* and *DEPI* were not included in this study as these variables had not yet been developed.

The protocols from the five groups were then rated by judges who also completed a questionnaire concerning participants' psychological characteristics and psychiatric diagnosis. Not surprisingly as the Rorschach has no validity indicators developed to detect malingering, judges could not reliably differentiate between valid and malingered protocols.

Perry and Kinder (1992) administered the Rorschach to college students under standard administration conditions and to college students instructed to simulate schizophrenia. Simulators were provided with a description of schizophrenia and instructed to respond as if they had this disorder. Because Perry and Kinder (1992) were concerned that group differences in response productivity might affect statistical analyses of group data, group comparisons were based on only the first or second response to each card. Consistent with the findings from previous research already discussed, simulators produced significantly fewer *Popular* responses than the control group. They also produced higher scores on the *SCZI*, *WSUM6*, *X−%*, and *M−%* and lower scores on the *X+%*. Schretlen (1997) pointed out that because Perry and Kinder's (1992) study did not include a group of schizophrenic patients, they could not determine whether protocols produced by simulators differed from protocols produced by actual patients. As only a selected set of responses were included in these analyses, the generalizability of these findings to clinical practice using complete Rorschach protocols is uncertain.

Netter and Viglione (1994) conducted a study in which the Rorschach was administered to 20 nonpatient adults using standard procedures, 20 patients with schizophrenia, and 20 nonpatients instructed to simulate schizophrenia. The simulators earned significantly higher scores than either nonpatient controls or schizophrenic patients on a self-report measure of unusual, deviant thought processes, the Eckblad–Chapman Scale of Magical Thinking (Eckblad & Chapman, 1983). This confirmed that simulators were making a concerted effort to convince others their thinking was abnormal.

Netter and Viglione (1994) compared the three groups on eight CS variables and on two experimental Rorschach measures. They found that when scores on the *SCZI* were examined, 3 nonpatient adults, 9 simulators, and 13 patients obtained positive scores. In other words, this showed that 45% of simulators produced Rorschach protocols that could be viewed as providing evidence of a psychotic disorder. They concluded that individuals informed about symptoms and behaviors associated with schizophrenia can successfully simulate schizophrenia when responding to the Rorschach, at least as measured by the *SCZI*. The extent to which this finding can be generalized to the Perception and Thinking Index, which replaced the *SCZI* on the CS Structural Summary (Exner, 2003), remains to be seen.

Based on responses to a postexperimental debriefing questionnaire and behavioral observations, Netter and Viglione (1994) identified several strategies used by simulators in their attempts to fake schizophrenia. These included pretending that the image on the card was alive, trying to appear withdrawn or confused, creating a dramatic story about the image, making references to personal distress, or making references to hearing voices in an atypical fashion.

Another simulation study investigated whether participants educated about the nature of the Rorschach test would be more successful at malingering schizophrenia than participants naive about the Rorschach. Sidhu (2000) compared scores on the Rorschach and the Personality Assessment Inventory (PAI; Morey, 1991) for two groups of graduate students in clinical psychology instructed to feign schizophrenia. One group of simulators was administered the Rorschach and PAI without any preparation, and the second group of simulators was coached about the Rorschach. As expected, both simulating groups produced elevations on the PAI Negative Impression Management scale, a validity scale developed to detect malingering. Although Sidhu (2002) predicted that the naive group would differ from the coached group, no differences were found on CS variables related to schizophrenia. These findings suggest that familiarity with the nature and procedure of the Rorschach does not increase the likelihood that one can successfully modify responses to produce a Rorschach profile characteristic of schizophrenia.

Clinical Studies

A different approach to investigation of malingering psychosis on the Rorschach was used by Ganellen, Wasyliw, Haywood, and Grossman (1996). Unlike previous studies that used college students or nonpatient adults instructed to simulate psychopathology, Ganellen et al. (1996) compared the Rorschach protocols of subjects referred for psychological evaluation while being tried for criminal offenses who faced the possibility of serious penalties if convicted. All participants in this study completed both the Rorschach and MMPI using standard administration and scoring procedures. Compared to volunteers who simulated psychological difficulties to obtain course credit or a small monetary reward, the defendants included in this study potentially had substantial motivation to claim a serious mental disorder that could skew their test data. For instance, a number of participants in this study were pursuing a NGRI (Not Guilty by Reason of Insanity) plea, whereas others claimed to be unfit to stand trial.

The criminal defendants in Ganellen et al.'s (1996) study were identified as responding in an honest or malingered manner on the basis of scores obtained on MMPI validity scales. Using guidelines derived from a meta-analysis of use of MMPI validity scales to detect malingering (Berry et al., 1991), participants who produced an *F* scale *T*-score greater than or equal to 90 were assigned to the malingering group, whereas participants who produced an *F* scale *T*-score less than 90 were classified as responding honestly. As predicted, highly significant differences were found when the honest and malingered groups were compared on MMPI scales related to psychosis (Scale 6 75.6 vs. 103.3, respectively, and Scale 8 78.5 vs. 116.6, respectively). This indicated that the malingered group reported significantly higher levels of psychotic symptomatology than the honest group on the MMPI. However, on the Rorschach, no between-group differences were found on the *SCZI* or for the total number of responses (*R*), the number of *Popular* responses, or variables related to psychotic disorders, including *X+%*, *X–%*, number of *Special Scores*, or the number of *Level 2 Special Scores*. Highly significant differences were found a measure of *Dramatic Content*, defined by Ganellen et al. (1996) as the number of responses containing *Blood*, *Sex*, *Fire*, or *Explosions* content plus the number of responses coded with *Aggressive* or *Morbid* special scores. This study used the *SCZI*, rather than the *PTI*, which recently replaced the *SCZI*. Future research needs to be done to see whether similar findings would be obtained using the *PTI*.

Ganellen et al. (1996) concluded that although defendants identified as malingering reported high levels of psychotic symptoms on the MMPI, they were not able to deliberately skew Rorschach variables empirically related to the presence of psychosis. They also observed that because no specific Rorschach variables distinguished between the honest and malingered groups, with the exception of *Dramatic Content*, Rorschach variables should not be used in isolation to identify intentional exaggeration of serious psychopathology. Ganellen et al. (1996) advised clinicians to weigh MMPI and Rorschach scores when an evaluation involves concerns about malingering and recommended that the index of suspicion for intentional malingering of a psychotic disorder should be considered to be high "when an individual produces MMPI validity scores in the malingering range, a marked discrepancy exists between indicators of psychosis on the MMPI and Rorschach, and responses on the Rorschach are overly dramatic" (p. 78).

MALINGERING OTHER DISORDERS: EMPIRICAL STUDIES

Simulation Studies

Meissner (1988) administered the Rorschach and Beck Depression Inventory to 29 college students using standard procedures and 29 college students informed about the clinical features and presentation of depression and instructed to respond as though they were severely depressed. An attempt was made to increase participants' motivation to simulate depression by offering a $50 cash reward for the most convincing portrayal of depression on assessment measures. Students were excluded from the study if they reported experiencing significant levels of depression on the MMPI Depression scale.

As expected, Meissner (1988) found that simulators earned significantly higher scores on the BDI than controls. The two groups were compared on 14 Rorschach variables conceptually related to a depressive disorder. These did not include the number of *Popular* responses or *Form Quality*. Consistent with findings from previous research, the simulators produced fewer responses than controls on the Rorschach and gave more responses with *Blood* or *Morbid* contents. It should be noted that these are two content categories identified in other research as reflecting *Dramatic Content*. No differences were found for other Rorschach variables. Schretlen (1997) pointed out that Meissner (1988) did not include a group of patients diagnosed with a depressive disorder. Thus, this study could not determine whether the malingered group responded to the BDI and Rorschach as depressed patients do.

Frueh and Kinder (1994) compared the MMPI and Rorschach protocols of 20 college students administered these tests under standard conditions, 20 Vietnam veterans diagnosed with combat-related Posttraumatic Stress Disorder (PTSD), and 20 college students who were informed about symptoms and problems associated with PTSD and instructed to simulate this disorder. As predicted, the role-informed simulators produced significant elevations on MMPI–2 validity indices signifying malingering and earned higher scores than controls or PTSD veterans on these scales. The role-informed simulators also produced significantly higher scores than controls and veterans on a self-report scale of symptoms of combat-related PTSD, the Mississippi Scale for Combat-Related PTSD (Keane, Caddell, & Taylor, 1988).

Consistent with findings from previous research, the simulators produced significantly higher scores than controls and veterans with PTSD on several Rorschach variables. These included a *Dramatic Content* score created by summing the number of responses that involved themes of depression, sex, blood, gore, aggression, hatred, or mutilation. The role-informed simulators also earned significantly higher scores than controls and patients on *X–%*, *Lambda*, and *SumC* and earned significantly lower scores on *X+%*. Contrary to predictions, the simulators did not differ from controls or veterans with PTSD on Rorschach variables related to emotional distress (e.g., *DEPI, D score, CDI*) or signs of withdrawal.

Frueh and Kinder (1994) concluded that role-informed simulators were able to intentionally alter responses when responding to the Rorschach. Although simulators skewed some Rorschach variables in a direction consistent with PTSD in some respects, they differed from veterans with PTSD in other respects. For example, Frueh and Kinder (1994) observed that simulators gave overly dramatic, excessively complex, and emotionally unrestrained responses in contrast to the "short, simple responses that were remarkably unexciting, devoid of melodramatic content or color, and relied primarily on pure form determinants" given by PTSD patients (p. 295).

Labott and Wallach (2002) investigated whether undergraduate women could skew their responses on psychological tests when instructed to simulate Dissociative Identity Disorder (DID). They administered a self-report inventory related to DID, the Dissociative Experiences scale II, and the Rorschach to two groups of undergraduate women. One group completed these measures under standard conditions and was told to respond honestly, whereas the second group was instructed to simulate DID. Although the simulators endorsed significantly more items related to dissociative symptoms on the DES than controls, indicating they made a deliberate effort to portray themselves as experiencing symptoms of DID, the two groups' scores on relevant Rorschach variables did not differ.

CLINICAL APPLICATIONS: DETECTION OF MALINGERING

Two general issues have been addressed in the literature reviewed earlier concerning malingering and the Rorschach. First, investigators have examined whether any Rorschach variable or constellation of variables effectively identifies individuals who consciously attempt to fake psychopathology or to overreport symptoms. Second, researchers have studied whether individuals who claim to have psychological problems they do not experience or who exaggerate existing psychological problems can skew responses on the Rorschach and produce significant values on Structural Summary variables that support these claims.

These issues are relevant to the position taken by Lilienfeld, Wood, and Garb (2000) in an article discussing forensic applications of the Rorschach. Lilienfeld et al. (2000) expressed concern that faking cannot be detected using existing Rorschach indexes and the Rorschach is susceptible to malingering. Both issues are addressed in the next sections.

Rorschach Indices of Malingering

With regard to the first issue, no specific indicators of malingering on the Rorschach have received enough empirical support to be considered an accurate, reliable marker of malingering. This is not surprising because the CS does not include validity indicators developed specifically to detect exaggeration of psychopathology.

One Rorschach variable associated with malingering that has received support in several studies is the Dramatic Content score (Frueh & Kinder, 1994; Ganellen et al., 1996; Meissner, 1988; Netter & Viglione, 1994). Before applying this score in clinical practice, however, one should be aware that the range of scores expected on *Dramatic Content* in clinical, nonclinical, and forensic samples responding honestly and in samples of simulating and actual malingerers has not been established, nor has a cutoff score differentiating between genuine and feigned protocols been determined. Furthermore, research has not examined the rates of accurate classification of examinees responding honestly and malingering. For these reasons, one would be in a precarious position if a determination of malingering was made on the basis of the *Dramatic Content* score alone.

Clinicians using the Rorschach should also be aware that the *Dramatic Content* score used in malingering research is quite similar to the Rorschach Trauma Content Index (TC/R) developed by Armstrong and Loewenstein (1990), a ratio of the sum of all *Blood, Anatomy, Sex, Morbid*, and *Aggressive* responses as compared to the total number of responses. The TC/R was originally developed to identify individuals who defend against traumatic memories using dissociative defenses, but has also been shown to be associated with a history of trauma, such as sexual and/or physical abuse, in patients who do not dissociate (Kamphuis, Kugeares, & Finn, 2000). Kamphuis et al. (2000) pointed out that none of the patients in their study were involved in litigation. Their finding raises the following caution for clinical use of the TC/R: In cases in which exaggeration of psychological difficulties is an issue, positive scores on the Trauma Content Index should be interpreted as providing support for a history of trauma only after the possibility of inflated report of symptoms and emotional problems has been objectively ruled out.

In short, in clinical practice one should not rely on the Rorschach as a stand-alone measure of malingering. Other, robust validity indicators shown to effectively discriminate between genuine and feigned accounts of psychological disturbance, such as the MMPI–2 validity scales or the Structured Interview of Reported Symptoms (SIRS; Rogers, 1992) should instead be relied on.

This should not be taken to mean, however, that the Rorschach plays no role in determinations of malingering. As pointed out by Rogers (1997, p. 392), no one method of detecting malingering, including the MMPI–2 and SIRS, is infallible. This occurs in part because two people motivated to malinger during a psychological evaluation may employ very different strategies as they attempt to convince others they have significant problems. Astute observers of malingering have identified multiple strategies used by malingerers, including reporting of rare symptoms; indiscriminate endorsement of a large array of symptoms; inconsistent, insufficient, or suboptimal effort; a high rate of claims of obvious, blatant features of a disorder; reporting nonsensical or extremely atypical symptoms or patterns of symptoms (Rogers, 1997; Sweet, 1999). Sweet (1999) also noted that malingering may be identified in some cases by comparing a patient's presentation against their real-life behavior. For instance, an individual I evaluated claimed to be unable to return to work in a position involving driving because of PTSD linked to a moving vehicle accident. During a break, the patient casually mentioned that he had enjoyed a recent family "road trip" to several national parks and, when I expressed some interest, described with some animation the highlights of the trip, the number of miles they had covered driving out West, and some of the sights they saw. His leisure activity while off work conflicted with his assertion of disability due to limitations driving or traveling in a vehicle. As there are multiple ways to malinger, one should not be surprised that specific clinical assessment methods may effectively identify some types of malingering, but not others.

Given the clinical reality that no one approach should be expected to accurately distinguish between individuals who respond honestly and those who exaggerate difficulties in all cases, it is incumbent on the responsible clinician to review relevant information obtained using different methods, including interview data, self-report data, and performance measures, such as the Rorschach. Rogers (1997) recommended that clinicians pay careful attention to the degree of consistency among different sources of information as consistencies and inconsistencies can provide critical evidence for or against a determination of malingering.

As noted by Ganellen et al. (1996), confidence in a determination that a particular individual is malingering can be strengthened by examining consistencies and inconsistencies among empirically validated indices of malingering, interview and self-report data, and patterns of Rorschach variables. In Ganellen et al.'s (1996) sample, the malingered group produced highly elevated scores on MMPI–2 scales related to psychosis, but did not obtain significant scores on Rorschach indices related to psychosis more frequently than the honest group. This is noteworthy, particularly as the Rorschach is a sensitive indicator of psychotic symptomatology (Ganellen et al., 1996). This suggests that, in legal cases in which psychosis is a central feature being investigated during a psychological evaluation, consistencies among self-report and Rorschach data concerning psychotic features should be examined carefully. In addition to elevated scores on validity scales sensitive to malingering, one pattern of malingering that may be observed among individuals invested in convincing others they suffer from a psychotic disorder may involve highly elevated scores on self-report scales relevant to psychosis (e.g., MMPI–2 Scales 8 and Bizarre Mentation) and within normal limits scores on Rorschach indices sensitive to psychosis, such as variables indicating disorganized or illogical thinking or impaired perceptual accuracy (e.g., *PTI, WSum6, X–%*).

Inconsistent findings from self-report measures and the Rorschach can occur in other ways. As discussed previously, some studies have suggested that individuals who deliberately exaggerate the symptoms they experience produce Rorschach protocols with low *R*. Although there is at present limited support for this guideline, confidence in a determination of malingering should be increased when an individual obtains significantly elevated scores on MMPI–2 validity indicators, such as the *F, FBack*, and *Fp* scales, which provide strong evidence of deliberate overstatement of psychological problems, and their responses to the Rorschach are characterized by low *R* (e.g., $R \leq 14$). A conclusion of deliberate overstatement of psychological difficulties would be strengthened if in addition to low *R*, scores on Rorschach indices conceptually related to the condition claimed by that individual (e.g., psychosis, depression, anxiety) are nonsignificant.

This pattern is illustrated by the evaluation of Mr. M, evaluated in the context of a dispute about his eligibility for disability benefits. Mr. M, a 45-year-old married man with a history of substantial achievement and academic and career success, owned and was the president of a company until he claimed that he was unable to work and manage the responsibilities of this position because of severe depression. He attributed the onset of depression to the embarrassment he experienced when he was forced to confess to his wife that he had continued visiting Internet pornography sites after promising he would stop. Mr. M explained that he had to inform his wife of these activities after his administrative assistant walked into his office while working late one evening without realizing Mr. M was there, discovered him masturbating, became flustered, and told him that either he had to tell his wife what had happened or she would. Needless to say, this compounded his sense of embarrassment. Shortly after this, he took a leave of absence from work. Mr. M's claim of disability was supported by the psychiatrist who had prescribed an SSRI more than a year before this incident when Mr. M first saw him at his wife's insistence when she initially found out he was visiting Web sites with pornographic content. He also was seeing a psychologist for psychotherapy once a month and characterized the sessions as talking about "sports, the stock market, and the weather."

MMPI–2 validity scales provide clear evidence that Mr. M was invested in convincing others he suffers from significant psychological difficulties ($F = 120$, $Fb = 112$, $Fp = 113$). The Rorschach Structural Summary is notable for the low number of responses ($R = 14$) and use of the most obvious features of the image ($Lambda = 1.33$; $W{:}D{:}Dd = 13{:}1{:}0$). Before concluding that some variables reflect emotional distress (e.g., D *score* $= -2$), one should take into account the extent to which the high number of *Pure F* and *W* responses likely skewed findings on other, relevant variables (e.g., $M = 1$; $EA = 2.0$; $3r + (2)/R = .07$). For instance, the low *EA*, an indication of an individual's psychological resources, is unexpectedly low given Mr. M's history of achievement, accomplishments, and demonstrated capacity throughout his life to respond to stress constructively and "turn lemons into lemonade." For these reasons, the Rorschach Structural Summary does not provide reliable, accurate information about Mr. M's psychological state. Overall, Rorschach and MMPI–2 findings provide convergent evidence of a deliberate attempt to make the point that he should be awarded disability benefits because psychological problems prevent him from returning to work.

Can Rorschach Findings Be Manipulated?

With regard to the second issue addressed in the literature, there are mixed findings concerning the possibility that individuals can deliberately alter scores on Rorschach indices of psychopathology. Some studies have suggested that, in both clinical and nonclinical samples, the Rorschach protocols of individuals identified as overreporting psychological difficulties do not differ from the Rorschach protocols of individuals responding honestly (Ganellen et al., 1996; Labott & Wallach, 2002; Sidhu, 2000). In contrast, other studies have raised concerns that some individuals motivated to feign a psychological disorder may indeed be able to produce Rorschach findings consistent with such claims (Netter & Viglione, 1994; Perry & Kinder, 1992). Simply put, the long-held belief that the Rorschach is impervious to conscious deception cannot be accepted unquestioningly.

To put this into perspective, however, studies have shown that other widely used measures, such as the MMPI–2, may also be susceptible to deliberate exaggeration and that some individuals who are motivated to do so may escape detection, particularly if they are informed about the presence and operating characteristics of validity scales (Rogers, Bagby, & Chakraborty, 1993; Storm & Graham, 2000). Rather than viewing this as a sign of concern (cf. Lilienfeld et al., 2002), the "take home" lesson for me is a sharp reminder that any and all psychological tests may be susceptible to deliberate efforts to skew findings in some situations, that clinicians involved in forensic practice should attempt to avoid becoming complacent, and that we should be aware of the strengths and weaknesses of the methods we use.

The possibility that some individuals may be able to manipulate responses to the Rorschach to simulate a psychological disorder is important to take into account in cases in which evidence of exaggeration is evident from other sources of data, such as the MMPI–2 validity scales, but the Rorschach protocol appears valid and contains signs of significant psychopathology. Guidelines for interpretation of the MMPI–2 (Greene, 2000) state that interpretation should stop if the validity scales indicate an individual is malingering and that the clinical scales should not be interpreted because one cannot have confidence they provide accurate, reliable information about the patient's psychological status. It is not clear that interpretation of the Rorschach should also stop if there is evidence an individual has overreported problems on a self-report measure as it is possible that valid information may still be obtained from the Rorschach even when response sets are present.

There are several interpretive possibilities a clinician should consider when there is evidence of malingering on the MMPI–2 or other self-report measure and the Rorschach protocol appears valid. This pattern may be seen in some cases of what Resnick (1977) labeled "pure malingering." As discussed earlier, *pure malingering* is a term that applies to cases in which patients feign symptoms of a specific disorder when in actuality that patient does not experience those symptoms. In cases of pure malingering, both MMPI–2 and Rorschach results are products of conscious attempts to convince others that significant psychopathology exists.

In other cases, a pattern involving an invalid MMPI–2 and an interpretable Rorschach protocol may be due to what Resnick (1977) labeled "partial malingering." As already discussed, *partial malingering* refers to cases in which an individual in actuality experiences some type of emotional or behavioral disturbance, but embellishes the nature or severity of these psychological problems and/or the extent of impairment caused by psychological difficulties. Findings from psychological evaluations in cases of partial malingering yield a mixture of information, which may include, on the one hand, an accurate description of psychological difficulties, as shown by Rorschach data, and, on the other, information alerting the clinician the patient deliberately provided an exaggerated account of psychological problems, as seen on the MMPI–2.

It can be challenging to distinguish between pure and partial malingering. Doing so requires the clinician to weigh the extent to which information obtained during the clinical interview, from record reviews, and contained in test data meshes. For instance, individuals charged with a criminal offense evaluated to determine whether they are fit to stand trial may report symptoms suggestive of a psychotic disorder during a clinical interview, obtain scores on MMPI–2 validity scales and the SIRS consistent with malingering, and obtain the following Rorschach values: $WSum6 = 45$, $X–\% = 64$, *Level 2 Special Scores* = 4. A determination that this defendant presents with a psychotic disorder, but was attempting to dramatize these problems, consistent with partial malingering, would be strengthened if the prisoner had a documented history of past treatment for a psychotic disorder and if prison staff noted that the prisoner frequently seemed to be responding to internal stimuli, stared off into space, and exhibited odd, unusual behavior.

In contrast, evidence that this defendant was engaged in pure malingering and attempting to "play" the role of a psychotic without actually experiencing the symptoms claimed during the clinical interview would be provided by non-test information and test findings. For example, in terms of non-test data, a determination of faking a psychotic disorder would be supported by reports provided by prison staff that the prisoner interacted comfortably and appropriately with both other prisoners and prison staff and only exhibited signs of inappropriate behavior or strained thinking and logic when meeting with mental health professionals or an attorney. Consistent with the findings discussed earlier, evidence of pure malingering would be provided in this instance by Rorschach findings of an elevated number of responses involving *Dramatic Content* or behavioral observations that during administration of the Rorschach the prisoner acted as though the image on the card was alive, produced responses involving dramatic stories about the images rather than reporting what it looked like, made repeated references to personal distress, fearfulness, panic, or other overdone emotional reactions "triggered" by looking at the inkblots, or insistently and repeatedly informed the examiner he was hearing voices in an unusual, melodramatic fashion (cf. Netter & Viglione, 1994).

The case of Mr. G meets the definition of partial malingering. Mr. G was evaluated in the context of a personal injury lawsuit based on a claim that he developed Posttraumatic Stress Disorder and depression while working as a guard stationed in a booth outside of an industrial facility. His job involved authorizing entrance of trucks into the industrial facility after the driver produced the proper documents and the truck was examined. Unfortunately, while working in this position, a truck rammed into the guard booth in which Mr. G was stationed. When this accident occurred, he was terrified he would be killed as the truck knocked the booth off its moorings and pushed it into the next lane. Fortunately, that lane was closed and had no traffic. He also reported that he had to be guided out of the guard booth to avoid being electrocuted because there were live power lines in the booth. He reported that he began to experience symptoms consistent with PTSD and an episode of Major Depression after this traumatic event. Following this accident, Mr. G began treatment at a community mental health center that included individual psychotherapy and medication management. He had been seeing a therapist regularly and receiving medication for approximately 2 years at the time he was evaluated at the request of the attorney for the defense.

Standard MMPI–2 validity scales indicated that although Mr. G was able to read and comprehend, and respond consistently to test items, there was reason to be concerned that he reported symptoms in an unrealistic, exaggerated manner (e.g., $F = 101$, $FBack = 108$, $Fp = 114$). These concerns were reinforced by scores on supplementary validity scales (e.g., $Ds = 99$; $O - S = +238$; $FBS = 37$). Overall, these scores are consistent with intentional exaggeration of symptoms of psychological disturbance and problems in functioning.

Although Mr. G claimed to be troubled by extremely high levels of emotional distress, anxiety, fearfulness, and tension when responding to the MMPI–2, variables from the Rorschach Structural Summary indicated he was able to adequately manage emotional demands in his life and was not bothered by high levels of distress, anxiety, helplessness, or depression ($D score = +1$; $DEPI = 3$; $Y = 2$; $m = 2$; $C' = 0$). Rorschach findings did highlight difficulties in interpersonal functioning, including a wary mistrust of others (a positive HVI; $T = 0$), a negative self-image ($3r + (2)/R = .21$), and difficulties in his capacity to modulate emotions ($FC:CF + C = 2:3$; $C = 2$; $Afr = .36$). Although one might argue that the issues identified by the Rorschach were caused by the traumatic accident, one might also plausibly link these findings to a childhood history of growing up in a household with an alcoholic, physically and emotionally abusive father who mistreated his wife and children and spent money on his mistress and the children he had with her. In addition, Mr. G described himself prior to the work-related accident as being "a recluse" who had never had a satisfying long-term relationship and who had experienced repeated past failures in his attempts to obtain full-time work in his chosen field and efforts to start his own business.

Subsequent investigation of events related to the accident obtained after the results of this psychological evaluation were conveyed to the attorney for the defense indicated that the account of the accident provided by Mr. G to the mental health professionals treating him and to myself contained considerable embellishment. For instance, these additional records showed, first, that the guard booth was not pushed off its moorings and shoved into another lane and, second, that there were no loose, live electrical wires hanging from the ceiling of the booth that presented a potential threat to his life. This information and the inconsistencies observed between MMPI–2 and Rorschach findings discussed previously do not indicate that Mr. G presented with no psychological issues or problems. Instead, consistent with a presentation of partial malingering, he clearly dramatized what happened during this unfortunate accident, described the emotional and behavioral problems he claimed were precipitated by this incident in an unrealistic, exaggerated manner, and gave the impression that all problems in his life were caused by the accident.

DEFENSIVE RESPONDING AND THE RORSCHACH: EMPIRICAL STUDIES

There have been studies conducted investigating whether a defensive approach to a psychological examination can alter responses to the Rorschach. Several early studies (Carp & Shavzin, 1950; Fosberg, 1941; Seamons, Howell, & Roe, 1981) used a similar research design to investigate this issue. In these studies, the Rorschach was administered to participants twice: when participants were instructed to make a "good" impression, and when instructed to make a "bad" impression. These studies yielded mixed results. One study (Fosberg, 1941) indicated these response sets did not affect the basic structural features of the protocol. Another (Seamons et al., 1981) found that participants instructed to appear well-adjusted produced more *Popular* responses and fewer responses involving *Dramatic Content* and inappropriate combinations than when instructed to convince others they suffered from a psychotic disorder. As Schretlen (1997) pointed out, however, because these studies did not include a control group and did not obtain protocols from participants instructed to respond honestly, it is difficult to determine whether these findings are a function of a defensive, minimizing or an exaggerating response set. In other words, given the design employed, it is difficult to determine whether individuals who are attempting to conceal emotional or behavioral problems produce elevated levels of *Popular* and fewer dramatic responses, whether individual who are trying to feign psychological disturbance produce fewer *Popular* and more dramatic responses, or whether the differences reflected both tendencies.

In an interesting series of studies, Bornstein, Rossner, Hill, and Stepanian (1994) investigated whether scores on a particular dimension of personality functioning, interpersonal dependence, could be consciously skewed. In these studies, dependence was measured using a self-report scale, the Interpersonal Dependence Inventory (IDI), and a scale developed to assess dependent characteristics based on clearly defined Rorschach variables, the Rorschach Oral Dependence scale (ROD). Bornstein et al. (1994) varied experimental conditions such that in some situations dependence was presented in positive terms as a desirable characteristic, whereas in others dependence was described as a negative, undesirable personality characteristic. Whereas scores on the IDI—a self-report scale—increased when dependence was described in positive terms and decreased when it was described in negative terms, scores on the ROD were not influenced by experimentally manipulated response sets. In other words, participants' conscious efforts to monitor and control how dependent or independent they appeared did not affect scores on the ROD. Bornstein et al. (1994) concluded that response sets and self-presentational pressures had little impact on responses to implicit measures of personality, such as the Rorschach, but did bias responses to explicit measures, such as the IDI.

A different approach to this issue was taken by Ganellen (1994), who administered the Rorschach and MMPI to commercial airline pilots who were mandated to undergo a fitness to return to work evaluation after their pilot's licenses had been revoked by the FAA because of a history of alcohol and/or substance abuse. The evaluation was conducted after the pilots had completed an inpatient substance abuse treatment program and were attempting to have their licenses reinstated. Realizing that all the pilots were highly motivated to return to work, Ganellen (1994) predicted they would produce elevated scores on MMPI validity scales of symptom minimization. He also examined the following Rorschach variables thought to be sensitive to a defensive response set: a decreased number of responses overall (low R), a constricted response style (*Lambda* > .99), an increased number of safe, conventional responses (elevated *Popular* responses), decreased effort (a low number of *Blend* and of *Zf* responses), and indications of defensiveness (elevated frequency of *Personalized* responses).

Ganellen (1994) compared pilots' Rorschach protocols with Exner's (1991) normative sample and found that pilots had a higher number of high *Lambda* protocols and produced approximately three times as many Personalized responses as subjects in the nonpatient reference sample. No differences were found for R, *Populars*, *Blends*, or *Zf*. Furthermore, although MMPI findings indicated that pilots were invested in creating a positive impression, indications of problems in psychological adjustment consistent with pilots' clinical history were observed in their Rorschach protocols. These findings were presented as being tentative as no control group was used.

Schretlen (1997) criticized Ganellen's (1994) findings on two grounds. Schretlen commented that Ganellen (1994), first, did not use the most effective MMPI indicators of defensiveness and, second, did not employ any indicators of denied substance abuse. It should be noted that the pilots in Ganellen's study had already acknowledged a history of alcohol and/or substance abuse, had completed an intensive inpatient substance treatment program, were actively involved in aftercare programs, and were seen to determine their readiness to return to work. For these reasons, use of indicators of substance abuse was irrelevant as the focus of the evaluation was not on determining whether the pilots had abused alcohol or other substances, but on whether any cognitive, emotional, or personality issues were present that could compromise a pilot's capacity to perform job-related duties that might constitute a threat to public safety.

Using a design conceptually similar to that employed in the Ganellen et al. (1996) study, Wasyliw, Benn, Grossman, and Haywood (1998) classified accused sex offenders seen for a forensic psychological evaluation as responding in an open or defensive manner based on their scores on MMPI validity scales. The population included in this study was heterogeneous, as some alleged sex offenders were clergymen and others were not and the victims of the alleged abuse involved children, adolescents, and adults. Although Wasyliw et al. (1998) examined standard MMPI validity scales (e.g., L and K), participants were grouped into open and minimizing groups based on their scores on the Obvious minus Subtle scales.

Based on findings from previous research, Wasyliw et al. (1998) compared the honest and minimizing groups on the following selected Rorschach variables: *R*, *Populars*, *Lambda*, *PER*, *Blends*, *Zf*, *D*, and *A*. No differences were found on any of these variables. Furthermore, no differences were found when participants who denied the allegations of sexual abuse were compared to participants who admitted committing sexual abuse on the same Rorschach variables. They concluded that the Rorschach protocols produced by alleged sexual offenders who adopted a defensive response set and were invested in "looking good" during a psychological evaluation did not differ from the Rorschach protocols produced by alleged sexual offenders who responded honestly.

In a follow-up to this study, Grossman, Wasyliw, Benn, and Gyoerkoe (2002) examined the MMPI and Rorschach protocols of a sample of clergymen and non-clergymen accused of sexual offenses who underwent forensic psychological evaluations. The authors did not specify whether this sample was independent of the sample used in the Wasyliw et al. (1998) study. It appeared that this sample incorporated into the expanded sample examined for the purposes of this study. Grossman et al. (2002) reasoned that individuals accused of sexual misconduct would be highly motivated to minimize or deny psychological problems, even though it would be understandable that they experienced a high degree of emotional distress given their predicament and the potential negative outcomes they faced. They examined whether alleged sexual offenders who responded honestly and those who denied psychological disturbance differed on Rorschach indicators of emotional distress, faulty judgment, poor interpersonal functioning, a predisposition of cognitive distortions, and sexual preoccupations.

Grossman et al. (2002) classified accused sexual offenders as responding openly or minimizing on the basis of MMPI validity scale. Parallel to the procedures used in their earlier study (Wasyliw et al., 1998), they selected the Obvious minus Subtle Index to make this determination. As predicted, participants who minimized psychopathology obtained significantly lower scores than those who responded openly on MMPI clinical scales. However, no differences between the open and minimizing groups were found for any Rorschach variables.

Grossman et al. (2002) concluded that although minimizers were able to produce MMPI clinical scale scores that fell within normal limits, they did not appear psychologically more healthy on the Rorschach than alleged sexual offenders who responded openly. To the contrary, when compared to Exner's normative sample, a substantial portion of the sample produced scores on Rorschach variables suggestive of psychological dysfunction, including indications of distress, unconventional judgment, and difficulties with interpersonal functioning. The conclusions that could be drawn from this comparison should be considered preliminary, however, as the authors acknowledged that no statistical comparisons of their groups and the normative sample could be conducted. This conclusion would have been strengthened if the study design included an appropriate control group. Furthermore, in both the Grossman et al. (2002) and Wasyliw et al. (1998) studies, participants were identified as responding openly or in a guarded, self-favorable way using scores on the Obvious minus Subtle scales. These are not the most widely used or well accepted MMPI indicators of defensiveness.

An unpublished dissertation provided partial support for the variables Ganellen (1994) suggested were characteristic of a guarded, minimizing response set. Kennelly (2002) administered the Rorschach to a sample of nonpatient adults who were instructed to respond either honestly or as though they were being evaluated in the context of a child custody evaluation and were invested in presenting themselves in the best possible light. Participants instructed to simulate a "fake good" response set produced fewer responses overall and fewer *Popular* responses than the group responding under standard administration conditions. These findings suggest that, in some instances, motivation to deliberately create a favorable impression and conceal psychological disturbance may constrict responses to the Rorschach and contribute to a decreased number of responses.

Singer, Hoppe, Lee, Oleson, and Walters (chap. 21, this vol.) presented Rorschach data on a large sample of individuals ($N = 728$) all of whom were evaluated in the context of a custody dispute. Singer et al. did not report MMPI–2 data for the individuals in their sample. However, as previous research provides strong evidence that the prototypical MMPI–2 profile for individuals embroiled in custody disputes reflect a defensive response set (Bagby et al., 1999; Bathurst et al., 1997; Medoff, 1999; Posthuma & Harper, 1998), it is reasonable to assume that the members of Singer et al.'s sample were similarly defensive.

In contrast to the findings reported by Kennelly (2002), participants in Singer et al.'s (chap. 21, this vol.) study produced an average number of responses ($R = 22.78$), as well as an average number of *Popular* responses (*Popular* = 4.93). Furthermore, although one would expect the participants in Singer et al.'s sample to try to portray themselves in a favorable light, Rorschach indicators of problems in psychological adjustment were readily apparent. For instance, 28% of this sample had a positive score on the *DEPI*, suggesting a vulnerability to periods of emotional distress, 38% earned a positive score on the *CDI*, indicating difficulties in interpersonal functioning and/or ineffective coping strategies, and 25% of the sample appeared to be mistrustful of others as shown by a significant score on the *HVI*.

Overall, Singer et al.'s (chap. 21, this vol.) findings suggest that, in contrast to the nonclinical individuals asked by Kennelly (2002) to respond to the Rorschach *as if* they were involved in a custody dispute, individuals actually engaged in a legal battle to determine custody issues and parental rights who had considerable, real-life motivation to create a favorable impression (a) produced average length Rorschach protocols, which (b) highlighted concerns about their psychological functioning. The differences in the results presented by Kennelly (2002) and Singer et al. (chap. 21, this vol.) may be a function of differences in the composition of the samples in each study and the motivations each group had. For instance, research strongly suggests that individuals who become involved in high conflict custody disputes tend to have significant psychological issues and high rates of personality disorders (cf. Singer et al., chap. 21, this vol., for a more detailed discussion of this issue). Thus, it should not be surprising that, although invested in "looking good," Rorschach data were consistent with difficulties in emotional regulation, coping skills, and interpersonal functioning in Singer et al.'s (chap. 21, this vol.) sample, in contrast to Kennelly's simulators, who were drawn from a nonclinical population.

Lilienfeld et al. (2000) commented that "there is virtually no methodologically sound research on the susceptibility of the Rorschach to impression management" or efforts to fake good (p. 57). The basis for this is unclear because they did not reference any of the studies discussed earlier. In fact, the only study Lilienfeld et al. (2000) cited involved simulating need for achievement on the TAT. The extent to which the finding of this study generalizes to the Rorschach, which involves different administration, scoring, and interpretation procedures than the TAT, is unclear.

CLINICAL APPLICATIONS: DETECTION OF DEFENSIVE RESPONDING

Similar to the literature investigating malingering and the Rorschach, the literature investigating defensive responding and the Rorschach has investigated two questions: First, is there a pattern of scores that characterizes defensive responding? And, second, can individuals responding defensively modify their responses to avoid revealing difficulties in psychological functioning? Some authors (Ganellen, 1994: Weiner, 2003) have suggested that Rorschach protocols produced by defensive responders are characterized by a low number of responses, a lack of engagement in the task as shown by elevated scores on *Lambda*, low scores on *Zf*, and a tendency to respond to the most obvious features of the stimuli (e.g., elevated number of *Populars*). As discussed earlier, limited empirical support for this characterization has been found.

Whereas this "guarded" pattern may not characterize all defensive responders, it does apply to a subset of defensive responders. In clinical forensic practice, some individuals approach an evaluation with the goal of protecting themselves from being judged negatively by guarding against revealing any information they think could be construed unfavorably. These individuals deliberately and consistently make an effort to withhold information. This is the psychological equivalent of "taking the fifth," or making an effort to avoid providing any information that could be used against them. Analogous to Resnick's label of pure malingering, this response set may be termed *deliberate defensiveness*. Strong support for a conclusion that an individual is responding in a guarded, defensive, nonrevealing manner would be found if an individual produced both an MMPI–2 with elevated scores on *L*, *K*, and *S* with low scores on *F*, and a Rorschach protocol with low *R*, low *Zf*, high *Lambda*, and high *Populars*. When this pattern is produced, the evaluator is limited in what they can learn about the individual's make-up and may not be able to reach sound conclusions about the presence or absence of psychological disturbance. Often, the most one can say is that patients were strongly invested in protecting the impression others formed of them and consciously attempted to avoid revealing information that could be viewed in a negative light, including minor personal shortcomings or foibles that most people would acknowledge.

The *deliberately defensive* response set is illustrated by the case of Mr. P, a 34-year-old pilot evaluated in order to assess his readiness to return to work after he had completed a 28-day inpatient alcohol treatment program. During the clinical interview Mr. P emphasized how enthusiastic he was about returning to work as soon as possible. He also repeatedly stated that, although he initially resented it when he was confronted by coworkers, a supervisor, and a union representative about his excessive use of alcohol during layovers, he now realized this intervention was "the best thing that ever happened to me." Given his obvious motivation to return to work, as well as his awareness that the results of the psychological evaluation would be seriously considered in reaching a decision about reinstating him, it is not surprising that Mr. P tried to reveal as little personal information as possible, particularly any information that might result in his being seen in a negative, unflattering light, when the Rorschach and MMPI–2 scores were administered. Given this guarded response set and self-protective strategy of deliberately "holding back," little could be learned about Mr. P's personal strengths and weaknesses during this evaluation. In my clinical experience, this pattern is not unusual in fitness to work evaluations when individuals are invested in being cleared to work.

Psychological "White Washing" and the Rorschach

Several studies have reported that the Rorschach profiles of defensive responders often contain scores indicating they present with significant psychological issues (Ganellen, 1994; Singer et al., chap. 21, this vol.) do not show less pathology than protocols produced by relevant comparison groups (Grossman et al., 2002; Wasyliw et al., 1998), and are not able to consciously control their responses or deliberately skew scores on specific dimensions of personality functioning (Bornstein et al., 1994). These findings indicate that individuals who approach an evaluation in a consciously guarded manner and try to create a positive impression, which is often evident on self-report measures, such as the MMPI–2, may still reveal signs of psychological difficulties when responding to the Rorschach. Further investigation is needed to determine whether findings from the Rorschach obtained under such conditions portray the full range of an individual's psychological issues or whether defensive responders may successfully guard against revealing specific concerns or the full range of psychopathology.

Instances in which an individual responds to an evaluation in a cautious manner and makes an effort to create a positive impression, as shown by elevated scores on MMPI–2 *L*, *K*, and/or *S* scales plus a low score on the *F* scale, but still produces a valid Rorschach that highlights concerns about the person's psychological condition may be considered a *consciously guarded but reluctantly revealing* pattern. This pattern is illustrated by test data from a bitterly contested child custody evaluation in which both parents portrayed the other in extremely unflattering terms.

In this case, claims and counterclaims and accusations and counteraccusations were made by Mr. and Mrs. D about each others' behavior and fitness to parent their children. In particular, Mr. D claimed that his estranged wife should not be awarded custody of their children because, in his view, she had a quick, explosive temper that he was afraid would damage the children. She adamantly denied this. I will focus on Mrs. D's test findings for the purposes of this discussion. Obviously, any determination in this case cannot be made based on information concerning Mrs. D alone; as a general principle, it would be unprofessional and unethical to reach a determination in a child custody evaluation without obtaining relevant information about both parents.

As might be expected under such circumstances, the MMPI–2 validity scales indicated that Mrs. D responded in a self-protective manner and tried to downplay, minimize, or deny any personal shortcomings in her psychological adjustment. She appeared to be invested in demonstrating that she was a reasonable, responsible, morally virtuous woman who adhered to conventional standards of behavior. The low scores on MMPI–2 clinical scales should be considered a function of this response set, rather than providing evidence for the absence of psychopathology.

In contrast to the MMPI–2 profile, there are no reasons to interpret the Rorschach profile as reflecting a defensive response set given the value for R ($R = 37$). Other findings underscored concerns about Mrs. D's ability to manage emotions in a mature manner ($FC: CF + C = 1:4$; $C = 1$) and the possibility that anger can be particularly disorganizing ($S = 6$; $S– = 3$). Concerns that she might be the kind of person who "shoots from the hip," acts on impulse without thinking, and does not recognize the impact of her actions were also suggested ($Zd = –4.0$; $FM = 1$; $FD = 0$). Although Mrs. D adamantly dismissed her husband's characterization of her, Rorschach findings line up with his description.

Contradictory Responding

Another pattern of responding involves indications of a careful, guarded attempt to downplay or deny psychological problems, on the one hand, at the same time an individual reports psychological difficulties openly. This may be identified on the MMPI–2 when there are indications of both defensiveness (e.g., elevated values on L, K, and/or S) and a realistic acknowledgment of symptoms, distress or problems functioning (e.g., F scale scores are greater than 65, but less than 100). In my experience, Rorschach protocols associated with this MMPI–2 validity scale pattern can either be brief and constricted, if the individual is making an effort to avoid revealing information, or can reflect an open, engaged response style.

The motivations identified by these contradictory response styles may be interpreted as signs, first, that these individuals have significant concerns about how the test findings will be interpreted and, second, that this apprehension leads them to readily report, if not try to call attention to, problems in certain areas of their life, while trying to conceal issues or concerns in other aspects of their life. Put differently, this response set should alert the clinician to the possibility that the individuals are engaging in "selective reporting" and most likely are presenting a biased account of their situation. For instance, the patients may manifest the self-protective strategies by failing to report symptoms, events in their lives, or other information, such as a history of treatment by mental health professionals, that are not consistent with the conclusions they are invested in demonstrating.

Although this contradictory response set can occur in forensic evaluations for a variety of reasons, one instance in which it occurs involves instances of what Resnick (1997) termed *false imputation*. As described previously, false imputation refers to situations in which individuals attribute causality for actual emotional or psychosocial difficulties to a specific event related to their legal case when their symptoms in actuality are not related to the event in question. This type of selective responding is illustrated by the case of Mrs. N, who claimed she developed symptoms of anxiety after she sustained minor physical injuries when she was punched in the face and abdomen, shoved, kicked, and forced to the floor at gunpoint when the fast food restaurant at which she worked as a cashier was robbed. She also reported that, as a result of the robbery, she developed multiple fears of being the victim of a future assault and had considerable difficulty leaving her home without someone accompanying her.

Mrs. N was evaluated in the context of personal injury litigation. The MMPI–2 validity scales are notable for a contradictory response style involving a guarded, self-protective response set, as shown by her scores on *L*, *K*, and *S*, on the one hand, and a ready willingness to report problems, on the other, as shown by the elevated score on *F* and multiple elevations on MMPI–2 clinical scales. Although *F* is elevated, the level of elevation provides no reason to think she is overreporting symptoms and concerns. The 278 codetype, as well as elevations on *ANX*, *DEP*, and *PK*, are consistent with Mrs. N's report of significant emotional distress, worry, repetitive, distressing, intrusive thoughts and fears.

Rorschach findings similarly portray Mrs. N experiencing considerable emotional distress and feeling overwhelmed and powerless given a positive *DEPI*, negative *D score*, and elevated number of shading responses. Several findings raise concerns, in addition, that Mrs. N has a chronic vulnerability to becoming unhappy, tense, and feeling emotionally troubled as the CDI is positive and the *Adjusted D score* is in the negative range. Other notable findings highlight longstanding struggles concerning her self-image (*Egocentricity Index* = .28), intensely self-critical attitudes, if not a sense of self-loathing (*V* = 3), and a distressing sense of isolation and feeling that she does not have meaningful connections with others (*Isolation Index* = .35). As several of these variables are highly stable over time, these findings raised questions as to whether the anxiety and depression Mrs. N reported were triggered by the events during the robbery or may have been due to other factors.

Review of records from the therapist who treated Mrs. N after the assault at work has a bearing on these questions. During the course of treatment, she revealed to the therapist that she had been repeatedly sexually and physically abused by her father starting in early adolescence. The abuse continued until she left home at age 18. Mrs. N also told the therapist that her father forced her to have sex with his drinking buddies on numerous occasions, became pregnant with her father's child at age 15, and was forced to give the child up for adoption. The therapist described Mrs. N as weeping inconsolably as she expressed aloud for the first time powerful feelings of guilt about putting her baby up for adoption, feelings that she had not revealed to over the 15 years since she left home.

The history of chronic, severe abuse, incest, and pregnancy was not disclosed to me during the clinical interview. To the contrary, Mrs. N had described her family life during childhood in generally positive terms and denied having been the victim of a sexual assault or abuse at any point in her life, even though asked specifically about this. This selective reporting of life events could plausibly be explained as being due to defensive attempts to deny, suppress, or disavow disturbing memories and feelings. However, in the context of litigation, this edited account of significant life experiences could also be reasonably construed as an attempt to claim that the emotional distress, negative views of herself, and problems in intimate relationships clearly apparent on the MMPI–2 and Rorschach reflected a deliberate attempt to "paint a picture" illustrating the connection between these problems and the trauma of the robbery, rather than to other factors. This should not be taken to imply that Mrs. N was not affected by the assault and robbery at her place of work. However, indications that Mrs. N deliberately provided a biased account of her history makes it difficult, if not impossible, to determine with accuracy what problems were caused by the trauma of the robbery; what emotional problems she experienced as a result of the trauma experienced during childhood and adolescence, problems that predated the robbery; and whether the impact of the robbery at work aggravated a preexisting condition.

Parenthetically, this case also highlights one of the challenges involved in interpretation of psychological test data both in clinical and forensic practice. Test findings provide information about an individual's psychological status and functioning, but do not, in and of themselves, explain the cause of that state. For example, someone evaluated shortly after the death of a family member may produce test data consistent with depression. However, those findings do not necessarily demonstrate that the depression was *caused* by that loss. The clinician's task is to consider whether there are any other causes of depression unrelated to the death, such as another stressful life event, whether the individual was depressed before the death occurred, and, if so, whether the loss intensified the depressive condition. Making a determination about the cause of depression in this example requires that the person provide an accurate, complete history so the clinician can reach an informed conclusion about the patient's emotional functioning and the factors contributing to it.

Similarly, in a legal case determining whether a psychological condition was caused by a specific cause, such as a traumatic incident, also requires that the clinician have the information necessary to weigh the contribution of one the events in question as opposed to the contribution of other factors. Different conclusions may be reached depending on what information is considered by the clinician and what information is available to consider. When defensive or contradictory response sets are in play, it is important for clinicians to be alert to the possibility that patients engaged in legal action may not only present their side of events in a self-serving manner that enhances their self-image, a traditional interpretation of elevated "fake good" validity scales, but may also steer away from, avoid discussing, omit, or "forget" to report information that does not support the claims they are making.

CONCLUSIONS

The literature summarized earlier indicates the following. First, the Rorschach does not yield robust information that can be used to reliably identify fake good or fake bad response sets. This is not surprising as no specific CS validity indices have been developed and validated to detect exaggeration or minimization of psychological problems.

The Rorschach variable most consistently associated with exaggeration of psychological disturbance has been labeled *Dramatic Content*. Over the years, different investigators have used somewhat different clusters of Rorschach variables to create a *Dramatic Content* score. It would be useful for researchers to establish an accepted set of CS variables to use to compute a *Dramatic Content* score, investigate the range of scores for this variable in different populations, examine how effectively it distinguishes between honest and malingering responders, and, if appropriate, establish cutting scores for use in clinical and forensic settings.

As already discussed, Rorschach data can make meaningful contributions to assessment of response sets, psychological functioning, and personality characteristics when used in conjunction with other instruments which do have sound validity scales, such as the MMPI–2. For instance, conclusions that a criminal defendant is malingering a psychotic condition may be strengthened by extreme elevations on MMPI–2 validity indicators in conjunction with a Rorschach protocol with little or no signs of disorganized, illogical thinking or inaccurate, distorted perception of events (Ganellen et al., 1996). This is most likely to occur in situations involving what Resnick (1997) terms pure malingering.

A determination that individual are deliberately attempting to avoid revealing information about their psychological functioning would be bolstered by test data showing elevated values for MMPI–2 defensive scales as well as a constricted, barren Rorschach (Ganellen, 1994; Kennelly, 2002; Seamons et al., 1981). This response style was characterized earlier as indicating a deliberately defensive approach to an evaluation in order to prevent the clinician from learning about the person's psychological functioning.

A more complicated situation exists when there are mixed findings, such as in cases of "partial malingering" (Resnick, 1977), false imputation, and contradictory responding. These cases may be identified when MMPI–2 validity scales are elevated, but the Rorschach findings appear interpretable and provide evidence of psychological disturbance. This may be a function of the fact that response sets, such as exaggeration of symptoms, are not necessarily all-or-none, dichotomous phenomena that are completely present or completely absent. In some cases, for instance, individuals whose MMPI–2 validity configuration shows they are overreporting problems do, indeed, have real emotional or behavior difficulties that are demonstrated on the Rorschach. This presentation obviously presents particular challenges in the context of a forensic evaluation.

In other cases, discrepancies between MMPI–2 validity scales and Rorschach data may be a signal that an individual selectively reported, divulged, or withheld information both when responding to psychological tests and during a clinical interview. Weighing whether this occurs because of a need to preserve self-esteem or a deliberate attempt to provide information that buttresses the position most favorable to the individual's position in the legal proceedings is the challenge the clinician faces in this situation.

REFERENCES

Albert, S., Fox, H. M., & Kahn, M. W. (1980). Faking psychosis on the Rorschach: Can expert judges detect malingering? *Journal of Personality Assessment, 44*, 115–119.

American Psychiatric Association. (1994). *Diagnostic and statistical manual of mental disorders* (4th ed.). Washington, DC: American Psychiatric Association.

Armstrong, J. G., & Loewenstein, R. J. (1990). Characteristics of patients with multiple personality and dissociative disorders on psychological testing. *Journal of Nervous and Mental Disorders, 178*, 448–454.

Bagby, M., Nicholson, R., Buis, T., Radovanic, H., & Fidler, B. (1999). Defensive responding on the MMPI–2 in child custody and access evaluations. *Psychological Assessment, 11*, 24–28.

Bathurst, K., Gottfried, A. W., & Gottfried, A. E. (1997). Normative data for the MMPI–2 in child custody litigation. *Psychological Assessment, 9*, 205–211.

Benton, A. L. (1945). Rorschach perfomances of suspected malingerers. *Journal of Abnormal and Social Psychology, 40*, 94–96.

Berry, D., Baer, R., & Harris, M. (1991). Detection of malingering on the MMPI: A meta- analysis. *Clinical Psychology Review, 11*, 585–598.

Bornstein, R. F., Rossner, S. C., Hill, E. L., & Stepanian, M. L. (1994). Face validity and fakability of objective and projective measures of dependency. *Journal of Personality Assessment, 63*, 363–386.

Bourg, S., Connor, E. J., & Landis, E. E. (1995) The impact of expertise and sufficient information on psychologists' ability to detect malingering. *Behavioral Sciences and the Law, 13*, 505–515

Butcher, J. N., Dahlstrom, W. G., Graham J. R., Tellegen, A., & Kaemmer, B. (1989). *Minnesota Multiphasic Personality Inventory–2 (MMPI–2): Manual for administration and scoring.* Minneapolis: University of Minnesota Press.

Carp, A. L., & Shavzin, A. R. (1950). The susceptibility to falsification of the Rorschach psychodiagnostic technique. *Journal of Counseling Psychology, 14*, 115–119.

Cohen, J. B. (1990). Misuse of computer software to detect faking on the Rorschach: A reply to Kahn, Fox, and Rhode. *Journal of Personality Assessment, 54*, 58–62.

Easton, K., & Feigenbaum, K. (1967). An examination of an experimental set to fake the Rorschach test. *Perceptual and Motor Skills, 24*, 871–874.

Eckblad, M., & Chapman, L. J. (1983). Magical ideation as an indicator of schizotypy. *Journal of Consulting and Clinical Psychology, 51*, 215–225.

Exner, J. E. (1991). *The Rorschach: A comprehensive system. Volume 2: Interpretation* (2nd ed.). New York: Wiley.

Exner, J. E. (2003). *The Rorschach: A comprehensive system. Volume 1: Basic foundations and principles of interpretation.* New York: Wiley.

Feldman, M. J., & Graley, J. (1954). The effects of an experimental set to simulate abnormality on group Rorschach performance. *Journal of Projective Techniques, 18*, 326–334.

Fosberg, I. A. (1938). Rorschach reactions under varied instructions. *Rorschach Research Exchange, 3*, 12–30.

Fosberg, I. A. (1941). An experimental study of the reliability of the Rorschach Psychodiagnostic Technique. *Rorschach Research Exchange, 5*, 72–84.

Fosberg, I. A. (1943). How do subjects attempt to fake results on the Rorschach test? *Rorschach Research Exchange, 7*, 119–121.

Frueh, B. C., & Kinder, B. N. (1994). The susceptibility of the Rorschach Inkblot Test to malingering of combat-related PTSD. *Journal of Personality Assessment, 62*, 280–298.

Ganellen, R. J. (1994). Attempting to conceal psychological disturbance: MMPI defensive response sets and the Rorschach. *Journal of Personality Assessment, 63*, 423–437.

Ganellen, R. J., Wasyliw, O. W., Haywood, T. W., & Grossman, L. S. (1996). Can psychosis be malingered on the Rorschach?: An empirical study. *Journal of Personality Assessment, 66*, 65–80.

Gough. H. G. (1954). Some common misperceptions about neuroticism. *Journal of Consulting Psychology, 18*, 287–292.

Greene, R. L. (2000). *The MMPI–2: An interpretive manual* (2nd ed.). Needham Heights, MA: Allyn & Bacon.

Grossman, L. S., Wasyliw, O. E., Benn, A. F., & Gyoerkoe, K. L. (2002). Can sex offenders who minimize on the MMPI conceal psychopathology on the Rorschach? *Journal of Personality Assessment, 78*, 484–501.

Haywood, T. W., Grossman, L. S., & Hardy, D. W. (1993). Denial and social desirability in clinical evaluations of alleged sexual offenders. *Journal of Nervous and Mental Disorders, 181*, 183–188.

Hunt, W. A. (1946). The detection of malingering: A further study. *Naval Medical Bulletin, 46*, 249–254.

Huprich, S. K., & Ganellen, R. J. (2006). The advantages of assessing personality disorders with the Rorschach. In S. K. Huprich (ed.), *Rorschach assessment of the personality disorders* (pp. 27–53). Mahwah, NJ: Lawrence Erlbaum Associates.

Kahn, M. W., Fox, H., & Rhode, R. (1988). Detecting faking on the Rorschach: Computer versus expert clinical judgment. *Journal of Personality Assessment, 52*, 516–523.

Kamphuis, J. H., Kugeares, S. L., & Finn, S. E. (2000). Rorschach correlates of sexual abuse: Trauma content and aggression indexes. *Journal of Personality Assessment, 75*, 212–224.

Keane, T. M., Cadell, J. M., & Taylor, K. L. (1988). Mississippi scale for combat-related post-traumatic stress disorder: Three studies in reliability and validity. *Journal of Counseling and Clinical Psychology, 56*, 85–90.

Kennelly, J. J. (2002). Rorschach responding and response sets in child custody evaluations. Dissertation Abstracts International, 63, 3034.

Labott, S. M., & Wallach, H. R. (2002). Malingering dissociative identity disorder: Objective and projective assessment. *Psychological Reports, 90*, 525–538.

Lees-Haley, P. R., English, L. T., & Glenn, W. J. (1991). A Fake Bad scale on the MMPI–2 for personal injury claimants. *Psychological Reports, 68*, 203–210.

Lilienfeld, S., Wood, J., & Garb, H. (2000). The scientific status of projective techniques. *Psychological Science in the Public Interest, 1*, 27–66.

Medhoff, D. (1999). MMPI–2 validity scales in child custody evaluations: Clinical versus statistical significance. Behavioral Sciences and the Law, 17, 409–411.

Meissner, S. (1988). Susceptibility of Rorschach distress correlates to malingering. *Journal of Personality Assessment, 52*, 564–571.

Mittenberg, W., Patton, C., Canyock, E. M., & Condit, D. C. (2002). Base rates of malingering and symptom exaggeration. *Journal of Clinical and Experimental Neuropsychology, 24*, 1094–1102.

Mittman, B. L. (1983). Judges ability to diagnose schizophrenia on the Rorschach: The effect of malingering (Doctoral Dissertation, California School of Professional Psychology). *Dissertation Abstracts International, 44*, 1248B.

Morey, L. C. (1991). *The Personality Assessment Inventory professional manual*. Odessa, FL: Psychological Assessment Resources.

Netter, B. E. C., & Viglione, D. J. (1994). An empirical study of malingering schizophrenia on the Rorschach. *Journal of Personality Assessment, 62*, 45–57.

Paulhus, D. L. (1986). Self-deception and impression management in test responses. In A. Angleitner & J. S. Wiggins (Eds.), *Personality assessment via questionnaire* (pp. 143–165). New York: Springer.

Perry, G. G., & Kinder, B. N. (1990). The susceptibility of the Rorschach to malingering: A critical review. *Journal of Personality Assessment, 54*, 47–57.

Perry, G. G., & Kinder, B. N. (1992). Susceptibility of the Rorschach to malingering: A schizophrenia analogue. In C. D. Spielberger & J. Butcher (Eds.), *Advances in personality assessment* (Vol. 9, pp. 127–140). Hillsdale, NJ: Lawrence Erlbaum Associates.

Pettigrew, C. G., Tuma, J. M., Pickering, J. W., & Whelton, J. (1983). Simulation of psychosis on a multiple-choice projective test. *Perceptual and Motor Skills, 57*, 463–469.

Posthuma, A., & Harper, J. (1998) Comparison of MMPI–2 responses of child custody and personal injury litigants. *Professional Psychology: Research and Practice, 29*, 437–443.

Resnick, P. J. (1997). Malingering of posttraumatic disorders. In R. Rogers (Ed.), *Clinical assessment of malingering and deception* (2nd ed., pp. 130–152). New York: Guilford.

Rogers, R. (1986). *Conducting insanity evaluations*. New York: Van Nostrand Reinhold.

Rogers, R. (1990). Development of a new classificatory model of malingering. *Bulletin of the American Academy of Psychiatry and the Law, 18*, 323–333.

Rogers, R. (1992). *Structured Interview of Reported Symptoms*. Odessa, FL: Psychological Assessment Resources.

Rogers, R. (1997). Researching dissimulation. In R. Rogers (Ed.), *Clinical assessment of malingering and deception* (2nd ed., pp. 309–327). New York: Guilford.

Rogers, R., Bagby, R. M., & Chakraborty, D. (1993). Feigning specific disorders on the MMPI–2. *Journal of Personality Assessment, 60*, 215–226.

Rogers, R. R., & McKee, G. R. (1995). Use of the MMPI–2 in the assessment of criminal responsibility. In Y. S. Ben-Porath, J. R. Graham, G. C. N. Hall, R. D. Hirschman, & M. S. Zaragoza (Eds.), *Forensic applications of the MMPI–2* (pp. 103–126). Thousand Oaks, CA: Sage.

Rogers, R., Sewell, K. W., & Goldstein, A. (1994). Explanatory models of malingering: A prototypical analysis. *Law and Human Behavior, 18*, 543–552.

Rogers, R., Sewell, K. W., & Salekin, R. T. (1994). A meta-analysis of malingering on the MMPI–2. *Assessment, 1*, 227–237.

Rosenberg, S. J., & Feldberg, T. M. (1944). Rorschach characteristics of a group of malingerers. *Rorschach Research Exchange, 8*, 141–158.

Schretlen, D. J. (1997). Dissimulation on the Rorschach and other projective measures. In R. Rogers (Ed.), *Clinical assessment of malingering and deception* (2nd ed., pp. 208–222). New York: Guilford.

Seamons, D. T., Howell, R. J., Carlisle, A. L., & Roe, A. V. (1981). Rorschach simulation of mental illness and normality by psychotic and nonpsychotic legal offenders. *Journal of Personality Assessment, 45*, 130–135.

Sidhu, L. S. (2000). Face validity: Implications for malingering. *Dissertation Abstracts International, 60*, 5791.

Slick, D. J., Sherman, E. M. S., & Iverson, G. L. (1999). Diagnostic criteria for malingered neurocognitive dysfunction: Proposed standards for clinical practice and research. *The Clinical Neuropsychologist, 13*, 545–561.

Storm, J., & Graham, J. R. (2000). Detection of coached general malingering on the MMPI–2. *Psychological Assessment, 12*, 158–166.

Sweet, J. J. (1999). Malingering: Differential diagnosis. In J. J. Sweet (Ed.), *Forensic neuropsychology: Fundamentals and practice* (pp. 255–286). The Netherlands: Swets & Zeitlinger.

Wasyliw. O. E., Benn, A. F., Grossman, L. S., & Haywood, T. W. (1998). Detection of minimization of psychopathology on the Rorschach in cleric and noncleric alleged sex offenders. *Assessment, 5*, 389–397.

Wachspress, M., Berenberg, A. N., & Jacobson, A. (1953). Simulation of psychosis. *Psychiatric Quarterly, 27*, 464–473.

Weiner, I. B. (2003). *Principles of Rorschach interpretation* (2nd ed.). Mahwah, NJ: Lawrence Erlbaum Associates.

Weiner, D. N. (1948). Subtle and obvious keys for the Minnesota Multiphasic Personality Inventory. *Journal of Consulting Psychology, 12*, 164–170.

6

PRESENTING AND DEFENDING
RORSCHACH TESTIMONY

Irving B. Weiner
University of South Florida

Psychologists seeking to become effective forensic consultants have much to learn. They must become familiar with the statutory and case law that defines psycholegal issues, including psychologically relevant criteria for determining competence, sanity, torts, and suitability to parent. They must become acquainted with rules of evidence, particularly as they apply to standards of admissibility. They must become knowledgeable about courtroom procedures and comfortable with the rigors of the adversarial process. Such legal learning is typically acquired through practical experience combined with educational programs and attention to the forensic psychology literature (e.g., Blau, 1998; Brodsky, 1991, 2004; Craig, 2005; Goldstein, 2003, 2007; Melton, Petrila, Poythress, & Slobogin, 1997; Weiner & Hess, 2006).

Along with legal sophistication, forensic psychologists must bring to their work a good grasp of clinical assessment. Those whose consultations include personality assessment with the Rorschach Inkblot Method (RIM) need, in particular, to understand the implications of Rorschach data for various personality characteristics, and they must also keep current with published research concerning the psychometric properties of this instrument. Rorschach interpretation and the reliability and validity of Rorschach assessment are discussed elsewhere in this volume and in an extensive contemporary literature (see Exner, 2003; Hilsenroth & Stricker, 2004; Mattlar, 2004, 2005; Meyer, 2004; Meyer & Archer, 2001; Society for Personality Assessment, 2005; Viglione & Hilsenroth, 2001; Weiner, 2001, 2003b, 2004a).

However, neither the legal knowledge gleaned from instructional and practical experiences nor mastery of assessment skills is of much avail unless forensic psychologists can translate their findings and conclusions into effective written reports and oral testimony. Guidelines for writing forensic reports can be found in contributions by Groth-Marnat and Horvath (2006), Harvey (1997), Heilbrun (2001, chap. 10), Melton et al. (1997, chap. 18), and Weiner (2006), among others. The chapter that follows addresses oral testimony, with a specific focus on effective presentation and defense of Rorschach-based testimony in the courtroom.

PRESENTING RORSCHACH TESTIMONY

Forensic psychologists who are familiar with assessment practices know how important it is to base their conclusions on an integrated interpretation of data from diverse sources, including a multimethod test battery (Beutler & Groth-Marnat, 2003; Weiner, 2005). In the courtroom, however, attorneys rarely allow expert witnesses to limit their testimony to an integrated summary of their impressions. Instead, especially if they intend to challenge the psychologist's impressions, attorneys are likely to require a description of each of the tests that has been used in evaluating a defendant or litigant, specification of the inferences derived from each of the tests, and justification either for the use of a particular test or for the inferences drawn from it.

Psychologists who use the RIM in a forensic examination should accordingly enter the courtroom prepared to describe the instrument clearly and explain how and why Rorschach assessment provides information about personality functioning. In addition, the following five tactics often enhance the effectiveness of Rorschach-based testimony and can reduce a forensic consultant's vulnerability to damaging or embarrassing cross-examination: (a) favoring structural over thematic data as the basis for inferences, (b) emphasizing summary scores rather than individual responses in formulating conclusions, (c) framing statements aptly in idiographic or nomothetic terms, (d) expressing views with appropriate levels of certainty, and (e) by managing computer-based test reports advisedly.

Describing Rorschach Assessment

Because the RIM is a complex and multifaceted assessment instrument, and because mastery of Rorschach assessment requires considerable study and practice, testifying psychologists may struggle to convey clearly how and why the instrument works. In communicating to judge and jury, as in teaching graduate students in their first Rorschach class, the best beginning is usually a simple formulation that skirts complexity for the moment and focuses instead on the basic premises of the instrument: For example, "The inkblot method takes a sample of how people look at the world, and how people look at their world says a lot about what kind of person they are and how they are likely to deal with events in their lives." An introductory statement of this kind leads easily into an elaboration of Rorschach administration, coding, and interpretive procedures along the following lines:

> The Rorschach method consists of 10 cards, and each card has a blot of ink on it. The inkblots aren't anything in particular, but people see various things in them when they look at them. The examiner shows the inkblots to the person taking the test one card at a time and asks the person, "What might this be?" On the first card, a person might use the whole blot for a response, and then the response would be coded as a *W*, for *Whole*. Or the person might use just a part or a detail of the blot for a response, and then the response would be coded as a *D*, for *Detail*. The person might say that this first card looks like a bat or a butterfly, which are things that many people report seeing in them, and such common responses are coded with *P*, for *Popular*.

After coding all of the responses given to the 10 cards, the examiner totals the number of these *W*'s, *D*'s and *P*'s in the record. People with a lot of *W*'s tend to be the kind of person who takes a global view of situations. Such people focus on the big picture, sometimes at the expense of overlooking details they should be paying attention to. People with a lot of *D*'s, on the other hand, tend to focus mainly on the details of situations, sometimes at the expense of losing sight of the forest for the trees and failing to grasp the overall significance of events. As for *Popular* responses, people with a lot of *P*'s in their record are seeing things in common ways, and they are consequently likely to be conventional in the opinions they form and how they conduct themselves. Persons whose records contain very few *P*'s, on the other hand, tend to be unconventional and perhaps nonconformimg in how they choose to think and act.

And that's a sample of how the Rorschach works. There are many other codes for various features of how people look at the blots, and the frequencies with which these different codes occur are yield well over 100 summary scores. The summary scores help to identify many aspects of personality functioning, including how people pay attention to what is going on around them, how they form concepts and ideas about events in their lives, how they experience and express feelings, how they manage stress, and how they view themselves and other people.

A description of Rorschach assessment in such terms usually suffices to establish the method as a sensible and understandable procedure. If an attorney attempts to muddle this message, adequately prepared Rorschach examiners should be able to respond effectively without having to give any ground. Asked, for example, "Isn't the Rorschach a pretty complicated test?", the witness can respond, "It's based on the simple premise I just mentioned, that how you look at the inkblots is a sample of how you look at the world, and how you look at the world is an indication of the kind of person you are." The courtroom is not the place to elaborate the multiple intervariable interactions that shape a sophisticated interpretation of Rorschach data.

With further respect to the interpretive process, an attorney may say, "As I understand it, Doctor, different examiners can interpret the same Rorschach protocol in different ways." A recommended response would be, "Examiners who are adequately familiar with the basic principles of Rorschach interpretation usually come to similar conclusions when then they look at the same Rorschach data." This statement is quite true, and the courtroom is not the place to elaborate the Beck–Klopfer argument or the interface between cognitive-perceptual and psychodynamic-object relations perspectives on Rorschach interpretation. As for the truth of the statement, it has been known at least since the work of Exner (1969) that skilled Rorschachists of diverse persuasions usually do arrive at similar personality descriptions when they look at a protocol, despite differences in their approach to the data and the theoretical language in which they prefer to express their conclusions.

Favoring Structural Over Thematic Data

The preceding description of how the RIM is administered, coded, and interpreted reflects a primarily structural approach to Rorschach assessment, without attention to the interpretive significance of the thematic imagery in a record. This structural emphasis does not signify any disregard for the utility of Rorschach imagery as a source of clinically valuable clues to respondents' underlying attitudes and concerns (see Lerner, 1998; Schafer, 1954; Weiner, 2003a, chap. 6). In the courtroom, however, there are at least four good reasons for favoring structural over thematic data as the basis for drawing conclusions from a Rorschach protocol:

1. Inferences based on the structural data are typically less speculative and more conclusive than inferences drawn from the thematic imagery in a Rorschach protocol. This difference reflects the fact that the structural data tend to be *representative* of behavior (e.g., a *W* response is an actual instance of a global approach to a situation), whereas the thematic data are primarily *symbolic* of behavior (e.g., the upper center detail on Card VI seen as "A long object that looks dangerous" could symbolize a spear and suggest concerns about aggression, or it could symbolize a penis and suggest concerns about sexuality, or it could symbolize and suggest something else entirely, depending on its meaning to the individual respondent).

2. Because the rationales for thematic interpretations are usually symbolic and likely to involve alternative possibilities, they are more complex and difficult to explain in the courtroom than the more definitive rationales for structural interpretations.

3. The validating data for interpretations based on the structural variables in a Rorschach protocol are more extensive than empirical confirmations of what thematic variables indicate. Impressions based on structure are therefore likely to impress judge and jury as being more objective and dependable than impressions based on imagery.

4. The interpretive implications of structural variables for respondents' functioning capacities, coping skills, and personal style are usually more relevant to the psychological issues in legal cases (e.g., Is this defendant competent to proceed to trial? Was the defendant sane at the time of his or her alleged offense? Has the plaintiff suffered psychic injury or some decline in functioning capacity from some previously higher level? Is this person capable of functioning effectively as a parent?) than are the interpretive implications of thematic variables for respondents' underlying attitudes and concerns.

Of further note, drawing their Rorschach conclusions mainly from structural features of the data gives expert witnesses an effective way of responding to attorneys who challenge the import of their testimony by saying, "Now all of this is just your *opinion,* Doctor, isn't that right?" Having favored the relatively objective structural data in a protocol, the witness can counter this challenge by replying, "No, it's not just my opinion, it's what the test shows." When buttressed by available reference data, this reply gives the psychologist's testimony a much closer relationship to objective fact than to subjective impression (e.g., "In the normative findings for the Rorschach, not one of the 600 persons in the nonpatient sample scored as high as Mr. A did on the Perceptual Thinking Index, which shows that his ways of thinking and perceiving events are outside the normal range").

This is not to say that informed opinion based on professional experience and clinical judgment lacks a respectable place in courtroom testimony. To the contrary, Sales and Shuman (2004) observed that widely cited Supreme Court rulings concerning standards for the admissibility of expert testimony in *Daubert v. Merrill Dow Pharmaceuticals* (1993), *General Electric v. Joiner* (1997), and *Kumho Tire v. Carmichael* (1999) have had little negative impact on the admissibility of testimony based on clinical opinions, despite concerns among forensic psychologists that the admissibility of such testimony might be in jeopardy. Nevertheless, attorneys who can lead witnesses into acknowledging that their testimony reflects their opinions may succeed in coloring this testimony as at least somewhat subjective in the eyes of judge and jury. Witnesses who are able to state that "This is what the test shows" are likely instead to enhance the effectiveness of their testimony, as just noted, by conveying to listeners that the testimony has an objective basis that goes beyond informed opinion.

As a final consideration with respect to favoring structural variables as the basis of their Rorschach conclusions, forensic examiners should keep in mind that recurrent content categories and repetitive content themes may in some instances be well worth bringing to bear on the issues in a case. For example, a record with four *Sex* responses, compared to a mean frequency of just 0.19 Sex responses in the records of nonpatients adults (Exner & Erdberg, 2005, Table 22.1), strongly suggests either sexual preoccupations or poor judgment on the part of the respondent. A record with numerous *Morbid* responses involving vivid scenes of bloody body parts points to heightened fearfulness of being injured in some way. Presented as evidence in a psychologist's testimony, dramatic imagery of this kind can be quite compelling and have sufficient face validity to speak for itself. As for the courtroom relevance of such imagery, imagine that the *Sex* responses were given by a parent in a contested custody case and the *Morbid* responses by a personal injury plaintiff claiming posttraumatic stress disorder.

Emphasizing Summary Scores Rather Than Individual Responses

Although vivid imagery of the kind just illustrated with bloody body parts can often speak for itself as evidence of a respondent's concerns, most individual responses lack such drama. Generally speaking, then, forensic consultants will do well to emphasize the summary scores in a record as the basis for their Rorschach testimony and avoid volunteering or being drawn into explanations of what individual responses might mean. As an illustration, consider a situation in which a cross-examining attorney reads aloud the following response to Card III: "On this one it looks like two people holding on to something, but I can't tell if they're fighting over it or helping each other do something with it." The attorney than asks, "Doctor, can you tell the court what this response means?"

Faced with this question, and having relied primarily on summary scores in arriving at conclusions, an expert witness can respond effectively to questions about what a particular response means by saying, "Taken by itself, it doesn't mean anything." The attorney may jump on this answer (e.g., "So your testimony is that what people say about these inkblots doesn't mean anything") or challenge the expert to account for it (e.g., "How is it possible that it doesn't mean anything?"). Should that occur, the examiner can explain that summary scores—for example, the previously mentioned total number of Ws, Ds, and Ps in a record—provide the main basis for Rorschach interpretations. The witness can note further that individual responses are important for their contribution to the total scores, but should not be considered out of context as a sole or definitive basis for drawing any inferences.

Forensic examiners who disregard this caution and discuss the meaning of individual responses can create problems for themselves. Readers who think otherwise should imagine a courtroom scene in which a Rorschach expert states that a male respondent's Card III response of people either fighting or helping each other "indicates a man who is indecisive and has a hard time making up his mind." The judge then asks to see Card III, looks at it a while, and says, "Well, I don't know, it looks that way to me too, like the people could be either fighting over this thing or helping each other lift it, and no one ever accused me of being indecisive or unable to make up my mind." The judge then chortles a bit and says, "Let's check out some more of these." At this point, matters can quickly go downhill for the witness and for Rorschach assessment, as the judge (and sometimes members of the jury as well) examine the cards, press the witness for interpretations of various answers given by the respondent, and compare these answers with their own impressions of what the inkblots look like and of their own personality characteristics. Lost in such regrettable shuffles are the credibility of the witness and any serious attention to the Rorschach testimony.

Framing Statements Aptly in Idiographic or Nomothetic Terms

Forensic examiners can usually enhance the effectiveness of their Rorschach testimony by choosing aptly between idiographic and nomothetic forms of framing their inferences. Idiographic statements describe the individual characteristics of a person without reference to what other people are like, as in "This man frequently forms inaccurate impressions of people and events" (inferred from a high $X-\%$) or "This woman appears to be experiencing a great deal of subjectively felt distress" (inferred from an elevated D score). Nomothetic statements, by contrast, compare the characteristics of a person to some relevant reference group, as in "His preoccupations resemble the kinds of concerns seen in people who have had a traumatic stress reaction" (inferred from an elevated Trauma Content Index) or "She shows some response patterns that are similar to patterns found in persons who later commit suicide" (inferred from an elevated *Suicide Constellation*).

Note that the idiographic examples just used describe the person's current characteristics, whereas the nomothetic examples refer to past or future events. Nomothetic statements can also prove effective in phrasing descriptions of current characteristics, as in "On a measure of illogical and incoherent thinking, Mr. X received a score far outside the normal range and at a level often associated with schizophrenic thought disorder." Idiographic statements, however, may not be effective in addressing how people are likely to behave in the future or what they are likely to have done or experienced in the past. Generally speaking, Rorschach and other personality assessment data can seldom be related to past and future events as definitively as they can be used to identify currently manifest personality characteristics. Hence, forensic consultants may forestall some unpleasant cross-examination by avoiding idiographic phrasing and opting for nomothetic statements when they are offering behavioral predictions and postdictions (see Weiner, 2003a).

This difference in suitability between idiographic and nomothetic framing of inferences in courtroom testimony derives from the generally acknowledged fact that behavior is an interactive function of a person's nature and the surrounding environmental circumstances. The more a particular behavior is determined by an individual's abiding dispositions, regardless of the circumstances, the more fully this behavior can be predicted or postdicted from measured personality characteristics. Additionally, the more fully environmental circumstances can be identified or controlled, the more dependably behavioral variations in those circumstances can be estimated from personality assessment data. Even so, the influence of environmental circumstances typically limits the extent to which personality characteristics can account for past or future behavior in the individual case.

Consider, for example, a Rorschach evaluation of violence risk potential in which the respondent appears to be an angry (numerous S), action oriented (extratensive EB), and self-centered ($Fr + rF > 0$, elevated *Egocentricity Index*) person who gives evidence of limited frustration tolerance (high *AdjD–* score), poor judgment (low *XA%*), and little interest in close, caring relationships with other people ($T = 0$, $COP = 0$). If asked what the inkblot test indicates about whether this person is dangerous, the expert witness can, with good support in the literature (e.g., Gacono & Meloy, 1994) say, "This person's Rorschach record is similar in many ways to the records given by people who are known to have behaved aggressively toward other people."

Based on information from multiple sources, including the respondent's behavioral history and profiles on other assessment instruments as well as the RIM, the expert witness in this example may have formed an overall opinion that the person "is showing considerable violence risk potential" or "is more likely than most people to become physically aggressive when provoked." As noted earlier, however, expert witnesses may be required to indicate the inferences they drew solely from the Rorschach, despite their psychologically sound preference for presenting an integrated summary of their findings. Given the limitations of predicting multiply determined behavior directly from a Rorschach protocol, witnesses will usually be on sounder ground if they reply to such requests with nomothetic resemblances than with idiographic assertions.

Expressing Appropriate Levels of Certainty

Rorschach examiners can enhance the effectiveness of their courtroom testimony by avoiding two temptations. One temptation is the urge to be cautious, even at the expense of offering only tentative hypotheses when fairly firm conclusions would be in order. The other temptation is the urge to be definitive, even at the expense of ascribing more certainty to inferences than is warranted by the available data. To be sure, both caution and definitiveness can be virtues, when exercised at opportune times. At less than opportune times, however, they can detract from the credibility and impact of Rorschach testimony.

Expressing tentative hypotheses, as in "There is some suggestion in Ms. A's test responses that she might at times be somewhat hasty and careless in deciding what to think and do," can be tempting to expert witnesses as a way of playing it safe, leaving their options open, and minimizing the risk of being pinned down on cross-examination. In reality, however, a steady dose of such cautious testimony may impress judge and jury as wishy-washy guesses by witnesses who are not very sure of themselves, and an attorney can easily fuel such impressions by remarking to an overly cautious witness, "So you're really not very sure about any of the things you have been saying, are you Doctor?" The testimony in this example would be particularly regrettable in the presence of a large minus Zd score, which would have warranted a fairly definitive version of the inference, as in "Ms. A's test responses indicate that she is the kind of person who often makes decisions about what to think and do in a careless and hasty way, without taking into account as much information as she should to make a good decision."

Expressing definitive conclusions, as in "This man's Rorschach clearly indicates that he is addicted to sensation-seeking behavior," can be tempting to expert witnesses as a way of demonstrating their self-assurance, the power of their assessment instruments, and their immunity to any damaging cross-examination. A definitive approach can backfire in each of these respects, however, especially when the expert's conclusion is based on sketchy data. Suppose in this example that the addiction to sensation-seeking behavior has been based on an $Xu\% = .25$. This $Xu\%$ is only modestly higher than the nonpatient mean, and levels even considerably higher than this are associated with several possibilities, of which a predilection for sensation-seeking behavior is just one (Weiner, 2003b).

Now comes the cross-examination, and the attorney poses such questions as "Do your findings *always* mean what you say they mean?" or "Isn't it true that there are *exceptions* to the way you are interpreting the tests or even *other possibilities* for what the findings might mean?" Ordinarily, the expert witness can reply to questions of this kind without losing any ground (e.g., "There are exceptions to just about anything"; "Although anything is possible, other possibilities seem unlikely"). However, experts who have been excessively definitive in presenting their conclusions run the risk in cross-examination of having to back off and temper their previous testimony. Having to back off from previous testimony can make experts appear cocky and overconfident, given to exaggeration and overgeneralization, and detract from their credibility as a witness.

To steer a middle ground between being overly cautious and excessively definitive, forensic consultants should express their conclusions with a level of certainty that is appropriate to the strength of the data. To begin with, examiners should keep in mind that even the most consistently accurate Rorschach inferences fall short of being absolute certainties. To avoid overstatement, expert witnesses should frequently qualify their conclusions with statements that their test findings are "usually indicative of," "often associated with," or "typical of" whatever is being inferred from them. Conclusions can also be qualified by preceding interpretations with statements that "the test data suggest" whatever is being inferred, or that persons being examined "seem to be" or "give evidence of having" whatever characteristics are being attributed to them.

To avoid understatement, expert witnesses should not hesitate to use data-based qualifiers to identify the probability of their conclusions and to speak in courtroom language to whether they have been drawn "with reasonable psychological certainty." A person with a Rorschach Depression Index (*DEPI*) of 4 is "showing some signs of depression," whereas someone with a *DEPI* of 7 is "giving considerable evidence of being depressed or being disposed to depressive episodes." Respondents with one $M-$ in their record "may be having difficulty forming accurate impressions of other people"; those with two $M-$ "are likely to be having difficulty forming accurate impressions of other people"; and someone with four *M−* is "very likely to be having difficulty forming accurate impressions of other people." In this way, then, forensic consultants should strive to phrase their inferences with a level of certainty that is appropriate to the strength of their data. Going as far as the data appear to allow, but not beyond what the data justify, meshes nicely with the previously mentioned advantage of being able to say, "This is not just my opinion; it is what the test data show."

In this last regard, Rorschach examiners should recognize and be prepared to acknowledge when their data are insufficient to warrant reasonably certain statements. Providing a litany of tentative inferences based on ambiguous test findings—although an honest way to proceed—rarely constitutes effective testimony. Examiners faced with uncertain findings concerning the psycholegal issues in a case should make it known to the attorney who has retained them that their testimony is unlikely to be helpful to the cause of the defendant or litigant whom the attorney is representing. When the expert testimony is nevertheless court ordered, consultants whose Rorschach data will support inferences of only limited certainty should testify to this effect, as in "The Rorschach findings are inconclusive."

Managing Computer Printouts Advisedly

Computer-generated test scores and narrative reports can enhance the psychodiagnostic process, but they can also pose a threat to the effectiveness of courtroom testimony concerning psychological test findings. In the case of the RIM, a computerized program saves considerable time in preparing the structural summary and arraying the data in ways that facilitate the interpretive process. In addition, a narrative Rorschach report generated by computer covers the full range of structural data that have implications for personality characteristics, including pieces of information that the examiner may otherwise have overlooked. As a further advantage, Weiner (2004b) has expanded the Rorschach Interpretation Assistance Program (RIAP5; Exner & Weiner, 2003) to include a Forensic Edition (RIAP5 FE). The RIAP5 FE narrative contains the basic personality descriptions provided by the RIAP5 and also offers special sections that discuss the specific relevance of the Rorschach findings to psycholegal issues in criminal, personal injury, and child custody cases.

Computer-generated narrative reports become problematic in forensic cases, however, because they cannot be left at home and they can be cross-examined in ways that detract from the effectiveness of a forensic consultant's testimony. To elaborate this first point, computer printouts become discoverable as soon as they are generated and the examiner is identified to the court as an expert in the case. This means that expert witnesses must make these printouts available when requested by the court to do so, whether directly or through an attorney acting as an officer of the court. Psychologists who generate a narrative test report and fail to include it with the reports and test data they provide in response to a subpoena can face considerable embarrassment in the courtroom. "Doctor," the cross-examining attorney intones, "I see in these papers the scores that you printed out for your Rorschach test, but I don't see any narrative report; did you print out a narrative report?" A "No" answer when such a report exists will constitute perjury. A "Yes" answer, although avoiding commission of a criminal act, identifies the witness as not having been fully forthcoming and perhaps not to be trusted or believed ("So, Doctor, when you were asked to provide all of your records, you provided only part of them and kept the rest hidden in your drawer, isn't that right?").

As for safeguarding the effectiveness of their testimony, Rorschach examiners should anticipate two types of challenge to computer-generated narratives. First, if they have generated a Rorschach report with the RIAP5 or RIAP5 FE, than they may be asked to indicate which data in the test protocol provided the basis for various statements in the report. Rorschach assessors who come to court unprepared to answer such questions are at risk for being made to look negligent or uninformed on the witness stand. This risk can be minimized by familiarity with the Exner (2003) and Weiner (2003a) texts, from which the RIAP personality descriptions are derived. Familiarity with these texts can help forensic examiners speak knowledgeably about the content of the interpretive printout and, by so doing, to enhance their appearance as a diligent and well-versed expert.

Second, forensic examiners may be asked to account for computer-generated statements that mischaracterize the person who took the test. At least a few inaccurate statements are almost inevitable in computer-based test interpretations, because these narrative reports describe the test protocol, not the individual respondent. If questioned about such statements, the expert witness should be prepared to explain that the descriptive statements in these computer printouts refer to characteristics shown by a group of people with a test protocol similar to the respondent's test protocol, and that some of these statements will consequently be more applicable than others to the person who has been examined. Most computerized test reports begin with a caveat to this effect, which in the RIAP5 printout reads as follows:

> The narrative statements produced by RIAP5 for Windows describe the implications of Rorschach findings among people in general, and do not necessarily apply in all respects to the functioning of any one person. To ensure a thorough and accurate description of a particular individual's personality characteristics and behavioral tendencies, examiners should … judge the applicability of RIAP5 interpretive hypotheses in light of information from other sources concerning the person's clinical status and past and present life circumstances. (Exner & Weiner, 2003, p. 1)

Even when clearly expressed, however, these explanations of seeming inaccuracies in a computer printout may have limited impact following an attorney's use of selected parts of the printout to "expose" the RIM as a misleading and undependable source of information. To minimize the negative fallout from inapplicable statements in a computer report, as in responding to questions about the data sources of various interpretations, forensic examiners should anticipate challenging cross-examination about such statements and coming to court prepared to explain the aforementioned caveat as clearly as possible. Additionally, the fact that interpretive statements are hypotheses to be verified in the process of a psychological assessment, through recourse to other relevant data sources, gives examiners a reasonable basis for explaining why some of these statements may be more accurate than others.

As a final note with respect to presenting Rorschach testimony, the courtroom appearances of forensic examiners are often preceded by a deposition. Depositions are designed to give attorneys fairly free rein to ask expert witnesses who have been retained by opposing counsel about their qualifications and their findings. To function effectively, forensic psychologists need to become familiar and comfortable with the deposition process as well as with courtroom procedures. Babitsky and Mangraviti (1999), two trial attorneys, provide some general advice to expert witnesses on how to give a good account of themselves in depositions. With specific respect to psychodiagnostic testimony, the guidelines presented in this chapter here for effective courtroom presentation of Rorschach procedures and findings apply equally to answering Rorschach questions that emerge during a deposition.

DEFENDING RORSCHACH TESTIMONY

Psychologists presenting Rorschach-based testimony in the courtroom may be challenged to defend either their qualifications as a Rorschach examiner, the dependability of the RIM as an assessment instrument, or the accuracy of the conclusions they have drawn from their Rorschach data. With respect to their qualifications, forensic consultants who include the RIM in their test battery should be confident that some combination of Rorschach-related education, supervision, workshop attendance, teaching assignments, practical experience, and published research in their background will suffice to quash any questions about their expertise. Psychologists with limited Rorschach credentials should defer using the instrument in forensic cases until they have increased their familiarity and involvement with it. As for defending the conclusions they have drawn from a Rorschach examination, knowledgeable psychologists who have interpreted their test data conservatively, and who have framed their findings along the lines recommended earlier in this chapter, should have little difficulty justifying the content of their testimony.

Given the usual ease with which cautious and well-prepared Rorschach examiners can defend their qualifications and conclusions, what remains as a potentially demanding challenge for an expert witness is defending Rorschach assessment itself. Attorneys' questions about the dependability of Rorschach-based testimony typically revolve around allegations of the following kind: "The Rorschach is an unreliable test of questionable validity, and it is not widely accepted in the scientific community. For these reasons, and also because the test is easy to fake, Rorschach testimony does not meet criteria for admissibility into evidence and is not welcome in the courtroom."

As documented by an extensive literature, each of these allegations is patently false, and Rorschach examiners should be prepared to discredit them whenever they surface during cross-examination. The documentation and relevant reference citations necessary for mounting this defense of forensic Rorschach assessment appear in chapters 2–5 of the present volume, which address the scientific status, admissibility, and authority of Rorschach data and their resistance to malingering and deception. Armed with the information in these chapters, expert witnesses can go to court fit for battle, should Rorschach assessment come under attack.

In addition to having a good grasp of the evidence and citations that affirm the propriety and utility of Rorschach-based testimony, forensic consultants should also be versed in specific tactics for responding effectively to what is called "learned treatise" cross-examination (see Brodsky, 1991, 2004; Poythress, 1980). As reviewed in chapters 2–5, the professional literature contains some harshly negative comments about the psychometric foundations and forensic suitability of Rorschach assessment, and some of these negative comments have been echoed in the popular press as well. Attorneys who have read or heard about these "treatises" may bring them into the courtroom in the form of "Isn't it true?" questions, as in "Isn't it true, Doctor, that the Rorschach method is highly controversial?" As for these treatises being "learned," attorneys often introduce this line of questioning by establishing the authority of the author: for example, "Are you familiar with the work of Dr. Garb?," followed by "He's a well respected psychologist, is he not?" and then by quoting some of Garb's disparaging remarks about Rorschach assessment, including his call for a moratorium on use of the instrument (Garb, 1999).

What recourse do expert witnesses have when confronted on cross-examination with statements by a respected psychologist that undercut the testimony they have given on direct examination? To begin with, Rorschach examiners under the learned treatise gun need to keep calm, be ready to stand their ground, and proceed with confidence that the facts are on their side. In this frame of mind, they should answer "Isn't it so?" and "Do you know?" questions as accurately as they can, but with nuances designed to deflate the obvious or implied criticisms in these questions and, in the process, to bolster the psychometric adequacy and practical utility of forensic Rorschach assessment.

To illustrate how such nuances can be injected into learned treatise responses, let us assume that Rorschach examiners giving testimony are familiar—as they should be—with relevant work of the respected psychologists who are quoted in cross examination. In this circumstance, witnesses should not hesitate to endorse the respectability of these professional colleagues. However, giving a general endorsement does not preclude qualifying the colleague's authority to the extent that the facts allow, as in "He is generally respected as a psychologist, but personality assessment is not one of his specialties" or "She has a good reputation in her field, but she has not published much original work on the Rorschach, and to my knowledge she has never made a Rorschach presentation at a major psychology meeting."

As for the content of learned treatise challenges, forensic consultants should keep in mind that harsh criticisms of Rorschach assessment quoted by a cross-examining attorney are likely with few exceptions to be irrelevant, out of date, unscientific, misleading, or erroneous. The following attorney questions and possible responses to them illustrate ways of capitalizing on these common shortcomings of learned treatise Rorschach challenges:

Attorney: Using the Rorschach is pretty controversial, isn't it Doctor?
Witness: Although there are some people who criticize use of the Rorschach, just as there are some critics of almost very procedure used in delivering health care services, the Rorschach is very widely used and taught, and the evidence supporting its use for appropriate purposes is very strong.

...

Attorney: This Rorschach test is really not very reliable, isn't that so, Doctor?

Witness: No. [A simple "No" answer to this type of question often proves effective, because it requires the attorney to choose between two unappealing alternatives. One alternative is to move on and allow the unchallenged "No" answer to convey implicitly to judge and jury that (a) Rorschach assessment is indeed a reliable procedure and (b) the attorney has gotten the facts wrong in suggesting otherwise. The attorney's other alternative is to question the "No" answer (e.g., "What basis do you have for saying that?"). This question gives the Rorschach expert the floor to expound on the ample research literature documenting the interscorer and retest reliability of Rorschach assessment.]

...

Attorney: As I understand it, the *Buros Mental Measurement Yearbook* is a highly regarded reference source, and Arthur Jensen is a distinguished psychologist, and what he had to say about the inkblot test in that yearbook was, and I quote, "The rate of scientific progress in clinical psychology might well be measured by the speed and thoroughness with which it gets over the Rorschach" [reference to Jensen, 1965]. So how can you come into this courtroom and ask us to base an important decision, even in small part, on such a discredited test?

Witness: With all due respect to Dr. Jensen, he said that back in 1965, and he was wrong then, because there has been a lot of scientific progress in clinical psychology over the last 40 years, and during that same time, the number of Rorschach tests being given around the world has increased substantially. And if Jensen were to say the same thing now, he would be wrong again. [The attorney could question the basis for saying that Jensen was wrong then or would be now. As in the previous example, the question would give a knowledgeable witness free rein to recount the many positive developments over the years in the science and practice of both clinical psychology and Rorschach assessment, including the growth of a thriving international Rorschach community.]

...

Attorney: [As in the previous example, pressing a "big book" attack] Well, I've got another important book here, a recently published book in which James Wood and some other professors devote 446 pages to reporting all the things that are wrong with the Rorschach [reference to Wood, Nezworski, Lilienfeld, & Garb, 2003]. A test with that much wrong with it is not a very good test, is it?

Witness: It's Dr. Wood and his co-authors who are wrong, because the best research shows that the Rorschach is really a good test. [Once more, the attorney, and not the witness, is left holding the bag. Unquestioned, the negation of Wood et al. conveys that the Rorschach is just fine and that the attorney has hitched the wagon to a faulty star. If questioned by the attorney ("How can you say that these widely published authors are wrong?"), the witness can then review the frequently noted flaws in much of contemporary Rorschach criticism].

With further respect to the flaws that characterize most negative commentaries on the RIM, prominent among those that can be identified by expert witnesses is selective and uncritical citation of the literature. As elaborated by Hibbard (2003), Hilsenroth and Stricker (2004), Meloy (2005), and Meyers (2001), among others, the authors who denigrate Rorschach assessment typically refer mainly to studies that support their point of view while ignoring or giving short shrift to research findings that contradict their conclusions. In being uncritical as well as selective, these authors often give unwarranted weight to poorly designed studies, without attending to the methodological limitations of these studies and the dubious significance of the results they yield.

Witnesses defending Rorschach assessment against published criticisms of its value may also find it helpful to note for the court that selective and uncritical citation of the literature has no respectable place in science. Science differs in this respect from advocacy, where it may be appropriate to cite only evidence in support of one's position without commenting on the dependability or preponderance of this evidence. Science, by contrast, calls for balanced review of all available evidence and conclusions based on the strength of this evidence. Because most Rorschach critiques are adversarial in nature, rather than scientific, they can lead to erroneous and misleading conclusions that give the appearance of being buttressed by research findings but do not in fact have such support. Meloy (2005), commenting on Wood, Nezworski, Lilienfeld, and Garb's (2003) *What's Wrong With the Rorschach?*, writes in this regard that "this is a tricky and crafty book that unfortunately sullies the scientific credibility of its authors" (p. 346):

Attorney: But in fairness, Doctor, aren't Wood and these other authorities correct when they say that the Rorschach is not yet fully validated, and that it often comes up with a wrong answer? [Now the attorney is showing considerable sophistication. Like all other personality assessment instruments, the RIM is not "fully validated," and there are many Rorschach variables for which the behavioral correlates are imperfectly understood or not yet empirically confirmed. As for wrong answers, neither the RIM nor any other personality assessment instruments has a perfect hit rate in identifying any personal characteristic or condition, and examiners must regularly take account of sensitivity and specificity indices and likely percentages of false negative and false positive findings. However, expert witnesses are in the courtroom, not the classroom or laboratory. Consistent with appropriate courtroom procedures, they should answer this attorney question honestly, but in a way that supports their testimony].

Witness: The Rorschach method generally shows the same level of validity as the MMPI, which is as good as can be expected for this kind of measure, and it is valid for the purposes for which I used it. As for being wrong, the test is not perfect, but when used properly for its intended purposes, it is rarely wrong.

As for the popular media, forensic consultants may be confronted in court with newspapers or magazine articles that echo Rorschach critics in disparaging the soundness and utility of the instrument. Adequately prepared witnesses should have little difficulty fending off this type of learned treatise challenge, simply by pointing out that journalism, like advocacy, is not science. The recent history of disgraced columnists and inaccurate or misleading new reports, although representing a small percentage of journalistic output, gives ample reason to take with a grain of salt popular media opinion presented in the guise of empirically supported fact.

Finally of note, forensic assessors will rarely be challenged to defend Rorschach assessment when giving testimony in a deposition. Psychologically informed attorneys may test out examiners a bit to see if they are conversant with the literature, as by asking, for example, "What books did you consult to help you interpret your Rorschach and write up your report?" or "Can you give me the names of some journals that publish articles on these inkblots?" They may even ask such apparently innocent questions as "Is the Rorschach a dependable test?" and then listen politely to the answer, perhaps even shaking their head in agreement. This type of question is intended to probe the expert witness' self-assurance and readiness to expound on the foundations of Rorschach assessment, not to obtain substantive information. The best answer to whether the Rorschach is a dependable test is a simple "Yes," assuming of course that the witness is adequately prepared to elaborate on the soundness and utility of the instrument if asked to do so. However, attorneys who are planning to challenge the relevance, reliability, or validity of Rorschach findings will ordinarily save this challenge for the courtroom. Raising such challenges in a deposition alerts experts to what they can expect during cross-examination in the courtroom and gives them an opportunity to prepare their responses. On the other hand, Rorschach examiners who are lulled into a false sense of security by attorneys who let them sail through a deposition without being challenged about their methods may be caught off guard when they are confronted in the courtroom with well-prepared and seemingly well-documented criticisms of Rorschach assessment that they did not anticipate and are not adequately prepared to refute.

CONCLUSIONS

Psychologists who use the Rorschach Inkblot Method (RIM) in their forensic evaluations must become skillful in presenting and defending Rorschach testimony in the courtroom. To help expert witnesses explain Rorschach assessment, this chapter provides a simple and easily understood description of how and why the instrument yields dependable information about personality characteristics. Five tactics are then recommended for enhancing the effectiveness of Rorschach-based testimony and reducing a forensic consultant's vulnerability to damaging or embarrassing cross-examination: (a) favoring structural over thematic data as the basis for inferences; (b) emphasizing summary scores rather than individual responses in formulating conclusions; (c) framing statements aptly in idiographic or nomothetic terms; (d) expressing views with appropriate levels of certainty; and (e) by managing computer-based test reports advisedly.

In defending Rorschach testimony in the courtroom, expert witnesses who are adequately informed and experienced and who formulate their statements along the lines recommended in this chapter should have little difficulty responding to cross-examination concerning their credentials or their conclusions. Nevertheless, aspersions on the value and propriety of Rorschach assessment, buttressed by harsh negative criticism of the instrument quoted from the professional and popular literature, can present the expert witness with a demanding challenge. Steadfastness, self-confidence, and familiarity with the extensive research findings documenting the soundness and utility of Rorschach assessment will assist adequately prepared witnesses in meeting this challenge effectively.

REFERENCES

Babitsky, S., & Mangraviti, J. J. (1999). *How to excel during depositions: Techniques for experts that work.* Falmouth, MA: Seak Inc.

Blau, T. H. (1998). *The psychologist as expert witness* (2nd ed.). New York: Wiley.

Beutler, L. E., & Groth-Marnat, G. (2003). *Integrative assessment of adult personality* (2nd ed.). New York: Guilford.

Brodsky, S. L. (1991). *Testifying in court.* Washington, DC: American Psychological Association.

Brodsky, S. L. (2004). *Coping with cross-examination and other pathways to effective testimony.* Washington, DC: American Psychological Association.

Craig, R. J. (2005). *Personality-guided forensic psychology.* Washington, DC: American Psychological Association.

Daubert v. Merrell Dow Pharmaceuticals, Inc., 509 U.S., 113 S. Ct. 2786 (1993).

Exner, J. E., Jr. (1969). *The Rorschach systems.* New York: Grune & Stratton.

Exner, J. E., Jr. (2003). *The Rorschach: A comprehensive system: Vol. 1. Basic foundations and principles of interpretation* (4th ed.). Hoboken, NJ: Wiley.

Exner, J. E., Jr., & Erdberg, P. (2005). *The Rorschach: A Comprehensive System: Vol. 2. Advanced interpretation* (3rd ed.). Hoboken, NJ: Wiley.

Exner, J. E., Jr., & Weiner, I. B. (2003). *Rorschach interpretation assistance program* (RIAP5). Lutz, FL: Psychological Assessment Resource.

Gacono, C., & Meloy, J. R. (1994). *The Rorschach assessment of aggressive and psychopathic personalities.* Hillsdale, NJ: Lawrence Erlbaum Associates.

Garb, H. N. (1999). Call for a moratorium on the use of the Rorschach Inkblot Test in clinical and forensic settings. *Assessment, 6,* 313–315.

General Electric C. v. Joiner, 526 U.S. 137 (1997).

Goldstein, A. M. (Ed.). (2003). *Forensic psychology.* In I. B. Weiner (Ed. in Chief), *Handbook of psychology* (Vol. 11). Hoboken, NJ: Wiley.

Goldstein, A. M. (Ed.). (2007). *Forensic psychology: Emerging topics and expanding roles.* Hoboken, NJ: Wiley.

Groth-Marnat, G., & Horvath, L. S. (2006). The psychological report: A review of current controversies. *Journal of Clinical Psychology, 62,* 73–82.

Harvey, V. S. (1997). Improving readability of psychological reports. *Professional Psychology: Research and Practice, 28,* 271–274.

Heilbrun, K. (2001). *Principles of forensic mental health assessment.* New York: Kluwer Academic/Plenum.

Hibbard, S. (203). A critique of Lilienfeld et al.'s (2000) "The scientific status of projective techniques." *Journal of Personality Assessment, 80,* 260–271.

Hilsenroth, M. J., & Stricker, G. (2004). A consideration of challenges to psychological assessment instruments used in forensic settings: Rorschach as exemplar. *Journal of Personality Assessment, 83,* 141–152.

Jensen, A. R. (1965). Review of the Rorschach Inkblot Test. In O. K. Buros (Ed.), *The sixth mental measurements yearbook* (pp. 501–509). Highland Park, NJ: Gryphon Press.

Kumho Tire Company, Ltd., v. Carmichael, 526 U.S. 137 (1999).

Lerner, P. M. (1998). *Psychoanalytic perspectives on the Rorschach.* Hillsdale, NJ: The Analytic Press.

Mattlar, C.-E. (2004). The Rorschach Comprehensive System is reliable, valid, and cost-effective. *Rorschachiana, 26,* 147–157.

Mattlar, C.-E. (2005). The utility of the Rorschach Comprehensive System: An increasing body of supportive research. *South African Rorschach Journal, 2,* 3–31.

Meloy, J. R. (2005). Some reflections on *What's wrong with the Rorschach? Journal of Personality Assessment, 85,* 344–346.

Melton, G. B., Petrila, J. R., Poythress, N. G., & Slobogin, C. (1997). *Psychological evaluations for the courts* (2nd ed.). New York: Guilford.

Meyer, G. J. (2001). Evidence to correct misperceptions about Rorschach norms. *Clinical Psychology: Science and Practice, 8,* 389–396.

Meyer, G. J. (2004). The reliability and validity of the Rorschach and Thematic Apperception Test (TAT) compared to other psychological and medical procedures: An analysis of systematically gathered evidence. In M. J. Hilsenroth & D. L. Segal (Eds.), *Personality assessment* (pp. 315–342). Hoboken, NJ: Wiley.

Meyer, G. J., & Archer, R. (2001). The hard science of Rorschach research: What do we know and where do we go? *Psychological Assessment, 13,* 486–502.

Poythress, N. G. (1980). Coping on the witness stand: Learned responses to "learned treatises." *Professional Psychology, 11,* 139–149.

Sales, B. D., & Shuman, D. W. (2004). *Experts in court: Reconciling law, science, and professional knowledge.* Washington, DC: American Psychological Association.

Schafer, R. (1954). *Psychoanalytic interpretation in Rorschach testing.* New York: Grune & Stratton.

Society for Personality Assessment. (2005). The status of the Rorschach in clinical and forensic practice: An official statement by the Board of Trustees of the Society for Personality Assessment. *Journal of Personality Assessment, 85,* 219–237.

Viglione, D. J., & Hilsenroth, M. J. (2001). The Rorschach: Facts, fictions, and future. *Psychological Assessment, 13,* 452–471.

Weiner, I. B. (2001). Advancing the science of psychological assessment: The Rorschach Inkblot Method as exemplar. *Psychological Assessment, 13,* 423–432.

Weiner, I. B. (2003a). Prediction and postdiction in clinical decision making. *Clinical Psychology: Science and Practice, 10,* 335–338.

Weiner, I. B. (2003b). *Principles of Rorschach interpretation* (2nd ed.). Mahwah, NJ: Lawrence Erlbaum Associates.

Weiner, I. B. (2004a). Rorschach assessment: Current status. In M J. Hilsenroth & D. L. Segal (Eds.), *Personality assessment* (Vol. 2, pp. 343–355). In M. Hersen (Editor-in-Chief), *Comprehensive handbook of psychological assessment.* Hoboken, NJ: Wiley.

Weiner, I. B. (2004b). *Rorschach interpretation assistance program: Forensic report (RIAP5 FE).* Lutz, FL: Psychological Assessment Resources.

Weiner, I. B. (2005). Integrative personality assessment with self-report and performance based measures. In S. Strack (Ed.), *Personology and psychopathology* (pp. 317–331). Hoboken, NJ: Wiley.

Weiner, I. B. (2006). Writing forensic reports. In I. B. Weiner & A. K. Hess (Eds.), *The handbook of forensic psychology* (3rd ed., pp. 631–651). Hoboken, NJ: Wiley.

Weiner, I. B., & Hess, A. K. (Eds.). (2006). *The handbook of forensic psychology* (3rd ed.). Hoboken, NJ: Wiley.

Wood, J. M., Nezworski, M. T., Lilienfeld, S. O., & Garb, H. N. (2003). *What's wrong with the Rorschach?* San Francisco: Jossey-Bass.

II

FORENSIC APPLICATIONS

7

THE USE OF THE RORSCHACH INKBLOT METHOD IN TRIAL COMPETENCY EVALUATIONS

B. Thomas Gray

North Texas State Hospital, Vernon, TX

Marvin W. Acklin

Private Practice, Honolulu, HI

Competency to stand trial (CST) evaluations are among the most commonly conducted forensic evaluations in the United States, annually affecting thousands of defendants and tens of thousands of hours of court and forensic assessment effort. Legal standards for evaluating trial competency are well established—most jurisdictions have adopted the U.S. Supreme Court *Dusky* standard—as the basis for determining whether defendants comprehend and are capable of effectively participating in their own defense.

A keystone of American jurisprudence is the premise that an accused individual must be competent to stand trial. The U.S. Supreme Court formally recognized the concept of competency to stand trial as early as 1899 in the case of *Youtsey v. U.S.*, when the court opined:

> It is fundamental that an insane person can neither plead to an arraignment, be subjected to a trial, or, after trial, receive judgment, or, after judgment, undergo punishment. ... If it appears after arraignment, and before trial, that the prisoner is probably not capable of making a rational defense, the proceedings should stop until the sanity of the prisoner is determined or restored. ... It is not "due process of law" to subject an insane person to trial upon an indictment involving liberty or life.

This decision asserted that defendants must be fully cognizant of their legal situation and the available legal options and capable of making reasoned choices among those options. Failing this represents a threat to the individuals' Sixth Amendment right to due process, which assumes defendants' ability to take full part in their own defense. Melton, Petrila, Poythress, and Slobogin (1997) cite two additional reasons underlying the critical importance of trial competency. First, trials will inevitably yield more accurate results when the defendant is productively engaged in the adversarial process; second, the process becomes undignified if carried on in the presence of a defendant who lacks ade-

---

Dr. Gray is currently at the Institute for Forensic Psychiatry at the Colorado Mental Health Institute at Pueblo.

quate understanding: "Even a proceeding that produces an accurate guilty verdict would be repugnant to our moral sense if the convicted individual were unaware of what was happening or why" (Melton et al., 1997, p. 121).

Questions of trial competency are among the most common forensic issues in which mental health professionals (MHPs) are asked to conduct assessments and offer opinions. CST evaluations are a mainstay in the practice of many forensic psychologists and psychiatrists (Hoge, Bonnie, Poythress, & Monahan, 1992; Steadman, Monahan, Hartstone, Davis, & Robbins, 1982). Because of the intertwining legal and clinical issues, MHPs must not only be knowledgeable of relevant legal standards, they must also be aware of the value and limitations of clinical and forensic instrumentation in developing valid and admissible information to the court.

This chapter reviews the legal foundations of trial competency, including legal standards, procedural strategies for assessment of competency to stand trial, and clinical and forensic tools for evaluating CST. The role and the value of the Rorschach test in CST evaluations are discussed in detail.

LEGAL STANDARDS FOR COMPETENCY TO STAND TRIAL[1]

English common law has recognized that a criminal defendant must be competent to ensure a fair and accurate trial since Frith's case in 1790 (Bardwell & Arrigo, 2002). This concept was tacitly acknowledged in the United States as early as 1835 when Richard Lawrence attempted to assassinate President Andrew Jackson. The court recognized Lawrence was seriously mentally ill and effectively refused to try him; he was placed in various facilities and spent the last several years of his life confined to Government Hospital for the Insane in Washington, DC.[2] Following the *Youtsey* decision, the courts reiterated the importance accorded of trial competence. For example, the Eighth District Court elucidated the issue in their jurisdiction by observing: "The court therefore must cause such an examination [of competency to stand trial] to be made in every case, where a motion is filed that cannot be declared to be without good faith or to be frivolous" *(Kenner v. U.S.,* 1960).

The issue of who may raise a question concerning competency was resolved with *Pate v. Robinson* (1966), when the Supreme Court ruled that any trial court must order a hearing *sua sponte* when any evidence is brought forth suggesting a defendant may be incompetent to stand trial (ICST), even if the issue is not raised by the defense. This finding was extended to include the prosecution's burden to raise the issue in *Drope v. Missouri* (1975).

Specific standards for competency to stand trial remained unarticulated until 1960 when the Supreme Court issued their opinion in *Dusky v. U.S* (1960). This opinion commented that "it is not enough for the district judge to find that 'the defendant is oriented to

---

[1]For a thorough consideration of case law pertaining to trial competency, see Frederick, DeMaier, & Tower (2004).

[2]The hospital was subsequently renamed St. Elizabeth's Hospital, the same facility where John Hinckley, the man who shot President Ronald Reagan in 1981, has been housed for more than 20 years.

time and place and has some recollection of events,'" and went on to define trial competency with this now-famous phrase: "The test must be whether he has sufficient present ability to consult with his lawyer with a reasonable degree of rational understanding and whether he has a rational as well as factual understanding of the proceedings against him" (*Dusky v. U.S.*, 1960). In *Cooper v. Oklahoma* (1966), the court established preponderance of the evidence as the standard of proof for demonstrating trial incompetency rather than the more rigorous clear and convincing evidence, the standard the state of Oklahoma had been using.

The *Dusky* formulation represents the basic standard for trial competency throughout the United States. Some jurisdictions have further elaborated the *Dusky* criteria, either legislatively or judicially. For example, in 1961 the Western District Court of Missouri outlined eight specific elements considered important to trial competency (*Wieter v. Settle*, 1961). A few states (notably Florida, Utah, and Texas) have included factors to be explicitly considered in evaluation of competency to stand trial (see Table 7–1). These factors make CST evaluations more straightforward because the defendant's functional psycholegal capacities are clearly specified.

Two points are important to note regarding these definitions. First, *trial competency* refers to the present functioning of the defendant. This is in direct contrast to mental state at the time of the offense (MSO) evaluations, which refer to the functioning of the individual *at the time of the offense* (Acklin, chap. 8, this vol.). These two issues, although often confused (note, e.g., reference to sanity in the quotation from the *Youtsey* case, cited earlier), are separate and distinct.

Second, the *Dusky* standards do not establish the threshold requirement that a defendant be suffering from a mental disorder. Although psychiatric problems, particularly psychotic disorders, are the most common barrier to competency, the *Dusky* standard refers only to the defendant's functional psycholegal capacities. Indeed, even before *Dusky*, the Supreme Court had effectively concluded that mental illness does not automatically indicate incompetency (*Higgins v. McGrath*, 1951). In other words, mental ill-

TABLE 7–1

Functional Abilities Related to Trial Competency in Three States' Statutes

Does the Defendant Have the Capacity to:	State		
	Texas	*Utah*	*Florida*
Appreciate the charges against him/her	✔	✔	✔
Appreciate the possible consequences s/he might face	✔	✔	✔
Disclose relevant information to an attorney	✔	✔	✔
Engage in a reasoned choice of legal strategies and options	✔	✔	
Appreciate the adversarial nature of the legal system	✔	✔	✔
Exhibit appropriate courtroom behavior	✔	✔	✔
Testify	✔	✔	✔

ness is not a sufficient criterion for whether or not an individual is competent to stand trial. A mentally ill individual can be competent to stand trial and an incompetent individual is not necessarily mentally ill (although usually that person is). Many state jurisdictions, however, have established the threshold condition of a mental disorder for an individual to be determined incompetent to stand trial (e.g., Hawaii).

FORENSIC EVALUATION OF COMPETENCY TO STAND TRIAL

Historical Background

Through the first decades of the 20th century, most defendants found incompetent to stand trial were sent to state psychiatric hospitals, where they were detained for extensive evaluation over lengthy, usually indeterminant periods (hence the famous 1972 Supreme Court decision in *Jackson v. Indiana*, 406 U.S. 715: "A person charged by a State ... who is committed solely on account of his incapacity to proceed to trial cannot be held more than a reasonable period of time necessary to determine whether there is a substantial probability that he will attain the capacity in the foreseeable future"). A routine part of the process was administration of a standard battery of psychological tests. With the movement toward deinstitutionalization that began in the 1970s, state hospital populations (and numbers of beds) were drastically reduced. In many locations, a model of community evaluation was adopted in which defendants were examined in jail or a clinician's private office (see Melton et al., 1997). Under this approach, the use of a battery of standard psychological tests was sometimes retained, although apparently less commonly than under the model of lengthy hospitalization.

In the 1980s, serious questions began to be raised concerning the quality of competency to stand trial evaluations that were being presented to attorneys and the courts (Grisso, 1988; Roesch & Golding, 1980). These issues were summarized in the first edition of the seminal work *Evaluating Competencies* (Grisso, 1986), where Grisso identified what have come to be known as his "five *I*'s": *Ignorance* of the legal process leads examiners to present *Irrelevant* psychological/psychiatric testimony, resulting in the *Intrusion* of psychological/psychiatric opinion into the legal arena. As a result, *Insufficient* evidence is often used to support the conclusions offered, and thus, evaluations are often seen as lacking *In credibility*.

Various jurisdictions have adopted legislative or judicial measures in attempting to improve the quality of CST evaluations. For a number of years, for example, Massachusetts has required evaluators to complete didactic training and mentoring program before being allowed to independently conduct competency evaluations, a move that has apparently been reasonably successful in improving the quality of work that has been done (Packer & Leavitt, 1998). A recent Texas statute pertaining to CST evaluations included two measures intended to achieve this goal: first, six factors to be considered in making a determination regarding trial competence were specifically identified that must be contained in reports (see Table 7–1); and second, the state mandated training requirements for forensic evaluators. Despite these legislative mandates, the level of adherence and quality in some situations remains dismally low (Gray, Black, Fulford, & Owen, 2005; Skeem & Golding, 1998). In a highly instructive study, Skeem and Golding (1998) surveyed forensic reports submitted by community examiners highlighting the weaknesses, limitations, and errors commonly encountered in community-based competency to stand trial evaluations. They make specific recommendations for improving the quality of forensic reports.

Conceptual and Procedural Approaches to Assessing Competency to Stand Trial

When evaluating competency to stand trial, forensic clinicians benefit from legal knowledge, conceptual tools, and a procedural framework. First, forensic clinicians must be aware of the statutory criteria for competency to stand trial in their jurisdiction. Second, the work of University of Virginia law professor Richard Bonnie and his colleagues (Bonnie, 1992; Poythress et al., 1999) provides valuable conceptual tools for assessing competency to stand trial.[3] The basic understanding that one is a defendant in a legal proceeding or has rudimentary knowledge of judicial terms is insufficient to establish competency to stand trial. Bonnie refers to this rudimentary level of comprehension as *minimal* competence. In contrast, in order to meet the *Dusky* standards criterion for factual as well as rational understanding, Bonnie asserts that *decisional* competence is also required, namely, the ability to distinguish between various legal alternatives and make reasoned choices. Awareness of the factors associated with judicial knowledge and underlying cognitive and clinical issues sets the framework for forensic psychological evaluation and permits a more descriptive assessment of the defendant's functional skills and deficits. It should be reiterated that competency to stand trial is not based on the individual's legal knowledge, but the *capacity* and *present ability* to rationally and factually understand their legal situation and assist in their defense (Melton et al., 1997, quoting *Dusky*). In *Godinez v. Moran* (1993), the U.S. Supreme Court rules that a defendant who is found competent to stand trial is also competent to waive any other constitutional rights, such as the right to counsel or to plead to a charge.

Grisso (1986, 1988, 2003) has been highly influential in promoting a conceptual and procedural framework for the evaluation of both civil and criminal competencies. Originally applied to competency to stand trial evaluations, Grisso has since extended the model to encompass a variety of other civil competencies (e.g., Grisso, 2003; Grisso & Appelbaum, 1998).

Grisso (2003) identified five specific domains for assessing competence in general:

1. *Functional*: the particular abilities or knowledge that the individual should have with respect to the specific competency in question. The original version of this model (Grisso, 1986) included a sixth component, Contextual, which was more recently subsumed into the Functional component (Grisso, 2003). From an evaluative perspective, this represents "what the individual can do or accomplish, as well as to the knowledge, understanding, or beliefs that may be necessary for the accomplishment" (Grisso, 2003, pp. 23–24). It is important to emphasize that this component can be related to, but is nonetheless distinct from, psychiatric diagnosis, level of intellectual functioning, personality traits, and other areas that are the target of standard psychological assessment.

---

[3]The prosecutor in one well-known case involving a seriously disturbed individual is reported to have stated, "somebody described competent once as 'knowing the difference between a grapefruit and a judge'" (Ewing & McCann, 2006, p. 195), thus indicating the rather low threshold for competency in many jurisdictions.

The relevant aspects of an individual's functioning vary according to the psycholegal question posed by the specific legal context.

2. *Causal*: the underlying causes for any functional abilities/deficits as identified in the Functional Component. A primary issue is identification of the factors that are causing deficits in functional capabilities.

3. *Interactive*: the person's level of functional ability in relation to the demands of the specific psycholegal situation involved. An oft-cited example of this is *Wilson v. U.S.* (1968) in which the Supreme Court ruled that a defendant's amnesia may not be sufficient to warrant a finding of ICST (see Melton et al., 1997, for a detailed discussion of this case).

4. The final two domains in Grisso's model are *Judgmental* and *Dispositional*. The former refers to the determination of whether the incongruence between person/context is sufficient to warrant a finding of ICST, and the latter to the consequences of a CST/ICST finding. Grisso (2003) contended that these domains are properly the purview of the court, not MHPs, and that MHPs should not offer an opinion on the ultimate issue, a controversial view that is shared by other authorities (e.g., Heilbrun, 2001; Melton, et al., 1997). Buchanan offers an insightful discussion of the history and controversy associated with ultimate opinion testimony, especially as it evolved in the Federal Rule of Evidence (Buchanan, 2006). In some jurisdictions, however, such as Texas, Colorado, and Hawaii, the statutes mandate that an opinion be offered.

In summary, Grisso's competency evaluation model establishes a firm conceptual and procedural structure for the conduct of competency to stand trial evaluations, including application of psychological data to relevant legal standards and clarification of the functional deficits and their underlying causes in relation to the particular legal issues.

As already noted, for many years it was common practice to include a battery of psychological tests during evaluation of trial competency. Over time, however, an increasing number of jurisdictions began to rely more on a model under which community-based MHPs were conducting CST assessments. Almost simultaneously, awareness increased among academic psychologists and MHPs that the instruments used in routine psychological evaluation were not adequate for such purposes because they were not designed to address essential psycholegal questions (e.g., Heilbrun, 1992; Lanyon, 1986). As forensic psychology has evolved and matured, Grisso (2003) and others (Otto & Heilbrun, 2002) have drawn distinctions between *forensic assessment instruments*, *forensically relevant instruments*, and *clinical measures and assessment techniques*. Intelligence scales, the Rorschach test, and other standard psychological tests fall into the latter category, the use of which requires the formulation of inferences between clinical assessment data and relevant legal constructs. Within Grisso's model of forensic psychological evaluation (2003), standard clinical measures make their strongest contribution in describing the functional abilities and weaknesses of the defendant.

Borum and Grisso (1995) surveyed board certified psychiatrists and psychologists in the early 1990s and found that approximately half used psychological testing at least some of the time. Predictably, psychiatrists made use of tests less often than psychologists. Most psychologists reported using tests at least some of the time. Personality inventories and intellectual testing were most commonly employed. Less than 15% of the psychologists used projective tests more than "sometimes." Since the mid–1990s, a series of articles critical of projective techniques, the Rorschach test in particular, have appeared in the professional assessment literature, igniting a controversy that has continued to the present (Board of Trustees, 2005; Grove, Barden, Garb, & Lilienfeld, 2002; Weiner, 2005; Wood, Nezworski, Garb, & Lilienfeld, 2006; Wood, Nezworski, Stejskal, & McKinzey, 2001). Perhaps reflecting the adverse impact of this controversy, Lally's (2003) survey of psychologists who had earned diplomate status with the American Board of Forensic Psychology indicated that over half (53%) considered the Rorschach test "unacceptable" for use in CST evaluations. This study focused only on board certified practitioners, and thus sampled only a small proportion of the MHPs who conduct such evaluations. Use of standards psychological assessment appears to be rarely utilized in CST evaluations, no doubt due to a combination of reasons based on policy, pragmatics, and concerns over scientific controversy. Similar results have been found in surveys of practitioners who evaluate CST with juveniles (Ryba, Cooper, & Zapf, 2003) and those working in other countries as well (Martin, Allan, & Allan, 2001). The reasons for this development are complex and deserve further attention. It seems likely that the decline of use of the Rorschach test in forensic psychological evaluations is the result of the controversies and criticisms of the test, unfounded timidity of Rorschach clinicians in understanding the controversy or the vigorous response of the Rorschach scholarly community (see Weiner, 2005), and perhaps, restraints imposed by time and economic concerns. No competent assessment psychologist would, however, use the Rorschach test, or presumably any other clinical instrument, as a sole basis for determining competency to stand trial.

In contrast to clinical assessment instruments, which describe functional capacities (e.g., attention, concentration, memory, thought organization), a number of forensic assessment instruments have been developed specifically to aid in evaluation of CST. Beginning in the early 1970s with the Competence to Stand Trial Instrument and Competence Screening Test (Laboratory of Community Psychiatry, Harvard Medical School, 1973), there has been continuous development of CST measures. In fact, a rather large and informative literature has grown up around the procedural, conceptual, and empirical aspects of CST evaluations. Subsequent efforts included the Georgia Court Competence Test (Nicholson, Briggs, & Robertson, 1988), and a specialized test designed for mentally retarded defendants, the Competence Assessment for Standing Trial for Defendants with Mental Retardation (Everington & Luckasson, 1992).

Tests that have received recent attention include the Evaluation of Competency to Stand Trial–Revised (ECST–R; Rogers, Jackson, Sewell, Tillbrook, & Martin, 2003), the Mac-Arthur Competence Assessment Tool–Adjudicative Competence (MacCAT– CA) (Poythress et al., 1999; Poythress, Bonnie, Monahan, Otto, & Hoge, 2002), and the Fitness Interview Test–Revised (FIT–R; Roesch, Zapf, Eaves, & Webster, 1998). Each of these instruments has a somewhat different orientation. Most of the earlier tests, for example, tend to focus primarily on issues relating to factual or minimal competency, providing little information concerning the individuals' rational understanding of their legal situation or ability to work with an attorney. The MacCAT–CA is based on Bonnie's (1992) previously mentioned model of adjudicative competence, which places substantial emphasis on "decisional competence," that is, the ability to make well-reasoned legal decisions. The

FIT–R was developed primarily with Canadian competency standards in mind, although there are many parallels to American-developed instruments. It has been amply demonstrated that most instruments specific to CST are susceptible to malingering (Rogers, Sewell, Grandjean, & Vitacco, 2002). Rogers's ECST–R, as an answer to previously developed measures, addresses both factual and decisional issues, and includes a series of scales designed to identify individuals who are malingering incompetence (Rogers, Jackson, Sewell, & Harrison, 2004).

The ECST–R uses an easel administered, structured interview format to assess the *Dusky* prongs: Consult with Counsel ("What do you expect your attorney to do for you?"), Factual Understanding of the Courtroom Proceedings ("Who is responsible for prosecuting the case?"), and Rational Understanding ("Putting aside the best and worst outcomes, what is the most likely outcome in your trial?"; Rogers, Tillbrook, & Sewell, 2004). The scale also permits assessment of Atypical Responding "by systematically screening a defendant for possible feigning" (Rogers, Tillbrook, & Sewell, 2004, p. 28). The issue of feigning or malingering on commonly used measures of competency has been well demonstrated (Rogers, Sewell, Grandjean, & Vitacco, 2002). Rogers and his colleagues have specifically assessed the vulnerability of the ECST–R to feigning or malingering (Rogers, Jackson, Sewell, & Harrison, 2004). ECST–R raw scores are transformed to standard scores based on a normative sample of competency referral and jail detainees.

The MacArthur Competence Assessment Tool–Criminal Adjudication (MacCAT–CA; Poythress et al., 1999) is the product of two major research initiatives sponsored by the MacArthur Foundation Research Network on Mental Health and the Law. The 22-item scale measures three competence-related abilities derived from the *Dusky* standard: Understanding, Reasoning, and Appreciation. In contrast to other competency assessment tools, the MacCAT–CA uses vignettes ("Fred and Reggie are playing pool in a bar and get into a fight") to illustrate factual and legal situations requiring more open-ended responses from the defendant, as well as items that assess the defendants' capacity to appreciate their own legal situation and circumstances ("We have talked a lot about Fred's case. I would like to ask you some questions about your situation."). The vignette-based semistructured interview format has the advantage of demonstrating the defendant's cognitive, language, and reasoning processes. The scale is normed on a sample of 729 defendants from three defendant groups: unscreened jail inmates, jail inmates receiving mental health services, and hospitalized incompetent defendants. The scoring summary permits normative interpretations of scores on the following scale: Minimal/no impairment, mild impairment, and clinically significant impairment. Clearly, the MacCAT–CA is a highly sophisticated tool in terms of its development and assessment of competency constructs.

The FIT–R is an interview-based rating scale using Canadian standards for fitness to stand trial (Roesch, Zapf, Eaves, & Webster, 1998) assessing Factual Knowledge of Criminal Procedure ("What happens in court to someone who pleads not guilty?"), Appreciation of Personal Involvement in and Importance of the Proceedings ("What do you think your lawyer should concentrate on in order to defend you best?"), and Ability to Participate in Defence ("Tell me how you got arrested."), with three levels of rated impairment (none, possible/mild, and definite serious). Although the FIT–R has been empirically developed, the range and quality of the reliability and validity foundations do not yet appear to measure up to either the ECST–R or MacCAT–CA.

Despite efforts to establish an empirical basis for inference and admissibility, forensic assessment instruments developed for evaluation of CST do not appear to be widely employed (Borum & Grisso, 1995; Lally, 2003). The normative assessment procedure continues to be interview data alone, without use of any sort of psychometrically validated instrument. In many cases, use of a structured or semistructured interview may yield acceptable results (see, e.g., Rogers, 2001), so long as the relevant conceptual issues are addressed (Grisso, 2003). However, in many other situations, including situations where a mental disease, disorder, or defect is the threshold basis for trial incompetence, and where psychometrically sound inferences concerning a defendant's functional deficits are needed, additional data is required that can only be provided by clinical measures such as intelligence scales, neuropsychological screening, and personality testing. The Rorschach test offers a unique contribution at this stage of the competency assessment process.

UTILITY OF THE RORSCHACH TEST IN CST ASSESSMENT

Given the likelihood that the forensic clinician may testify in court on the issue of a defendant's current mental state (competency), some consideration of admissibility issues should be kept in mind. Depending on the jurisdiction, the court may rely on either *Frye* (1923) and *Daubert* (1993) tests, and/or Federal Rules of Evidence (2004) for admissibility. As noted earlier, the most common causes for the determination of incompetency to stand trial are psychotic disorders and mental deficiency. Fortunately, the Rorschach assessment of psychotic disorders rests on a robust behavioral science foundation (Acklin, 1999; chap. 8, this vol.). As already noted, in contrast to mental state at the time of the offense evaluations (MSO), CST evaluations are concerned about functional abilities and deficits at the time of the evaluation. There are a number of situations in which the Rorschach test is potentially valuable and may even be the only instrument that can adequately elucidate requisite information, particularly information concerning thought organization and pathology and malingering.

The Rorschach test takes its proper place in a psychological assessment methodology using multiple sources of information: self report, cross-informant and clinician observation, cognitive/neuropsychological performance measures, self-report personality tests, and performance measures (Acklin, Li, & Tyson, 2006). Gacono and Evans note that "the Rorschach provides an open structured, performance based cognitive perceptual problem solving task that is quite different from more closed structured instruments" (Gacono & Evans, preface, this vol.). The Rorschach test is of particular value in relation to the problems with self-report where individuals may feign, exaggerate, or malinger psychopathology (Ganellen, 1994, 1996; Ganellen, Wasyliw, Haywood, & Grossman, 1996; Grossman, Wasyliw, , Benn, & Gyoerkoe, 2002; Gacono, Evans, & Viglione, 2002). Increasingly, research has focused on obtaining base rate data on a variety of relevant forensic groups, making the Rorschach more valuable as a forensic assessment tool. Despite criticisms from established method critics, surveys continue to support the appropriate forensic use of the Rorschach test (Acklin, chap. 8, this vol.; Meloy, Hansen, & Weiner, 1997; Weiner, 2005).

It has been noted that a large majority of individuals who are found ICST are diagnosed with some sort of psychotic disorder (Roesch & Golding, 1980; Viljoen, Roesch, & Zapf, 2002; Viljoen, Zapf, & Roesch, 2003), with the resultant clinical impairment contributing substantially to an inability to meet one or more of the functional requirements of trial competency. The Rorschach test has been shown to be particularly helpful in identifying psychotic illness, a point that is sometimes even conceded by the test's harshest critics. Acklin (1992, 1999, chap. 8, this vol.) provides comprehensive coverage of factors associated with psychosis in the clinical and forensic application of Rorschach data. The Thought Disorder Index (TDI), in particular (Johnston & Holzman, 1979), has been especially useful for such purposes (see Holtzman, Levy, & Johnston, 2005; also Acklin chap. 8, this vol.). This was well illustrated by the case of a man in his mid-thirties who was facing two counts of capital murder, and who by virtue of his family/cultural background, considered mental illness to be an indication of a lack of religious faith. He was therefore incensed at the thought that he would be considered ICST. Although he was reluctant to participate in formal evaluation ("I have no need for this, my way his His way ..."), he produced an interpretable Rorschach that included important elevations on *WSum6* and *TDI*. This confirmed the opinion that he did indeed have a psychotic illness, and highlighted the disturbed thinking that interfered with the requisite functional abilities involved in trial competency. It should be recalled not all psychotic individuals are necessarily ICST. Indeed, we often see people who remain manifestly ill, yet meet the basic requirements to be considered CST.[3] Such individuals may, for example, manifest delusional/psychotic thinking that is sufficiently circumscribed to allow them adequate functioning to make reasoned choices within the legal arena.

The Rorschach test has unique utility to assist in clarifying functional abilities and deficits with relevance to trial competency. As observed by Skeem and Golding (1998), clinicians may provide an opinion concerning a defendant's diagnosis or competency to stand trial without describing the reasoning underlying their opinion, that is, failing to link functional deficits and causal components of Grisso's assessment model (2003). Rorschach test data offers the potential of helping to fill in this missing element by assisting in establishing the functional deficits that result from mental health issues, in turn allowing the clinician to more effectively document what is causing the defendant to be ICST. For example, we know of cases in which the person presents with obvious symptoms of psychosis and has been diagnosed with Schizophrenia, yet the Rorschach test has demonstrated a substantial affective component to the illness. In such cases, not only was a more accurate diagnosis clarified and more effective treatment made possible, but the functional deficits causing the person to be ICST were more clearly elucidated. A Rorschach assessment of personality also aids the examiner in providing information concerning problematic courtroom behavior, and/or in formulating recommendations for maintaining trial competency once it has been achieved (including elucidating the potential impact of continued incarceration on the individual's mental stability).

Gacono and Evans (preface, this vol.) provide a useful assessment scenario that demonstrates the Rorschach Inkblot Method's (RIM) role in ICST evaluations. In the case of an identified psychopath (PCL–R $\geq$ 30) suspected of malingering Schizophrenia, the evaluation of competency to stand trial would be aided by a strategy that incorporates the Rorschach, the Structured Interview of Reported Symptoms (SIRS), the PCL–R, and collateral data. Whereas the assessment of malingering may necessitate administration of the SIRS (Rogers, Bagy, & Dickens, 1992), an observation of ward behavior, the assessment of thought disorder (with the Rorschach), and an evaluation of psychopathy level would add weight to the examiner's conclusions. First, the context of the evaluation suggests potentially high motivation for feigning a mental illness. Second, ward observations might reveal inconsistencies in the patient's presentation, such as interacting in a normal manner when he doesn't realize staff is observing him. Third, Rorschach indices of disturbed thinking, perception, and reality testing may be inconsistent with psychosis, but consistent with character disordered or nonpatient samples. Finally, the elevated PCL–R total score along with a substantiated history of lying, conning, and manipulation (scores of 2 on PCL items 4 & 5) adds additional data to the hypothesis that the patient may be malingering. Knowledge of the Rorschach malingering literature is, of course, essential in assessing the validity of feigned, exaggerated, and malingered psychosis (Netter & Viglione, 1994). Thus, in a multisource assessment database, the Rorschach test provides unique and invaluable information describing functional clinical and forensic deficits.

Finally, in cases where functional deficits are clearly present, for example, in documenting clinical psychosis that interferes with reasoning, the Rorschach test can be utilized in re-testing after treatment or restoration efforts have been initiated. Such data are also of value in determinations of the proper level of disposition and management (Jumes, Oropeza, Gray, & Gacono, 2002; Weiner, 2004, 2005).

CONCLUSIONS

It is a foundational element of American jurisprudence that a criminal defendant be competent to stand trial. This is supported by hundreds of years of common law, an abundance of case law, as well as legislative efforts to define and clarify the psycholegal issues involved. Various legislative, judicial, and scholarly initiatives have encouraged careful and comprehensive evaluation when the question is raised. Unfortunately, however, MHPs have not always lived up to the challenge posed by the judicial system in applying empirically developed psychological/psychiatric evidence pertaining to the CST issue (e.g., Nicholson & Norwood, 2000; Skeem & Golding, 1998).

For many years, it was standard practice to administer batteries of psychological tests, often including a Rorschach test, to individuals who were hospitalized for extensive evaluation after being found incompetent to stand trial. This is no longer the most common approach, however, in large part because of social policy and institutional changes in the management of criminal defendants (i.e., a shift from hospital-based to community-based evaluation in many jurisdictions) and a more refined and delimited understanding of the strengths and weaknesses of psychological tests, including their direct relevance to legal statutes. As forensic psychological assessment has matured as a discipline, forensic assessment instruments have been developed for the specific purpose of evaluating competency to stand trial. A burgeoning empirical literature provides guidance to forensic behavioral scientists and clinicians. Nevertheless, clinical instrumentation that effectively evaluates self-reported symptoms, cognitive skills and deficits, thought organization, and reality testing remain essential to the clinical and forensic task.

Psychological evaluation instruments, however, remain invaluable in articulating the functional abilities and deficits that underlie trial competency or other criminal competencies, particularly when linked to forensic assessment instruments. The Rorschach test is of particular value where issues related to the defendant's reality testing, thought organization, and reasoning are of interest. The Rorschach test remains the premier instrument for detection and elucidation of the nature of psychotic processes (Acklin, 1992, 1999, chap. 8, this vol.). In addition, malingering of mental illness is not uncommon in populations where questions of competency to stand trial are raised, and standardized tests, including the Rorschach test, can be quite helpful in uncovering cases of feigned symptoms or inconsistent effort. Rorschach clinicians must not only be knowledgeable of relevant legal standards in their jurisdiction, but they must also have a sophisticated understanding of the technical utility and limitations of their instruments.

Consistent with feedback from jurists and attorneys as well as community surveys (Skeem & Golding, 1998), the most common criticism of CST evaluations has focused on the failure to explain how observed deficits (e.g., symptoms of serious mental illness) cause the individual to be ICST. This is precisely where clinical assessment tools, including the Rorschach test, are of greatest potential value, in that clinical assessment tools specifically address the functional and causal domains of Grisso's competency evaluation model. Grisso summarizes the point thusly: "The causal component of legal competence constructs focuses on explanations for an individual's apparent deficits in relevant functional abilities, in order to assure that the consequences of a finding of incompetence are not misapplied" (Grisso, 2003, p. 30).

Despite criticisms and controversy, clinical assessment measures, including the Rorschach test, remain the most valuable tools in the forensic clinician's armamentarium, particularly with respect to issues of methodological rigor, scientific certainty, and admissibility in court (whether *Frye* or *Daubert*). The clinical and behavioral science of psychological evaluation in general is the foundation of empirically-based and validated efforts to assess human skills and deficits, particularly when vulnerable individuals find themselves in legal jeopardy.

REFERENCES

Acklin, M. W., Li, S., & Tyson, J. (2006). Rorschach assessment of personality disorders: Applied clinical science and psychoanalytic theory. In S. Huprich (Ed.), *Rorschach assessment of personality disorders* (pp. 423–444). Mahwah, NJ: Lawrence Erlbaum Associates.

Acklin, M. W. (1992). Psychodiagnosis of personality structure: Psychotic personality organization. *Journal of Personality Assessment, 58*(3), 454–463.

Acklin, M. W. (1999). Behavioral science foundations of the Rorschach test: Research and clinical applications. *Assessment, 6*(4), 319–326.

Acklin, M. W., Li, S., & Tyson, J. (2006). Rorschach assessment of personality disorders: Applied clinical science and psychoanalytic theory. In S. Huprich (Ed.). *Rorschach assessment of personality disorders*. Mahwah, NJ: Lawrence Erlbaum Associates.

Bardwell, M., & Arrigo, B. (2002). Competency to stand trial: A law, psychology, and policy assessment. *Journal of Psychiatry & Law, 30*, 147–269.

Board of Trustees of the Society for Personality Assessment. (2005). The status of the Rorschach in clinical and forensic practice: An official statement by the Board of Trustees of the Society for Personality Assessment. *Journal of Personality Assessment, 85*, 219–237.

Bonnie, R. (1992). The competence of criminal defendants: A theoretical reformulation. *Behavioral Sciences and the Law, 10*, 291–316.

Borum, R., & Grisso, T. (1995). Psychological test use in criminal forensic evaluations. *Professional Psychology: Research and Practice, 26*, 465–473.

Buchanan, A. (2006). Psychiatric evidence on the ultimate issue. *Journal of the American Academy of Psychiatry and the Law, 34*(1), 14–21.

Committee on the Judiciary, U.S. House of Representatives. (2004). *Federal rules of evidence*. Washington, DC: U.S. Government Printing Office.

Cooper vs. Oklahoma, 517 U.S. 348 (1996).

Daubert v. Merrill Dow Pharmaceuticals, Inc., 509 U.S. 579 (1993).

Drope v. Missouri, 420 U.S. 162 (1975).

Dusky v. U.S., 362 U.S. 402 (1960).

Everington, C., & Luckasson, R. (1992). *Competence Assessment for Standing Trial for Defendants with Mental Retardation: Test manual*. Worthington, OH: IDS Publishing.

Ewing, C. P., & McCann, J. T. (2006). *Minds on trial: Great cases in law and psychology*. New York: Oxford University Press.

Frederick, R. I., DeMier, R. L., & Towers, K. (2004). *Examinations of competency to stand trial: Foundations in mental health case law*. Sarasota, FL: Professional Resource Press.

Frye v. U.S., 293 F 1013 (D.C. Cir., 1923).

Gacono, C., Evans, B., & Viglione, D. (2002). The Rorschach in forensic practice. *Journal of Forensic Psychological Practice, 2*(3), 33–52.

Ganellen, R. J. (1994). Attempting to conceal psychological disturbance: MMPI defensive response sets and the Rorschach. *Journal of Personality Assessment, 63*, 423–437.

Ganellen, R. J. (1996). Exploring MMPI–Rorschach relationships. *Journal of Personality Assessment, 67*, 529–542.

Ganellen, R. J., Wasyliw, O. E., Haywood, T. W., & Grossman, L. S. (1996). Can psychosis be malingered on the Rorschach: An empirical study. *Journal of Personality Assessment, 66*, 65–80.

Godinez v. Moran, 509, US 389 (1993).

Gray, B. T., Black, J. A., Fulford, L. K., & Owen, A. D. (2005). Evaluating trial competency evaluations: Impact of Article 46B. *Texas Psychologist, 56*(1), 18–23.

Grisso, T. (1986). *Evaluating competencies: Forensic assessments and instruments*. New York: Plenum.

Grisso, T. (1988). *Competence to stand trial evaluations: A manual for practice*. Sarasota, FL: Professional Resource Press.

Grisso, T. (2003). *Evaluating competencies: Forensic assessments and instruments* (2nd ed.). New York: Kluwer Academic.

Grisso, T., & Appelbaum, P. (1998). Assessing competence to consent to treatment: A guide for physicians and other health professionals. New York: Oxford University Press.

Grossman, L. S., Wasyliw, O. E., Benn, A. F., & Gyoerkoe, K. L. (2002). Can sex offenders who minimize on the MMPI conceal psychopathology on the Rorschach? *Journal of Personality Assessment, 78*, 484–501.

Grove, W. M., Barden, R. C., Garb, H. N., & Lilienfeld, S. O. (2002). Failure of Rorschach- comprehensive-system-based testimony to be admissible under the *Daubert–Joiner–Kumho* standard. *Psychology, Public Policy, and Law, 8*(2), 216–234.

Heilbrun, K. (1992). The role of psychological testing in forensic assessment. *Law and Human Behavior, 16*, 257–272.

Heilbrun, K. (2001). *Principles of forensic mental health assessment.* New York: Kluwer.

Higgins v. McGrath, 98 F. Supp. 670 (D. Mo. 1951).

Hoge, S. K., Bonnie, R. J., Poythress, N., & Monahan, J. (1992). Attorney–client decision-making in criminal cases: Client competence and participation as perceived by their attorneys. *Behavioral Sciences and the Law, 10*, 385–394.

Holzman, P. S., Levy, D. L., & Johnston, M. H. (2005). The use of the Rorschach technique for assessing formal thought disorder. In R. Bornstein & J. Masling (Eds.), *Scoring the Rorschach: Seven validated systems* (pp. 55–95). Mahwah, NJ: Lawrence Erlbaum Associates.

Jackson v. Indiana, 113 S. Ct. 1424 (1993).

Johnston, M. H., & Holzman, P. S. (1979). *Assessing schizophrenic thinking.* San Francisco: Jossey-Bass.

Jumes, M. T., Oropeza, P. P., Gray, B. T., & Gacono, C. B. (2002). Use of the Rorschach in forensic settings for treatment planning and monitoring. *International Journal of Offender and Comparative Criminology, 46*, 294–307.

Kenner v. United States, 286 F .2d 208 (8th Cir., 1960).

Laboratory of Community Psychiatry, Harvard Medical School. (1973). *Competence to stand trial and mental illness* (DHEW Pub. No. ADM 77–103). Rockville, MD: NIMH, Department of Health, Education, and Welfare).

Lally, S. J. (2003). What tests are acceptable for use in forensic evaluations? A survey of experts. *Professional Psychology: Research and Practice, 34*, 491–498.

Lanyon, R. I. (1986). Psychological assessment procedures in court-related settings. *Professional Psychology: Research and Practice, 17*, 260–268.

Martin, M. A., Allan, A., & Allan, M. M. (2001). The use of psychological tests by Australian psychologists who do assessments for the courts. *Australian Journal of Psychology, 53*(2), 77–82.

Melton, G., Petrila, J., Poythress, N., & Slobogin, C. (1997). *Psychological evaluations for the courts: A handbook for mental health professionals* (2nd ed.). New York: Guilford.

Meloy, J., Hansen, T., & Weiner, I. (1997). Authority of the Rorschach: Legal citations during the past 50 years. *Journal of Personality Assessment, 69*(1), 53–62.

Netter, B. E. C., & Viglione, D. J. (1994). An empirical study of malingering schizophrenia on the Rorschach. *Journal of Personality Assessment, 62*, 45–57.

Nicholson, R., Briggs, S., & Robertson, H. (1988). Instruments for assessing competence to stand trial: How do they work? *Professional Psychology: Research and Practice, 19*, 383–294.

Nicholson, R. A., & Norwood, S. (2000). The quality of forensic psychological assessments, reports, and testimony: Acknowledging the gap between promise and practice. *Law and Human Behavior, 24*, 9–44.

Otto, R., & Heilbrun K. (2002). The practice of forensic psychology: A look toward the future in light of the past. *American Psychologist, 57*, 5–18.

Packer, I. K., & Leavitt, M. (1998). *Designing and implementing a quality assurance process for forensic evaluations.* Paper presented at the biennial meeting of the American Psychology-Law Society.

Pate v. Robinson, 383 U.S. 375 (1966).

Poythress, N. G., Bonnie, R. J., Monahan, J., Otto, R., & Hoge, S. J. (2002). *Adjudicative competence: The MacArthur studies.* New York: Kluwer Academic.

Poythress, N., Nicholson, R., Otto, R., Edens, J., Bonnie, R., Monahan, J., & Hoge, S. (1999). *The MacArthur Competence Assessment Tool–Criminal Adjudication: Professional manual.* Odessa, FL: Psychological Assessment Resources.

Roesch, R., & Golding, S. L. (1980). *Competency to stand trial.* Urbana: University of Illinois Press.

Roesch, R., Zapf, P., Eaves, D., & Webster, C. (1998). *Fitness Interview Test* (rev. ed.). Burnaby, British Columbia, Canada: Mental Health, Law and Policy Institute, Simon Fraser Univ.

Rogers, R. (2001). *Handbook of diagnostic and structured interviewing.* New York: Guilford.

Rogers, R., Bagby, R. M., & Dickens, S. E. (1992). *Structured Interview of Reported Symptoms: Professional manual*. Odessa, FL: Psychological Assessment Resources.

Rogers, R., Jackson, R. L., Sewell, K. W., & Harrison, K. S. (2004). An examination of the ECST–R as a screen for feigned incompetency to stand trial. *Psychological Assessment, 16*(2), 139–145.

Rogers, R., Jackson, R. L., Sewell, K. W., Tillbrook, C. E., & Martin, M. A. (2003). Assessing dimensions of competency to stand trial: Construct validation of the ECST–R. *Assessment, 10*, 344–351.

Rogers, R., Sewell, K. W., Grandjean, N., & Vitacco, M. (2002). The detection of feigned mental disorders on specific competency measures. *Psychological Assessment, 14*(2), 177–183.

Rogers, R., Tillbrook, C. E., & Sewell, K. W. (2004). *ECST–R: Evaluation of Competency to Stand Trial–Revised. Professional manual*. Odessa, FL: Psychological Assessment Resources.

Ryba, N. L., Cooper, V. G., & Zapf, P. A. (2003). Juvenile competence to stand trial evaluations: A survey of current practices and test usage among psychologists. *Professional Psychology: Research and Practice, 34*, 499–507.

Skeem, J. L., & Golding, S. L. (1998). Community examiners' evaluations of competence to stand trial: Common problems and suggestions for improvement. *Professional Psychology: Research and Practice, 29*, 357–367.

Steadman, H., Monahan, J., Hartstone, E., Davis, S., & Robbins, P. (1982). Mentally disordered offenders: A national survey of patients and facilities. *Law and Human Behavior, 6*, 31–38.

Viljoen, J. L., Roesch, R., & Zapf, P. A. (2002). An examination of the relationship between competency to stand trial, competency to waive interrogation rights, and psychopathology. *Law and Human Behavior, 26*, 481–506.

Viljoen, J. L., Zapf, P. A., & Roesch, R. (2003). Diagnosis, current symptomatology, and the ability to stand trial. *Journal of Forensic Psychology Practice, 3*, 23–37.

Weiner, I. B. (2004). Monitoring psychotherapy with performance-based measures of personality functioning. *Journal of Personality Assessment, 83*(2), 323–331.

Weiner, I. B (2005, Spring). The utility of Rorschach assessment in clinical and forensic practice. *Independent Practitioner, 25*(2),76–83.

Weiner, I. B., Exner, J. E., & Sciara, T. (1996). Is the Rorschach welcome in the courtroom? *Journal of Personality Assessment, 67*, 422–424.

Wieter v. Settle, 193 F. Supp. 318 (W.D. Mo. 1961).

Wilson v. U.S., 391 F.2d 460 (D.C. Cir. 1968).

Wood, J. M., Nezworski, M.T., Stejskal, W.J, & McKinzey, R.K. (2001). Problems of the comprehensive system for the Rorschach in forensic settings: Recent developments. *Journal of Forensic Psychology Practice, 1*(3), 89–103.

Wood, J. M., Nezworski, M. T., Garb, H. N., & Lilienfeld, S. O. (2006, Spring). The controversy over Exner's Comprehensive System for the Rorschach: The critics speak. *Independent Practitioner*, 73–82.

Youtsey v. U.S., 97 F.937 (6th Cir. 1899).

8

THE RORSCHACH TEST AND FORENSIC PSYCHOLOGICAL EVALUATION: PSYCHOSIS AND THE INSANITY DEFENSE

Marvin W. Acklin
Private Practice, Honolulu, HI

No area of the legal system and mental health law is more controversial than the question of criminal responsibility and the insanity defense. Societies have wrestled with how to hold individuals responsible for actions who have committed crimes when they were "out of their mind." The commission of a criminal act, particularly a heinous crime that outrages the sensibilities of the community, generates demands for retribution. Nevertheless, legal systems since antiquity have made allowances for individuals who were "insane," by whatever definition was culturally relevant and current at the time. Because the majority of criminal defendants acquitted by reason of insanity are diagnosed as psychotic (Melton, Petrila, Poythress, & Slobogin, 1997), the chief focus here is on "psychosis." It needs to be emphasized that psychosis is not simply tantamount to insanity, as will be seen in the discussion of criteria for the insanity defense.

This chapter reviews fundamental legal constructs concerning criminal responsibility, describes psychosis as a clinical and forensically relevant phenomenon, reviews clinical and theoretical constructs relevant to understanding psychosis, reviews the utility of the Rorschach test in the assessment of psychotic mental states, and provides tactical and strategic issues in the forensic assessment of psychosis when the question of criminal responsibility is raised.

THE INSANITY DEFENSE

Historically, societies have developed a variety of "tests" for determining basic principles of rationality and moral responsibility. Criminal codes from the ancient Middle East, Greek and Roman antiquity, medieval Europe, pre-Norman England, and more recently, in Anglo-American law have defined the basic parameters of what constitutes sanity and definitional criteria for excusing individuals of criminal responsibility when their actions were manifestly irrational (Robinson, 1996).

Modern jurisprudence on the insanity defense can be traced at least as far back as a 1505 case, which recorded a jury verdict of insanity (Perlin, 1989, p. 285). Since that time, judicial systems have struggled to define and refine standards of criminal responsibility necessary to exculpate individuals from guilt in the commission of a criminal act when they were "not in their right mind." In the early 18th-century, English judges began attempting to define for juries mental conditions that would excuse, as a matter of law, otherwise criminal behavior (Perlin, 1989, p. 286). The most significant case in the history of the insanity defense in England (1843) arose out of the shooting by Daniel M'Naghten of Robert Drummond, the secretary of Prime Minister Robert Peel, M'Naghten's intended victim. Based on his delusion that he had been persecuted by Peel and the Tory party, the jury found M'Naghten not guilty by reason of insanity. The M'Naghten decision established the fundamental conceptual basis for most subsequent insanity defense formulations, including the necessity of a threshold "mental disease or defect," questions about the defendant's *knowledge* or *appreciation* of the "nature and quality of the act," and later, whether the individual was capable of fundamental self-control. Bonnie (1983) asserts the foundational moral basis of the insanity defense and the centrality of the cognitive/rational impairment: "It is fundamentally wrong to condemn and punish a person whose rational control over his or her behavior was impaired by the incapacitating effects of severe mental illness" (pp. 194–195).

Forensic mental health evaluations where there is a question of an insanity defense "require an investigation of the defendant's mental state at the time of the offense (MSO)—a reconstruction of the defendant's thought processes and behavior before and during the alleged crime (Giorgi, Guarnieri, Janotsky, et al., 2002; Melton et al., 1997, p. 186). The logic and process of forensic mental health evaluations has been definitively established by Grisso, where empirically developed mental health constructs and procedures are applied to legal standards (Grisso, 2003; Otto & Heilbrun 2002). Grisso distinguishes between *forensic assessment instruments*, *forensically relevant instruments*, and *clinical measures and assessment techniques* that assess psychopathology, intelligence, personality, and academic achievement, but require "the examiner to exercise a greater level of inference to move from the construct assessed to the issue before the court" (Otto & Heilbrun, 2002, p. 9; Otto, Edens, & Barcus, 2000). The Rorschach test and other psychological evaluation measures are useful in this context.

Understanding the insanity defense requires understanding criminal responsibility in relation to the associated notions of "just deserts" or "blame" for violations of society's laws:

> The Anglo-American legal system is grounded on the premise that persons are normally capable of free and rational choice between alternative acts and that one who chooses to harm another is thus morally accountable and liable to punishment. If, however, a person for any reason lacks the capacity to make rational choices or to conform his behavior to the moral and legal demands of society, traditionally he has been relieved of criminal responsibility and liability for his actions. (Brakel, Parry & Weiner, 1985, p. 707, cited in *Clark vs. Arizona,* amicus brief, p. 25)

Based on the fundamental notions that the law's objectives are retribution and deterrence, "a person lacking the required intelligence, reasoning ability and foresight capacity to understand the [criminal] code or its sanctions will not be deterred by them …" (Brakel, Parry, & Weiner, 1985, p. 707, cited in *Clark vs. Arizona*, amicus brief, p. 25).

The American Law Institute (ALI) Model Penal Code test—foundational in the United States and developed in the mid-1950s to avoid pitfalls of earlier tests until revision prompted by the 1984 shooting of President Reagan—states that a defendant "is not responsible for his or her criminal conduct if, as a result of mental disease or defect, he or she lacked a *substantial* capacity either to *appreciate* [italics added] the criminality [*wrongfulness*] of his conduct [cognitive prong] or to conform his or her conduct to the requirements of the law [volitional prong]." The Federal Code and many state legislatures revised the standard in 1984 as a result of public outrage about President Reagan's shooting by John Hinckley (*United States v. Hinckley*, 1981) removing the volitional prong and essentially reverting to the more restrictive M'Naghten right–wrong standard. A number of states have abolished the insanity defense entirely (e.g., Utah). By 1995, the full ALI test was being used by about 20 states "down from its peak of 25 states in the early 1980s. Some variation of the M'Naghten cognitive impairment only test held sway in about half the states" (Melton et al., 1997, p. 193). During the controversy following Reagan's shooting, proposals by the American Bar Association (ABA), expressing an unwillingness to return to the strict M'Naghten test, proposed another test: "A person is not responsible for criminal conduct if, at the time of such conduct, and as a result of mental disease or defect, that person was unable to *appreciate* the wrongfulness of such conduct" (ABA, 1984, p. 118).

U.S. commentaries and case law on the insanity defense have refined definitional criteria for the "cognitive" and, where the ALI standard still holds, "volitional" prongs of insanity statutes. The M'Naghten rule is more restrictive than the ALI/ABA test. The M'Naghten rule provides for exculpation on two grounds: when the defendant did not know the nature and quality of the criminal act, or when the defendant did not know that the act was wrong (cited in Melton et al., 1997, p. 198). The ALI test combines the cognitive component of the M'Naghten test with the volitional component associated with the irresistible impulse test, an earlier and ultimately unsuccessful formulation. Under the ALI test, in contrast, the concept of "appreciation" of the wrongfulness or legality of the criminal conduct is of central importance in MSO evaluations.

Distinctions between *knowing* versus *appreciation* are critical in conceptualizing mental state at the time of offense assessments (*Hawaii v. Uyesugi*, 2002); *appreciation* represents a more complex weighing and consideration of facts. Many prosecutors feel that criminal conduct that is "organized" cannot by definition be "insane," resorting to a standard for insanity that states "he knew what he was doing" (M'Naghten) or approximating the "wild beast test of 1724" (Robinson, 1996; Perlin, 2000, p. 225) as the criterion for mental conditions that exculpate criminal responsibility. (The wild beast test itself is of clinical, forensic, and historical interest: The 19th-century wild beast test of insanity is exemplified in Benjamin Rush's description of moral derangement: "A wild and ferocious countenance; enlarged and rolling eyes; constant singing; whistling and hallowing; imitations of the voices of different animals; walking with a quick step; or standing still with hands and eyes elevated towards the heavens the madman, or maniac, is in a rage" (cited in Faigman, Kaye, Saks, & Sanders, 2002, p. 335). In this context, for example, the planned, cold blooded mass killing of seven individuals in a workplace violence incident by a Xerox repair man, who was delusionally convinced that his coworkers conspired to sabotage his photocopy machines, was not be considered insane.

Courts and legal philosophers have struggled with a refinement of the concepts of "substantial impairment," "appreciation," and "wrongfulness" (Schopp, 1991), particularly when the criminal action is delusional but not necessarily disorganized. The ALI standard does not require a showing of total lack of knowledge but only the lack of "substantial capacity" (American Psychiatric Association, 1982, p. 2). Definition of the cognitive core of the culpability concept has focused on the words "know" (M'Naghten) and "appreciate" (ALI). Despite controversy (*Connecticut vs. Wilson, Hawaii vs. Uyesugi, Kelley vs. Tennessee*) "to know" has been more narrowly construed than "to appreciate" with respect to the breadth of the cognitive skill involved. Appreciation has been preferred by Congress, the American Law Institute, the American Bar Association, and the American Psychiatric Association. The American Psychiatric Association (APA) observed that *appreciation* has "an affective, more emotional, more personalized approach for evaluating the nature of a defendant's knowledge and understanding" (APA, 1982, p. 2). Finagerette (1972) observed that appreciation is "the capacity to rationally assess—define and evaluate—his own particular act in the light of the relevant public standards of wrong."

In *Kelley vs. Tennessee* (2005), the Tennessee Criminal Court of Appeals wrestled with the meaning of the term *wrongfulness* as opposed to *criminality*, parsing wrongfulness into legal, moral, and personal wrongfulness. In *State of Connecticut v. Wilson* (1997), the Connecticut Supreme Court sought to give content to the "appreciation of wrongfulness" language of the ALI standard, particularly the implied moral aspect of the term *wrongfulness*. In *Wilson*, the defendant argued that "morality must be defined in purely personal terms." The state, in contrast, argued that "morality must be defined by societal standards." Under such a reading, "a defendant is not responsible for his criminal acts as long as his mental disease or defect causes him personally to believe that those acts are morally justified, even though he may appreciate that his conduct is wrong in the sense that it is both illegal and contrary to societal standards of morality." Attempting to find a middle way, the Connecticut court offered the following opinion (cited in Faigman et al., 2002, p. 340):

> We conclude ... that a defendant does not truly "appreciate the wrongfulness of his conduct" ... if a mental disease or defect causes him both to harbor a distorted perception of reality and to believe that, under the circumstances as he honestly believes them, his actions do not offend societal morality even though he may be aware that society, on the basis of the criminal code, does not condone his action. Thus, a defendant would be entitled to prevail ... if as a result of his mental disease or defect, *he sincerely believes that society would approve of his conduct if it shared his understanding of the circumstances underlying his actions* (italics added; *State v. Wilson*, 700 A, 2d at 643, 1997).

This formulation permits the forensic mental health examiner to address the perceptions, reasoning, and beliefs that underlie the criminal conduct.

In most jurisdictions, the insanity defense is considered an affirmative defense (a defense which negates criminal responsibility) and, in most jurisdictions, including the federal courts, the burden of proof is placed on the defendant with a preponderance of the evidence standard of proof. Others, including the federal courts, requite clear and convincing evidence (Parry & Gilliam, 2002). Rogers and Schuman (2000) note the numerous social and political factors that affect the adjudication of severely disturbed defendants, including public reactivity and misperceptions of the (rare) frequency and (limited) success with which the insanity defense is used.

As noted earlier, many states either abolished the insanity defense or adopted "guilty but mentally ill" standards. In this instance, juries may find that the defendant suffers from a "substantial disorder of thought or mood which significantly impairs judgment, behavior, capacity to recognize reality or ability to cope with the ordinary demands of life" (Michigan Comp. Laws, paragraph 330.1400a (1980). Nevertheless, these conditions remain centrally pertinent to an inquiry and evaluation of the defendant's mental state at the time of the offense (MSO), regardless of the ultimate legal disposition.

FORENSIC RELEVANCE OF PSYCHOSIS

Psychotic disorders have been described in great detail since the origins of clinical psychiatry at the end of the 19th century (Gottesman, 1990). Kraepelin and Bleuler, two pioneering psychiatrists, catalogued the characteristic symptoms of schizophrenia and the major psychoses, including hallucinations, delusions, thought disorder, mood disturbances, affective blunting, and social withdrawal. The major psychoses include schizophrenia, delusional disorders, major depressive disorder, and bipolar disorder. Psychotic disorders may also be the result of medical disorders (e.g., Huntington's chorea or Parkinsonism) or substance-induced (methamphetamine-induced psychotic disorder). Causes of "schizophrenia-like" symptoms can involve general medical conditions, neurological and metabolic disorders, psychoactive substances, medications, and toxins. For example, I once examined a former police officer who delusionally believed that he was being "airbombed" by an electronic apparatus in his neighbor's attic. He terrified the family by storming into the house with a shotgun. His delusions were the result of a hypertensive crisis that miraculously did not cause a massive stroke. His symptoms remitted almost immediately upon receiving emergency medical attention. My elderly grandmother was committed to a state hospital after she attempted to buy a pistol at the local gun shop in order to shoot her next door neighbor because she believed that her neighbor was pumping poisonous gases through her open windows, most likely the result of a vascular dementia.

The major psychoses embrace a variety of clinical symptoms involving thinking (errant basic assumptions, illogical thinking, disorganization or confusion of thought or speech), perception (inaccurate input through auditory, visual, or other senses), and mood (extreme dampening or excitation of emotional responding; Kirkpatrick & Tek, 2005; Poythress, Slobogin, Stevens, & Heilbrun, 2002, p. 353; Woods & McGlashan, 2005). The term *psychotic* is reserved where symptoms, particularly perception and thinking, cause *impaired reality testing*. Weiner (1966) refers to the disturbed relation to reality observed in psychosis, namely, the sense of reality and reality testing. The most common symptoms of psychosis include delusions (inaccurate but firmly held beliefs, e.g., the mother's belief that she and her children are being subjected to a remote body scan by government agents) auditory hallucinations (hearing voices), and ideas of reference (feelings that the radio is sending personally significant messages or that a camera in the bathroom, according to one patient, was broadcasting pictures of her on "worldwide TV").

Psychotic individuals may have a distorted sense of their personal importance: "The most intimate thoughts, feelings, and acts are often felt to be known to or shared by others, and explanatory delusions may develop, to the effect that natural or supernatural forces are at work to influence the afflicted individual's thoughts and actions in ways that are often bizarre. The individual may see himself or herself as the pivot of all that happens" (World Health Organization, 1992). The psychotic individual frequently feels caught up in mythic or predestined events: "Events seem to occur not by chance or at random, but because they are preordained" (Arieti, 1974, p. 31). The ICD–10 diagnostic criteria note the frequent presence of the following:

> thought echo, insertion, or broadcasting; delusions of control, influence or passivity; hallucinatory voices giving a running commentary on the patient's daily experiences; persistent delusions that are culturally inappropriate or completely impossible (such as religious or political identities or superhuman powers and abilities); persistent hallucinations in any modality; breaks in thought, incoherence, irrelevance, or neologisms; catatonic behavior; negative symptoms such as apathy, poverty of speech, mood incongruity; and deterioration of personal behavior: aimlessness, idleness, self-absorption, and social withdrawal. (WHO, 1992, cited in Sadock & Sadock, 2005, p. 1417)

A key psychotic symptom is "thought disorder," a disturbance in the form and organization of thought and language (loosening of associations, incoherence, word salad, blocking), for which the Rorschach test has demonstrated unique sensitivity, even in the absence of obvious clinical disturbance (Kleiger, 1999). Psychosis often involves a severe disturbance and impairment of self-awareness and self-reference. It is a rare instance that psychotic individuals have "insight" into their nonsocially consensual perceptions and thoughts.

The primary forensic relevance of psychotic disorders is the fact that individuals may act on their experiences as if they were real. Sometimes these actions may involve violations of the law. In these cases, the issue of criminal responsibility may arise. Of central importance is that psychosis may play a role in either the cognitive (more likely) or volitional prongs (less likely) of pertinent insanity statutes. "The fact that the [psychotic] defendant's symptoms diminish the ability to 'know' or 'appreciate' the nature of criminal behavior or 'conform' conduct to objective legal mandates provides a potential basis for the judge or jury to determine that the individual should not be held morally responsible" (Poythress et al., 2002, p. 354).

As noted earlier, psychosis is the most common basis for the insanity defense (data from New York, California, and Georgia indicate that major psychoses were diagnosed in 82%–97%, 84%, and 85%–86% of successful insanity cases, cited in Poythress et al., 2002, p. 354), although the insanity defense is rarely used and even less frequently successful (raised in less than 1% of cases and successful in less than one quarter of the cases:

Steadman, Keitner, Braff, & Arvanites, 1983; Steadman, McGreevy, Morrisey, & Callahan, 1993). Most jurisdictions require a diagnosable mental disorder as a threshold for the impairment criterion, whether know, appreciate, or in the case of volitional cases, self-control.

RORSCACH ASSESSMENT OF PSYCHOSIS: STRATEGIC CONSIDERATIONS

The forensic psychological evaluation of psychosis in insanity defense cases is based on an assessment strategy that aims to assess the defendant's mental state at the time of the offense (MSO; Melton et al., 1997) relevant to the pertinent legal standard. It is not typically the case, however, that a clinician with a set of Rorschach cards or a Wechlser scale just happens to be present at the time of a criminal offense to examine the defendant's state of mind! Except for those rare, fortunate coincidences where a clinical examination occurs proximate to the commission of a crime, most evaluations take place at some temporal distance from the offense, sometimes preceding, but most typically, at a time following the offense. As noted by Melton and his colleagues, "Psychological tests provide information about *current* functioning, whereas an MSO examination seeks to reconstruct the defendant's *prior* mental state" (p. 241). Consequently, the assessment of criminal responsibility is commonly a *retrospective* task in which a reconstruction of the defendant's behavior and state of mind is necessary (Melton et al., 1997). Melton and his colleagues refer to these evaluations as "investigations" noting that "a typical MSO examination illustrates the forensic evaluation *par excellence*" (Melton et al., 1997, p. 234; see Figure 8–1 and Tables 8–5 and 8–6 in Melton et al.'s text for a detailed flow chart and outlines for the conduct of an MSO evaluation).

There are a number of tools and procedures that may assist the clinician in reconstructing the defendant's state of mind: defendant interviews to obtain offense-related information; observations of eye witnesses; reports of other third parties (e.g., family members or employers who had contact with the defendant prior to an following the offense); police reports; reports of treating clinicians prior to, at the time of, and following the offense; and clinical methods/techniques such as the Rogers Criminal Responsibility Scales (R–CRAS; 1984), which organize a number of factors relevant to an ultimate opinion concerning MSO.

The use of psychological tests in MSO is a particularly sensitive issue for a variety of reasons. As noted earlier (Otto & Heilbrun 2002), the use of clinical techniques that are unvalidated for specific forensic constructs demands clinician inferences that are subject to a variety of clinical and methodological criticisms, including malingering and problems with clinical judgment described by Meehl, Garb (1998), and others. Otto and Heilbrun noted, "The professional literature is barren in terms of sound empirical studies demonstrating either that psychological test data are useful as a means of establishing a link between particular diagnostic conditions and legally relevant behavior in individual cases or that they are useful for assigning individuals to discrete legal categories" (e.g., sane vs. insane; Melton et al., 1997, p. 241). Westen and Weinberger's recent response to Garb et al. (Westen & Weinberger, 2004), however, strengthens the confidence of clinicians in the disciplined use of clinical techniques.

In many cases, nevertheless, observations of witnesses or statements of defendants may suggest the presence of psychosis at the time of the offense. Some defendants will remain psychotic at the time of the examination, particularly if treatment efforts have been absent, avoided, or ineffective. Frequently, I have been fortunate enough to have family reports, reports of treating clinicians, other eye witnesses (including victims), first responder reports, emergency room reports, police reports, or clinicians in jails that document the presence of bizarre, disorganized behavior suggesting clinical psychosis, and the defendant remains psychotic at the time of the clinical and forensic examination. The administration of psychological tests, in particular the Rorschach test, then, has a solid basis on which to inform a clinical and forensic opinion, namely, detecting the clinical indicia of psychosis.

THE UTILITY OF THE RORSCHACH THE FORENSIC ASSESSMENT OF PSYCHOSIS

Given the likelihood that the forensic clinician may testify in court on the issue of a defendant's mental state at the time of the offense, some consideration of admissibility issues should be kept in mind. Depending on the jurisdiction, the court may rely on either *Frye* (1923), *Daubert* (1993) tests, or Federal Rules of Evidence (Committee on the Judiciary, 2004) for admissibility. This topic is considered later in the discussion of admissibility and testimony at court. Fortunately, the Rorschach assessment of psychotic disorders rests on a robust behavioral science foundation, which has been immune to attacks by Rorschach critics (Acklin, 1999). Gacono and Evans note that "the Rorschach provides an open structured, performance based cognitive perceptual problem solving task that is quite different from more close structured instruments" (Gacono & Evans, preface, this vol.). The Rorschach test is of particular value in relation to the problems with self-report where individual attempts to underreport or exacerbate or malinger psychopathology (Gacono, Evans, & Viglione, 2002; Ganellen, 1994, 1996; Ganellen, Wasyliw, Haywood, & Grossman, 1996; Grossman, Wasyliw et al., 2002). Increasingly, research has focused on obtaining base rate data on a variety of relevant forensic groups, making it even more desirable as a forensic assessment tool (Gacono & Meloy, 1994).

Rorschach noted the characteristic aspects of "schizophrenic" thinking in his seminal monograph (Rorschach, 1942). Rorschach noted the influence of E. Bleuler in his conceptualization of schizophrenia, although it should be remembered that schizophrenia as a clinical entity, until the *DSM–III*, was often used synonymously with psychosis ("acute schizophrenic reactions"). Rorschach observed the boundary disturbances and combinatory thinking frequently noted in psychotic records, including the Contamination response, observing that schizophrenics "give many interpretations in which confabulation, combination, and contamination are mixed in together" (Rorschach, 1942, p. 38).

Subsequent understanding of thought disturbance on the Rorschach test was strongly influenced by David Rapaport (Rapaport, 1951; Rapaport, Gill, & Schafer, 1968). On the basis of the verbalizations to the cards, Rapaport wrote that "one can infer the presence of thinking which does not adhere to the reality of the testing situation, as defined by attitudes, responses, and verbalizations of the normal population." Rapaport referred to "autistic thinking" (p. 426, referring to Bleuler's notions, 1911, of schizophrenic thought disturbance in his massive chapter in Rapaport, 1951). Rapaport referred to "deviant verbalizations" as indicative of thought disturbance (e.g., fabulized combinations, confabulations, and contaminations), the examination of which was "the highway for investigating disorders of thinking" (p. 431, cited in Kleiger, 1999, p. 46).

Watkins and Stauffacher (1952) attempted to quantify Rapaport's categories by means of the Index of Pathological thinking or Delta Index (d for deviant), which was later revised and developed into the Thought Disorder Index (TDI; Johnston & Holzman, 1979). The Delta Index, like the TDI that followed it, included 15 coding categories, including all of Rapaport's categories, with a weighting scheme to indicate level of severity: minor deviations receiving the lowest weights (.25), moderate instance receiving intermediate weights (.5 and .75), and severe instance of pathological verbalization receiving the highest weights (1.0). A number of studies have demonstrated the strengths and weaknesses of the Delta Index, but Kleiger notes "the Delta Index must be heralded as the first carefully constructed quantifiable scale focused exclusively on measuring thought pathology per se ...," advancing "a degree closer to a more sophisticated conceptual approach to identifying schizophrenia on the Rorschach" (Kleiger, 1999, p. 37).

Perhaps the most comprehensive and sensitive approach to assessing thought disorder on the Rorschach test was developed by Johnston and Holzman—the Thought Disorder Index (TDI; 1979). They combined earlier systems for the detection of thought disorder into a reliable coding system. A revised version of the index was published in 1986 (Solovay et al., 1986). The TDI, derived from standard administration of the Rorschach test, can be used to quantify the amount and severity of disordered thinking, and to identify qualitative features of thought disorder. The TDI includes 23 categories of thought slippage at four levels of severity (.25, .50, .75, 1.0). Examples of mild of thought slippage include peculiar verbalizations and mild combinatory thinking. Moderately disordered thinking includes phenomena such as looseness, idiosyncratic symbolism, and queer use of language. At the more severe end of the spectrum, one finds autistic logic, more serious forms of combinatory thinking, neologisms, and incoherence. The TDI has been shown to be a reliable and valid measure for assessing thought disorder in adults, children, and adolescents. Originally developed for clinical use, the Rorschach TDI has been extensively studied in contemporary schizophrenic research.

A large number of TDI research articles have appeared in peer-reviewed journals since the early 1980s. The TDI has been shown to discriminate between hospitalized schizophrenic patients, first-degree relatives of schizophrenics, and normal controls (Haimo & Holzman, 1979). In studies of thought disorder in children, the TDI was able to discriminate psychotic and high-risk children from normal controls and nonpsychotic hospitalized children (Arboleda & Holzman, 1985). Adolescent schizophrenic patients showed the same characteristics of thought disorder as adult schizophrenics (Makowski et al., 1997). A number of studies have used the TDI in distinguishing types of thought disorder as they apply to the differential diagnosis of schizophrenia and bipolar disorder. Holzman, Solovay, and Shenton (1985) provided evidence that the TDI reflected thought disorder across a continuum of severity. Holzman, Shenton, and Solovay (1986) used the TDI to differentiate between quantity and quality of thought disorder in manic, schizophrenic, schizoaffective manic, and schizoaffective depressed patients. They found that quality of thought disorder differs in schizophrenia and mania, and the thought disorder in schizoaffective conditions resembles that of schizophrenia. Shenton, Solovay, and Holzman (1987) and Solovay, Shenton, and Holzman (1987) examined thought disorder in patients with schizoaffective disorder, manic conditions, and schizophrenia to determine whether the TDI could differentiate between diagnostic groups. They demonstrated similarities and distinctions between the diagnostic groupings using the TDI. The thought disorder of manic patients was extravagantly combinatory, usually with humor, flippancy, and playfulness. The thought disorder of schizophrenic patients on the other hand, was disorganized, confused, and ideationally fluid, with many peculiar words and phrases.

Coleman, Levy, Lezenweger, and Holzman (1996) used the TDI to quantify and classify thought disorder in individuals with schizotypal characteristics (schizophrenia-spectrum disorders). They found that individuals psychometrically identified as schizotypal displayed thought disorder similar to that shown by schizophrenic patients and some of their first-degree relatives. Hurt, Holzman, and Davis (1983) examined the usefulness of the TDI in distinguishing thought disorder across a range from subtle to flagrant. The TDI charted changes in thought disorder upon administration of antipsychotic medications and showed a high congruence with concurrently administered scales of thought disorder. Gold and Hurt (1990) found the TDI was sensitive enough to detect subtle changes in disturbed thinking following the administration of antipsychotic medications to psychiatric in-patients. Shenton, Solovay, Holzman, Coleman, and Gale (1989) used the TDI to examine first-degree relatives of schizophrenic, manic, and schizoaffective patients. In all three groups, there was a tendency for probands with higher thought disorder to have first-degree relatives with higher thought disorder.

All of the studies cited here have reported adequate to excellent interrater reliability (e.g., Coleman et al., 1993). An extensive study of reliability and clinical validity studies (effects of treatment, distinguishing mania from schizophrenia, studies of schizoaffective disorder, thought disorder in biological relatives, TDI in children and adolescents, schizophrenia spectrum disorders, right hemisphere cortical damage, and other schizophrenia research) is summarized in Holzman, Levy, and Johnston (2005).

Kleiger (1999) summarizes the Rorschach TDI research noting that it rests on a sturdy empirical foundation and has solid clinical applications. After mastering the TDI, the clinician is sensitized to the detection of the most subtle disturbances in language and thinking. Kleiger noted that the TDI shows promise "as a focal diagnostic tool to help clinicians discriminate among different types of psychotic disorders" (1999, p. 99).

Exner developed the Comprehensive System (CS) for the Rorschach (originally published in 1974) after reviewing and integrating the splintered Rorschach scoring approaches extant in the late 1960s (Exner, 1969). The Comprehensive System has been in continuous revision since the 1970s to refine its psychometric properties. A primary motivation was to establish codes and categories with strong interrater reliability. Exner gathered a group of codes for unusual verbalizations that became the basis for several clusters reflecting thought disturbance: *Deviant Verbalizations* (*DV*), *Deviant Responses* (*DR*), *Incongruous Combinations* (*INCOM*), *Fabulized Combinations* (*FABCOM*), *Contamina-*

tions (*CONTAM*), and *Autistic Logic* (*ALOG*), which are weighted and summarized into the *WSUM6*, a gross measure of the amount of thought disorder present in the record. Out of these codes emerged a composite index to detect "schizophrenia" (the Schizophrenia Index [*SCZI*]: *M*–, weighted special scores, low *X*+ and *F* + %, *CF* + *C*), high *X*–%, and absence of whole human responses. The *SCZI* showed reasonably good clinical sensitivity but also a rather high false positive rate. "Examiners using the SCZI to identify schizophrenia need to be alert to the distinct possibility of obtaining a 'false positive 4' (see Exner & Weiner, 1995, pp. 148–153; Weiner, 1998b). For this reason, the *SCZI* was replaced in the Comprehensive System by the PTI" (cited in Weiner, 2003). In 1990, Exner added Level 1 and Level 2 distinctions to responses based on their deviancy which improved the discriminatory power of the *SCZI* Index.

Exner replaced the Schizophrenia Index with the *Perceptual Thinking Index* (*PTI*) to further improve the conceptual and psychometric properties. The *PTI* is a nine variable index with five criterion tests:

1. *XA%* < .70 and *WDA%* < .75%.
2. *X*–% > .29.
3. *LV2* > 2 and *FAB2* > 0.
4. *R* < 17 and *WSUM6* > 12 or *R* > 16 and *WSUM6* > 17 (Adjust for age 13 and younger: If *R* > 16: 5 to 7 equals 20; 8 to 10 = 19; 11 to 13 = 18 and if *R* < 17:5 to 7 = 16; 8 to 10 = 15; 11 to 13 = 14).
5. *M*– > 1 or *X*–% > .40.

These changes have considerably reduced the relatively high false-positive rate that had characterized the *SCZI*. A *PTI* of 3 or greater "usually identifies serious adjustment problems attributable to ideational dysfunction. It is not possible for *PTI* to exceed 3 without there being an elevation of *WSum6* … a measure of disordered thinking" (Weiner, 2003, p. 280). The *PTI* is a more sensitive CS measure of psychosis "… the more *WSUM6* exceeds the minimum criterion for a point on the *PTI*, is dominated by the more serious *Special Scores*, and includes *Level 2 Special Scores*, the more likely a respondent is to have the type of thought disorder typically observed in schizophrenia, schizoaffective disorder, delusional disorder, and paranoid and schizotypal personality disorder" (Weiner, 2003, p. 128).

One recent study investigated the *PTI* with 42 inpatient children and adolescents in a private psychiatric hospital specializing in acute short-term treatment (Smith et al., 2001). Using a greater than 4 cutoff for the five-item *PTI,* the authors found that patients with higher *PTI* scores has significantly higher findings on measures of atypicality, reality distortion, hallucinations and delusions, feelings of alienation, and social withdrawal derived from either from a parenting scale or from a self-report measure. The authors conclude that "the PTI may be a more pure measure of thought disorder in children and adolescents than the SCZI" and that it "may be assessing a more severe thought disturbance that not only has characteristics of cognitive slippage but may be marked by behavioral disturbance as well" (p. 458). The *PTI* is an indicator of the kinds of difficulties in perceptual accuracy and thinking that can have a pervasive impact on perception, thought, reasoning, and judgment. *PTI* scores of four or five signal difficulties in perceptual accuracy and thinking and suggest that findings from the *Processing*, *Mediation*, and *Ideation* clusters (Weiner, 2003) will play an important role in aspects of the individual's functioning.

Acklin (1992) integrated innovations and developments in clinical psychoanalytic theory (Blatt's concept of the object, Urist's Mutuality of Autonomy scale, Lerner Defense scales, and Otto Kernberg's tripartite classification of personality organization: Neurotic, borderline, and psychotic personality organization (Kernberg, 1986) with CS approaches to Rorschach psychodiagnosis. Translated into contemporary Rorschach psychology, which integrates nomothetic and idiographic approaches, the psychodiagnostician examining an individual with suspected psychosis or psychotic personality organization might expect to find the following Rorschach characteristics: Loading up of *Special Scores* especially, *Level 2 Special Scores*; a heavily *Weighted Sum6*; and the *SCZI* at 4 or 5, or the *PTI* at 4 or 5; disturbances and oddities of syntax and representation indicative of thought disorder; deterioration of form level: especially human percepts; disturbances in the structural features of percepts; failure of defensive operations and utilization of primitive defenses; expression of raw, drive-laden, primary process material (Dudek, 1980; Holt, 2005) and themes of bareness, emptiness, and malevolent interaction. In his classic textbook of clinical cases, writing about the quality of verbalizations, Schafer (1948) notes that "instability of appearances" in psychotic records indicates "confusion and feelings of unreality … this type of verbalization refers to perceptual fluidity in a setting of disorganization" (p. 309).

As this survey of the literature on the Rorschach assessment of psychosis demonstrates, the test is highly sensitive to the presence of perceptual and thought disturbance with a strong and long-standing behavioral science foundation. In conjunction with the sort of information noted previously (retrospective self-reports, police and witness reports, and treatment reports, if any), the test provides the forensic clinician with the best possible tools to determine a defendant's MSO and the degree to which psychosis played a role in the defendant's conduct.

FORENSIC OPINIONS AND COURT TESTIMONY

As noted earlier, the determination of a defendant's MSO requires careful coordination of sources of information: retrospective reports of the defendant, eye witness accounts, collateral and police observations, treatment records, and results of a psychological evaluation conducted at some time after the offense. In most respects, evaluation procedures that examine the temporal and causal associations between state of mind and psychological evaluation data to validate a forensic opinion resemble an applied clinical research design—a mini-research project (Stricker & Trierweiler, 1995; Stricker, 2006)— where hypotheses are formulated, evaluated, and results described in a disciplined scientist-practitioner methodology. This forms the basis of the expert's opinions, which may be proffered to the referring attorney or court. This raises the likelihood that forensic evaluators may have to present and defend their findings at trial.

The Rorschach test has never been without its critics. Academic psychologists (Jensen, 1965), method critics, and, more recently, informed critics of the Comprehensive System have severely criticized aspects of the test's psychometrics. During the past 10 years, Wood, Garb, and their colleagues have leveled strong and consistent criticism of the Comprehensive System (Wood, Nezworski, Lilienfeld, & Garb, 2003). Garb (1999), who completely ignores much of the literature reviewed here, called for a moratorium on the use of the test in clinical and forensic settings. Serious attacks on the Comprehensive System's credibility have come from Grove and his colleagues (Grove & Barden, 1999; Grove, Barden, Garb, & Lilienfeld, 2002; with rejoinders by Ritzler, Erard, & Pettigrew, 2002a, 2002b; Wood, Nezworski, Stejskal, & McKinzey, 2001). The response from the Rorschach community has been a vigorous, thorough-going examination of the test's reliability, validity, norms, and basis for admissibility of Rorschach testimony to court. The result has been a wave of research studies that has strengthened the test's basis, but critics, although recognizing the developments, remain unconvinced (Wood, Nezworski, Garb, & Lilienfeld, 2006).

With respect to the forensic assessment of psychosis, in contrast to criticisms of the Comprehensive System, the behavioral foundations are close to unimpeachable. The forensic clinician, however, must not only be able to use the test clinically, but also be knowledgeable and prepared to present and defend challenges to the admissibility of Rorschach testimony in court. Typically, this requires a through understanding of the behavioral science foundations of the testimony and recognition of the strengths and limitations of the findings.

As noted earlier, the *Frye* and *Daubert* tests and Federal Rules of Evidence (Committee on the Judiciary, 2004) are used across most jurisdictions. A review of the legal literature by Meloy, Hansen, and Weiner (1997) examined 7,934 cases in which psychologists presented Rorschach testimony, Weiner, Exner, and Sciara (1996) found only six incidents (.08%) when the test was seriously challenged, and only one time (.01%) when the testimony was declared inadmissible as evidence. A computer-based search of Rorschach legal citations between 1945 and 1995 was conducted by the authors. The Rorschach test was cited in 247 cases in state, federal, and military courts of appeal, averaging 5 times per year. Twenty-six cases were identified in which the reliability or validity of the Rorschach findings were an issue (10.5%). Despite occasional disparagement by prosecutors, the majority of the courts found the test findings to be both reliable and valid. When Rorschach testimony was limited or excluded, it was usually due to invalid inferences that the expert had made from the test data.

In a summary response to criticisms of the Rorschach, the Society for Personality Assessment (2005) recently published a "white paper" addressing the clinical and forensic use of the Rorschach, summarizing the scientific literature and examining issues of reliability, validity, and ethical use with an extensive reference list covering a whole range of psychometric, research design, and forensic issues. Weiner (chap. 6, this vol.) provides an overview for presenting Rorschach testimony in court with behavioral science resources to provide the necessary foundation for admissibility. Hilsenroth and Stricker (2004) describe in great detail the information a forensic clinician may rely on in preparing, presenting, and defending Rorschach testimony (Gacono, Evans, & Viglione, 2002). Aside from expert knowledge on the Rorschach's strengths and contribution to the forensic assessment of psychosis, the clinician needs to understand and master aspects of effective testimony (e.g., Brodsky, 1991, 2004).

CONCLUSIONS

The Rorschach test has a lengthy and sturdy history demonstrating its sensitivity and efficacy in the detection of thought disturbance associated with the major psychoses and schizophrenia-spectrum disorders. The behavioral science basis of the Rorschach's sensitivity to psychosis is one of its sturdiest scientific foundations. The skilled, disciplined Rorschach clinician who is informed and knowledgeable of the test's strengths and weaknesses is capable of making a significant contribution to the resolution of legal issues where a defendant's state of mind is in question.

REFERENCES

Acklin, M. W. (1992). Psychodiagnosis of personality structure: Psychotic personality organization. *Journal of Personality Assessment, 58*, 3, 454–463.

Acklin, M. W. (1999). Behavioral science foundations of the Rorschach test: Research and clinical applications. *Assessment, 6*(4), 319–326.

American Bar Association. (1984). *Criminal justice mental health standards IV*. Washington, DC: American Bar Association.

American Psychiatric Association. (1982). The insanity defense: Position statement. *APA Document Reference 82002*. Washington, DC: American Psychiatric Association.

Arboleda, C., & Holzman, P. (1985). Thought disorder in children at risk for psychosis. *Archives of General Psychiatry, 42*, 1004–1013.

Arieti, S. (1974). *Interpretation of schizophrenia* (2nd ed.). New York: Basic Books.

Bleuler, E. (1911). *Dementia praecox or the group of schizophrenias*. New York: International Universities Press.

Bonnie, R. J. (1983). The moral basis of the insanity defense. *American Bar Association Journal, 69*, 26.

Brakel, S., Parry, J., & Weiner, B. (1985). *The mentally disabled and the law*. Chicago: American Bar Foundation.

Brodsky, S. L. (1991). *Testifying in court*. Washington, DC: American Psychological Association.

Brodsky, S. L. (2004). *Coping with cross-examination and other pathways to effective testimony*. Washington, DC: American Psychological Association.

Clark vs. Arizona. (2006). Brief amicus curiae for the American Psychiatric Association, American Psychological Association, and the American Academy of Psychiatry and the Law S Petitioner.

Coleman, M., Carpenter, J., Waternaux, C., Levy, D., Shenton, M., Perry, J., Medoff, D., Wong, H., Monoach, D., Meyer, P., O'Brian, C., Valention, C., Robinson, D., Smith, M., Makowski, D., & Holzman, P. (1993). The Thought Disorder Index: A reliability study. *Psychological Assessment, 5*(3), 336–342.

Coleman, M., Levy, D., Lezenweger, M., & Holzman, P. (1996). Thought disorder, perceptual aberrations, and schizotypy. *Journal of Abnormal Psychology, 105*(3), 469–473.

Committee on the Judiciary, U.S. House of Representatives. (2004). *Federal rules of evidence*. Washington, DC: U.S. Government Printing Office.

Daubert vs. Merrill Dow Pharmaceuticals, Inc. 509 US 579 (1993).

Dudek, S. (1980). Primary process ideation. In R. H. Woody (Ed.), *Encyclopedia of clinical assessment* (Vol. 1, pp. 520–539). San Francisco: Jossey-Bass.

Exner, J. (1969). *The Rorschach systems*. New York: Grunne & Stratton.

Exner, J., & Weiner, I. (1995). *The Rorschach: A Comprehensive System: Vol. 3. Assessment of children and adolescents* (2nd ed.). New York: Wiley.

Faigman, D. L., Kaye, D. H., Saks, M. J., & Sanders, J. (2002). *Modern scientific evidence: The law and science of expert testimony* (Vol. 1). St. Paul, MN: West Publishing.

Finagerette, H (1972). *The meaning of criminal insanity.* Berkeley: University of California Press.

Frye vs. United States 293F 1013 (DC Cir 1923).

Gacono, C., & Meloy, J. (1994). *The Rorschach assessment of aggressive and psychopathic personalities.* Hillsdale, NJ: Lawrence Erlbaum Associates.

Gacono, C., Evans, B., & Viglione, D. (2002). The Rorschach in forensic practice. *Journal of Forensic Psychological Practice, 2*(3), 33–52.

Ganellan, R. J. (1994). Attempting to conceal psychological disturbance: MMPI defensive response sets and the Rorschach. *Journal of Personality Assessment, 63*, 423–437.

Ganellan, R. J. (1996). Exploring MMPI–Rorschach relationships. *Journal of Personality Assessment, 67*, 529–542.

Ganellen, R. J., Wasyliw, O. E., Haywood, T. W., & Grossman, L. S. (1996). Can psychosis be malingered on the Rorschach: An empirical study. *Journal of Personality Assessment, 66*, 65–80.

Garb, H. (1998). *Studying the clinician: Judgment research and psychological assessment.* Washington, DC: American Psychological Association.

Garb, H. N. (1999). Call for a moratorium on the use of the Rorschach Inkblot Test in clinical and forensic settings. *Assessment, 6*, 313–315.

Gold, J., & Hurt, S. (1990). The effect of haloperidol on thought disorder and IQ and schizophrenia. *Journal of Personality Assessment, 54*, 390–400.

Gottesman, I. (1990). *Schizophrenia genesis: The origins of madness.* New York: Henry Holt & Company.

Grisso, T. (2003). *Evaluating competencies: Forensic assessments and instruments* (2nd ed.). New York: Kluwer Plenum.

Giorgi-Guarnieri, D., Janofsky, J., Keram, E., Lawsky, S., Merideth, P., Mossman, D., Schwartz-Watts, D., Scott, C., Thompson, J., & Zonana, H. (2002). AAPL practice guideline for forensic psychiatric evaluation of defendants raising the insanity defense. *Journal of the American Academy of Psychiatry and the Law, 30*(2 Suppl.), 3–40.

Grossman, L., Wasyliw, O., Benn, A., & Gyoerkoe, K. (2002). Can sex offenders who minimize on the MMPI conceal psychopathology on the Rorschach? *Journal of Personality Assessment, 78*(3), 484–501.

Grove, W. M., & Barden, R. C. (1999). Protecting the integrity of the legal system: The admissibility of testimony from mental health experts under *Daubert/Kumho* analyses. *Psychology, Public Policy, and Law, 5*, 224–242.

Grove, W. M., Barden, R. C., Garb, H. N., & Lilienfeld, S. O. (2002). Failure of Rorschach-Comprehensive-System-based testimony to be admissible under the Daubert–Joiner–Kumho standard. *Psychology, Public Policy, and Law, 8*(2), 216–234.

Haimo, S., & Holzman, p. (1979). Thought disorder in schizophrenics and normal controls: Social class and race differences. *Journal of Consulting and Clinical Psychology, 47*(5), 963–967.

Hawaii vs. Byran Uyesugi, 100 Hawaii 442, P. 3d 843 (2002).

Hilsenroth, M. J., & Stricker, G. (2004). A consideration of challenges to psychological assessment instruments used in forensic settings: Rorschach as exemplar. *Journal of Personality Assessment, 83*, 141–152.

Holt, R. (2005). The Pripro scoring system. In R. Bornstein & J. Masling (Eds.), *Scoring the Rorschach: Seven validated systems* (pp. 191–235). Mahwah, NJ: Lawrence Erlbaum Associates.

Holzman, P., Levy, D., & Johnston, M. (2005). The use of the Rorschach technique for assessing formal thought disorder. In R. Bornstein & J. Masling (Eds.), *Scoring the Rorschach: Seven validated systems* (pp. 55–95). Mahwah, NJ: Lawrence Erlbaum Associates.

Holzman, P., Solovay, M., & Shenton, M. (1985). Thought disorder specificity and functional psychoses. In M. Alpert (Ed.), *Controversies in schizophrenia* (pp. 228–245). New York: Guilford.

Holzman, P., Shenton, M., & Solovay, M. (1986). Quality of thought disorder in differential diagnosis. *Schizophrenia Bulletin, 12*(3), 360–373.

Hurt, S., Holzman, P., & Davis, J. (1983). Thought disorder: The measurement of its changes. *Archives of General Psychiatry, 40*, 1281–1285.

Jensen, A. R. (1965). Review of the Rorschach Inkblot Test. In O. K. Buros (Ed.), *The sixth mental measurements yearbook* (pp. 501–509). Highland Park, NJ: Gryphon Press.

Johnston, M. H., & Holzman, P. S. (1979). *Assessing schizophrenic thinking.* San Francisco: Jossey-Bass.

Kelley vs. Tennessee, 2005 WL 2255854 Tenn. Criminal App. (2005).

Kernberg, O. (1986). *Object relations in clinical psychoanalysis.* New York: Aronson.

Kirkpatrick, B., & Tek, C. (2005). Schizophrenia: Clinical features and psychopathology concepts. In B. J. Sadock & Virginia A. Sadock (Eds.), *Comprehensive textbook of psychiatry* (Vol. 1, 8th ed., pp. 1412–1436). Philadelphia: Lippincott Williams & Wilkins.

Kleiger, J. H. (1999). *Disordered thinking and the Rorschach: Theory, research, and differential diagnosis.* Hillsdale, NJ: Analytic Press.

Makowski, D., Waternaux, C., Lajonchere, C., Dicker, R., Smoke, N., Koplewicz, H., Min, D., Mendell, N., & Levy, D. (1997). Thought disorder in adolescent-onset schizophrenia. *Schizophrenia Research, 23*, 147–165.

Meloy, J., Hansen, T., & Weiner, I. (1997). Authority of the Rorschach: Legal citations during the past 50 years. *Journal of Personality Assessment, 69*, 1, 53–62.

Melton, G. B., Petrila, J., Poythress, N. G., & Slobogin, C. (1997). *Psychological evaluations for the courts: A handbook for mental health professionals and lawyers* (2nd ed.). New York: Guilford.

Otto, R., Edens, J., & Barcus, E. (2000). The use of psychological testing in child custody evaluations. *Family and Conciliation Court Review, 38*, 312–340.

Otto, R., & Heilbrun K. (2002). The practice of forensic psychology: A look toward the future in light of the past. *American Psychologist, 57*, 5–18.

Parry, J., & Gilliam, F. P. (2002). *Handbook on mental disability law.* Washington, DC: American Bar Association.

Perlin, M. (1989). *Mental disability law: Civil and criminal* (Vol. 3). Charlottesville, VA: The Michie Company.

Perlin, M. L. (2000). *The hidden prejudice: Mental disability on trial.* Washington, DC: American Psychological Association.

Poythress, N., Slobogin, C., Stevens, T., & Heilbrun, K. (2002). The scientific status of research on insanity and diminished capacity. In D. Faigman, D. Kaye, M. Saks, & J. Sanders (Eds.), *Modern scientific evidence: The law and science of expert testimony* (pp. 353–408). St. Paul, MN: West Publishing.

Rapaport, D. (1951). *Organization and pathology of thought: Selected sources.* New York: Columbia University Press.

Rapaport, D., Gill, M., & Schafer, R. (1968). *Diagnostic psychological testing.* New York: International Universities Press.

Ritzler, B., Erard, R., & Pettigrew, G. (2002). Protecting the integrity of Rorschach expert witnesses: A reply to Grove and Barden (1999) Re: The admissibility of testimony under Daubert/Kumho Analyses. *Psychology, Public Policy, and Law, 8*(2), 201–215.

Ritzler, B., Erard, R., & Pettigrew (2002). A final reply to Grove and Barden: The relevance of the Rorschach Comprehensive System for expert testimony. *Psychology, Public Policy, and Law, 8*(2), 235–246.

Robinson, D. N. (1996). *Wild beasts & idle humors: The insanity defense from antiquity to the present.* Cambridge, MA: Harvard University Press.

Rogers, R. (1984). *Manual for the Rogers Criminal Responsibility Scales (R–CRAS).* Odessa, FL: Psychological Assessment Resources.

Rogers, R., & Shuman, D. W. (2000). *Conducting insanity evaluations* (2nd ed.). New York: Guilford.

Rorschach, H. (1942). *Psychodiagnostics: A diagnostic test based on perception* (P. Lemkau & B. Kronenberg, Trans., 7th ed.). New York: Grune & Stratton.

Sadock, G., & Dadock, V. (2005). *Comprehensive textbook of psychiatry* (Vol. 1, 8th ed.). Philadelphia: Lippincott Williams & Wilkins.

Schafer, R. (1948). *The clinical application of psychological tests: Diagnostic summaries and case studies*. New York: International Universities Press.

Schopp, R. F. (1991). *Automatism, insanity, and the psychology of criminal responsibility*. New York: Cambridge University Press.

Shenton, M., Solovay, M., & Holzman, P. (1987). Comparative studies of thought disorder: II. Schizoaffective disorder. *Archives of General Psychiatry, 44,* 21–30.

Shenton, M., Solovay, M., Holzman, P., Coleman, M., & Gale, H. (1989). Thought disorder in the relatives of psychotic patients. *Archives of General Psychiatry, 46,* 897–901.

Smith, S., Baity, M., Knowles, E., & Hilsenroth, M. (2001). Assessment of disorder thinking in children and adolescents: The Rorschach Perceptual-Thinking Index. *Journal of Personality Assessment, 77*(3), 447–463.

Society for Personality Assessment (2005). The status of the Rorschach in clinical and forensic practice: An official statement by the Board of Trustees of the Society for Personality Assessment. *Journal of Personality Assessment, 85,* 219–237.

Solovay, M., Shenton, M., & Holzman, P. (1987). Comparative studies of thought disorder: I. Mania in schizophrenia. *Archives of General Psychiatry, 44,* 13–20.

Solovay, M., Shenton, M., Gasperetti, C., Coleman, M., Daniels, E., Carpenter, J., & Holzman, P. (1986). Scoring manual for the Thought Disorder Index. *Schizophrenia Bulletin, 12*(3), 483–496.

State of Connecticut v. Wilson 242 Conn. 605, 700 A.2d 633 (1997).

Steadman, H., Keitner, L., Braff, J., & Arvanites, T. (1983). Factors associated with a successful insanity defense plea. *American Journal of Psychiatry, 140,* 401–405.

Steadman, H., McGreevy, M. A., Morrissey, J. P., Callahan, L. A., Robbins, P. C., & Cirincione, C. (1993). *Before and after Hinckley: Evaluating insanity defense reform*. New York: Guilford Press.

Stricker, G. (2006). The local clinical scientist, evidence-based practice, and personality assessment. *Journal of Personality Assessment, 86*(1), 4–9.

Stricker, G., & Trierweiler, S. (1995). The local clinical scientist: A bridge between science and practice. *American Psychologist, 50*(12), 995–1002.

United States v. Hinckley, 525, F. Suppl. 1342. DDC. (1981).

Watkins, J., & Stauffacher, J. (1952). An index of pathological thinking in the Rorschach. *Journal of Projective Techniques, 16,* 276–286.

Weiner, I. B. (1966). *Psychodiagnosis in schizophrenia*. New York: Wiley.

Weiner, I. (1998). Rorschach differentiation of schizophrenia and affective disorder. In G. P. Koocher, J. C. Norcross, & S. S. Hill (Eds.), *Psychologist–s desk reference* (pp. 151–154). New York: Oxford University Press.

Weiner, I. B. (2003). *Principles of Rorschach interpretation* (2nd ed.). Mahwah, NJ: Lawrence Erlbaum Associates.

Weiner, I., Exner, J., & Sciara, T. (1996). Is the Rorschach welcome in the courtroom? *Journal of Personality Assessment, 67,* 422–424.

Westen, D., & Weinberger, J. (2004). When clinical description becomes statistical prediction. *American Psychologist, 59*(7), 595–613.

Wood, J., Nezworski, M., Garb, H., & Lilienfeld, S. (2006). The controversy over Exner's Comprehensive System for the Rorschach: The critics speak. *Independent Practitioner, 26*(2), 73–82.

Wood, J., Nezworski, T., Lilienfeld, S., & Garb, H. (2003). *What's wrong with the Rorschach?: Science confronts the controversial inkblot test*. San Francisco: Jossey-Bass.

Wood, J. M., Nezworski, M.T., Stejskal, W. J., & McKinzey, R. K. (2001). Problems of the Comprehensive System for the Rorschach in forensic settings: Recent developments. *Journal of Forensic Psychology Practice, 1*(3), 89–103.

Woods, S., & McGlashan, T. (2005). Schizophrenia and other psychotic disorders: Special issues in early detection and intervention. In B. J. Sadock & V. A. Sadock (Eds.), *Comprehensive textbook of psychiatry* (Vol. 1, 8th ed., pp. 1550–1558). Philadelphia: Lipppincott Williams & Wilkins.

World Health Organization. (1992). *The ICD–10 classification of mental and behavioural disorders: Diagnostic criteria for research.* Geneva: World Health Organization.

9

DANGEROUSNESS RISK ASSESSMENT

B. Thomas Gray
North Texas State Hospital, Vernon, TX

J. Reid Meloy
University of California, San Diego

Michael T. Jumes
North Texas State Hospital, Vernon, TX

Issues of dangerousness arise in a variety of forensic contexts, including the commitment and release of patients to and from psychiatric hospitals, the management of defendants found not guilty by reason of insanity, death penalty cases, the evaluation of criminally violent predators (e.g., *Kansas v. Hendricks*, 1997), and decisions concerning probation and parole. There is a widespread notion that violence toward others is typically linked with mental illness. Such a perception is not without foundation; population surveys have consistently revealed a higher base rate of interpersonal aggression in persons with mental illness than in the population as a whole (Swanson, Holzer, Ganzu, & Jono, 1990; Swanson et al., 2006), although a critical aggravating variable among the mentally ill who are violent is alcohol or illicit drug use (Steadman et al., 1998). Often characters in the media are portrayed as engaging in a type of violence described as *predatory,* defined by a planned attack during which the aggressor is emotionless and often quite calm. This is distinguished from the other and more common type of violence, often labeled *affective*. In this latter mode, the actor responds to a perceived threat in an emotion-laden fashion with intense autonomic arousal, only intending to reduce or eliminate the perceived threat (Meloy, 2006). The psychosocial differences between these two modes of violence—notwithstanding their striking biological distinctions—are often clinically obvious through careful scrutiny of the violence history and behaviors at the time of the offense. Understanding the differences in modes of violence is essential when opining about an individual's dangerousness.

Given the apparent relationship between mental state and dangerousness, it is not surprising that the opinions of mental health professionals (MHPs) concerning the risk of future acts of dangerousness are often a crucial component in the decisions that are made.

This is true even with the diversity of situations in which assessment of dangerousness arises. This chapter reviews information pertaining to dangerousness risk assessment, with special reference to forensic settings, and discusses the important contribution of the Rorschach to such assessments.[1]

RISK ASSESSMENT

Actuarial Versus Clinical Prediction

For many years, clinical judgment was considered the sine qua non of mental health practice, including that within forensic contexts. For almost as many years, questions concerning the accuracy of clinical judgement have been raised (Dawes, Faust, & Meehl, 2002; Meehl, 1954). A number of studies have demonstrated the increased accuracy of actuarial instruments when compared with the judgment of even well-trained and experienced clinicians (e.g., Gardner, Lidz, Mulvey, & Shaw, 1996; Grove & Meehl, 1996; McNiel, Gregory, Lam, Binder, & Sullivan, 2003). An extreme position was taken by Quinsey, Harris, Rice, and Cormier (1998) in *Violent Offenders*. These authors argued for the exclusive virtues of actuarial assessment: "What we are advising is not the addition of actuarial methods to existing practice, but rather the complete replacement of existing practice with actuarial methods" (p. 171).

Such a radical stance has effectively renewed the controversy, and no clear consensus has yet emerged. Litwack (2001), for example, argued that the distinction between clinical judgment and the actuarial approach is, in fact, rather blurred. He noted that much of the scoring used in actuarial assessment involves at least a reasonable degree of clinical judgment (see Douglas, Cox, & Webster, 1999). Despite considerable evidence supporting the utility of actuarially oriented instruments, a growing number of clinicians have argued for inclusion of more clinical data in risk assessment (e.g., Douglas & Skeem, 2005). Indeed, placing an emphasis on the nomothetic while ignoring idiographic information eliminates valuable information. As Parry and Drogin (2001) have observed, "Despite the number of variables that can be addressed [using actuarial instruments], the aggregate determination does not wholly account for the individual involved" (p. 24).

We support such an integrated approach, which takes into account both nomothetic and idiographic data (Stricker & Gold, 1999). Furthermore, Rorschach results are in many instances ideal for assisting the trier of fact in understanding how the subject in question operates internally. Rorschach data are intensely personal, and help us know the permutation of an individual's internal psychology that may be related to violence risk. There are Rorschach indices that provide better understanding of such variables as an individual's ability to modulate affect, control impulses, represent others, and organize their thinking, as well as to identify any tendency toward hypervigilance, mood disorder, or psychosis. Use of such data allows the MHP to elucidate more fully the exact nature of a subject's risk of potential dangerousness, as well as how best to manage that risk

---

[1]Use of the Rorschach in evaluating for suicidality is beyond the scope of this chapter. Fowler and his colleagues (Fowler, Hilsenroth, & Piers, 2001; Fowler, Piers, Hilsenroth, & Padawer, 2001) have reviewed this topic.

(Heilbrun, 1997). Although the Rorschach does not improve the incremental validity of a probability estimate of risk based on a large group of individuals, it is idiographically sensitive—which actuarial instruments are not—to the unique characteristics of a subject that may be related to violence risk. To assume otherwise is to wrongfully conclude that all individuals within a nomothetic validation group are exactly the same.

Previous Research

Johnny Baxtrom was one of many offenders being held in hospitals for the criminally insane during the 1960s. Despite the fact that they were at or near the ends of their criminal sentences, Baxtrom and his peers were being confined because they were considered too dangerous (presumably as a result of their mental illnesses) to be released to the public. Suit was filed by Baxtrom, which eventually reached the U.S. Supreme Court. The Justices ruled such a system of confinement to be unconstitutional (*Baxtrom v. Herold,* 1966), and Baxtrom and 100 others were released to the community or transferred to other, less secure hospitals. The fact that they had been restricted to a maximum security facility clearly implied that these individuals had been determined to be dangerous, yet the actual rate of aggression over the next 4 years was only about 20% (Steadman, 1973; Steadman & Keveles, 1972).[2] As an aside, this finding also serves to illustrate the strong tendency in most, if not all, predictions of violence risk to err on the side of caution by incorrectly identifying nondangerous individuals as potentially dangerous (a false positive error with minimal consequence), rather than mistakenly labeling dangerous individuals as not dangerous (a false negative error with maximal consequence). This emotional bias is primarily due to the simple fact that it is virtually impossible to demonstrate that a false positive prediction has occurred, whereas a false negative error can yield results that are salient and potentially horrific.

The results of the Baxtrom studies were part of the evidence that led an American Psychological Association (APA, 1978) task force to state that "the validity of psychological predictions of dangerous behavior, at least in the sentencing and release situation ... is extremely poor" (p. 1110). Similarly dismal commentary was found in an *amicus curie* American Psychiatric Association brief filed in *Barefoot v. Estelle* (1983). At the beginning of the 1980s, Monahan (1981) reviewed the five existing studies that had evaluated clinical judgement. He concluded: "We know very little about how accurately violent behavior may be predicted under many circumstances" (p. 37). He reiterated this point in 1984 when he observed that MHPs' predictions about violence among individuals with mental illness were correct in only about one of three cases (Monahan, 1984).

Such negative views about violence prediction could have led to the abandonment of mental health testimony in cases of dangerousness. The dilemma, however, was legally put to rest by the U.S. Supreme Court in *Barefoot v. Estelle* (1983). The most widely quoted element of the opinion likened denial of psychiatric testimony concerning a de-

---

[2]Although lower than predicted, it is important to note that a 20% rate of aggression is distinctly higher than that of the U. S. population as a whole. This figure is almost identical to the frequency of self-reported violence found in the survey of Swanson and his colleagues (Swanson et al., 2006).

fendant's potential dangerousness to "disinventing the wheel." A more appropriate metaphor may have been to "disinvent the Szondi test." The logic was that juries composed of laypersons are routinely asked to make decisions involving potential dangerousness. Thus, to disallow information that might be offered by mental health experts made no sense.

Reframing the Question

The extensive and negative commentary of the 1970s and early 1980s regarding MHPs' accuracy in predicting dangerousness had the beneficial effect of stimulating research, ultimately improving the way in which risk assessment is conducted. This was greatly enhanced by two important changes in the way these issues are conceptualized. First, dangerousness is more effectively characterized in terms of relative risk rather than as a simple "yes or no" decision. In other words, rather than determining whether an individual is potentially dangerous (a dichotomous answer), the question is, "What is the relative likelihood that the person may commit a particular kind of violent act within a specified time frame in the future?" This has been extended to include the nature of the risk being assessed, the time frame involved, and the psycholegal context (i.e., release to the community, inpatient hospitalization, incarceration, etc.). In other words, it is more accurate and achievable to predict that an individual is at high, moderate, or low risk of a specific sort of violent behavior within a specific environment and over a specified period of time.

Violence Risk Research

Numerous studies of factors contributing to risk of violent behavior have been conducted in a variety of settings over the past 30 years. These include examination of the risk of recidivism and violence committed by mentally ill inmates released to the community from prison settings (Bonta, Law, & Hanson, 1998; Gagliardi, Lovell, Peterson, & Jemelka, 2004); potential violence committed by psychiatric patients who presented to a hospital emergency room (Lidz, Mulvey, & Gardner, 1993); aggression by patients within psychiatric facilities (e.g., Daffern, Howells, Ogloff, & Lee, 2005; McNiel & Binder, 1994); and, especially, violence committed by patients released to the community from psychiatric hospitals (Douglas, Ogloff, Nicholls, & Grant, 1999; Monahan et al., 2001, 2005).

One of the most important studies focusing on the violence of the civilly committed mentally ill was conducted in the 1990s under the auspices of the MacArthur Foundation (Monahan et al., 2001, 2005). Directed by John Monahan and Henry Steadman, a total of 1,316 English-speaking patients with diagnoses of thought, mood, substance use, or personality disorder, and ranging in age from 18 to 40 years, were followed carefully for a year after being discharged from one of three psychiatric hospitals. Official records were consulted to document arrests and mental health contacts, and each patient was interviewed 10 weeks postdischarge, and every 10 weeks thereafter for a year. In addition, at the time of enrollment, each patient identified a close relative or friend to serve as a collateral informant, and these individuals were also interviewed regularly as a means of validating the patients' self-reports. A battery of diagnostic tests was also administered to each individual. Variables measured were grouped into four broad categories (Monahan & Steadman, 1994): Dispositional (demographics, personality functioning including impulsivity and psychopathy, and cognitive functioning); Historical (social, psychiatric, criminal, and violence histories); Contextual (stress, social supports, means for violence); and Clinical (psychiatric issues, including substance abuse; also see Gacono & Evans, preface, this vol.).

Almost one in five (18.7%) of the subjects committed one or more violent acts (defined as assault causing injury, sexual assault, or assault or threat involving a weapon[3]) within the first 20 weeks of their hospital discharge. Psychopathy, as measured by the Psychopathy Checklist: Screening Version (Hart, Cox, & Hare, 1995; Hart, Hare, & Forth, 1994) was the single best predictor of postdischarge violence. Prior violence, regardless of the way it was measured, was also a strong predictor, as was substance abuse/dependence. At first blush, ethnicity appeared to have at least moderate predictive value, with African Americans exhibiting a notably higher level of violence. However, when socioeconomic status was controlled, this effect disappeared, indicating that what was being seen was the impact of poverty.

Despite the variety of contexts in which violence risk has been studied, a few general conclusions can be drawn. It is commonly said that past behavior is the best predictor of future behavior and, indeed, a history of aggression is one of the strongest indicators of increased dangerousness risk. This is a finding that has been consistently found across most, if not all, settings. Substance use represents a significant risk factor as well, particularly use of alcohol and/or psychostimulants (especially cocaine and amphetamine). This finding is also robust across most settings, although the extent to which substance use may be moderated in institutions such as prisons or psychiatric hospitals, where access to alcohol and other drugs is (at least in theory) more limited, is not entirely clear.

Finally, psychopathy, as measured by Psychopathy Checklist–Revised (PCL–R; Hare, 1991, 2003), appears to be the strongest predictor of greater risk for violence toward others (Gacono & Bodholdt, 2001; Hare, 2003; Salekin, Rogers, & Sewell, 1996; Serin & Brown, 2000) if strength is measured in proportion of explainable variance. This finding is consistent with theoretical and empirical data demonstrating substantially higher rates of interpersonal violence, especially predatory or instrumental violence, among psychopaths (Meloy, 2006; Serin & Brown, 2000). It has also been consistently shown that Factor II of the PCL–R (chronic antisocial behavior) has more predictive value for aggression than does Factor I (aggressive narcissism), although variance accounted for is typically less than 10% (Belfrage, Fransson, & Strand, 2000; Grann, Långström, Tengström, & Kullgren, 1999; Gray et al., 2003; Salekin et al., 1996).

Although yielding data of great value, use of the PCL–R does require specialized training (Gacono, 2000, 2005). Adequate records documenting the individual's personal history are also a prerequisite, yet these are unfortunately not always available. Perhaps

---

[3]This outcome variable, like that used in most research pertaining to violence risk, is characterized as a dichotomy; this has the unfortunate effect of equating acts such as a passing threat as opposed to a homicidal attack. Although such an approach facilitates calculation of many actuarial statistics, the variance in the outcome measure is reduced, making it more difficult to demonstrate accuracy in prediction.

in part for these reasons, psychopathy has not always been well evaluated in studies of violence risk.

PSYCHOLOGICAL TESTING IN RISK ASSESSMENT

Psychological instruments have been developed for the purpose of evaluating general violence risk, and the two most widely used of these, the Violence Risk Appraisal Guide (VRAG) and the HCR–20 Version 2, are briefly reviewed here. Several additional instruments have been designed specifically for sex offender populations, such as the Sex Offender Risk Appraisal Guide (Quinsey et al., 1998), a younger sibling of the VRAG (see later); the STATIC–99 (Hanson & Thornton, 2000); and the Minnesota Sex Offender Screening Tool–Revised (Hanlon, Larson, & Zacher, 1999). These are not considered in this discussion (see Campbell, 2004; DeClue, 2002, 2005).

Both the VRAG and the HCR–20 rely heavily on variables from the historical domain of Monahan and Steadman's (1994; Monahan et al., 2001) model, as well as psychopathy and related personality factors (dispositional domain) such as impulsivity (see Gacono, 2000). This is disturbing in that by definition, historical variables are fixed and unchangeable (i.e., static), and psychopathy is widely regarded as essentially untreatable and therefore also static. Dynamic variables, on the other hand, located in the clinical and contextual domains, are often amenable to change, and therefore have potential implications for treatment and management. The latter are frequently more readily evaluated with traditional psychological tests, including the Rorschach. As Gacono and Evans (preface, this vol.) have observed:

> In the process of choosing assessment methods for forensic evaluations, we emphasize the need for using multiple assessment methods, such as review of collateral materials and records, clinical and semistructured interviewing, standardized psychological testing, and so forth. For example, some methods, such as the PCL–R (Hare, 2003) and other semistructured interviews, are useful for collecting and quantifying certain dispositional and historical variables, whereas other methods, such as the RIM and MMPI–2, add to understanding certain clinical and dispositional variables.

For example, a subject being evaluated for risk may have a score of 23 on the PCL–R, locating him nomothetically in the range of moderate psychopathy. Yet, his violence history indicates that it is almost always preceded by an agitated depression, which he attempts to self-medicate with amphetamine, but instead results in a psychotic decompensation with paranoid features. The *dynamic* evaluation of this subject's risk would clinically benefit from indices on the MMPI–2 that indicate his current level of depression, energy, and paranoia (Scales 2, 6 and 9, and other relevant subscales, such as the Harris and Lingoes and other content scales); as well as Rorschach indices of psychotic decompensation ($M-$, $X-\%$, *WSum6 Special Scores, PTI,* and other cognitive processing variables). Both tests, when used over a period of time if the subject were incarcerated and drug free, would also help to determine whether his depression and subsequent psychotic decompensation were solely attributable to a history of amphetamine use, or the drug use was secondary to a naturally occurring major mental disorder.

Violence Risk Appraisal Guide (VRAG)

The Violence Risk Appraisal Guide (VRAG) was under development at about the same time the MacArthur violence study was initiated. The initial validation study included 866 mentally disordered men, mostly White, after they had been released from confinement in a maximum security forensic hospital or a prison in Canada. The criterion variable was defined as a violent act that led to the individual either facing a new charge or being returned to the forensic hospital in lieu of being charged (Quinsey et al., 1998). This is a rather restrictive outcome measure, as acts of aggression that escaped the notice of authorities could not be accounted for in any way.

The VRAG model is entirely probabilistic. The instrument consists of 12 items, including a PCL–R rating of psychopathy. Each item is weighted (full scoring criteria were first published in Quinsey et al, 1998), and the scores summed. Total scores are divided into nine groups, and actuarial data is provided showing the probabilities of violent recidivism for each risk group at 7 and 10 years postrelease. The developmental study yielded a recidivism base rate of .31, with a modest sensitivity of .40. The overall hit rate was.74, however. Using ROC analyses, six additional studies have yielded consistent results, with areas under the curve ranging between .72 and .77 (see Quinsey, Harris, Rice, & Cormier, 2005, for a review).

HCR–20 Version 2

Like the VRAG, the HCR–20 was developed in Canada using forensic psychiatric patients. The name is an acronym based on the content of the 20 items that constitute the instrument: Ten are Historical (past) variables, five are Clinical (present), and five relate to Risk Management (future), lending a nice chronological flavor to the process. Each item is coded on a 3-point Likert scale ranging from 0 to 2, much like the PCL–R. The HCR–20 has been used in a wide variety of studies across different settings, and in several different countries in North America and Europe (Douglas & Webster, 1999; Grann, Belfrage, & Tengström, 2000; Gray et al., 2003).

At the outset the authors comment, "This manual for the HCR–20 is a guide to assessment, and not a formal psychological test" (Webster, Douglas, Eaves, & Hart, 1997, p. 1). And, indeed, it is important to note that no norms for this instrument have been published. Nonetheless, a number of studies in several countries have adopted an actuarial approach in evaluating the performance of the instrument, including comparison with the VRAG and the PCL–R (Belfrage et al., 2000; Douglas & Webster, 1999; Grann et al., 2000; Gray et al., 2003). Results for all three instruments have been generally positive, with all showing good predictive validity, and no clear consensus emerging as to which might be most accurate. Indeed, there is a good deal of evidence showing that the HCR–20 and the PCL have considerable shared variance between them (Douglas & Webster, 1999; Gray et al., 2003), particularly between the PCL–R and the HCR–20 Historical and Clinical scales. Given that psychopathy is one of the HCR–20 Historical scale items, and other HCR–20 items, such as impulsivity, also appear as criteria on the PCL–R, such a result is not surprising. One might expect similar results with respect to the VRAG as well.

Personality Tests: The MMPI/MMPI–2 and the PAI

Despite the lengthy and extensive history of research associated with the MMPI and its more recent offspring, the MMPI–2, little has been done linking MMPI–2 scales with aggression, violence, or dangerousness risk (see Heilbrun & Heilbrun, 1995, for a review). Some evidence was presented suggesting that the Anger Content scale, and a composite of Scales F, 4, and 9, might be correlated with aggressive tendencies, although the predictive value was slight (O'Laughlin & Schill, 1994). Verona and Carbonell (2000) found the Overcontrolled Hostility scale useful in discriminating women offenders categorized as violent on a single occasion from those who showed repeated violence or no violence. This finding has apparently not been replicated, however.

Development of the new Personality Psychopathology Five (PSY–5) scales for the MMPI–2 (Harkness, McNulty, Ben-Porath, & Graham, 2002) included an Aggressiveness (*AGGR*) scale. The scale "focuses on offensive and instrumental aggression. Persons high on PSY–5 Aggressiveness may enjoy intimidating others and may use aggression as a tool to accomplish goals" (Harkness et al., 2002, p. 3). Although Sharpe and Desai (2001) found some utility of *AGGR* in predicting aggression with a sample of college students, the empirical support for this scale thus far remains rather scant.

Several studies have examined the use of the Personality Assessment Inventory (PAI) in identifying potential aggression, and thus increased risk for violence. Focusing primarily on the Antisocial and Aggression scales, much of the extant research appears to have been in the context of correctional settings (e.g., Caperton, Edens, & Johnson, 2004; Morey & Quigley, 2002). Although the generalizability of this research beyond these settings is unknown, Douglas, Hart, and Kropp (2001) found sufficient evidence to warrant consideration of the PAI in forensic settings.

APPLICATIONS OF THE RORSCHACH

There is a growing data base of literature incorporating Rorschach data in responding to psycholegal questions (Cunliffe & Gacono, chap. 17, this vol.; Gacono, Gacono, & Evans, chap. 16, this vol; Gacono, Meloy, & Bridges, chap. 18, this vol.; Gacono & Gacono, chap. 20, this vol.; Singer et al., chap. 21, this vol.). Information from the Rorschach Comprehensive System (Exner, 1993, 2001), together with that accumulated using other assessment methods, is of great value in clarifying an individual's present clinical functioning and the influence it has on potential for violence risk.

For example, reality testing and perceptual accuracy indices ($X-\%$, $F + \%$, $X+\%$) provide clues as to degree to which the subject perceives reality in conventional ways and how the individual discriminates between internal and external stimuli. In a violence risk context, these data help us understand the subject's propensity to override others' actual behaviors and intents with their own fantasies and idiosyncractic interpretations.

To what degree a subject experiences conscious emotion, the nature of their emotional experiences, how well they modulate emotions, their ability to organize behavior despite emotions, the presence of anxiety and the nature of an individual's capacity to bond to others (*FC:CF + C, Y, V, C', Afr, S, T, Blends, Pure C, AdjD*) are all relevant to violence risk formulation. These RIM indices provide suggestions as to whether violence is more likely to be affective rather than predatory, and therefore whether it can be modulated through various psychopharmacological interventions. For example, subjects largely devoid of socialized emotion (Meloy, 1988) and chronically detached will have no inhibitions to their aggression toward objects and are unlikely to be treatable from a risk management perspective.

The RIM provides information about interpersonal relationships. To what degree do the subjects have an interest in others, expect cooperation, depend on or remains detached from others, and how do they internally represent others as objects? (*COP, AG, GHR:PHR, Food, T, Human Content, Pure H, PER, Isolation Index*). Most of these variables, if within the normal range, would inhibit risk of violence. If the subject had been violent, and produced normative interpersonal indices, then it would suggest an ego-dystonic aggressive act and would implicate external factors and situational circumstances as the precipitants of the violence (Revitch & Schlesinger, 1981). Individuals devoid of such interest and impaired in their ability to internally represent others in whole, real, and meaningful ways—psychopathology that occurs along a schizoid-psychopathic dimension—would suggest the absence of internal constraints against violence. The presence of paranoia (*HVI*) would add a dimension of hypervigilance, and could suggest the psychodynamic projection of persecutory objects onto others. Conflicting Rorschach variables (e.g., *Food* responses and an elevated *Isolation Index*) suggest intrapsychic dilemmas concerning dependency and avoidance.

Self-perception or the degree to which individuals realistically appraise themselves and value themselves in relation to others (*Egocentricity Index, Rf, SumV, FD*) contributes to violence risk. Is there a perception of self as deeply injured (*MOR*)? Are psychosomatic preoccupation and dysphoric feeling predominant characteristics of the personality structure (*An + Xy*)? Are they self-absorbed and pathologically narcissistic? Is there a sense of failed narcissism or grandiosity (*Rf + MOR*)? Is there a capacity for insight despite the self-focus? Do they unrealistically devalue or aggrandize their sense of self as a defense against other emotional states? Were any of these characteristics motivating factors in their past violent behavior, and therefore predictive of motivation in the future? Or has treatment modified some of these characteristics when Rorschach data are compared over time?

Finally, the RIM provides clues to the degree to which subjects organize their behavior, demonstrate controls over impulses, volitionally modify behavior, and adapt to changing circumstance (*D, AdjD, CDI, EA, EBPer*). A history of violence in the absence of such normative data suggests impulsive, reactive, and perhaps affective aggression. A history of violence in the presence of such normative data suggests a pattern of Rorschach variables apparent among psychopaths (Gacono & Meloy, 1994), and suggests violence that is deliberate, planned, perhaps premeditated, and modally predatory (see Young, Justice, & Erdberg, 1999).

Measures such as the PCL–R, the VRAG, and the HCR–20 provide information that correlates with Rorschach data regarding behaviors and attitudes. "Simply stated, multiple methods assess different but complementary personality dimensions" (Gacono, Jumes, & Gray, chap. 11, this vol.).

As with other widely used tests of personality, such as the MMPI, the Rorschach was initially developed with purposes in mind other than prediction of aggression or other forms of dangerousness risk. Nevertheless, a number of early workers recognized potential applications in this area, and either implicitly or explicitly identified Rorschach variables that pertained to constructs related to aggression in general, and dangerousness risk in particular (see Gacono & Meloy, 1994, esp. pp. 260–263, for a brief review).

White Space

White Space (S) responses have traditionally been considered to indicate anger and hostility, oppositional attitudes, and potential for aggression. Ingram (1954) found that S had limited predictive value for aggressive behavior under certain circumstances, and work by Carlson and Drehmer (1984) lent some support to this interpretation. Bandura (1954) also found that S responses were linked to some extent with oppositional behavior in a sample of high school students. More recently, however, Frank (1993) concluded that using S as an indicator of oppositionality was not supported, and that $CF + C > FC$ was a much better predictor of aggression (Frank, 1994).

AG and *Extended Aggression* Scores

The *Aggressive Movement* (*AG*) score was developed by Exner (1986) as part of the Comprehensive System of Rorschach scoring, representing an amalgam of various prior efforts to characterize responses that included aggressive content. *AG* is limited to aggressive actions occurring in the present tense in the response. Citing research that was, for the most part, unpublished, and with relatively limited empirical support, Exner (1993) suggested that an increased frequency of *AG* scores was correlated with a greater likelihood of aggressive behavior. However, this relationship has not been found in forensic populations (Gacono, Gacono, Meloy, & Baity, 2005).

Meloy and Gacono (1992a) concluded that Exner's (1986) practice of limiting the characterization of expressions of aggression in Rorschach responses to only one score "has grossly reduced the usefulness of aggression responses to the Rorschach as a source of nomothetic comparison and idiographic understanding" (Gacono & Meloy, 1994, p. 263). Based in no small part on the earlier works of authorities such as Rapaport, Schafer, and Holt, they proposed four additional special scores in addition to traditional Comprehensive System scores: *Aggressive Potential* (*AgPot*), *Aggressive Content* (*AgC*), *Aggressive Past* (*AgPast*), and *Sado Masochism* (*SM*; see Gacono et al., 2005).

Comparative studies have revealed that antisocial and psychopathic offenders, for whom aggression is presumably more ego-syntonic, tend to produce fewer *AG* responses than other groups. However, individuals with *DSM* Axis II diagnoses often associated with increased rates of aggression (i.e., Antisocial, Borderline, and Narcissistic Personality Disorders) generally produced more *AgC* and *AgPast* (Gacono

& Meloy, 1994; Gacono, Meloy, & Berg, 1992; Meloy & Gacono, 1992a; Gacono et al., 2005).[4] Other studies have also generally supported the utility of the expanded set of Aggression scores (Baity & Hilsenroth, 2002; Mihura & Nathan-Montano, 2001), although some of the research has been reported in unpublished dissertations (e.g., Pointkowski, 2001; White, 1999). Hartmann, Norbech, and Gronnerod (2006) found that *AgPast* responses accumulated incrementally in the prediction of violent offenders being either psychopathic or nonpsychopathic, and *AgC* accumulated incrementally in the prediction of subjects being either violent offenders or inpatient schizophrenics when entered into a logistic regression equation after other CS variables. They also found that there was no significant difference in *AG* scores among the violent offenders, inpatient schizophrenics, and university students, supporting the notion that *AG* alone is not a useful predictor of risk of aggression.

Gacono and Meloy (1994) have further developed applications of the *Extended Aggression* scores within the context of the CS to include idiographic interpretation. Ratios of *Ma:Mp* may be informative with respect to the use of fantasy in rehearsing aggressive acts (see Meloy, 1988). Extreme *FM* elevations among serial murderers are likely measuring certain aspects of the obsessive-compulsive nature of their killings (Gacono, Meloy, & Bridges, chap. 18, this vol.; Meloy, Gacono, & Kenney, 1994). *AgPot* responses absent color or shading determinants may be more indicative of predatory (as opposed to affective) aggressive drives. Further, some cases have been documented in which individuals gave *AgC* responses that were representations of weapons they had used in committing assaultive acts (Gacono & Meloy, 1994). There have also been a few anecdotal cases in which Card II has evoked images and memories of an actual homicide in the subject's history.

Psychopathy

Gacono and Meloy (1994, 2002; Meloy & Gacono, 2000) have suggested a modal Rorschach profile for psychopaths. This included features such as: a simplistic, well-defended problem-solving style (*Lambda* >1), no indication of behavioral disorganization (*D* and *AdjD* $\geq$ 0), poor modulation of affect (*FC* < *CF* + *C*), pathological narcissism (*Rf* > 0), chronic emotional detachment (*T* = 0), a predominance of part object representations of others (*Hd* + *[Hd]* > *H* + *[H]*), grandiosity (*W:M* > 3:1), formal thought disorder (elevated *Wsum6*), and borderline reality testing (*X–%* > 25). Although separately these indices are not specific to psychopathy, and were not statistically derived like other CS constellations, the picture that emerges is consistent with the prototypical psychopath (Hare, 2003): an angry and detached individual who experiences relatively little emotion of any depth, exploits others, is quite narcissistic, and thinks and perceives in unusual and odd ways.

---

[4]Research on the *SM* score has been distinctly limited due to the requirement that the subject be observed during administration of the Rorschach. Thus, it obviously cannot be scored retrospectively.

Additional Scales

Standard CS scoring, including *Extended Aggression* scores, have been used together with special scales developed by Kwawer (1979, 1980; Kwawer, P. Lerner, H. Lerner, & Sugarman, 1980) and the Defense scales of Cooper and Arnow (1986; Cooper, Perry, & Arnow, 1988) in a series of studies demonstrating their utility in gaining a deeper understanding of the individual being examined, as well as groups of such individuals (see Meloy, Acklin, Gacono, Murray, & Peterson, 1997). Gacono reported an idiographic Rorschach study of a sexual homicide perpetrator, and Meloy (1992) did so on Sirhan Sirhan. Meloy and Gacono have similarly examined in detail the dynamics of a borderline psychopath (Meloy & Gacono, 1993) and a psychotic and psychopathic sex offender (Meloy & Gacono, 1992b). More nomothetically oriented studies have included offenders convicted of sexual homicides (Meloy et al., 1994); Antisocial Personalities (Gacono & Meloy, 1991; Gacono, Meloy, & Heaven, 1990); psychopaths (Gacono & Meloy, 1993, 2002; Meloy & Gacono, 1998, 2000); and a comparison of psychopaths, sexual homicide perpetrators, and pedophiles (Gacono, Meloy, & Bridges, 2000, 2007; Huprich, Gacono, Schneider, & Bridges, 2004).

CASE EXAMPLE

Stanley[5] is a never-married White male who was in his early 40s at the time he was arrested on a misdemeanor charge of stalking.[6] He was evaluated for trial competency on three occasions by the same examiner, and was later referred by his treating psychiatrist for assessment of dangerousness risk. Considerable psychological test data was accumulated during the course of these evaluations.

Little was known concerning his birth, early development, or family background. It appeared, however, that his parents divorced when Stanley was 6 years old. His mother subsequently remarried twice, both times to men with serious alcohol problems. He completed high school in a timely fashion, and a few years later went on to attend a technical school, funded by his mother; he did not complete the course. He has no record of sustained employment, and at the time of his arrest he was living alone in a small house paid for by his mother.

Some 10 years earlier, he had apparently developed a "friendly" relationship with a couple living nearby, which in short order led to him becoming obsessed with the wife. The woman's husband confronted him about the time and attention Stanley was devoting to her. Stanley became enraged, and one report indicates that he retrieved a handgun with which he threatened the husband. This may have been the precipitating event that led to his first known mental health care, a state hospital placement that yielded a diagnosis of Schizophrenia. He was discharged after less than 2 weeks, and there is no indication that he received any follow-up care.

---

[5]Identifying features of this case have been masked to protect the confidentiality of the individuals involved.

[6]Legislative actions since the time of Stanley's arrest have raised the severity of the charge to the felony level.

At some point over the next several years, he developed an obsession with a media personality, and eventually began habitually showing up at her scheduled public appearances. He was arrested after he simultaneously sent flowers to her and to his first victim, with whom he had apparently maintained some (unwanted) contact, as well. He was found incompetent to stand trial, and eventually the charges against him were dropped as he had already been held for a period longer than the maximum sentence he could have received. However, before he could be released from jail, he was committed to a state hospital on grounds of dangerousness to others, and was quickly transferred to a maximum security hospital.

Testing conducted while he was being held on the competency issue was most helpful in elucidating the question of Stanley's risk for engaging in future acts of violence, either in a less restrictive hospital or in the community if he were to be released. His intellectual functioning was measured in the Low Average range (WAIS–III Full Scale IQ = 82). He produced a self-serving MMPI–2 protocol (*L* scale *T*-score = 78), consistent with an elevated Desirability scale (*BR* = 89) on his MCMI–III profile. There were no clinically significant MMPI–2 elevations (3–1 codetype), and his MCMI–III produced a spike on the Narcissism scale. The latter was clarified by his PCL–R and Rorschach results. On the former, he attained a high score on Factor I (90th percentile), but not on Factor II (12th percentile), and his Total Score was slightly below average for male forensic patients (33rd percentile).

Our understanding of Stanley was more fully appreciated with inclusion of data from his valid Rorschach (*R* = 28, *L* = 1.15). The most striking features were the disordered thinking (W*Sum6* = 38), and a marked degree of self-involvement (*Egocentricity Index* = 0.68). *Special scores* included several Level 2 *DV*s and *DR*s, as well as a Level 1 *INC*. Given this, it was not surprising to find poor reality testing (*X–%* = 36), as well, which was particularly disturbing given that both of his *S* responses were *FQ–*. This was likely also related to an inability to adequately read and interpret social cues and a tendency for inappropriate behavior (*GHR:PHR* = 2:6). He maintained a rather narrow focus of attention (*W:D* = 4:17), which perhaps helped him to maintain a sense of control, yet also contributed to the apparent deficits in his interactions with others.

Stanley's elevated *Egocentricity Index* was not unexpected given his MCMI–III and PCL–R Factor I scores. The *Egocentricity Index* score derived entirely from the presence of 19 pairs in a 28 response protocol, which somewhat surprisingly contained no reflections. However, he provided two responses that might be considered "spoiled reflections," such as the following on Card X:

Free Association: Two Mexicos, real Mexicos (D9)

Inquiry: ... Oh, the red right here, and this'd be where California hooks on to it, and this [points to other side] would be backwards. ... That's the way the land travels, it looks like that on a globe, dipping down south from a north area.

Had one or even both of those responses fully met the criteria to be scored as reflections, his Egocentricity Index would have been even more elevated.

Within the context of a high degree of narcissism, it is no surprise that he was apparently experiencing little or no subjective distress, either chronically ($AdjD = -1$) or situationally ($D = -1$). His developmental history of inconsistent primary attachments suggests that Stanley's protocol may well demonstrate a self-focus based principally on simplifying a detached, unpredictable, and quite chaotic interpersonal sphere, the need for which could have been exacerbated by his disordered thinking.

He produced 3 *COP* and no *AG* responses, which might indicate that his limited known history of aggression was ego-syntonic. However, his protocol contained none of the *Extended Aggression* scores, suggesting a reduced likelihood of violent behavior. There was a strong indication that Stanley often retreats into fantasy ($Ma:Mp = 1:3$), and we postulate that he is primarily at risk for danger to others only when someone intrudes into his fantasy world, at which time his affective processes fuel harm-producing behaviors. Indeed, during the several years he has been confined in the maximum security setting, he has been rude and unpleasant on numerous occasions, usually when confronted about (nonaggressive) inappropriate behavior. However, during that time, he has never aggressed toward either staff or other patients, nor has he made any attempt to contact any of his victims.

His VRAG score was between 2 and 3 (the range due to uncertainties concerning his early history), which placed him in VRAG category 5 (56th percentile). Compared with a group of predominately White Canadian males, the probability of violent recidivism for individuals with scores equivalent to Stanley's was .35 over 7 years, and .48 over 10 years (Quinsey et al., 1998). Likewise, his HCR–20 data showed an important but not overwhelming history of factors contributing to violence risk (11 of 20 possible points), and important clinical (lack of insight, active symptoms, and unresponsive to treatment) and risk (unfeasible plans, no personal support, and stress) factors. Both of these instruments suggested a moderate degree of dangerousness risk. However, it was only through use of other testing, the Rorschach, in particular, that the psychodynamic underpinnings of his potential for harm to others could be elucidated.

CONCLUSIONS

The question of an individual's risk of committing violent acts arises in a variety of situations, many of them forensic, and MHPs are typically accorded considerable respect in formulating opinions on these issues. Some have argued that only actuarial tools should be used in developing and rendering such opinions, without any influence from clinical judgement (e.g., Quinsey et al., 1998). It is critical to keep in mind that doing so effectively eliminates from consideration a wealth of data that can be used in developing a more thorough understanding of the individual involved, of what may cause that individual to behave dangerously, and how best to manage such behaviors. As Parry and Drogin (2000) have observed, "No matter how carefully a forensic expert assembles the available information, there is still going to be a significant leap in reaching conclusions about a particular individual" (pp. 24–25).

Actuarial data ultimately provide estimates of violence risk for groups of people, not for individuals. As an example, it would be an egregious error for us to have asserted that, based on his VRAG score, Stanley had a 35% chance of violent recidivism within a 7-year period. We could only realistically opine that Stanley fits within a group of individuals who have a 35% chance of violent recidivism within a 7-year period. His idiographic Rorschach data, however, assisted us in understanding the permutations of his internal operations of potential value in risk managing his potential for violence. Without such individual data, actuarial estimates truncate our knowledge. Consider two offenders with the same VRAG scores, one psychopathic and with a history of predatory violence, the other nonpsychopathic but with a lengthy history of affective violence. Absent data beyond the VRAG, we would have no way of knowing that very different risk management approaches would be in order: for the psychopath, intensive supervision would be the rule; for the nonpsychopath, medication to help reduce his impulsivity might be of great value. In both cases, the Rorschach would inform us about the internal structure and dynamics of the individual, particularly when integrated with other clinical testing.

Heilbrun and Heilbrun (1995) concluded, "The integration of the MMPI–2 into risk assessment presently shows promise but little actualization" (p. 173). A decade ago, the same might have been said concerning the Rorschach. The situation has substantially improved, and approaches have been developed to enhance the utility of the Rorschach in the assessment and risk management of violence.

REFERENCES

American Psychological Association. (1978). Report of the task force on the role of psychology in the criminal justice system. *American Psychologist, 33*, 1099–1133.

Baity, M. R., & Hilsenroth, M. J. (1999). Rorschach aggression variables: A study of reliability and validity. *Journal of Personality Assessment, 72*, 93–110.

Bandura, A. (1954). The Rorschach white space response and "oppositional" behavior. *Journal of Consulting Psychology, 18*, 17–21.

Barefoot v. Estelle, 463 U.S. 880 (1983).

Baxtrom v. Herold, 383 U.S. 107 (1966).

Belfrage, H., Fransson, G., & Strand, S. (2000). Prediction of violence using the HCR–20: A prospective study in two maximum security correctional institutions. *Journal of Forensic Psychiatry, 11*, 167–175.

Bonta, J., Law, M., & Hanson, K. (1998). The prediction of criminal and violent recidivism among mentally disordered offenders: A meta-analysis. *Psychological Bulletin, 123*, 123–142.

Campbell, T. W. (2004). *Assessing sex offenders: Problems and pitfalls*. Springfield, IL: Charles C. Thomas.

Caperton, J. D., Edens, J. F., & Johnson, J. K. (2004). Predicting sex offender institutional adjustment and treatment compliance using the Personality Assessment Inventory. *Psychological Assessment, 16*, 187–191.

Carlson, R. W., & Drehmer, D. E. (1984). Rorschach space response and aggression. *Perceptual and Motor Skills, 58*, 987–988.

Cooper, S., & Arnow, D. (1986). An object relations view of the borderline defenses: A Rorschach analysis. In M. Kissen (Ed.), *Assessing object relations phenomena* (pp. 143–171). Madison, CT: International Universities Press.

Cooper, S., Perry, J., & Arnow, D. (1988). An empirical approach to the study of defense mechanisms: I. Reliability and preliminary validity of the Rorschach defense scale. *Journal of Personality Assessment, 52*, 187–203.

Daffern, M., Howells, K., Ogloff, J., & Lee, J. (2005). Individual characteristics predisposing patients to aggression in a forensic psychiatric hospital. *Journal of Forensic Psychiatry & Psychology, 16*, 729–746.

Dawes, R. M., Faust, D., & Meehl, P. E. (2002). Clinical versus actuarial judgment. In T. Gilovich, D. Griffin, & D. Kahneman (Eds.), *Heuristics and biases: The psychology of intuitive judgment* (pp. 716–729). New York: Cambridge University Press.

DeClue, G. (2002). Avoiding garbage in sex offender re-offense risk assessment: A case study. *Journal of Threat Assessment, 2*(2), 73–92.

DeClue, G. (2005) Avoiding garbage 2: Assessment of risk for sexual violence after long-term treatment. *Journal of Psychiatry & Law, 33*, 179–204.

Douglas, K. S., Cox, D. N., & Webster, C. D. (1999). Violence risk assessment: Science and practice. *Legal and Criminological Psychology, 4*, 149–184.

Douglas, K. S., Hart, S. D., & Kropp, P. R. (2001). Validity of the Personality Assessment Inventory for forensic assessments. *International Journal of Offender Therapy and Comparative Criminology, 45*, 183–197.

Douglas, K. S., Ogloff, J. R. P., Nicholls, T. L., & Grant, I. (1999). Assessing risk for violence among psychiatric patients: The HCR–20 violence risk assessment scheme and the Psychopathy Checklist: Screening Version. *Journal of Consulting and Clinical Psychology, 67*, 917–930.

Douglas, K. S., & Skeem, J. L. (2005). Violence risk assessment: Getting specific about being dynamic. *Psychology, Public Policy, and Law, 11*, 347–383.

Douglas, K. S., & Webster, C. D. (1999). The HCR–20 violence risk assessment scheme: Concurrent validity in a sample of incarcerated offenders. *Criminal Justice and Behavior, 26*, 3–19.

Exner, J. E. (1986). *The Rorschach: A Comprehensive System: Vol. 1. Basic foundations* (2nd ed.). New York: Wiley.

Exner, J. E. (1993). *The Rorschach: A Comprehensive System: Vol. 1. Basic foundations* (3rd ed.). New York: Wiley.

Fowler, J. C., Hilsenroth, M. J., & Piers, C. (2001). An empirical study of seriously disturbed suicidal patients. *Journal of the American Psychoanalytic Association, 49*, 161–186.

Fowler, J. C., Piers, C., Hilsenroth, M. J., Holdwick, D. J., Jr., & Padawer, J. R. (2001). The Rorschach suicide constellation: Assessing various degrees of lethality. *Journal of Personality Assessment. 76*, 333–351.

Frank, G. (1993). On the validity of Rorschach's hypotheses: The relationship of space responses (*S*) to oppositionalism. *Psychological Reports, 72*(3, Pt. 2), 1111–1114.

Frank, G. (1994). On the prediction of aggressive behavior from the Rorschach. *Psychological Reports, 75*(1, Pt. 1), 183–191.

Gacono, C. B. (2000). *The clinical and forensic assessment of psychopathy: A practitioner's guide.* Mahwah, NJ: Lawrence Erlbaum Associates.

Gacono, C. B. (2002). Forensic psychodiagnostic testing. *Journal of Forensic Psychology Practice, 2*(3), 1–10.

Gacono, C. B. (2005). *The clinical and forensic interview schedule for the Hare Psychopathy Checklist: Revised and screening version.* Mahwah, NJ: Lawrence Erlbaum Associates.

Gacono, C. B., Bannatyne-Gacono, L. A., Meloy, J. R., & Baity, M. R. (2005). The Rorschach extended aggression scores. *Rorschachiana, 18*, 164–190.

Gacono, C. B., & Bodholdt, R. (2001). The role of the Psychopathy Checklist–Revised (PCL–R) in risk assessment. *Journal of Threat Assessment, 1*(4), 65–79,

Gacono, C. B., & Meloy, J. R. (1991). A Rorschach investigation of attachment and anxiety in antisocial personality. *Journal of Nervous and Mental Disease, 179*, 546–552.

Gacono, C. B., & Meloy, J. R. (1993). Some thoughts on Rorschach findings and psychophysiology in the psychopath. *British Journal of Projective Psychology, 38*, 42–52.

Gacono, C. B., & Meloy, J. R. (1994). *The Rorschach assessment of aggressive and psychopathic personalities.* Hillsdale, NJ: Lawrence Erlbaum Associates.

Gacono, C. B., & Meloy, J. R. (2002). Assessing antisocial and psychopathic personalities. In J. N. Butcher (Ed.), *Clinical personality assessment: Practical approaches* (pp. 361–375). New York: Oxford University Press.

Gacono, C. B., Meloy, J. R., & Berg, J. (1992). Object relations, defensive operations, and affective states in narcissistic, borderline, and antisocial personality. *Journal of Personality Assessment, 59,* 32–49.

Gacono, C. B., Meloy, J. R., & Bridges, M. R. (2000). A Rorschach comparison of psychopaths, sexual homicide perpetrators, and nonviolent pedophiles: Where angels fear to tread. *Journal of Clinical Psychology, 56,* 757–777.

Gacono, C. B., Meloy, J. R., & Heaven, T. (1990). A Rorschach investigation of narcissism and hysteria in antisocial personality disorder. *Journal of Personality Assessment, 55,* 270–279.

Gagliardi, G. J., Lovell, D., Peterson, P. D., & Jemelka, R. (2004). Forecasting recidivism in mentally ill offenders released from prison. *Law and Human Behavior, 28,* 133–155.

Gardner, W., Lidz, C. W., Mulvey, E. P., & Shaw, E. C. (1996). Clinical versus actuarial predictions of violence in patients with mental illnesses. *Journal of Consulting and Clinical Psychology, 64,* 602–609.

Grann, M., Belfrage, H., & Tengström, A. (2000). Actuarial assessment of risk for violence: Predictive validity of the VRAG and the historical part of the HCR–20. *Criminal Justice and Behavior, 27,* 97–114.

Grann, M., Långström, N., Tengström, A., & Kullgren, G. (1999). Psychopathy (PCL–R) predicts violent recidivism among criminal offenders with personality disorders in Sweden. *Law and Human Behavior, 23,* 205–217.

Gray, N. S., Hill, C., McGleish, A., Timmons, D., MacCulloch, M. J., & Snowden, R. J. (2003). Prediction of violence and self-harm in mentally disordered offenders: A prospective study of the efficacy of HCR–20, PCL–R, and psychiatric symptomatology. *Journal of Consulting and Clinical Psychology, 71,* 443–451.

Grove, W. M., & Meehl, P. E. (1996). Comparative efficiency of informal (subject, impressionistic) and formal (mechanical, algorithmic) prediction procedures: The clinical-statistical controversy. *Psychology, Public Policy, and Law, 2,* 293–323.

Hanlon, M. J., Larson, S., & Zacher, S. (1999). The Minnesota SOST and sexual reoffending in North Dakota: A retrospective study.

Hanson, R. K., & Thornton, D. (2000). Improving risk assessments for sex offenders: A comparison of three actuarial scales. *Law and Human Behavior, 24,* 119–136.

Hare, R. (1991). *Manual for the Revised Psychopathy Checklist.* Toronto: Multi-Health Systems.

Hare, R. (2003). *The Hare Psychopathy Checklist–Revised* (2nd ed.). Toronto: Multi-Health Systems.

Harkness, A. R., McNulty, J. L., Ben-Porath, Y. S., & Graham, J. R. (2002). MMPI–2 Personality Psychopathology Five (PSY–5) Scales: Gainini an overview for case conceptualization and treatment planning. *MMPI–2/MMPI–A test reports, 5.* Minneapolis, MN: Univ. Minnesota Press.

Hart, S., Cox, D., & Hare, R. (1995). *The Hare Psychopathy Checklist: Screening version.* Toronto: Multi-Health Systems.

Hart, S., Hare, R., & Forth, A. (1994). Psychopathy as a risk marker for violence: Development and validation of a screening version of the Revised Psychopathy Checklist. In J. Monahan & H. Steadman (Eds.), *Violence and mental disorder: Developments in risk assessment* (pp. 81–98). Chicago: University of Chicago Press.

Hartmann, E., Norbech, P., & Gronnerod, C. (2006). Psychopathic and nonpsychopathic violent offenders on the Rorschach: Discriminative features and comparisons with schizophrenic inpatient and university student samples. *Journal of Personality Assessment, 86,* 291–305.

Heilbrun, K. (1997). Prediction versus management models relevant to risk assessment: The importance of legal decision-making context. *Law and Human Behavior, 21,* 347–359.

Heilbrun, K., & Heilbrun, A. B. (1995). Risk assessment with the MMPI–2 in forensic evaluations. In Y. S. Ben-Porath, J. R. Graham, G. C. N. Hall, R. D. Hirschman, & M. S. Zaragoza (Eds.), *Forensic applications of the MMPI–2* (pp. 160–178). Thousand Oaks, CA: Sage.

Huprich, S. K., Gacono, C. B., Schneider, R. B., & Bridges, M. R. (2004). Rorschach oral dependency in psychopaths, sexual homicide perpetrators, and nonviolent pedophiles. *Behavioral Sciences & the Law, 22*, 345–356.

Ingram, W. (1954). Prediction of aggression from the Rorschach. *Journal of Consulting Psychology, 18*, 23–28.

Kansas v. Hendricks, 521 U.S. 346 (1997).

Kwawer, J. (1979). Borderline phenomena, interpersonal relations, and the Rorschach test. *Bulletin of the Menninger Clinic, 43*, 515–524.

Kwawer, J. (1980). Primitive interpersonal modes, borderline phenomena and Rorschach content. In J. Kwawer, A. Sugarman, P. Lerner, & H. Lerner (Eds.), *Borderline phenomena and the Rorschach test*. New York: International Universities Press.

Kwawer, J., Lerner, P., Lerner, H., & Sugarman, A. (1980). *Borderline phenomena and the Rorschach test*. New York: International Universities Press.

Lidz, C., Mulvey, E., & Gardner, W. (1993). The accuracy of predictions of violence to others. *Journal of the American Medical Association, 269*, 1007–1011.

Litwack, T. R. (2001). Actuarial versus clinical assessments of dangerousness. *Psychology, Public Policy, and Law, 7*, 409–443.

McNiel, D., & Binder, R. (1994). Screening for risk of inpatient violence: Validation of an actuarial tool. *Law and Human Behavior, 18*, 579–586.

McNiel, D. E., Gregory, A. L., Lam, J. N., Binder, R. L., & Sullivan, G. R. (2003). Utility of decision support tools for assessing acute risk of violence. *Journal of Consulting and Clinical Psychology, 71*, 945–953.

Meehl, P. (1954). *Clinical versus statistical prediction: A theoretical analysis and a review of the evidence*. Minneapolis: University of Minnesota.

Meloy, J. R. (1988). *The psychopathic mind: Origins, dynamics and treatment*. Northvale, NJ: Aronson.

Meloy, J. R. (1992) Revisiting the Rorschach of Sirhan Sirhan. *Journal of Personality Assessment, 58*, 548–570.

Meloy, J. R. (2006). The empirical basis and forensic application of affective and predatory violence. *Australian and New Zealand Journal of Psychiatry , 40*, 539–547.

Meloy, J. R., Acklin, M. W., Gacono, C. B., Murray, J. F., & Peterson, C. A. (Eds.). (1997). *Contemporary Rorschach interpretation*. Mahwah, NJ: Lawrence Erlbaum Associates.

Meloy, J. R., & Gacono, C. B. (1992a). The aggression response and the Rorschach. *Journal of Clinical Psychology, 48*, 104–114.

Meloy, J. R. & Gacono, C. B. (1992b). A psychotic (sexual) psychopath: "I just had a violent thought ..." *Journal of Personality Assessment, 58*, 480–493.

Meloy, J. R., & Gacono, C. B. (1993). A borderline psychopath: "I was basically maladjusted ..." *Journal of Personality Assessment, 61*, 358–373.

Meloy, J. R., & Gacono, C. B. (1998) The internal world of the psychopath. In T. Millon, E. Simonsen, M. Birket-Smith, & R. D. Davis (Eds.), *Psychopathy: Antisocial, criminal, and violent behavior* (pp. 95–109). New York: Guilford

Meloy, J. R., & Gacono, C. B. (2000). Assessing psychopathy: Psychological testing and report writing. In C. B. Gacono (Ed.), *The clinical and forensic assessment of psychopathy: A practitioner's guide* (pp. 231–249). Mahwah, NJ: Lawrence Erlbaum Associates.

Meloy, J. R., Gacono, C. B., & Kenney, L. (1994). A Rorschach investigation of sexual homicide. *Journal of Personality Assessment, 62*, 58–67.

Mihura, J. L., & Nathan-Montano, E. (2001). An interpersonal analysis of Rorschach aggression variables in a normal sample. *Psychological Reports, 89*, 617–623.

Monahan, J. (1981). *Predicting violent behavior: An assessment of clinical techniques*. Beverly Hill, CA: Sage.

Monahan, J. (1984). The prediction of violent behavior: Toward a second generation of theory and policy. *American Journal of Psychology, 141*, 10–15.

Monahan, J., & Steadman, H. J. (Eds.). (1994). *Violence and mental disorder: Developments in risk assessment*. Chicago: University of Chicago Press.

Monahan, J, Steadman, H., Robbins, P., Appelbaum, P., Banks, S., Grisso, T., Heilbrun, K., Mulvey, E., Roth, L., & Silver, E. (2005). An actuarial model of violence risk assessment for persons with mental disorders. *Psychiatric Services, 56*, 810–815.

Monahan, J., Steadman, H. J., Silver, E., Appelbaum, P. S., Robbins, P. C., Mulvey, E. P., Roth, L. H., Grisso, T., & Banks, S. (2001). *Rethinking risk assessment: The MacArthur study of mental disorder and violence*. New York: Oxford.

Morey, L. C., & Quigley, B. D. (2002). The use of the Personality Assessment Inventory (PAI) in assessing offenders. *International Journal of Offender Therapy and Comparative Criminology, 46*, 333–349.

O'Laughlin, S., & Schill, T. (1994). The relationship between self-monitored aggression and the MMPI–2 F, 4, 9 composite and anger content scale scores. *Psychological Reports, 74*, 733–734.

Parry, J., & Drogin, E. Y. (2000). *Criminal law handbook on psychiatric and psychological evidence and testimony*. Washington, DC: American Bar Association.

Parry, J., & Drogin, E. Y. (2001). *Civil law handbook on psychiatric and psychological evidence and testimony*. Washington, DC: American Bar Association.

Pointkowski, S. R. (2001). The Rorschach aggressive categories of Meloy and Gacono in a nonpatient sample: An exploratory study (J. R. Meloy, C. B. Gacono). *Dissertation Abstracts International, 62*(3-B), 1593.

Quinsey, V. L., Harris, G. T., Rice, M. E., & Cormier, C. A. (1998). *Violent offenders: Appraising and managing risk*. Washington, DC: American Psychological Association.

Quinsey, V. L., Harris, G. T., Rice, M. E., & Cormier, C. A. (2005). *Violent offenders: Appraising and managing risk* (2nd ed.). Washington, DC: American Psychological Association.

Revitch, E., & Schlesinger, L. (1981). *Psychopathology of homicide*. Springfield, IL: Charles C. Thomas.

Salekin, R., Rogers, R., & Sewell, K. (1996). A review and meta-analysis of the Psychopathy Checklist and Psychopathy Checklist–Revised: Predictive validity of dangerousness. *Clinical Psychology: Science and Practice, 3*, 203–215.

Serin, R. C., & Brown, S. L. (2000). The clinical use of the Hare Psychopathy Checklist-Revised in contemporary risk assessment. In C. B. Gacono (Ed.), *The clinical and forensic assessment of psychopathy* (pp. 251–268). Mahwah, NJ: Lawrence Erlbaum Associates.

Sharpe, J. P., & Desai, S. (2001). The revised NEO Personality Inventory and the MMPI–2 Psychopathology Five in the prediction of aggression. *Personality and Individual Differences, 31*, 505–518.

Steadman, H. J. (1973). Implications from the Baxstrom experience. *Bulletin of the American Academy of Psychiatry and the Law, 1*(3), 189–196.

Steadman, H. J., & Keveles, G. (1972). The community adjustment and criminal activity of the Baxstrom patients: 1966–1970. *American Journal of Psychiatry, 129*, 304–310.

Steadman, H., Mulvey, E. P., Monahan, J., Robbins, P. C., Appelbaum, P. S., Grisso, T., Roth, L. H., & Silver, E. (1998). Violence by people discharged from acute psychiatric inpatient facilities and by others in the same neighborhoods. *Archives of General Psychiatry, 55*, 393–401.

Stricker, G., & Gold, J. R. (1999). The Rorschach: Toward a nomothetically based, idiographically applicable configurational model. *Psychological Assessment, 11*, 240–250.

Swanson, J. W., Holzer, C. E., Ganju, V. K., & Jono, R. T. (1990). Violence and psychiatric disorder in the community: Evidence from the Epidemiological Catchment Area surveys. *Hospital and Community Psychiatry, 41*, 761–770.

Swanson, J. W., Swartz, M. S., Van Dorn, R. A., Elbogen, E. B., Wagner, H. R., Rosenheck, R. A., Stroup, T. S., McEvoy, J. P., & Lieberman, J. A. (2006). A national study of violent behavior in persons with schizophrenia. *Archives of General Psychiatry, 63*, 490–499.

Verona, E., & Carbonell, J. L. (2000). Female violence and personality: Evidence for a pattern of overcontrolled hostility among one-time violent female offenders. *Criminal Justice and Behavior, 27*, 176–195.

Webster, C. D., Douglas, K. S., Eaves, D., & Hart, S. D. (1997). *HCR–20: Assessing risk for violence* (Version 2). Burnaby, British Columbia: Mental Health, Law, and Policy Institute, Simon Fraser University.

White, D. O. (1999). A concurrent validity study of the Rorschach extended aggression scoring categories. *Dissertation Abstracts International, 59*(9-B), 5152.

10

DEATH PENALTY AND MITIGATION

Nancy Kaser-Boyd
Geffen School of Medicine, UCLA

When the death penalty was reinstituted, psychologists found themselves called on for their expertise in understanding the multiple causes of violence, and also to answer questions about competence to be executed. Prompted by the greater involvement of psychologists in capital cases, and by news of death row inmates exonerated through the use of DNA evidence, the American Psychological Association (2006) passed a resolution urging caution in implementing the death penalty. The Resolution notes:

- Recent application of DNA technology has resulted in 62 postconviction determinations of actual innocence, with 8 having been sentenced to death at trial (APA, 2006).
- Across the United States, two thirds of death penalty cases from 1973 to 1995 were overturned on appeal, with the most common reasons cited as incompetent counsel, inadequate investigative services, or police and prosecutors withholding exculpatory evidence.
- Race and ethnicity have been shown to affect the likelihood of being charged with a capital crime and therefore of being sentenced to die by the jury. Those who kill European American victims are more likely to receive the death penalty, even after the differences such as the heinousness of the crime, prior convictions, and the relationship between the victim and the perpetrator are considered. This is especially true for African Americans (e.g., Keil & Vito, 1995; Thomson, 1997) and Hispanic Americans who kill European Americans (Thomson, 1997).
- Capital punishment appears statistically neither to exert a deterrent effect nor save a significant number of lives through the prevention of repeat offenses. Further, research shows that the murder rate increases just after state-sanctioned executions (APA, 2006).
- Jurors who survive the "death-qualifying" process are more conviction-prone than jurors who have reservations about the death penalty.
- Jurors often misunderstand the concept of mitigation and its intended application so that mitigation factors, for example, the defendant's previous life circumstances, mental and emotional difficulties, and age have little or no relationship to penalty phase verdicts.

Ethical issues clearly arise when the outcome of an evaluation forms the basis of a decision for execution. One board of the American Psychological Association has opposed the participation of psychologists in "routine certification of competency for execution" and has stated that justification for participation should be based solely on the possibility of bringing new information that might change the legal verdict and subsequent death sentence (APA, 1989; Melton, Petrilla, Poythress, & Slobogin, 1995). Many psychologists will undoubtedly participate in capital cases, in some form of consultation. Melton et al. (1995) advise that the psychologist determine whether personal beliefs will make an objective assessment difficult.

ESTABLISHING GUIDELINES

On the surface, this may seem like an odd chapter for inclusion in a book on the Rorschach. For some, the use of a Rorschach might be the last thing to consider in the extensive work-up that has come to characterize mitigation investigations. This chapter reviews the scope of psychological evidence presented in penalty phase proceedings, and illustrates how a Rorschach might be integrated with other mitigation evidence to support and illustrate the impairments of the defendant. It discusses the potential relevance of Rorschach data to evaluations of competence for execution.

Case law establishing guidelines for legal proceedings in capital cases has been refined over a series of cases. In *Gregg v. Georgia* (1956), the Supreme Court outlined a bifurcated proceeding where the sentencer(s) learns of information concerning the crime and the offender and is given standards to guide its discretion in using this information to recommend the appropriate sentence. The court indicated that the jury should hear factors in aggravation and factors in mitigation. Factors in aggravation are those that are said to justify the imposition of a more severe sentence on the defendant, compared to others found guilty of murder (*Zant v. Stephens*, 1983), and the law requires, for eligibility for the death penalty, the state must prove the existence of at least one aggravating factor (*Zant v. Stephens*). *Woodson v. North Carolina* (1976) defined mitigating factors as those "compassionate factors stemming from the diverse frailties of human kind" (Haney, 2005, p. 24). *Woodson* established the principle that the penalty of death is qualitatively different from a sentence of imprisonment, however long. Because of this, the Constitution requires that capital defendants be treated as uniquely individual human beings with punishment related directly to the personal culpability of the defendant and the unique nature of his character and record (Tully, 2003).

In a death penalty hearing that follows the law, the jurors should be allowed to hear any and all evidence that might help them understand, although not excuse, the crime. *Lockett v. Ohio* (1978) defines mitigation broadly, stating that the sentencer may not be precluded from considering "any aspect of a defendant's character or record and any of the circumstances of the offense that the defendant proffers as a basis for a sentence less than death" (p. 604). The sentencer must be permitted to give "independent mitigating weight" (p. 604) to all evidence proffered in mitigation. *Mills v. Maryland* (1988) states that an individual juror must be allowed to consider any factor in mitigation found to exist from the evidence in the case, whether or not any other jurors agree to its existence or its importance in determining punishment. The court has ruled that the death penalty is unconstitutional for someone 15 years or younger (*Thompson v. Oklahoma,* 1988), and that execution of the mentally retarded constitutes cruel and unusual punishment (*Atkins v. Virginia,* 2002).

Haney (2005) critically reviews the history of the implementation of *Gregg* and subsequent cases, stating:

> Aggravation—evidence that would incline jurors toward death sentences—usually comes in the form of heinous facts about the crime itself and evidence of criminal behavior in which the defendant engaged in the past. Typically, this kind of evidence is straightforward for prosecutors to find and present, and it often represents powerful evidence in favor of a death verdict. Indeed, graphic details about the crime for which the defendant is being tried usually are introduced in the guilt phase of the case. Similarly, if the defendant has a criminal history, it usually is well documented and readily accessible though law enforcement records.
>
> On the other hand, mitigation—evidence that would incline jurors toward life sentences—is often difficult to obtain and requires special effort on the part of defense attorneys to locate, analyze, and present. Unlike a criminal history, mitigation is less often well documented and rarely is found in an easily accessed, centralized location. Instead, it requires painstaking and time-consuming investigation to acquire. Defense team members must locate and interview an often large number of potential witnesses and comb through diverse sources of information. This kind of mitigation is critical to the outcome of a capital case and to any semblance of fair and reliable death sentencing. In most cases, it represents the only real hope defendants have of avoiding the death penalty. (p. 20)

Following this case law, the preparation of capital cases for the death penalty hearing is a time-consuming and careful process that usually starts long before an expert is contacted. In fact, early preparation of mitigation evidence could convince the prosecution to drop its argument for death; this would avoid a "death-qualified" jury,[1] which could give the client a better chance in the guilt phase of the case. The American Bar Association issued revised "Guidelines for the Appointment and Performance of Defense Counsel in Death Penalty Cases" setting a high standard for professional representation in capital cases (Schaye & Schaye-Glos, 2005). A recent case—*Wiggins v. Smith* (2003)—clearly and conclusively established the necessity of extensive mitigation work and the persuasive authority of the ABA guidelines that apply to every stage of a case from the time of arrest through clemency proceedings (Schaye & Schaye-Glos, 2005). The ABA guidelines (ABA, 1984) call for the presence on a defense team of a "mitigation specialist." This is not necessarily a psychologist or a lawyer, but someone who possesses clinical and information-gathering skills and training, and the time and ability to search records and conduct sensitive interviews. The exploration of mitigating factors is a process that should begin at the very beginning of a case, because it may take time for institu-

---

[1] A "Death-Qualified Juror" is one who has survived the *voir dire* questioning because that person has said there would be no reservations about putting the defendant to death.

tions to respond to records requests and the records will provide new clues about possible mitigation witnesses who should be interviewed. Typical records collected include: birth and death records, dependency and delinquency court records, adult arrest records, court proceedings, employment, marriage, physical or mental health, military, probation or parole, school, social services, immigration, and Social Security Administration (Schaye & Schaye-Glos, 2005). The search through a client's history will likely produce positive and negative facts, but the goal is not to edit reality, but to develop a cohesive analysis of the cause of problem behavior. Evaluation of possible mitigation factors involves collecting a well-documented psychosocial history of the client, analyzing the significance of the information in terms of development (including the effect on personality and behavior) and finding mitigating themes in the client's life history. The goal is not to justify the crime but to help explain it.

Mitigation evidence is varied and every case is different. As a general rule, the following areas are places to begin:

1. Unusual conditions of gestation or birth, such as exposure to drugs *in utero*, prematurity, mother battered while pregnant.
2. Family history of mental disorder or substance abuse.
3. Extreme family circumstances, such as extreme poverty, child abuse or neglect, father in prison, severe childhood illness.
4. Learning disabilities, such as ADHD, sojourns in special education, or a learning history that qualified for special education but didn't receive any intervention.
5. Exposure to extreme neighborhood violence; for example, witnessing other youths die, sleeping where gunfire erupts or bullets enter houses.
6. Victimization by violence, such as beatings by other youths, siblings shot or killed, personal trauma such as shot or stabbed.
7. Mental health history, such as records of treatment for behavioral problems, depression, or psychotic symptoms.
8. Substance abuse history and interventions.
9. Areas of prosocial functioning.

Inquiry into these areas will provide a large amount of information for psychological analysis. If the legal team is working according to the guidelines discussed earlier, these individuals will have accumulated much of this history and the psychologist's job will consist of reading this material with a psychologist's eye. This will allow the psychologist to develop a cohesive theory of mitigation and delineate new areas of psychological inquiry that may include interviewing crucial individuals in the defendant's background. In reality, a review of the real behavior in the life history takes precedence over psychological testing. Psychological testing can be done to generate hypotheses about mitigation, but capital defense teams have become wary of the use of psychological tests on their clients. One widely expressed view is summarized by Schaye and Schaye-Glos (2005):

> Psychiatrists and psychologists use personality testing to aid in diagnostic testing, using instruments like the Minnesota Multiphasic Personality Inventory to provide helpful treatment tools,

but they can be extremely damaging for a capital penalty trial and should virtually never be administered to a client. ... Suffice it to say that the purpose of a thorough evaluation is not to diagnose but to understand how the client's symptoms led to the capital crime. More than one psychologist has claimed—contrary to the teachings of endless prior cases—the evaluation would have no credibility if personality testing was not done. Experts have used such tests after being specifically told not to do so. (p. 7)

Although psychological experts are not likely to appreciate being told what not to do in conducting their job, the forensic expert is aware that both prosecution and defense make decisions about what to present in a trial. Both may be entirely within their ethical guidelines, as the criminal defense attorney is expected to protect his client's civil rights, whereas the prosecutor's ethics require the disclosure of material that may be exculpatory.

There is an inherent problem in relying on psychological tests, in any event, to evaluate "personality" in a capital defendant. Many intervening variables have occurred since the client's crime and detention. By the time the forensic psychologist arrives at the jail to interview and conduct tests, the client may have been on a medication regimen, may have been assaulted in the jail or had a serious illness, or may be in a different phase of a cycling or biphasic disorder (Bipolar Disorder and Posttraumatic Stress Disorder, to name two). The MMPI–2 is quite sensitive to "state," and should not be considered a simple measure of "personality."[2] Elevations on Scale 4, for example, may reflect the interpersonal mistrust and authority problems that occur during long periods of incarceration.

An ideal compromise between the psychologist's interest in psychological test data and the attorney's concerns about the misuse of this data is the bifurcation of experts. The defense team can call in a psychologist, whose role is strictly to conduct a battery of psychological tests, and a second psychologist, whose role is primarily to review the client's history, integrate data, and outline mitigating factors. The second expert may integrate psychological test data, if the defense team elects to make this "discoverable."

THE RORSCHACH AND PREPARATION OF MITIGATION EVIDENCE

The Rorschach may sidestep the problems noted with an MMPI–2 (e.g., there is no Scale 4, with all the misconceptions that surround Scale 4 interpretations) and it has many features that commend it in an evaluation of mitigation evidence. Not strictly diagnostic in its purpose, as it is a sample of the way the client views the world, including impairments in thinking and problem solving, dealing with emotion, distortions in his self-concept, and impairments in interpersonal relationships. The Rorschach is particularly sensitive to trauma disorders (see Armstrong & Kaser-Boyd, 2003; Kaser-Boyd, & Evans, chap. 13, this vol.), and it can elegantly illustrate just how thinking goes awry. Unlike tests that rely on the defendant's self-report, where manipulation (e.g., faking mental illness, or de-

---

[2]Asked if an MMPI collected 2 years after a homicide could be an accurate representation of the mental state of a criminal defendant who had killed his children while in a psychotic depressed state, Dr. Alex Caldwell said that some scales are quite stable (e.g., Scale 0), but the MMPI profile should be expected to change, in various ways, over time, and commented that he once knew a psychologist who took the MMPI every day for some time and found fluctuations in the profile from day to day.

fensively denying pathology) is often alleged, the Rorschach bypasses an individual's volitional controls to collect data about personality (Meloy, 1991). Rogers and Cavanaugh (1983) note that the Rorschach is mostly likely to be used to answer questions about mental state during the commission of the crime, to assess dangerousness, and to discuss treatability. It is assumed that the expert will score and interpret the Rorschach according to the Exner Comprehensive Scoring System (Exner 2003), because this is the most widely taught and used scoring and interpretation method, with the most current research on reliability and validity.

The Rorschach is generally admissible in Court (Gacono, Evans, & Viglione, 2002; Meloy, chap. 4, this vol.; Meloy, Hanson & Weiner, 1997; Weiner et. al, 1996). McCann (1998; McCann, Evans, chap. 3, this vol.) notes that legal admissibility does not require that all scientific issues be completely resolved to the satisfaction of all members of the professional community, and expert testimony should rest on methodology that is generally accepted, testable, standardized, relevant, and helpful. The expert witness should be ready to apply the Rorschach to the practical points to be made in testimony and to answer questions about the Rorschach's reliability and validity. Research has found that most Rorschach variables achieve an acceptable level of scoring agreement (Acklin, McDowell, & Verschell, 2000; Gacono et al., 2002; Viglione & Meyer, chap. 2, this vol.). Validity issues should usually be focused on the scores on the defendant's protocol, that is, on the scores that seem significant. Not all of the scores available from computer interpretation will be relevant and, in fact, a pedantic and overly inclusive survey of many variables will be exhausting for a group of laypeople (e.g., the jury). The variables chosen to illustrate the defendant's personality should have sufficient validity to withstand questioning (Viglione & Meyer, chap. 2, this vol.). The case example will illustrate how the Rorschach was used and how it was defended in court.

CASE EXAMPLE

The capital defendant, Mr. D, was a 33-year-old Anglo man from a rural part of the West, a community that largely migrated West during the 1940s from the Bible Belt of Oklahoma, which was relatively poverty stricken and very religious. His childhood could be described as painful and frightening. When he was very young, his father was sent to a mental institution. Although diagnosed with Schizophrenia, this admission came during a time in the United States when both Bipolar and Schizophrenic patients frequently received the same label and his father's symptoms seemed much more clearly Bipolar. To have any mental disorder at all, however, was stigmatizing in his uneducated community, and Mr. D often heard, as a child, "You're crazy, just like your Daddy." It was not entirely clear what behavior led to this label.

Mr. D's mother remarried when he was in middle childhood and his stepfather proved to be both psychologically and physically brutal. He was singled out in many of these attacks, which his half-sisters witnessed. He was regularly denigrated and often beaten. In one such beating, the belt buckle inadvertently hit his penis, requiring medical treatment. Mr. D seemed much brighter than his half-siblings, which caused additional resentment and rejection. He also suffered from a seizure disorder that began somewhere in adolescence, which may have been caused by a beating. Mr. D coped with this difficult family environment by throwing himself into his studies and by pretending he belonged somewhere else. He constructed an elaborate life history that was different than his own and told others that his family on his father's side were wealthy and educated.

When he was barely 19, Mr. D married a woman who was somewhat older and somewhat maternal. Deeply religious, she helped him graduate from college and then a seminary, where he became an ordained minister in a fundamentalist Christian church. Unfortunately, Mr. D had what seemed like an insatiable sexual drive. While married, he had multiple affairs with other women, both in and outside of his church. He sometimes had sexual relations with more than one woman a day and he fathered at least one child out of wedlock. When he was not consummating a relationship, he was trying to meet new women and he often made himself seem even more educated and accomplished than he was. He wrote to women in other cities where he had no plans to travel.

Mr. D's wife was found shot to death on a county road. A witness had seen part of a car and license plate that was later traced to Mr. D. Shortly before the homicide, he took out a large insurance policy on his wife. This, plus evidence of his substantial extracurricular sex life, provided evidence for a charge of first degree murder. Nevertheless, when Mr. D was told of his wife's death, he "fell out," a moment that was captured on videotape. Murder for financial gain is a capital offense in the state where the murder occurred, and the expert was called to assist with the penalty phase of the trial.

The preparation of the case began with interviews with family members and then with the collection of records from various sources. As is often the case, Mr. D's mother and stepfather denied that Mr. D was subjected to physical or emotional abuse. They said that he had always been a "weird kid" and they seemed like they would make very poor penalty phase witnesses. Mr. D's half-sisters, however, told another story. They had felt horrified and guilty about being witness to their older half-brother's abuse and they proved to be articulate in describing the rejection, humiliation, and overt physical abuse that Mr. D suffered. Mental health records for his father were sought and fortuitously, they were received. They proved to be quite useful in documenting the biological history. Interestingly, hospital handwritten notes discussed his father's obsession with sex, as well as a number of other symptoms now more likely to be seen as manic. Records from the Department of Children's Services were also found and they documented physical abuse Mr. D received as a child and adolescent. School records from college, seminary, and early years indicated that Mr. D was quite bright and there was nothing in his school or behavioral history to predict a cold-blooded killing. Although he had lived a double life as a pastor, no one in his parish suspected this, and many people spoke highly of Mr. D.

Early in the case, Mr. D received a complete neuropsychological test battery, and he also had an MRI. Neither neurological nor neuropsychological evaluations yielded any solid data about brain impairment, despite the history of seizure disorder.

The mitigation team had done a good job of gathering important life history, family history, school and behavioral records, and there were a number of people who could serve as witnesses to Mr. D's character and the fact that the crime seemed very out of character. There was little, however, to explain how this intelligent man had walked down the path to a badly planned murder and left so much evidence along the way. He had clearly been engaged in a fantastic and elaborate reconstruction of himself. During preparation for the trial, he continued to seem out of touch with reality. He enrolled in a correspondence course that would lead to a master's degree in business and he preferred to talk about the businesses he would start when he was acquitted. In his interviews, Mr. D seemed very pressured and intense. He spoke rapidly and seemed annoyed if the expert seemed puzzled about something he said. He could be described as abrasive, rarely failing to express his disdain for his legal team. He was somewhat tangential, but his movement from one topic to another was generally logical. What useful data could the Rorschach provide?

Mr. D delivered 34 responses to the Rorschach, which illustrated an abundance of associations (e.g., beginning his record by noting that he saw "a multiplicity of things"), even though he was somewhat defensive, with a Lambda of 1.62. He sometimes made reference to having seen the percept "in a book," which underscored his defensiveness. Many of his responses were part object, both human and animals. For example, he saw frog's eyes, a skull, a pelvis with ovaries, an elephant head, an animal hide (with no texture), shoulder blades, a human nose, and another pelvis. There was no *Whole H*, no *Human Movement*, and, not surprisingly, no *Cooperative Movement*. His *H: Hd + (H) + (Hd)* was 0:4, and his *Isolation Index* was .24. Weiner (1998) discusses these two scores under his heading "Sustaining Interpersonal Interest, Involvement, and Comfort." He states:

> People live in an interpersonal world, and the common experience of all people attests the vital role of company and companionship in keeping one's peace of mind and sense of well-being. Few punishments are more harsh than solitary confinement, few characters are more sympathetic than Robinson Crusoe before he found Friday, and few individuals are more removed from living the good life than those who by design or misfortune must pass their days in seclusion. (p. 162)

Here, the "seclusion" in question is not the seclusion of incarceration, but the seclusion of Mr. D's tortured childhood and his inability to connect and get comfort from others as an adult. Mr. D's *H:Hd + (H) + (Hd)* score illustrates his social discomfort, his inability to get comfort from or identify with others. He shows little expectation of engaging in collaborative relationships with other people and, as a result, he may seem indifferent or aversive and strike others as distant and aloof. Weiner (1998, p. 163) continues,

> People with this imbalance in their human contents typically experience uneasiness in dealing with people who are real, live, and fully functional. ... At a fantasy level, such individuals may well be attempting to minimize feelings of threat or inadequacy.

This description goes a long way toward explaining Mr. D's creation of a "fantasy self" with unlimited ideas of success and his inability to relate to women as whole and fully functional people. It also recasts his sexual obsession as an obsessive search for comfort. Unlike a psychopath, who may engage in impersonal, trivial, and poorly integrated sexual relationships (Cleckley, 1976), he had two Texture responses, Gacono, Loving, and Bodholdt (2001) and Gacono and Meloy (1994) note that Texture is usually absent in the psychopath.

The cluster examining self-perception adds additional insight about his feelings about himself and his relationships with others. (See Table 10–1.)

He compares himself unfavorably to other people. He lacks self-esteem and confidence. His tendency to judge himself unfavorably may result in feelings of futility, especially if he is kept from usual modes of ego repair. His low $3r + (2)/R$ may also come from purposely avoiding self-focusing, but his 2 FD are not consistent with this hypothesis. His FD score indicates a capacity for, and interest in, being introspective. He has a moderate level of self-awareness. In a death penalty hearing, this score has particular importance, as it indicates a capacity to participate in psychotherapy and positive personality change, in other words, a reason to vote for life rather than death. Still examining the Self-Perception Cluster, Mr. D has an abundance of *Anatomy* and *X-ray* responses ($An + Xy = 5$). This indicates that he is unusually concerned about his body. He was young and in good health at the time of the evaluation, but a focus on anatomy is not uncommon for adults who were abused as children, a fact consistent with the CS interpretive statement that similar individuals experience themselves as fragile and vulnerable. It is hard to picture a more vulnerable situation than having one's penis injured by an abusive parent.

Mr. D also had many features associated with Manic Depressive illness or a mood disorder. Table 10–2 summarizes important variables from the Affect Cluster of the Rorschach.

In sentences derived from the Affect Cluster, the computer-generated narrative states:

1. This person appears to be susceptible to episodes of affective disturbance that are likely to involve features of depression. The client may not necessarily complain of feeling depressed or emotionally upset, but he nevertheless gives evidence of being disposed to affective malaise that interferes with his being able to function effectively.

2. He appears to be at considerable risk for being flooded by affect and overwhelmed by more emotion that he can tolerate. This emotional overload is likely to be interfering with his ability to think before he acts, and difficulties in maintaining

TABLE 10–1

Self-perception Cluster

$H: (H) + Hd + (Hd) = 0:4$
$An + Xy = 4$
$FD = 2$
$3r + (2)/R = 0.18$

TABLE 10–2

Affective Cluster

$DEPI = 5$
$SCON = 7$
$S = 7$
$EB = 0:3.5$
$eb = 1:5$
Sum Shading $= 5$
One Color-Shading Blend

attention may also be impairing the adequacy of his decision making. He is, consequently, susceptible to losing self-control and behaving in an impulsive manner.

It would be hard to ignore the fact that a significant part of Mr. D's intense affect is anger. His $S = 7$ and his $Su\%$ of 57% indicate that he is more angry and resentful than the average person and anger interferes with accurate perception. Anger and resentment are not unusual in an adult who has experienced significant child abuse.

Additionally, the narrative notes, that Mr. D shows less psychological complexity than most people (i.e., that he functions in a more simplistic and psychologically impoverished way than most people). Usually this means that the person employs rather simplistic and primitive psychological defenses, the very nature of which make the person less able to cope with demands, and makes it more likely that stress elicits strong affect or dysfunctional behavior. He is positive on the Coping Deficit Index, which supports statements about his poor ability to cope with life's demands.

Finally, Mr. D is not very well grounded in reality. The clusters concerning Cognitive Mediation and Ideation (see Table 10–3) indicate that his reality testing is poor. Almost half of his record is composed of unusual *Form Quality*. His $X + \%$ of .56 and his $F + \%$ of .48 indicate that his perceptual accuracy is poor even when emotion is not tapped in his response. He would be considered idiosyncratic in his world view and the CS computer narrative states that he would be "at risk" for "behaving in ways that others regard as odd or eccentric."

Mr. D's Rorschach demonstrates the kind of impairment to personality that is seen in adults from very abusive backgrounds. This set of impairments to personality functioning has been variously called Complex Posttraumatic Stress Disorder (Herman, 1992), Disorders of Extreme Stress (van der Kolk, 2005), and Personality Disorders Resulting from Extreme Stress (van der Kolk, Roth, Pelcovitz, Sunday, & Spinazzola, 2005). Impairments are described in six domains:

1. Alterations in regulation of affect and impulses. Deficits of affect regulation are illustrated by difficulty modulating affect, including anger, self-destructive behavior, deficits of modulation of sexual involvement, and excessive risk-taking.

2. Alterations in attention or consciousness. Here, there may be transient dissociative episodes or derealization and depersonalization.

3. Alterations in self-perception. These are exemplified by a sense of having been permanently damaged, shame, feelings of ineffectiveness, excessive guilt, and other indicators of an impaired sense of self.

TABLE 10–3

Cognitive Mediation and Ideation

$P = 4$
$FQxo = 19$
$FQxu = 13$
$X + \% = .56$
$F + \% = .48$
$Xu\% = .38$
Weighted Sum6 = 2

4. Alterations in perception of others. These individuals develop distorted beliefs about others as the result of their "distorted" experiences of childhood. They swing from idealizing others, to devaluation. They have a pervasive inability to trust and may be preoccupied with hurting those who have hurt them. In their adult lives, they may be revictimized, or may revictimize others (with some gender differences here).

5. Somatization. Although they may not have chronic pain or illness, this somatic preoccupation is more common than in normal individuals. They may have compromised functioning in one domain (e.g., cardiopulmonary or digestive). They often have sexual symptoms and also often have conversion symptoms.

6. Alterations in systems of meaning. They have difficulty sustaining hope and quickly feel helpless and despairing in crises.

Table 10–4 illustrates how Rorschach findings support these impairments to Mr. D's personality functioning. These problematic personality dynamics were energized by underlying Mood Disorder, which is the biological legacy of his father.

PREPARING FOR TESTIMONY ON THE RORSCHACH

Given the nature of the crime, it might be assumed that Mr. D had psychopathic personality features. In fact, the prosecution asserted that Mr. D was a clever psychopath who had been good at manipulating people and presenting a false front. Although Mr. D clearly had a need for power and admiration, his Rorschach did not exhibit the scores typically associated with psychopathy. Reflections were absent from the record. Perhaps more important, he had two Texture responses and two *FD* responses. The prosecution had collected a number of witnesses who testified that Mr. D was arrogant and argumentative, and that he had been dishonest in other domains than the sexual. Some witnesses indicated that Mr. D seemed to think of himself as better and smarter than the other pastors in the region. This, at a minimum, suggested Narcissistic Personality Disorder. The expert must focus on the

TABLE 10–4

Disorders of Extreme Stress Criteria and Rorschach Indices

1. Alterations in regulation of affect and impulses

$DEPI = 5$	$Y = 3$
$S = 7$	$T = 2$
$EB = 0: 3.5$	
$eb - 1:5$	

2. Alterations in attention or consciousness

3. Alterations in self-perception

$3r + (2)/R = 0.18$

$FD = 2$

$An + Xy = 5$

4. Alterations in perception of others

$H: (H) + Hd + (Hd) = 0:4$

$Isolate/R = 0.24$

$COP = 0$

$T = 2$

5. Somatization

$An + Xy = 5$

6. Alterations in systems of meaning

$DEPI = 5$

$SCON = 7$

negative things that can be said about the defendant. In some cases, these are accurate depictions of him; in other cases, they are not, or they clearly result from understandable and perhaps sympathetic causes (e.g., severe child abuse).

Mr. D probably could be diagnosed with Narcissistic Personality Disorder (NPD). The defense team and the expert witness acknowledged that he had a number of traits of NPD, including grandiosity, fantasies of unlimited success and power, the belief that he is "special," a sense of entitlement, and arrogance. Expert testimony explained how this was a defense to his underlying sense of himself as damaged, weak, and worthless—the sense of self internalized from childhood. The expert agreed that Mr. D had a personality disorder (i.e., a chronic maladaptive way of thinking, feeling, and behaving), but testified that this was a predictable outcome of the type of child abuse he experienced, serious physical abuse, and brutal psychological assaults. He did not exhibit a necessary number of features to warrant a designation of psychopathy (e.g., no parasitic lifestyle, no early behavioral problems, no lack of long-term goals, no juvenile delinquency, no criminal versatility).

Preparation for testimony included:

1. A thorough review of the research on the developmental consequences of serious child abuse.
2. A review of the defendant's father's psychiatric records and updating research on the risk of biologically based mental disorders.
3. A review of both prosecution and defense evidence about Mr. D's personality and behavior.
4. A review of the Rorschach research on psychopaths and on adults with childhood histories of serious abuse.
5. A review of Rorschach reliability and validity studies, with special focus on the scores that were significant in Mr. D's Rorschach.

The last item requires further comment. The death penalty phase of a trial is not as much of a battle as the trial in chief. Many times, the prosecution seems to be sliding into home base, having already won a conviction that will carry a sentence of life without parole or death. They have put on a significant amount of evidence of a crime and the jury has voted for conviction. This means that there may be no battle over Rorschach data. The expert is well-advised to prepare as if there will be the most rigorous challenge to the validity of the Rorschach, and be prepared to answer questions in simple, everyday language, while focusing on the big picture. In a death penalty hearing, the "big picture" is the integration of all of the data into a narrative that explains how this particular defendant ended up convicted of this particular crime. It is always essential to remember that Rorschach is only a part of this overall picture (see Erdberg, chap. 27, this vol.).

Mr. D was convicted of murder, but the jury did not vote for execution. Instead, he received a sentence of life without parole. One of his half-sisters made a powerful witness to his childhood of psychological and physical abuse. The expert testimony, utilizing many pieces of data from the mitigation investigation, and using the Rorschach to illustrate the personality impairments likely a result of child abuse, explained how an elaborate fantasy life and impaired judgment develop and how they direct a crime.

COMPETENCE FOR EXECUTION

The concept of "competence for execution" is defined by statute and states vary in how competence is defined. No state, however, allows the execution of a prisoner who is incompetent. A brief but cogent discussion of competence for execution occurs in Melton et al. (1995):

> Constitutionalizing [the] centuries-old common-law rule, the Supreme Court's 1986 decision in *Ford v. Wainwright [477 U.S. 399 (1986)]* held that the Eighth Amendment, banning cruel and unusual punishment prohibits the execution of an "insane" person. While the Court did not formulate a definition of competency to be executed, Justice Powell, in a concurring opinion, suggested that the Eighth Amendment "forbids the execution only of those who are unaware of the punishment they are about to suffer and why they are to suffer it." (p. 182)

The American Bar Association has articulated a provisional standard that defines incompetence in death penalty cases as follows: "… an inability on the part of the defendant to understand the nature of the proceedings against him, what he was tried for, the purpose of the punishment, or the nature of the punishment, as well as an inability to recognize or understand any fact which might exist which would make his punishment unjust or unlawful, or … to convey such information to counsel or the court" (Melton et al., 1985, p. 182).

A determination about competence usually surrounds cognitive functioning, as the ABA standard suggests. "Knowing," "understanding," and "recognizing" are related to intelligence, although in practice, intelligence must be quite impaired for the capital defendant to be unable to understand these points. A more likely situation is that where significant mental illness impairs rational thinking and therefore impairs "understanding." Mentally ill capital defendants may have psychotic illness, or psychotic episodes, with delusional thinking or a formal thought disorder that interferes with their ability to "understand." The Rorschach can be particularly useful in these situations. The Rorschach's Information Processing, Mediation, and Ideation Clusters assess accurate perception and adequate reality testing, which are fundamental to accurate understanding of the charges and the legal system. Paranoid or psychotic defendants may be quite intelligent and have the intellectual capacity to grasp the relatively simple concepts that are required for competence, but they are often unable to cooperate because their distorted thinking interferes with their ability to be rational. In many such cases, the defendant has specific paranoid beliefs about their attorney or about "the system," which interfere with their ability to assist counsel in preparing their defense. The Rorschach can illustrate how their thinking goes awry. There are many comparison samples of thought disordered patients that can buttress such testimony (see Exner & Erdberg, 2005).

REFERENCES

Acklin, M. W., McDowell II, C. J., Vershell, M. S., & Chan, D. (2000). Inter-observer agreement, intra-observer reliability, and the Rorschach Comprehensive System. *Journal of Personality Assessment, 74*, 15–47.

American Bar Association. (1984). *Criminal Justice Mental Health Standards, Standard 7–5.2.*

American Psychological Association. (2006). *The death penalty in the United States: A resolution.* Washington, DC: American Psychological Association.

American Psychological Association, Board of Social and Ethical Responsibility in Psychology. (1989, May). *Agenda,* at 117.

Armstrong, J., & Kaser-Boyd, N. (2003). Projective assessment of trauma. In M. Hilsenroth & D. Segal (Eds.), *Comprehensive handbook of psychological assessment: Vol. 2. Objective and projective assessment of personality and psychopathology* (pp. 500–512). New York: Wiley.

Atkins v. Virginia, 122 S. Ct. 2242, 153 L. Ed. 2d 335 (2002).

Cleckley, H. (1976). *The mask of sanity* (6th ed.). St. Louis, MO: Mosby.

Exner, J. E. (2003). *The Rorschach: A comprehensive system* (4th ed.). New York: Wiley.

Exner, J. E., & Erdberg, P. (2005). *The Rorschach: A Comprehensive System* (3rd ed). Hoboken, NJ: Wiley.

Gacono, C. B., Evans, F. B., & Viglione, D. J. (2002). The Rorschach in forensic practice. *Journal of Forensic Psychology Practice, 2*(3), 33–54.

Gacono, C. B., Loving, J. L., & Bodholdt, R. H. (2001) The Rorschach and psychopathy: Toward a more accurate understanding of the research findings. *Journal of Personality Assessment, 77*, 16–38.

Gacono, C., & Meloy, J. R. (1994). *The Rorschach assessment of aggressive and psychopathic person-alities.* Hillsdale, NJ: Lawrence Erlbaum Associates.

Haney, C. (2005). *Death by design: Capital punishment as a social psychological system.* New York: Oxford University Press.

Gregg v. Georgia, 428 U.S. 153 (1956).

Herman, J. L. (1992). Complex Posttraumatic Stress Disorder: A syndrome in survivors of prolonged and repeated trauma. *Journal of Traumatic Stress, 5*(3), 377–391.

Keil, T. J., & Vito, G. F. (1995). Race and the death penalty in Kentucky murder trials: 1976–1991. *American Journal of Criminal Justice, 20*(1), 17–36.

Lockett v. Ohio, 438 U.S. 586 (1978).

McCann, J. (1998). Defending the Rorschach in court: An analysis of admissibility using legal and professional standards. *Journal of Personality Assessment, 70*(1), 125–144.

Melton, G., Petrilla, J., Poythress, N. G., & Slobogin, C. (1995). *Psychological evaluation for the courts* (2nd ed.). New York: Guilford.

Meloy, J., Hansen, T., & Weiner, I. (1997). Authority of the Rorschach: Legal citations during the past 50 years. *Journal of Personality Assessment, 69*, 53–62.

Meloy, J. R. (1991, Fall/Winter). Rorschach testimony. *Journal of Psychiatry and the Law,* 221–235.

Mills v. Maryland, 486 U.S. 367 (1988).

Rogers, R., & Cavanaugh, J. (1983). Usefulness of the Rorschach: A survey of forensic psychiatrists. *Journal of Psychiatry and the Law, 11*, 55–67.

Schaye, N., & Schaye-Glos, R. (2005). Mitigation in the death belt—twelve steps to saving clients' lives. In *The Champion* (pp. 18–27). Washington, DC: National Association of Criminal Defense Lawyers.

Thomson, E. (1997). Research note: Discrimination and the death penalty in Arizona. *Criminal Justice Review, 22*(1), 65–76.

Thompson v. Oklahoma, 487 U. S. 815 (1988).

Tully, M. A. (2003, February). *Penalty phase law: Mitigation and its consideration.* Paper presented at the California Attorneys for Criminal Justice Capital Case Seminar, Monterey, CA.

van der Kolk, B. A. (2005). Developmental trauma disorder: Towards a rational diagnosis for chronically traumatized children. *Psychiatric Annals, 35*(5), 401–408.

van der Kolk, B. A, Roth, S., Pelcovitz, D., Sunday, S., & Spinazzola, J. (2005). Disorders of extreme stress: The empirical foundation of a complex adaptation to trauma. *Journal of Traumatic Stress, 18*(5), 389–399.

Wiggins v. Smith, 539 U. S. 510, 123 S. Ct. 2527, 156 L. E. D. 2d 471 (2003).

Woodson v. North Carolina , 428 U.S. 280 (1976).

Zant v. Stephens, 462 U. S. 862 (1983).

11

USE OF THE RORSCHACH IN FORENSIC TREATMENT PLANNING

Carl B. Gacono
Private Practice, Austin, TX

Michael T. Jumes
North Texas State Hospital, Vernon, TX

B. Thomas Gray
North Texas State Hospital, Vernon, TX

As mental health resources dwindle, efficient use of available services becomes an economic and ethical necessity. Integral to the efficient use of resources are screening, assessment, and treatment planning (Maruish, 2004; Mortimer & Smith, 1983; Weiner, 2004). Treatment planning is especially critical in correctional settings where change resistant Antisocial Personality Disordered (ASPD) individuals comprise a disproportionate percent of the population. ASPDs are not homogeneous; some are treatable, and some are not. Psychological assessment is invaluable when evaluating the treatment amenability within this population (Gacono, 1998).

Likewise, treatment planning is important in forensic mental health settings where a significant number of patients have serious mental illness (Davison, Leese, & Taylor, 2001; Swanson et al., 2001). The forensic hospital's high degree of structure and security are intended to control a patient's behavior. However, high levels of structure can mask or suppress psychopathology, leading forensic treatment providers to overestimate a patient's actual psychological resources and controls (Bannatyne, Gacono & Greene, 1999; Gacono & Gacono, chap. 20, this vol.). This "misattribution of psychological health" (Kosson, Gacono, & Bodholdt, 2000) is likely to impede effective treatment, misguide postrelease and community-based treatment planning and, at worst, may contribute to re-offense. By providing an understanding of the patient's psychology, the Rorschach Inkblot Method (RIM) forms one cornerstone for effective forensic treatment planning.

Within the forensic evaluation, the RIM adds to and refines hypotheses generated from history, behavioral observations, and other assessment methods (Gacono, 2002a, 2002b;

Gacono & Meloy, 1994, 2002; Meloy, 1991).[1] It provides information concerning problem-solving and response style (*Lambda, introversive, extratensive*), processing (*Zd*), reality testing (*X–%*), perceptual accuracy (*F+, X+*), controls and current stress levels (*D/AdjD*), levels of emotionality and how the patient deals with them (*FC:CF + C, Afr*; i.e., avoidance), self-perceptions (*W:M, Fr + rF, MOR*), coping resources (*EA, CDI*), desire for affectional relatedness (*T*), and interpersonal interest, maturity, and expectations (*H, [H], COP, AG*). Other measures, such as the PCL–R, quantify observable attitudes and behaviors while Rorschach data correlates with them. Simply stated, multiple methods assess different but complementary personality dimensions.

This chapter describes how the RIM adds incrementally to forensic treatment evaluations. Case examples are used to illustrate how RIM is used to guide treatment planning and monitoring.

FORENSIC TREATMENT EVALUATION—ARREST THROUGH INSTITUTIONAL RELEASE

The criminal process moves through a sequence that involves arrest, adjudication, and disposition. At any phase, the forensic evaluator may be called on to make treatment recommendations. At the pre-trial phase, odd verbalizations, unconventional behavior, or a documented psychiatric history may raise mental health and/or legal concerns (Acklin, chap. 8, this vol.; Gray & Acklin, chap. 7, this vol.). Detention centers sometimes provide rapid screening, stabilization, and crisis management, but leave in-depth psychological assessment to other settings.

A minority of criminal defendants are found incompetent to stand trial (Gray & Acklin, chap. 7, this vol.; Grisso, 1988; Shapiro, 1984). Whereas assessment of trial competency considers diagnosis, identifies relative psychological strengths and weaknesses, and aids in monitoring patients' current mental state, it specifically assesses their factual and rational understanding of the proceedings, and their ability to consult with counsel (cf. *Dusky*, 1960; Grisso, 1988; Shapiro, 1984). In-depth personality assessment is more frequently conducted after the patient has been found incompetent to stand trial or acquitted by insanity and remanded to a forensic psychiatric institution for treatment. Whereas competency evaluations address current mental state, sanity evaluations involve an assessment of mental status at the time of offense (*mens rea*, diminished capacity; Acklin, chap. 8, this vol.; Melton, Petrila, Poythress, & Slobogin, 1997).

At the sentencing phase, in-depth psychological evaluation is used to elucidate the contribution of psychosocial history to the offense. Assessment information is offered to aid the trier of fact in determining what factors were mitigating or aggravating, and whether the offender requires and/or is amenable to treatment. According to Melton et al. (1997), the typical sentencing evaluation will review a number of areas: whether the defendant has a serious mental health condition, and if so, its functional implications; history of substance abuse or dependence; intellectual and adaptive abilities; educational

---

[1]Choosing a battery of tests to address a referral question is pragmatic, responsible, and ethically sound (McCann, 1998). Selected items must be cost-effective and incrementally valid.

and vocational experience; and range of interpersonal skills. Also assessed are the defendant's present motivation for treatment and history of mental health treatment response. Once the motivations and circumstances of the offense have been clarified, treatment recommendations can be made to maximize the likelihood of reducing future offending.

Once sentenced to a correctional institution, psychological assessment provides useful information concerning the offender's treatment needs and treatment progress. Within a forensic hospital, treatment evaluations can be useful treatment planning, monitoring, and case management (Gacono, Meloy, Sheppard, Speth, & Roske, 1995; Gacono, Meloy, Speth, & Roske, 1997). Comprehensive psychological assessment is also useful in postrelease treatment planning whether the individual is an inmate or patient (Bannatyne et al., 1999; Gacono & Gacono, chap. 20, this vol.; Neiberding, Moore, & Dematatis, 2002).

The typical forensic assessment battery is comprised of multiple methods (Jumes et al., 2002). Semi-structured clinical interviews (e.g., Gacono, 2001, 2005) facilitate diagnosis and ratings for actuarial instruments, such as the PCL–R (Hare, 2003). They also provide information related to lifestyle, interpersonal context, and long-standing behavior patterns of the individual (historical and clinical factors). Personality measures provide rich information about dimensional and interpersonal aspects of the patient's clinical presentation (dispositional factors). Additionally, consideration of family conflicts and other interpersonal issues (contextual factors) guide decisions about placement and probation.

FORENSIC TREATMENT EVALUATION—PSYCHOLOGICAL ASSESSMENT

Given the obvious incentives for image management, access to collateral information is essential to all forensic evaluations (Melton et al., 1997; Rogers, 1997). In conducting the forensic examination, it is recommended that information be obtained from three sources: collateral information, interview, and psychological testing (Meloy, 1997); and be relevant to one or more of four domains: *Dispositional Factors* (including anger, impulsivity, psychopathy, and personality disorders), *Clinical or Psychopathological Factors* (including diagnosis of mental disorder, alcohol or substance abuse, and the presence of delusions, hallucinations, or violent fantasies), *Historical or Case History Variables* (including previous violence, arrest history, treatment history, history of self-harm, as well as social, work, and family history), and *Contextual Factors* (including perceived stress, social support, and means for violence).[2] This framework aids the examiner in first, deciding relevant assessment issues, and second, in selecting methods for obtaining the information (Gacono & Evans, preface, this vol.). The forensic examiner chooses all assessment measures with an awareness of the requirements of admissibility (McCann, 1998).

The forensic evaluation is always conducted within a legal context. The forensic work product (consultation, report, and/or testimony) objectively links opinions to a psycholegal question. Because forensic treatment evaluations may not be voluntary, the foren-

---

[2]Monohan et al.'s (2001) model for risk assessment has been adapted for forensic treatment evaluations (Gacono, 2002b); Gacono & Evans, preface, this vol.).

sic evaluator's client is likely to be an institution, court, or an attorney. This creates potential role conflicts. Rather than taking the traditional role of "collaborative helper" operating in the best interest of the patient, the forensic evaluator maintains a more neutral and skeptical stance to preserve objectivity (Greenberg & Shuman, 1997). Recommendations may seem inconsistent with the defendant's point of view (see Greenburg & Shuman, 1997).

FORENSIC TREATMENT EVALUATION AND THE RORSCHACH

Although the Rorschach literature provides a growing forensic database (Cunliffe & Gacono, chap. 17, this vol.; Gacono, Gacono, & Evans, chap. 16, this vol.; Gacono, Meloy, & Bridges, chap. 18, this vol.; Gacono & Gacono, chap. 20, this vol.; Singer, Lee, & Hoppe, chap. 21, this vol.), there have been few studies reviewing the contributions of the RIM in forensic evaluations. Rorschach Comprehensive System data (Exner, 1993, 2001; Exner et al., 1995), in concert with other assessment methods, elucidates the individual's current clinical presentation and likelihood for favorable psychotherapy response.

Most readily apparent with respect to treatment evaluations, the Rorschach's capacity to bypass volitional processes helps clarify test-taking approaches that may support, or alternatively discount, the validity of other assessment methods (Gacono & Gacono, chap. 20, this vol.). That is, the relationship between validity configurations for self-report personality inventories and Rorschach variables help establish degrees of defensiveness (*Lambda, R, Sequence of Scores*), stress (*D, Adjusted D*), qualities of inner tension (*C', V, m*) and together, provide a more complete description of motivations for change. Self-report data suggesting current mental health stability, coupled with Rorschach data suggesting rigid defensiveness, is immediately suspect. In light of recommendations by Melton et al. (1997), RIM findings in context with other data are best suited to formulating opinions concerning treatment amenability.

The RIM Comprehensive System (Exner, 1993, 2001) evaluates Rorschach data in several clusters and constellations useful for formulating treatment strategies. Consequently, these are readily organized within the framework described earlier (Monahan et al., 2001). *Mediation Variables* assess the extent to which an individual is oriented toward making conventional or acceptable responses. These relate behavioral and personality data consistent with *Dispositional* or *Characterological Factors. Ideation variables* address how inputs become conceptualized and used, and elucidate *Clinical Factors* associated with florid and subtle thought disorder symptoms. *Processing* reveals processing effort, motivation, and processing efficiency and corresponds to elements of *Clinical* and *Dispositional Factors*. The *Affect Cluster* examines the role of emotion in psychology and functioning, and may likewise relate to *Clinical* and *Dispositional Factors*, and assist with identifying the degree of controls and coping strategies employed to contend with stress. The *Self-Perception Cluster* provides a picture of self-image and self-worth and considered with *Interpersonal Variables* reveals how an individual perceives and relates to others (Exner, 1993, 2001), elucidating aspects of the intersection between the *Individual* and *Contextual Factors*.

Treatment response is dependent on treatment retention. Hilsenroth, Handler, Toman, and Padawer (1995) found that subjects remaining in treatment tended to have more *Aggressive Movement* (*AG*) and *Texture* (*T*), but less *Cooperative Movement* (*COP*) relative to subjects who terminated early. Subjects who remained in psychotherapy appeared more disturbed and interpersonally needy, although this trend was not statistically significant. Comparatively, Gacono and Meloy (1994) found that psychopaths, as a group, showed elevated narcissistic self-interest (elevated reflection, *Fr* + *rF*, and personalization, *PER*, responses), and percepts included more primitive modes of interpersonal relatedness relative to nonpsychopathic persons with Antisocial Personality Disorder (ASPD). However, psychopaths tended to show relative absences of both needs for interpersonal closeness (shading *Texture*, *T*) and *Ego-dystonic Aggression* (*AG*; Gacono, Gacono, Meloy, & Baity, 2005). Given that psychopathy is commonly associated with poor prognosis (Gacono, 2000; Young, Justice, Erdberg, & Gacono, 2000), these findings appear to compliment and extend those of Hilsenroth et al. (1995).

Other work has examined RIM treatment outcome correlates. Weiner and Exner (1991) compared treatment outcomes for groups of patients in short- versus long-term psychodynamic therapy. CS variables included markers of acute and chronic distress (*D*, *AdjD*, respectively), organized coping resources and problem-solving approaches (*EA*, *CDI*, *Ambitent*, *Lambda*, *Zd*), reality testing (*X+%*, *X–%*), affect regulation and controls (*SumShad:FM + m*, *DEPI*, *Afr*, *CF:FC + C*), formal thought process and organization (*Sum6*, *M–*), defensive operations and self-inspecting (*Intellect*, *Reflections*, *Pairs*, *FD*), rigidity (*a:p*), and attachments and interpersonal qualities (*T*, *H:Hd + (H) + (Hd)*). For both groups, more than half of these variables marked clinical improvement after the first year, and roughly 75% of the selected variables measured gains after 4 years. With respect to forensic treatment, Gacono (1998) found that certain nonpsychopathic ASPD individuals in forensic settings, who were willing to engage in ambiguous, emotionally salient situations *(low Lambda)*, and who tended to be introversive (*M* > *WsumC*) while maintaining potential for attachment (*T* = 1), appeared reasonably amenable to therapeutic change.

These studies provide important foundations for forensic treatment planning. Forensic treatment obstacles deserve special consideration. Careful consideration during treatment planning and monitoring should be given to image management (Bannatyne et al., 1999; Meloy, 1988; Gacono & Gacono, chap. 20, this vol.) and transference-countertransference reactions (Kosson et al., 2000; Meloy, 1988). The forensic patient may feign or minimize psychopathology for a variety of reasons, such as to avoid anticipated consequences or to influence disposition planning. Additionally, the visceral qualities associated with certain crime types (e.g., serial sex murder) and the complexities inherent in the multiple roles commonly encountered in forensic settings (e.g., seemingly competing roles of corrections vs. rehabilitation) stimulate powerful transference and countertransference reactions (Kosson et al., 2000) that may impact treatment.

CASE EXAMPLES

We now present four cases to illustrate the role of the RIM in treatment planning and monitoring. Each subject is housed in a forensic institution. Cases 1 and 2 are forensic psychiatric patients. Cases 3 and 4 are Antisocial Personality Disordered offenders referred for institutional treatment. Monahan and colleague's (2001) model for risk assessment, adapted for the forensic treatment evaluation (Gacono & Bodholdt, 2002; Gacono & Evans, preface, this vol.), is used to organize the discussion of Cases 1 and 2.

Cases 1 and 2: Forensic Psychiatric Inpatients

Case 1: Mr. Jones

Mr. Jones was a 20-year-old White male committed to the hospital under an extended commitment. He was evaluated near the time of admission using the Kaufman Brief Intelligence Test (Kaufman & Kaufman, 1990), the Psychopathy Checklist–Revised (Hare, 2003), MMPI–2 (Hathaway & McKinley, 1989), and RIM. The purpose of Mr. Jones's evaluation was to determine dangerousness risk factors. The goal of Mr. Jones's treatment was to reduce his risk of future dangerousness. At the time of his assessment, Mr. Jones was committed to a forensic hospital after assault charges were dropped.

Historical Factors. Mr. Jones's parents divorced during his early childhood. His mother remarried, and his stepfather eventually committed suicide. Following release from his first psychiatric hospitalization at age 19, Mr. Jones was arrested for assaulting his father. Upon arrest, Mr. Jones attempted suicide by hanging. He was then transferred to a psychiatric facility, where he assaulted a female patient, ostensibly in an attempt to "save her." Several months after that episode, he was arrested for a minor traffic violation, culminating in his alleged assault of two officers (the instant offense).

Clinical and Dispositional Factors. Mr. Jones's family history includes Bipolar Disorder. He showed atypical motor skills in early development involving repetitive hand gestures. Mr. Jones began using marijuana, hallucinogens, intravenous amphetamines, and cocaine in his early adolescence.

Mr. Jones's psychiatric symptoms included paranoid, grandiose delusions and command hallucinations. He maintained idiosyncratic religious ideation involving an assignment from God to kill someone. He became socially withdrawn at age 19, with his adaptive living skills diminishing markedly.

Mr. Jones's violence history was impulsive, ego-syntonic, and affectively charged. Delusional thinking led Mr. Jones to believe he "saved" an immobile woman when he attacked her without warning; in other instances, he struck out violently when arguments escalated.

Mr. Jones is diagnosed with Schizoaffective Disorder, Bipolar Type, Cannabis Dependence, Hallucinogen Abuse, Amphetamine Abuse, and Cocaine Abuse (APA, 2000).

Contextual Factors.   Mr. Jones's victims were vulnerable, and his attacks opportunistic and fueled by active psychosis. He was unsuccessful in college. His aggressive behavior while in the community was affectively motivated and precipitated by perceived threats that resonated with delusional themes. It is likely substance use contributed to this violent behavior. While hospitalized (and more readily observed), his violence appears to have been precipitated by delusional ideas and command hallucinations.

Integrating Psychological Test Data.   Mr. Jones's intellectual functioning was estimated to fall within the low Average range, with a significant discrepancy between the Verbal (low Average range) and Performance (Borderline range) scores. He evidenced notable memory deficits. His MMPI–2 (Hathaway & McKinley, 1989) profile was marked by a considerable elevation on the F scale (> 95), reflecting severe thinking problems. Combined with his 2–8 codetype, indicating dysphoria, confusion, and alienation, Scale F was consistent with his Schizoaffective Disorder. His low PCL–R score (Total score = 15; Hare, 2003) indicated an absence of psychopathy. This total score fell below the average male forensic hospital patient mean ($M = 21.1$; $SD = 7.0$) and was consistent with his pattern of affective, rather than predatory, violence.

Mr. Jones produced 23 Rorschach responses. This, coupled with a *Lambda* of .22, suggests a valid protocol (see Table 11–1). His problem solving style ($EB = 10:5.5$) is *introversive*, marked by a pervasive tendency to rely on ideational coping strategies. The effectiveness of an *introversive* style rests in large part on the accuracy of the information that is being internally processed. Several factors from Mr. Jones's protocol ($PTI = 4$; $X+\% = 0.17$; $X–\%$; = 0.39; $M– = 2$; $WSum\ 6 = 46$) suggest that his internal world is not reality based. His processing is severely impacted by personality issues as well as a functional psychosis. His profile is similar to Exner's (2001) typical Schizophrenic inpatient with low *Lambda* ($PTI \geq 4$; *Mean X–%* = .36). Special Scores (*Sum 6* = 12, *WSum6* = 46) suggest that derailed thinking ($DR = 5$; $DR2 = 4$) contributes to his impaired judgment.

These cognitive problems are coupled with affective regulation problems. Together, they are consistent with MMPI–2 data ($F > 95$, 2–8 codetype) and a diagnosis of Schizoaffective Disorder. His strong *introversive* coping style ($M > Sum\ C$; *EB Per* = 1.8) is overworked in its attempts to hold emotions at bay ($Afr = 0.64$), and maintain impulses ($FC:CF + C = 0:5$; *Blends* = 12). The RIM adds to understanding his affective violence, as he becomes overwhelmed with strong emotions ($FC:CF + C = 0:5$; *Blends* = 12:23; multiple *color-shading blends*) that impact his perceptual accuracy ($XA\% = .61$).

Higher level defenses, such as intellectualization ($2AB + Art + Ay = 11$), are used in an attempt to stay organized and distant from his affect. Higher level defenses, however, give way to more primitive ones such as omnipotence/projective identification (*PER*) and isolation (*IsolateR* = .30). Mr. Jones's defenses and self-worth ($3[r] + 2/R = .22$) are tenuous at best. His sense of being damaged is pervasive (*MOR* = 6). Justifiably, Mr. Jones harbors pessimism about himself, his future, and interpersonal relationships (*COP* = 0; *GPR:PPR* = 3:7; *H:[H]* = 5:8). These expectations have likely been reinforced by

TABLE 11–1

Summary of Select Rorschach Variables and PCL–R Scores for Case Examples 1 and 2

Variable	"Critical" Level	Mr. Jones Adm. 1	Mr. Jones Adm. 2	Ms. Smith
R	< 14	23	35	19
Lambda	> .99	0.21	0.67	0.58
CDI	> 3	1	3	1
D	< 0	+1	**–3**	0
AdjD	< 0	+2	**–1**	0
EA	< 7	15.5	8.5	7
EB	Ambitent	10:5.5	**4:4.5**	**3:4.0**
eb	FM + m < Sum Shading	**4:7**	10:7	**1:4**
Zd	< –3.0	+0.5	–1.0	**–5.5**
DEPI	≥ 5	**6**	**6**	5
Afr	< .50	.64	.94	**.46**
FC:CF + C	CF + C > FC + 1	0:5	**3:2**	**3:2**
X + %	< .70	**.17**	**.20**	**.53**
X – %	> .20	**.39**	**.31**	**.21**
Sum 6 Sp Sc	> 6	**12**	6	9
M–	> 0	2	**4**	1
Ma:Mp	Ma < Mp	7:3	2:2	2:1
a:p	a + 1 < p	10:4	6:8	2:2
Intellect	> 5	**11**	3	1
Fr + rF	> 0	0	0	0
3r + (2)/R	< .33 or > .43	**.22**	**.03**	**.32**
FD	> 2	**8**	**3**	0
T	< 1 or > 1	1	**0**	**0**
H:(H) + Hd + (Hd)	Pure H < 2	5	3	4
	H < (H) + Hd + (Hd)	**5:8**	**3:6**	4:1
GHR:PHR	GHR + 1 < PHR	**3:7**	**0:9**	2:2
PCL–R Factor 1		4		11
PCL–R Factor 2		11		9
PCL–R Total Score	PCL–R ≥ 30	15		20

Note. Values at or above "Critical" level are in bold.

218

real-world relational experiences and are likely defended against by his delusional grandiosity.

This combination of introversiveness, grandiosity, malevolent internalized objects, difficulties regulating affect (*DEPI, Afr, Blends*), and inability to separate from the environment (*Lambda* = .21) is particularly distressing in an individual organized at a psychotic level. These RIM patterns help the clinician to understand Mr. Jones's propensity for affective violence. Despite his natural tendency to process information in fantasy (*Introversive*; Rorschach content) in an affect free state, he finds himself attracted to and even "pulled" into the emotionality of others. This stimulates emotions that exacerbate poor judgment and impulsivity. Feeling overwhelmed and out of control increases his feelings of paranoia and his propensity to "attack rather than be attacked."

Metaphorically, the goal of Mr. Jones's treatment is to (a) Increase his *Lambda*; that is, to achieve better separation from and tolerance of his emotions, as well as those of others; and (b) to increase his reality testing and cognitive slippage (lower his *Special Scores* and *X–%*, and increase his *X+%*). More concretely, psychoactive medications and an array of psychosocial programming would aid in increasing his thought organization, mood stability, and, in turn, increase impulse controls. Mr. Jones's difficulties forming and maintaining relationships (*Isolate* = .30; *GHR:PHR* = 3:7) would necessitate considerable time and energy for establishing a therapeutic alliance.

Treatment Progress. Following initial treatment gains, a second Rorschach was administered to assist with treatment monitoring and planning. At first glance (see Table 11–1), changes evident in Mr. Jones's clinical profile suggest regression. By the second assessment, Mr. Jones was in considerable discomfort (*D* = –3, *AdjD* = –1). Data suggest unmet need states (*FM* = 6) and painful introspection (*V* = 1; *FD* = 3) contributed to inner distress (*eb* = 10:7; *C'* = 3). Containing, rather than acting on, his distress likely motivated his treatment involvement. His thinking became increasingly flexible (*a:p* = 6:8), as he was more open to therapeutic challenges. Despite inner discomfort, Rorschach data suggest improved emotional controls. He was less internally oriented (*EB* = 4:4.5), likely due to improvement in affect regulation (*FC > CF + C*) and reality testing (decreased *X–%* and *Sum 6*). His increased *Lambda* (0.67) also indicates improved ability to separate his thoughts from feelings, making interpersonal relationships less frightening.

Motivated for therapeutic change, Mr. Jones required a supportive psychotherapeutic approach. Individual psychotherapy was enlisted to further increase affective controls while reducing his historic vulnerability to situational stress (*D* = –3; *FM + m* = 10; *FD* = 3). An important secondary goal would be to improve his self-worth (*3r + (2)/R* = .03). This necessitated improving his self (*3r + 2/R* = .03) and other (*GHR:PHR* = 0:9; *H:all [H]* = 3:6) appraisal skills. In concert with individual therapy, the treatment milieu would be organized in a fashion to facilitate generalization of therapeutic gains to various social settings.

During an initial and lengthy alliance-building phase, Mr. Jones was slow to engage in the psychotherapy process despite inner discomfort (*D* = –3; *AdjD* = –1). After 20 sessions, he began identifying core deficits in interpersonal skills. He developed skills for basic conversation, as well as for coping without withdrawal to fantasy. After 10 more sessions, in concert with changes to his mood stabilizing medication, Mr. Jones began to examine his own feelings of worth, and he briefly considered his chronic delusional thinking. He acknowledged that by giving up his grandiose delusions connecting him to supernatural powers, he would be giving up his special position in the world. Looking past his grandiosity put him in touch with underlying dysphoric affect (*MOR*; *3r + 2/R*). Predictably then, Mr. Jones's tendency to withdraw from others would reappear. Here, Rorschach data reflected relevant defensive operations that figured prominently in the dynamics underpinning his violence, and helped guide additional psychotherapeutic work.

Case 2: Ms. Smith

Ms. Smith was a 42-year-old Caucasian committed to the hospital as NGRI. She was evaluated at the time of admission using the K–BIT, MMPI–2, PCL–R, and RIM. The purpose of evaluation was to determine institutional violence risk factors and make recommendations about her treatment. At the time of assessment, Ms. Smith had been acquitted by reason of insanity for an attempted assault.

Historical Factors.   Ms. Smith completed high school. She has no record of sustained employment and was fired from her most recent job. She was married at age 26 and had two children by that union. She experienced considerable marital turbulence, and was divorced after 15 years. She was briefly hospitalized on several occasions for threats of self-harm. Her legal history includes acquittal by insanity for an attempt to harm her husband with a motor vehicle.

Clinical and Dispositional Factors.   Ms. Smith's psychiatric problems included dysphoric and irritable mood, as well as moderate levels of thought disorder. She developed idiosyncratic, overvalued ideas that her husband was having an affair. Her mode of violence involved passivity, in that she attempted to have her vehicle struck by another driver. Strong tendencies to control interpersonal exchanges and externalize blame were evident. She has no history of substance abuse. She carried diagnoses of Schizoaffective Disorder, Bipolar Type and Borderline Personality Disorder (APA, 2000).

Contextual Factors.   Ms. Smith has two children by her marriage. She experienced considerable marital turbulence and was divorced after 15 years. After she lost custody of her children, she made daily harassing phone calls and wrote threatening letters to her husband. She also began following her children. The combined losses of her marriage and of her children appear to have precipitated the instant offense.

Integrating Psychological Test Data.   Ms. Smith's intellectual functioning fell within the average range without significant differences between verbal and nonverbal reasoning skills. Her PCL–R profile was marked by a moderately elevated Factor 1 score (11), suggesting a callous disregard for others, remorselessness, failure to take responsibility for her behavior, and manipulative behavior. Her total score (PCL – R = 20) was below the threshold for psychopathy, and similar to the mean for female offenders (*M* = 19.0, *SD* = 7.5; Hare, 2003).[3] Her Factor 2 score of 9 indicated chronic impulsivity, irresponsibility, and considerable problems with behavior controls.

The MMPI–2 suggested a tendency to present herself in a favorable light (*L* = 66; *F* = 44). Her approach is not uncommon in individuals with limited psychological insight, and who engage in positive image management (Bannatyne et al., 1999; Gacono & Gacono, chap. 20, this vol.). Despite her denial, Ms. Smith's MMPI–2 markedly elevated 6–4 code type (81, 73, respectively), coupled with low scores on Scales 5 (43) and 3 (51), appears highly consistent with her history of hostility and impulsivity. Demanding and dependent persons, like Ms. Smith, often alienate significant others, from whom they crave admiration. Such dynamics would reinforce a tendency to externalize blame.

Turning to Rorschach findings (see Table 11–1), Ms. Smith produced 19 responses, which when combined with a *Lambda* of 0.58 suggest a valid protocol. Most notable is the clinical elevation on the *Depression Index* (*DEPI* = 5). This is consistent with her diagnosis and provides clues to the instant offense, which involved elements of affective violence precipitated by situational stress (i.e., divorce and loss of child custody amid chronic unemployment and interpersonal turmoil). When feeling stressed, Ms. Smith is without a consistent problem-solving style (*EB* = 3:4.0, *Ambitent*). Having less than average psychological resources (*EA* = 7), she becomes overwhelmed and prone to poor judgment (*X+%* = .53, *X–%* = .21; *Xu%* = .26, *F + %* = .43). Her judgment is further impacted by her difficulties assessing important interpersonal information (*Zd* = –5.5; *M–* = 1).

Ms. Smith does not seem to form significant attachments (*T* = 0). Her history suggests her interpersonal relationships tend to be maladaptive and chaotic. Her self-worth is lower than average (*3r + (2)/R* = .32), and is likely compensated with grandiosity (PCL–R Item 16 = 2; Item 2 = 1). Her aspirations far outstrip the resources needed to meet her aims (*W:M* = 11:3), a pattern that may contribute to poor self appraisal and feelings of frustration (*C'* = 2).

Ms. Smith portrays herself as healthy (*D* = 0, *AdjD* = 0). Despite her present circumstances, she lacks or minimizes distress. This is consistent with her tendency to externalize blame (PCL–R Item 16 = 2). Her lack of distress would appear inconsistent with her cognitive vulnerabilities (*Zd* = –5.5; *X–%* = .21). Coupled with positive image management (elevated MMPI–2 *L, K*), her profile suggested she was a poor candidate for traditional, insight-oriented therapies. Without the RIM data, which is consistent with her behavioral history, the evaluator might overestimate Ms. Smith's psychological resources.

Treatment Planning.   The hospital structure helped to organize and contain Ms. Smith's behavior. Recommendations based solely on her institutional presentation or self-report measures would contribute to the "misattribution of psychological health" (Kosson et al., 2000) and result in premature release. Given her lack of insight (MMPI–2

---

[3]Hare's published normative data does not include samples comprised of female forensic inpatients; data are interpreted with reasonable caution.

$L = 66$; $FD = 0$) and treatment motivation, the milieu was expected to play a key role in monitoring her stabilization. With gradual reduction in staff supervision, she would face increasing interpersonal challenges. Her reactions to increased stress would provide a measure of any treatment gains.

The goal of treatment was to develop skills for more independent and effective interpersonal functioning. Careful reassessment of gains would be essential to community re-entry, as situational factors were significantly related to her violence. Rorschach variables of interest in Ms. Smith's case would include those reflecting affective regulation (e.g., *DEPI*; *EB*; *FC:CF* + *C*; *Afr*), judgment and decision making (*Zd*; *W:M*; *X+%*; *X–%*; *M–*), and self- and interpersonal relatedness (*IsolateR*; *FD*; *3r* + *[2]/R*; *GHR:PHR*). Coupled with behavioral observation, RIM data were expected to elucidate true therapeutic gains and identify areas for continued treatment.

Cases 3 and 4: Two Incarcerated Antisocial Personality Disordered Offenders

Steve and Dave were incarcerated, Caucasion males in their mid to late 20s carrying a diagnosis of Antisocial Personality Disorder (APA, 2000). Consistent with treating severe character pathology, Steve and Dave began treatment within an institutional setting (Gacono, 1985; Kernberg, 1984). They were voluntary participants in a state offender treatment program. Group treatment was based on Reality Therapy (Glasser, 1966) and included Rational Behavior Training (RBT; Maultsby, 1979), criminal thinking (Yochelson & Samenow, 1977), anger management, and relapse prevention (Marlatt & Gordon, 1985).

Concurrent to group participation, both subjects participated in one-to-one counseling. Steve completed 9 months of short-term psychodynamic therapy (Strupp & Binder, 1984). His treatment focused on grief work and identity issues related to a history of sexual abuse. Dave attended 16 months of supportive counseling, which included problem-solving and assertiveness training. Both were rated as improved by their treating therapists.

PCL–Rs and initial Rorschachs were administered prior to treatment as a routine part of admissions testing (see Tables 11–2 through 11–5). PCL–Rs were administered and independently scored by two experienced raters with final item scores being determined by rater consensus. The second Rorschach was administered after 10 months of treatment. A third Rorschach was administered to Dave 16 months into treatment. These latter Rorschachs were administered by a clinical psychologist or advanced graduate psychology intern as a routine part of program evaluation. All 5 Rorschachs were rescored by CBG for reliability with rater consensus between CBG and the test administrator determining final scores. All protocols were then rescored independently by LAG (an experienced, PhD level rater) and yielded the following reliabilities: *Location*—99%, *Space*—100%, *Developmental Quality*—92%, *Determinants*—87%, *a/p*—100%, *Form Quality*—94%, *Pairs*—96%, *Content*—96%, *Populars*—100%, *Z scores*—91%, and *Special Scores*—67%.[4]

---

[4]Reliability was determined by comparing every response from CBG's final sequence of scores with LAG's corresponding independently coded sequence response scores. To be counted as a "hit" (agreement) determinants had to have achieved the same level of form domination (*FC*, *CF*, *C*), whereas special scores needed the same level (1 or 2); any deviation was counted as a "miss" (no agreement). Lowered % agreement for determinants and special scores reflect this stringent procedure. When agreement was adjusted for special scores without considering level, agreement rose to the acceptable 80% cutoff.

TABLE 11–2

Steve's PCL-R Protocol

Item	Factor 1	Factor 2	Total Score
1. Glibness/superficial charm	1		1
2. Grandiose sense of self worth	1		1
3. Need for stimulation/ proneness to boredom		1	1
4. Pathological lying	1		1
5. Conning/manipulative	1		1
6. Lack of remorse or guilt	1		1
7. Shallow affect	1		1 (0–1)
8. Callous/lack of empathy	1		1
9. Parasitic lifestyle		1	1
10. Poor behavioral controls		2	2
11. Promiscuous sexual behavior			2
12. Early behavioral problems		1	1
13. Lack of realistic, long-term goals		1	1
14. Impulsivity		1	1
15. Irresponsibility		1	1
16. Failure to accept responsibility for own actions	1		1
17. Many short-term marital relationships			2
18. Juvenile delinquency		0	0
19. Revocation of conditional release		2	2
20. Criminal versatility			1
Total	8	10	23

Case 3: Steve

Steve's PCL–R score was 23 (see Table 11–2) placing him in the low end of the moderate range (Gacono & Hutton, 1994). He is not a psychopath. None of his Factor 1 items are prototypic (scored 2). Despite narcissistic traits, he is not an arrogant narcissist, not a pathological liar, has some capacity for affective experience, attachment, empathy, and remorse, and accepts some responsibility for his antisocial behavior (Items 6, 7, 8, & 16). Despite attachment difficulties (Items 11 & 17), one *T* response and 2 *COP*s on the Rorschach (see Table 11–3) support attachment potential and "expectations of cooperative human interaction," even in the context of self-focus (*Fr* = 1).[5]

---

[5]*Texture* (*T*) responses indicate desire for affectional relatedness; a prognostically positive but unusual finding in ASPDs (while 79% of adult ASPD males are *T*-less [Gacono & Meloy, 1994], only 11% of nonpatient adults are [Exner, 1995]) and a likely contributor to Steve's request for one-to-one counseling.

Given above-average intelligence (Zachary, 1986), high levels of treatment motivation, and the absence of a sexual deviation, Steve's prognosis is favorable, despite his ASPD diagnosis. Had Items 1 and 2 (narcissism) and Items 6, 7, and 8 (shallow affect) been prototypic (2s), concurrent to a T-less Rorschach protocol with $Fr = 1$, treatment prognosis would have been dismal.

Factor 2 items indicate a "later" rather than early onset for antisocial behavior (early behavior problems = 1, juvenile delinquency = 0), prognostically a positive sign. One point scores on Items 3, 14, 15, indicate some impulse control, coping resources, and capacity for delay ($M = 3$). However, as indicated by 1 point scores, instead of 0s, and supported by Rorschach data (EA, M), Steve is in need of comprehensive skills training (Ross, Fabiano, & Ewles, 1988), including anger management (PCL–R Item 10 = 2; $S-\%$ = .25). Concurrent to an ASPD diagnosis, a Cluster B personality style containing narcissistic, histrionic, and borderline traits is suggested.

Steve's low *Lambda* is consistent with his elevated Zd, indicating an inefficient problem-solving style and a tendency to become overinvolved with stimuli (Exner, 1993). Low *Lambda* combined with a tendency toward introversion[6] (EB) suggest that *Overincorporation* (Zd) may be due in part to self-criticism associated with the need "to avoid error or failure" (Exner, 1993, p. 409). In ASPD patients, this pattern relates to suspiciousness and can correlate with an early history of abuse induced vigilance. Other cognitive deficits include perceptual accuracy problems ($X+\%$, $F+\%$), unconventional thinking ($Xu\%$, P), reality testing difficulties ($X-\%$), and cognitive slippage ($WSum6$, $SCZI$). The pervasiveness of these thinking problems suggests the need for cognitive-behavioral group therapy augmented by psychodynamic therapy.[7] Due to Steve's history, range of affect, and testing data suggesting bonding potential ($T = 1$; PCL–R Item 7), introversion, and the capacity for empathy ($M = 3$; PCL–R Item 8) and remorse ($V = 1$; PCL–R Item 6), a short-term psychodynamic therapy was included in his treatment.

Treatment Progress.   Successful treatment should reveal increases in coping resources, reality testing, conventional thinking, emotional control, emotional tolerance, accurate perceptions of self and others, and interpersonal relatedness. Steve's Rorschach supports treatment gains. Organized resources (EA) increased (4.5 to 9.5) without subsequent decreases in controls ($D/AdjD = 0/1$). Coping resources increased (CDI, 3 to 1) to within normative range (Exner, 1993). Capacity for delay and perhaps empathy increased (M doubles) and a predominant introversive problem-solving style surfaces.

Lambda remained similar but now organizing is more efficient, less strained, and more accurate ($X-\%$, .31 to .13). Perceptual accuracy without affect ($F+\%$) remains constant, however, improvement in $X+\%$ (.46 to .63) may suggest less emotionally caused disruptions. Perhaps the disruptive effects of anger on thinking has lessened ($S-\% = .00$). Al-

---

[6]Reduced R ($R = 13$) results in an *Ambitent* style on Protocol 1. Steve's predominant *Introversive* style surfaces on the second 16 response protocol.

[7]The combination of cognitive-behavioral techniques within a psychodynamic framework (Gacono & Meloy, 1988) would be an example of prescribed or technical eclecticism (Lazarus, 1989; Stricker, 1994). Cognitive restructuring and life skills can increase the ASPD patient's ability to tolerate deeper therapeutic work.

TABLE 11–3

Select Rorschach Variables for Steve

		PRE	*POST*
	R	13	16
	Lambda	.44	.33
	EA	4.5	9.5
	EB	3:1.5	6:3.5
	D/AdjD	0/0	0/1
Ideation	**Ma:Mp**	3:0	6:0
	M–	0	1
	M	3	6
	WSum6	30	30
Mediation	**P**	4	7
	X+%	.46	.63
	F+%	.50	.50
	X–%	.31	.13
	Xu%	.23	.25
	S–%	.25	.00
Affect	**FC:CF + C**	1:1	1:3
	PureC	0	0
	Afr	.30	.45
	T	1	1
	Y	0	1
	V	1	2
Processing	**Zd**	+4.5	−1.5
	W:M	10:3	8:6
Self Perception	**3r + (2)/R**	.46	.56
	Fr+rF	1	1
	FD	0	2
	MOR	1	0
Interpersonal	**COP**	2	2
	AG	0	0
	H	1	2
	(H)	1	2
	Hd:(Hd)	1:0	1:0
Constellations	**SCZI**	4	1
	DEPI	3	4
	CDI	3	1
	S-CON	7	6

though the level of cognitive slippage (*WSum6*) remains stable, Steve was better able to identify what is "popularly" seen by others (*P* = 4 to 7). Not unexpected for an ASPD individual, unusual perceptual accuracy remains pervasive (*Xu%*). Observable gains in Steve's judgment and problem-solving skills accompanied these Rorschach changes.

Despite continued difficulties with affect modulation (*FC:CF* + *C*), Steve is more tolerable of affect (*FC:CF* + *C* = 1:3, *Afr*) and now allowing "new" affective states, such as anxiety (*Y*). Increased emotional tolerance is essential, as negative emotions comprise "high risk situations." Although self-focused (*EgoC* = .56), Steve's self-appraisal lacks grandiosity and is more realistic (*W:M* = 8:6). He has increased psychological mindedness with some objectivity (*FD* = 2), but ruminates painfully (*V* = 2; perhaps guilt). His self-focus, absent the malignant narcissism, may even be a source of "ego strength." Interest in others has increased (*M, H, (H)*). Combined observable behaviors and Rorschach data suggest improvement to a *maintenance stage* (Prochaska et al., 1992).[8]

Case 4: Dave

Given above-average intelligence (Shipley; Zachary, 1986), high levels of treatment motivation (*action stage*), and the absence of a sexual deviation, Dave's low PCL–R score (PCL–R = 15; see Table 11–4) is prognostically promising. Zero scores on glibness and grandiosity (Items 1 & 2), 1 point on failure to accept responsibility for own actions (Item 16), and low scores on lack of remorse (Item 6 = 1), shallow affect (Item 7 = 0) and callous lack of empathy (Item 8 = 1) rule out a narcissistic or psychopathic disorder and are consistent with his below average *Egocentricity Ratio* (*3r + [2]/R*; as noted in Table 11–4). A low Egocentricity Ratio, 4 *MOR* responses, and the absence of a reflection response suggests a damaged rather than grandiose sense of self.[9]

Dave's *T* response, coupled with low scores on PCL–R Items 6, 7, and 8, indicate a desire and capacity for attachment. Like Steve and other nonpsychopathic ASPD patients, Dave is not without affect, but intolerant of it (*Afr* = .38). The absence of points on Items 11 (*promiscuous sexual behavior*) and 17 (*short-term marital relationships*) also support bonding capacity. Dave has been exclusively involved with one sexual partner, his wife, for approximately a decade. The composite data suggested a Cluster C personality disorder with an avoidant style concurrent to an ASPD diagnosis (additional data also support a passive-aggressive personality; *Mp* > *Ma* + 1, *S* = 3).

Factor 2 scores indicate behavioral problems originating in childhood (PCL–R Items 12 & 18). Early onset of antisocial behavior coupled with elevated Factor 1 scores are consistent with a psychopathy diagnosis (Smith, Gacono, & Kaufman, 1997). Fortunately, this is not the case. Dave's impulse controls are deficient but not absent (PCL–R Items 3, 14, 15; *D/AdjD* = 0/0). A source of strength, Item 9 (*Parasitic Lifestyle* = 0) reflected that Dave held legal employment the majority of his adult life. Despite vacillation by CBG on scoring Item 10 (*Poor Behavioral Controls*, anger problems) 1 or 2, any

---

[8]The maintenance stage is designated by "the stage in which people work to prevent relapse and consolidate the gains attained during action" (Prochaska, DiClemente, & Norcross, 1992, p. 1104).

[9]Only the first and third Rorschach are discussed. The second "transitional" Rorschach is presented for the reader's review. Dave remains in the latter phases of the Action stage.

TABLE 11–4
Dave's *PCL–R* Protocol

Item	Factor 1	Factor 2	Total Score
1. Glibness/superficial charm	0		0
2. Grandiose sense of self worth	0		0
3. Need of stimulation/ proneness to boredom		1	1
4. Pathological lying	1		1
5. Conning/manipulative	0		0
6. Lack of remorse of guilt	1		1
7. Shallow affect	0		0 (0–1)
8. Callous/lack of empathy	1		1
9. Parasitic lifestyle		0	0
10. Poor behavioral controls		1	1 (1–2)
11. Promiscuous sexual behavior			0
12. Early behavioral problems		2	2 (1–2)
13. Lack of realistic, long-term goals		1	1
14. Impulsivity		1	1
15. Irresponsibility		1	1
16. Failure to accept responsibility for own actions	1		1
17. Many short-term marital relationships			0
18. Juvenile delinquency		1	1
19. Revocation of conditional release		2	2
20. Criminal versatility			1
Total	4	10	15

points for an incarcerated ASPD felon on this item alert the clinician to needed anger management skills.

Dave's low *Lambda* suggests difficulties identifying the most economical means for confronting a task, and is consistent with him being easily overwhelmed by emotionally laden stimuli. His Rorschach suggests moderate to severe problems with perceptual accuracy (*Mediation*, $X+\%$, $F+\%$), unusual thinking ($Xu\%$), reality testing ($X-\%$; $M-$), coping (*CDI*), affect modulation and tolerance ($FC:CF + C$; $C' = 2$; *Afr*), hostility ($S = 3$), and depression (*DEPI*).[10] A comprehensive life skills training program is recommended to: (a) begin to address these deficits (Ross, Fabiano, Ewles, 1988), (b) orient him to the treatment process, and (c) further assess his treatment amenability.

---

[10]Like many other ASPD patients who manifest borderline personality organization and elevate on DEPI, Dave described his "depression" as boredom and emptiness.

TABLE 11–5

Select Rorschach Variables for Dave

		1st	2nd	3rd
	R	22	28	24
	Lambda	.22	.56	.33
	EA	12	8.5	10.0
	EB	7:5	7:1.5	8:2
	D/AdjD	0/0	0/0	0/0
Ideation	Ma:Mp	1:6	2:5	1:7
	M–	1	1	1
	M	7	6	8
	WSum6	12	25	10
Mediation	P	6	5	5
	X + %	.41	.43	.46
	F + %	.25	.50	.50
	X – %	.14	.07	.04
	Xu%	.45	.43	.50
	S – %	.00	.00	.00
Affect	FC:CF + C	0:4	1:2	0:2
	PureC	2	0	0
	Afr	.38	.47	.41
	S	3	4	3
	T	1	1	1
	C'	3	1	1
	Y	1	0	0
	V	2	1	4
Processing	Zd	+2.5	−1.5	−2.0
	W:M	6:7	6:7	3:8
Self Perception	3r + (2)/R	.36	.43	.50
	Fr + rF	0	0	0
	FD	1	2	0
	MOR	4	4	3
Interpersonal	COP	0	2	2
	AG	0	0	2
	H	3	3	2
	(H)	0	1	1
	Hd:(Hd)	3:3	6:1	5:2
Constellations	SCZI	1	2	1
	DEPI	6	4	6
	CDI	3	2	2
	S-CON	5	5	5

Dave's combination of hostility ($S = 3$), passivity ($Mp > Ma + 1$), and damaged sense of self ($MOR = 4$) manifest in a diagnosable passive-aggressive disorder and identify another area for treatment intervention (i.e., assertiveness training). Although interested in others ($M = 7, H = 3$), his past relationships including his childhood have been toxic and resulted in the lack of expectations for positive human interaction ($COP = 0$).

Dave's initial Rorschach is consistent with an avoidant, passive, inadequate, individual who would "peddle his bicycle" in order to sell drugs. Unlike Steve, who demonstrated high levels of self-focus and some "narcissism," Dave's inadequacy requires direct intervention, as a basic sense of being damaged underlies his avoidant, passive-aggressive style.

Treatment Progress.   Successful treatment should result in improved perceptual accuracy and reality testing, better affect tolerance, less hostility, increased self-worth (but less self absorption and grandiosity), greater assertiveness, more interest in others, and better skills for assessing interpersonal relationships (judgment, self and other appraisal). Dave's Rorschach suggests treatment gains, but also highlights areas for continued work.

Still an unconventional thinker ($Xu\%$), Dave produced significant gains in perceptual accuracy ($X+\%$, $F+\%$) and reality testing ($X-\%$). Although not perfect ($M- = 1$), Dave can now exercise "better judgment" in interpersonal relationships, one of several factors contributing to his avoidant/passive-aggressive style.

Growing confidence, both personally (handling emotions) and interpersonally, has contributed to his increased self-worth ($3r + [2]/R$, .36 to .50). However, his self-image is still tarnished by a basic sense of damage ($MOR = 3$), residue from a neglectful and deprived childhood. Dave now associates positive attributes with interpersonal interactions ($COP = 2$), possibly a byproduct of his therapeutic alliance and certainly an avenue through which his damaged self might, overtime, be modified. Although test data and self-report confirm increased confidence in managing emotions, affect tolerance ($FC:CF + C = 0:2$; $Afr = .41$), depression ($DEPI = 6$), and anger ($S = 3$) remain problematic. His passive-aggressiveness ($Mp > Ma + 1$; $S = 3$) continues to be a treatment focus.

CONCLUSIONS

Taken together, available literature indicates the RIM is a psychometrically well-established instrument when appropriately administered, scored, and interpreted. It is well-suited for treatment planning and monitoring within forensic settings and at various stages of the criminal process. The RIM's capacity to bypass volitional controls and assess personality processes renders it uniquely invaluable in forensic settings where image management is typical. Often, forensic assessments are requested to obtain information used to make recommendations concerning disposition and placement; such assessments usually pit the forensic patient's personal liberty against the safety and interest of the public. Rorschach science should continue to sharpen focus on clinical applications, rather than on "pseudo-debates" that cloud its uses (Gacono, Loving, & Bodholdt, 2001; Gacono & Evans, preface, this vol.).

A patient's characteristic problem-solving approaches and defensive operations, as well his or her relatedness to self and others, are helpful points of focus when applying Rorschach data to forensic treatment planning. Further, by integrating RIM and other data within the framework recommended by Monahan et al. (2001), the interplay between personality and behavior becomes clear. In particular, the relative influences of contextual and dispositional factors can be more readily observed through multiple methods of assessment (cf. Bannatyne et al., 1999). From this vantage point, the evaluator is better prepared to view the full set of factors bearing on a case, and to employ the forensic treatment or corrections environment itself, in creative, individualized and effective ways to maximize treatment outcomes.

ACKNOWLEDGMENTS

This chapter is adapted from "Use of the Rorschach in Forensic Settings for Treatment Planning and Monitoring." *International Journal of Offender Therapy and Comparative Criminology, 46*(3), 294, 2002; and "The Use of the Psychopathology Checklist–Revised (PCL–R) and Rorschach in Treatment Planning With Antisocial Personality Disordered Patients." *International Journal of Offender Therapy and Comparative Criminology, 42*(1), 49–64, 1998.

REFERENCES

American Psychiatric Association (2000). *Diagnostic and statistical manual of mental disorders* (4th rev. ed.).Washington, DC: Author.

Bannatyne, L. A., Gacono, C. B., & Greene, R.L. (1999). Differential patterns of responding among three groups of chronic, psychotic, forensic outpatients. *Journal of Clinical Psychology, 55*(12), 1553–1565.

Davison, S., Leese, M., & Taylor, P. J. (2001). Examination of the screening properties of the personality diagnostic questionnaire 4+ (PDQ–4+) in a prison population. *Journal of Personality Disorders, 15*(2),180–194.

Dusky v. U.S., 362 U.S. 402 (1960).

Exner, J. E. (1993). *The Rorschach: A Comprehensive System: Vol. 1. Basic foundations* (3rd ed.). New York: Wiley.

Exner, J. E. (2001). *A Rorschach workbook for the Comprehensive System* (5th ed.). North Carolina: Rorschach Workshops.

Exner, J. E., Colligan, S., Hillman, L., Ritzler, B., Sciara, A., & Viglione, D. (1995). *A Rorschach workbook for the Comprehensive System* (4th ed.). North Carolina: Rorschach Workshops.

Gacono, C. B. (1985, April). Mental health work in a county jail: A heuristic model. *Journal of Offender Counseling, 5*(1), 16–22.

Gacono, C. B. (1998). The use of the Hare Psychopathy Checklist–Revised (PCL–R) and Rorschach in treatment planning with Antisocial Personality Disordered patients. *International Journal of Offender Therapy and Comparative Criminology, 42*(1), 49–64.

Gacono, C. B. (Ed.). (2000). *The clinical and forensic assessment of psychopathy: A practitioner's guide.* Mahwah, NJ: Lawrence Erlbaum Associates.

Gacono, C. B. (2002a). Guest editorial: Why there is a need for the personality assessment of offenders. *International Journal of Offender Therapy and Comparative Criminology, 46*(3), 271–273.

Gacono, C. B. (2002b). Introduction to a special series: Psychological testing in forensic settings. *International Journal of Offender Therapy and Comparative Criminology, 46*(3), 274–280.

Gacono, C. B. (2005). *The clinical and forensic interview schedule for the Hare Psychopathy Check-list: Revised and screening version*. Mahwah, NJ: Lawrence Erlbaum Associates.

Gacono, C. B., & Bodholdt, R. (2002). The role of the Psychopathy Checklist–Revised (PCL–R) in violence and risk assessment. *Journal of Threat Assessment, 1*(4), 65–79.

Gacono, C., & Hutton, H. (1994). Suggestions for the clinical and forensic use of the Hare Psychopathy Checklist–Revised (PCL–R). *International Journal of Law and Psychiatry, 17*(3), 303–317.

Gacono, C. B., Loving, J. & Bodholt, R. (2001). The Rorschach and psychopathy: Toward a more accurate understanding of the research findings. *Journal of Personality Assessment, 7*(1), 16–38.

Gacono, C. B., & Meloy, J. R. (1988). The relationship between cognitive style and defensive process in the psychopath. *Criminal Justice and Behavior, 15*(4), 472–483.

Gacono, C. B., & Meloy, J. R. (1994). *The Rorschach assessment of aggressive and psychopathic personalities*. Hillsdale, NJ: Lawrence Erlbaum Associates.

Gacono, C. B., & Meloy, J. R. (2002). Assessing antisocial and psychopathic personalities. In J. Butcher (Ed.), *Clinical personality assessment: Practical approaches* (2nd ed., pp. 361–375). New York: Oxford University Press.

Gacono, C. B, Meloy, J. R., Sheppard, K., Speth, E., & Roske, A. (1995). A clinical investigation of malingering and psychopathy in hospitalized insanity acquittees. *Bulletin of the American Academy of Psychiatry and the Law, 23*(3), 1–11.

Gacono, C. B, Meloy, J. R., Speth, E., & Roske, A. (1997).Above the law: Escapes from a maximum security forensic hospital and psychopathy. *American Academy of Psychiatry and the Law, 25*(4), 1–4.

Glasser, W. (1966). *Reality therapy: A new approach to psychiatry*. New York: Harper & Row.

Greenburg, S., & Shuman, D. (1997). Irreconcilable conflict between therapeutic and forensic roles. *Professional: Psychology: Research and Practice, 23*(1), 50–57.

Grisso, T. (1988). *Competency to stand trial evaluations: A manual for practice*. Sarasota, FL: Professional Resource Exchange, Inc.

Hare, R. (2003). *The Hare Psychopathy Checklist–Revised* (2nd ed.). Toronto: Multi-Health Systems.

Hathaway, S. R., & McKinley, J. C. (1989). *MMPI–2*. Minneapolis: University of Minnesota Press.

Hilsenroth, M. J., Handler, L., Toman, K. M., & Padawer, J. R. (1995). Rorschach and MMPI–2 indices of early psychotherapy termination. *Journal of Consulting and Clinical Psychology, 63*(6), 956–965.

Jumes, M. T., Oropeza, P. P., Gray, B. T., & Gacono, C. B. (2002). Use of the Rorschach in forensic settings for treatment planning and monitoring. *International Journal of Offender Therapy and Comparative Criminology, 46*(3), 294–308.

Kaufman, A. S., & Kaufman, N. L. (1990). *Kaufman Brief Intelligence Test*. Circle Pines, MN: American Guidance Service, Inc.

Kernberg, O. (1984). *Severe personality disorders:psychotherapeutic strategies*. London: Yale University Press.

Kosson, D., Gacono, C., & Bodholdt, R. (2000). Assessing psychopathy: Interpersonal aspect and clinical interviewing. In C. B. Gacono (Ed.), *The clinical and forensic assessment of psychopathy: A practitioner's guide* (pp. 203–229). Mahwah: NJ. Lawrence Erlbaum Associates.

Lazarus, A. (1989). *The practice of multimodal therapy*. Baltimore: Johns Hopkins University Press.

Marlatt, G., & Gordon, J. (1985). *Relapse prevention: A self-control strategy for the maintenance of behavioral change*. New York: Guilford.

Maruish, M. E. (2004). *The use of psychological testing for treatment planning and outcome assessment* (3rd ed.). Mahwah, NJ: Lawrence Erlbaum Associates.

Maultsby, M. (1979). *Freedom from alcohol and tranquilizers*. Lexington, KY: Rational Self-Help Books.

McCann, J. T. (1998). Defending the Rorschach in court: An analysis of admissibility using legal and professional standards. *Journal of Personality Assessment, 70*, 125–144.

Meloy, J. R. (1988). *The psychopathic mind: Origins, dynamics, and treatment*. Northvale, NJ: Aronson.

Meloy, J. R. (1991). Rorschach testimony. *Journal of Psychiatry & Law, 19*, 221–235.

Meloy, J. R. (1997). *Violent attachments.* Northvale, NJ: Aronson.

Melton, G. B., Petrila, J., Poythress, N. G., & Slobogin, C. (1997). *Psychological evaluations for the courts: A handbook for mental health professionals and lawyers* (2nd ed.). New York: Guilford.

Monahan, J., Steadman, H., Silver, E., Appelbaum, P., Robbins, P., Mulvey, E., Roth, L., Grisso, T., & Banks, S. (2001). *Rethinking risk assessment: The MacArthur study of mental disorder and violence.* New York: Oxford University Press.

Mortimer, R., & Smith, W. (1983). The use of the psychological test report in setting the focus of psychotherapy. *Journal of Personality Assessment, 47*(2), 134–138.

Nieberding, R. J., Moore, III, J. T., & Dematatis, A. P. (2002). Psychological assessment of forensic psychiatric outpatients. *International Journal of Offender Therapy and Comparative Criminology, 46*(3), 294–308.

Prochaska, J., DiClemente, C., & Norcross, J. (1992). In search of how people change: Application to addictive behaviors. *American Psychologist, 47*(9), 1102–1114.

Rogers, R. (1997). Current status of clinical methods. In R. Rogers (Ed), *Clinical assessment of malingering and deception* (2nd ed., pp. 373–397). New York: Guilford.

Ross, R., Fabiano, E., & Ewles, C. (1988). Reasoning and Rehabilitation. *International Journal of Offender Therapy, 32*, 29–35.

Shapiro, D. (1984). *Psychological evaluation and expert testimony: A practical guide to forensic work.* New York: Van Nostrand Reinhold.

Smith, A., Gacono, C. B., & Kaufman, L. (1997). A Rorschach comparison of psychopathic and nonpsychopathic conduct disordered adolescents. *Journal of Clinical Psychology, 53*(4), 1–12.

Stricker, G. (1994). Reflections on psychotherapy integration. *Clinical Psychology: Science and Practice, 1*(1), 3–12.

Strupp, H., & Binder, J. (1984). *Psychotherapy in a new key: A guide to time-limited dynamic psychotherapy.* New York: Basic Books.

Swanson, J. W., Borum, R., Swartz, M. S., Hiday, V. A., Wagner, H. R., & Burns, B. J. (2001). Can involuntary outpatient commitment reduce arrest among persons with severe mental illness? *Criminal Justice and Behavior, 28*, 156–189.

Weiner, I. B. (2004). Rorschach Inkblot Method. In M. Maruish (Ed.), *The use of psychological testing for treatment planning and outcome assessment* (pp. 553–587). Mahwah, NJ: Lawrence Erlbaum Associates.

Weiner, I. B., & Exner, J. E., Jr. (1991). Rorschach changes in long-term and short-term psychotherapy. *Journal of Personality Assessment, 56*, 453–465.

Yochelson, S., & Samenow, S. (1977). *The criminal personality: Vol. 1. A profile for change.* New York: Aronson.

Young, M., Justice, J., Erdberg, P., & Gacono, C. (2000). The incarcerated psychopathy in psychiatric treatment: management or treatment? In C. B. Gacono (Ed.), *The clinical and forensic assessment of psychopathy: A practitioner's guide* (pp. 313–331). Mahwah: NJ. Lawrence Erlbaum Associates.

Zachary, R. (1986). *Shipley Institute of Living Scale: Revised manual.* Los Angles: Western Psychological Service.

12

THE RORSCHACH IN CHILD CUSTODY AND PARENTING PLAN EVALUATIONS: A NEW CONCEPTUALIZATION

F. Barton Evans
Private Practice, Bozeman, MT

Benjamin M. Schutz
Private Practice, Springfield, VA

As *The Handbook of Forensic Rorschach Assessment* amply demonstrates, the Rorschach Inkblot Method (RIM)[1] enjoys broad acceptance and usage in forensic psychological assessment, including Child Custody and Parenting Plan Evaluations (CCPPE).[2] The goal of this chapter is to propose a new, systematic model in CCPPEs; to conceptualize how the RIM might fit best in this model; to offer a systematic protocol for RIM use in CCPPE; and to provide the reader a review of proposed central RIM variables within this new model. We examine the research on how frequent the RIM is currently used in CCPPE, its role in the generally accepted model (GAM) for CCPPE, and its legal sufficiency in doing so. We also review the relevant case law on the RIM in CCPPE.

Although there have been unprecedented calls for the ban of the Rorschach in court (Grove, Barden, Garb, & Lilienfeld, 2002; Wood et al., 2003), it is beyond the scope of this chapter to fully respond to this general challenge. We refer the reader to chapters 1 through 5 of this book for a thorough coverage of the scientific and legal foundations of the Rorschach in forensic evaluations. In particular, however, Wood et al. (2003) level a specific criticism of the Rorschach in CCPPE, stating the Rorschach caused a parent to lose custody of a child to a well-known child abuser based largely on the results of the Rorschach inkblot test, suggesting the CCPPE commonly ignore other test information

---

[1]Throughout this chapter, all references to the Rorschach are to the CS (Exner, 2003), the only Rorschach system with sufficient empirical validity to be admissible in court (Gacono, Evans, & Viglione, chap. 1, this vol.; McCann, Evans, chap. 3, this vol.).

[2]We include the term *parenting plan evaluations* along with the more traditional term *child custody evaluations*. We do so to reflect the changing legal climate emphasizing parenting plans in the best interest of the child over the more possession-oriented term *custody*, as well as acknowledging states like Montana, which have statutorily substituted parenting plan evaluations for custody evaluations.

in favor of the Rorschach. In response, we wish clearly to reiterate something that perhaps seems obvious to forensic evaluators: The Rorschach should never be the sole data source in any psychological evaluation, but rather part of a comprehensive, multimethod evaluation (see Erdberg, chap. 27, this vol.; Schutz, Dixon, Lindenberger, & Ruther, 1989). Indeed, to do so is unethical (Code of Ethics, American Psychological Association, 2002) and falls below standards of practice in psychological testing in general (Educational Research Association, 1999), in forensic psychological assessment (Committee on Ethical Guidelines for Forensic Psychologists, 1991) and for the use of the Rorschach in particular (Board of Trustees of the Society for Personality Assessment, 2005). Further, research on clinical judgment and psychological testing finds that single method assessment vastly increases error rate and bias in forming valid judgments (Garb, 1998).

USE OF THE RIM IN CCPPE: TWENTY YEARS OF PRACTICE SURVEYS

There have been a number of studies that have surveyed experienced CCPPE evaluators on their practices, including their use of psychological tests. Keilin and Bloom (1986) found the Rorschach the second (behind the Minnesota Multiphasic Personality Inventory, MMPI) most commonly used test with adults (41.5% of respondents used the test a mean of 67.3% of their cases). Following Hagen and Castagna's (2001) use calculations, overall percent use in child custody evaluations is (41.5 × 67.3) = 27.9%. With children, the Rorschach was the third most frequently used personality measure, behind the TAT/CAT and miscellaneous projective drawings. (29.2% of respondents used the test a mean of 77.9% in their cases. Overall % use (29.2 × 77.9) = 22.7). Ackerman and Ackerman (1996) again found the Rorschach in the same position, second to the MMPI, in use with adults (47.8% of respondents use the test a mean of 63.6% of their cases). Overall, the percent usage in CCPPE is 47.8 × 63.6 = 30.4%, up 2.5% since 1986. For children, the Rorschach was now the sixth most often used personality measure behind the TAT/CAT, then sentence completion, miscellaneous projective drawings, HTP, KFD (27.4% of respondents used it a mean 47.9% of the time). Overall, use was 13.1% (27.4 × 47.9), indicating Rorschach use with children fell by 43%. It is unclear why RIM use with children has dropped so dramatically.

In terms of use in general personality assessment, Archer and Newsome (2000) and Piotrowski and Keller (1989) found that the Rorschach is the second most widely used personality assessment technique in clinical practice with adults and adolescents (also see Butcher & Rouse, 1996). Reviewing Piotrowski et al.'s (1998) research on the impact of managed care on the decreased use of projective techniques, Lilienfeld, Wood, and Garb (2000) report that several projective techniques, such as the Rorschach and TAT, "have been abandoned by a sizeable minority of users" and that "at least some of the decline may also stem from the cumulative impact of criticisms leveled at these techniques over the past several decades." Apparently, the fact that Piotrowski et al. concluded that most managed care companies refuse to pay for the Rorschach for purely financial reasons and they do not mention criticisms of the Rorschach did not seem to enter Lilienfeld et al.'s (2000) analysis when assessing the meaning of the article. Moreover, Quinnell and Bow (2001) reported the Rorschach to be the third most frequently used personality measure with adults, behind the MMPI–2 and the Millon Clinical Multiaxial Inventory—III (MCMI–III; 44% of respondents used it a mean of 64% of their cases; overall use, 44 × 64 = 28.2%). There is remarkably stable use of the RIM over the 15-year period of those three surveys; roughly 44% of practitioners use it 65% of the time. Whatever the controversy over the Rorschach Inkblot Method, the aforementioned studies indicate that practitioners have consistently found it to be one of the most useful personality measures for adults, even though the RIM is a far more challenging instrument to administer, score, and interpret when compared to self-report measures.

With children, Quinnell and Bow (2001) report the Rorschach to be the sixth most often used personality measure behind the Kinetic Figure Drawing, Draw A Person, Sentence Completion, House Tree Person, and TAT/CAT. Twenty-three percent of respondents used this test on a mean of 64% of their cases (overall use, 23 × 64 = 14.7%). Rorschach use with children seems to have stabilized after a significant decline from 1986 to 1996. One reason statistically for its lower frequency of use with children than with adults may be that the CS cannot be used with children younger than 6 years, thus curtailing the range of applicability for children in custody disputes. The more frequently used drawings, apperception tests, and sentence completion may be the instruments of choice with younger children. The next practice survey should collect test usage data for children of different ages to see if this hypothesis is correct. Another reason is that CCPP evaluators may find the formal assessment of children's mental health to be less often at issue before the court than their parents.

REVIEW OF LEGAL DECISIONS

In terms of overall legal decisions involving the Rorschach, Meloy (chap. 4, this vol.) updated the 10 years since Meloy, Hansen, and Weiner (1997) reported on the authority of the Rorschach in court. Together these studies of 60 years of legal citations that appeared in federal, state, and military courts of appeal concerning the Rorschach found that the test was cited in 247 published cases (1945–1995) and 150 appellate cases between 1996 and 2005 (nearly three times the rate of citation than during the previous half century). Meloy concluded that "it is clear that the test continues to have authority, or weight, in higher courts of appeal throughout the United States" (p. 85).

To supplement Meloy's work, a Lexis Nexis search using "Rorschach and Child Custody" was conducted, which produced 43 hits from 1956 to 2005.[3] Before discussing relevant cases, it should be remembered that these citations represent only the very tip of the iceberg regarding the use of the RIM and CCPPEs, because most CCPPEs result in settlement of the dispute. Roughly 10% of these evaluations are presented as evidence at a hearing (Ash & Guyer, 1984). We do not know of any statistics on the percentage of litigated child custody disputes that are appealed. Anecdotal reports suggest that the number is quite small, perhaps as low as 1%. Therefore, the reported cases—our only (therefore best) source of data—may not be an accurate picture of the courts' reception of RIM data in child custody disputes.

---

[3]Thanks go to attorneys Wendy N. Schwartz and Kristen A. Parillo, who conducted this search and retrieval for the authors.

A review of the appellate decisions produced only five cases that touched on the admissibility or scientific status of the RIM. They fall into three of Meloy's categories—the inappropriate use of the RIM, qualified use of the RIM, and criticism of the RIM. In terms of inappropriate use, in *Metzger, Bradt, & Izen Jr. v. Sebek et al.* (1994), appellants raised the issue that the psychologist's conclusions about child sexual abuse were based on the interpretation of card 3 of the RIM. The court did not address this overall issue of the use of the Rorschach, because the court record acknowledged that the conclusions were not based on any single response.

In terms of qualified use of the RIM, in the matter of *DSS v. Hamlet* (1997), the appellant argued that the trial court inappropriately relied on the RIM because it is not a reliable determiner of narcissism. The court did not directly respond to this assertion. Instead, it concluded that, even if this was true, it was harmless error, because the outcome would have been the same even if the entirety of the psychologist's report was eliminated from the record. In *The People of the State of Illinois v. Tonya L. and Clayton J.* (2004), appellants argued that the RIM and other tests were subjective, severely criticized, and open to any interpretation by the interviewer. The court noted that, whereas the psychological examiner characterized the tests as subjective, nothing in the record indicated that the tests have been severely criticized. This determination suggests that there was no rebuttal expert at the original hearing criticizing the use of the RIM.

With regard to criticism of the RIM, two cases yielded opposing decisions. In *Ford v. Ford* (pseudonyms, 2000), the court admitted and gave weight to the RIM data. In its opinion the court wrote: "The court is especially concerned with Dr. Romirowsky's findings regarding Susan's response to the Rorschach Test (and the TAT) because they showed a different side of Susan." In *Mayo v. Mayo* (2000), the trial court did not find the testimony of one of the psychologists credible because the bases of his opinions were not reliable, valid tests. They were described as highly subjective and lacked generally recognized scientific validity and reliability as predictive tests. One of the tests so described was the RIM. The decision included comments by the dissenting North Dakota Supreme Court justice on the handling of the case by the trial court. This judge noted that there were already two precedent opinions admitting the Rorschach in North Dakota courts. These comments indicate that at trial the court did not find the RIM to pass a Daubert-Frye analysis, even though there were previous opinions admitting the test.

In conclusion, out of 43 cases in 50 years, there were only 5 cases addressing the admissibility or scientific status of the RIM. The court understood bad practice when they saw it (*Metzger, Bradt, & Izen Jr. v. Sebek et al.*) and recognized that possible problems with the Rorschach did not by itself constitute appealable grounds (*DSS v. Hamlet* and *People of the State of Illinois v. Tonya L. & Clayton J.*). In the two remaining cases, the court was split on whether or not the RIM was useful (*Ford v. Ford*) or unreliable (*Mayo v. Mayo*). Interestingly, in *Mayo*, a published dissent from one of the state appellate judges noted that the RIM had been admitted two previous times in that state, suggesting a further split in the opinion about the RIM. Unfortunately, we were not privy to the quality of expert opinion in any of these cases.

CHILD CUSTODY EVALUATIONS: CONTENT

The first step in demonstrating the Rorschach Inkblot Method's (RIM) utility in child custody evaluations is to show that it measures aspects of psychological functioning known to be related to children's postdivorce adjustment. These are the content areas or factors that a child custody evaluation assesses.

Determinations of child custody are—absent a constitutional issue—overwhelmingly left to each state to decide according to their own rules of evidence. Admissibility of expert scientific testimony is governed on a state-by-state basis by the Daubert test, the Frye test, or other state-specific reliability tests for evidence (Giannelli & Imwinkelried, 1999). We use the Daubert test for our analysis because it incorporates the Frye test and therefore provides the most widespread guidance. It is possible in the dozen or so states that are neither Frye nor Daubert that their reliability test is more rigorous than Daubert, although we have not found mention of this in the legal or psychological literature.

Daubert v. Merrell Dow Pharmaceuticals, Inc. (1993) created a multiprong "test" to establish the minimum necessary conditions for scientific expert testimony to be considered reliable (the legal term for valid) and therefore admissible. Ironically, the Daubert test, as an example of legal thinking at the highest level, produced a test that embodies most of the flaws in the scientific testimony that it was meant to keep out. Its terms are vaguely defined; it lacks weighting or combinatorial rules; it vests decision making in a single individual, untrained in areas relevant to the decisions they make; it grants them discretionary authority to construct the "test" as they see fit on a case-by-case basis; it has never been subjected to empirical testing; and it has no known error rates. Four prongs do not necessarily produce a useful fork. Indeed, Gatowski et al. (2001) found that, although judges strongly endorse (91%) the utility of *Daubert/Kumho* guidelines, they failed to demonstrate a credible understanding of the two prongs of falsifiability (95% error rate) and error rate (96% error rate). Indeed, it could be argued that, applying *Daubert* standards to this study, judges themselves do not pass *Daubert* standards for reliability in understanding one half of *Daubert*.

In regard to the content of the evaluation, the test requires that the underlying theory of the child custody evaluation be published in peer-reviewed literature, be empirically testable and tested, and generally accepted by the relevant professional community. There have been four statements from psychological (APA, 1994), psychiatric (AACAP, 1997), interdisciplinary (Association of Family and Conciliation Courts; AFCC, 1994), and social work (Luftman et al., 2005)[4] organizations that we believe provide the content areas that would meet a *Daubert* test. An analysis of the guidance for CCPPE provided by psychology, psychiatry, and social work (Schutz, forthcoming) produced the proposed content for a generally accepted (GA) model of CCPPEs in Figure 12–1.

Current professional guidance only provides a list of factors to consider, nothing about how they interact with each other. Their arrangement within/between individuals and the directions of the arrows of influence in the figure are the product of one author's review of the empirical literature (Schutz, in press) to provide an empirical anchor and thus greater elaboration and specificity to the currently generally accepted content for a CCPPE. The boxes under Father

---

[4]The 2006 version was published after this was written.

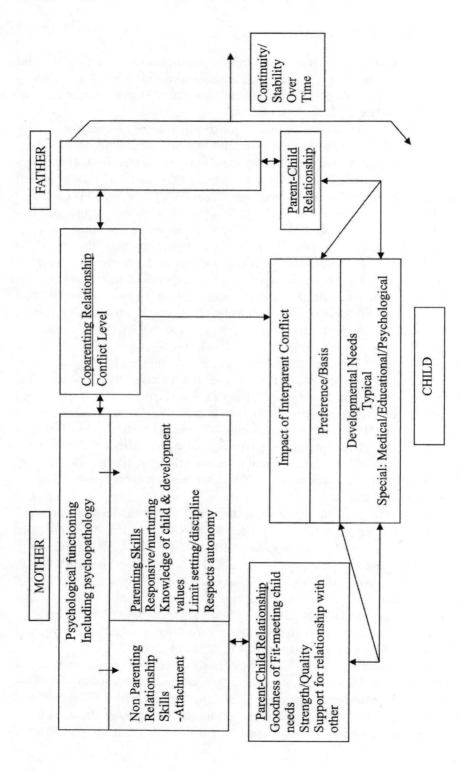

Figure 12–1. Proposed factors for a generally accepted (GA) child custody evaluation.

contain the same information as under Mother. Once such a model was generally accepted, all the prongs of *Daubert* would be met for the content of a CCPPE.

The review of the literature (Schutz, in press) produced the following further specification of the content of the GA model:

1. Stresses and Coping Styles: including self-efficacy, locus of control and specific coping styles (problem solving, support seeking, emotional regulation, and avoidance).
2. Normal Psychological Functioning/Psychopathology: Specific diagnoses known to impact parenting are affective disorders, psychosis/schizophrenia, substance abuse, antisocial personality disorders, and anxiety disorders. Problems with emotional availability/responsiveness and affect regulation characterize inept parenting in both normal and clinical populations and are seen in all diagnostic categories.
3. Quality of Parent–Child Relationship: Research has focused on the following dimensions, especially as they are experienced and evaluated by the child: attachment security, closeness/estrangement (including alienation), conflict/harmony, warmth/hostility, role reversal (including parentification), individuation/boundary problems (including intrusiveness, enmeshment, rejection), triangulation/coalitions.
4. Parenting: Including sensitive responding, behavioral/psychological controls; monitoring; styles, including authoritarian, authoritative, permissive, and indifferent.
5. Child Temperament and Other Coping Resources: Such as intelligence, social skills, and positive peer relationships.
6. Child Special Needs: Including medical, educational, psychological—specifically internalizing/externalizing disorders.
7. Coparenting Relationship: Similarity/inconsistency in parenting, disagreement and gatekeeping, conflict type, history and tactics.

CHILD CUSTODY EVALUATION METHODS

There are only four methods available to the child custody evaluator for collecting data: interviews with the caretakers and their children, interviews with third parties and/or review of their records, direct observation of the interactions of family members, and psychological testing of family members (Schutz, in press). The *Daubert* prongs identified earlier also apply to the methods used in a child custody evaluation. They need to be published in peer-reviewed literature, empirically testable and tested, generally accepted by the relevant professional community, administered according to professional standards, and with known error rates.

The methodology that best meets these criteria is psychological testing. All of the other methodologies have been generally referred to and occasionally described in peer-reviewed publications (Halon, 1990; Schutz et al., 1989), are potentially empirically testable, and their utility is generally accepted. However, no specific interview format for parents, children, or third parties, or for observations of parents and children, has ever been empirically tested. None have been generally accepted or have known error rates.

Of all the psychological tests used in child custody evaluations, the two with the best child custody evaluation specific research underpinnings are the Minnesota Multiphasic

Personality Inventory (MMPI/MMPI–2; Schutz, in press) and the RIM. The practice surveys reviewed earlier show that the RIM has been the most frequently used nonobjective personality measure for adults in child custody evaluators over the last 20 years. It is the most frequently used nondrawing/storytelling personality measure for children.

It may be argued that the Rorschach Inkblot Method is not "generally accepted" because it is not used by more than one half of the surveyed evaluations in over one half of their cases. The only test that has met that threshold is the MMPI/MMPI–2. The unique incrementally valid contribution of the Rorschach beyond what the MMPI–2 offers in this and other contexts is the subject of other chapters in this volume (see Viglione & Meyer, chap. 2, this vol.; Ganellen, chap. 5, this vol.). It is the authors' practice to use both instruments in child custody evaluations when appropriate issues have been raised in the dispute.

As a psychological test, the administration, scoring, and interpretation are subject to the *Standards for Educational and Psychological Testing* (Educational Research Association, 1999). Figure 12–2 is a decision tree on the use of psychological tests in CCPPEs (Schutz, in press). To be appropriate, a test must meet the following criteria:

1. Must be incrementally valid. It must add information to the assessment process not available from other personality tests or interview.
2. Must have reliability and validity evidence for its proposed use.
3. The evidence must be applicable to all proposed test takers.
4. The mean test score differences between relevant subgroups are not due to construct irrelevant variance.
5. Differentiate normal from abnormal.
6. Have evidence beyond size of group means.
7. If qualitative test taking behaviors or other factors affect performance, are the effects known? Can they be corrected for?
8. Is a computer-generated interpretation appropriate?

Clearly, as noted by McCann (1998) and Evans (chap. 23, this vol.), the Rorschach has been empirically tested and the results published in peer-reviewed journals. It has clear standards for administration that are required for scoring and interpretation (Exner, 2003) and the RIM is generally accepted as useful in CCPPEs. Even though its previously mentioned overall use is less than 50%, this may reflect the fact that personality testing was not appropriate or necessary in all cases. Finally, if there were known error rates for the test in identifying individuals on dimensions known to be relevant to child custody determinations, then it would meet all the prongs of the *Daubert* test.

THE ROLE OF THE RORSCHACH IN CHILD CUSTODY EVALUATIONS: A PROTOCOL

Although Erard (2005) has addressed what the Rorschach can contribute to CCPPE, to date, there has been no standard model for how the RIM is to be incorporated into such an evaluation, leaving it to evaluators to determine their own approach, systematically or otherwise. In forensic settings, transparent and replicable procedures for administration and interpretation of psychological assessment offer a substantial advantage, providing the trier of fact with a clear rationale for the methodology.

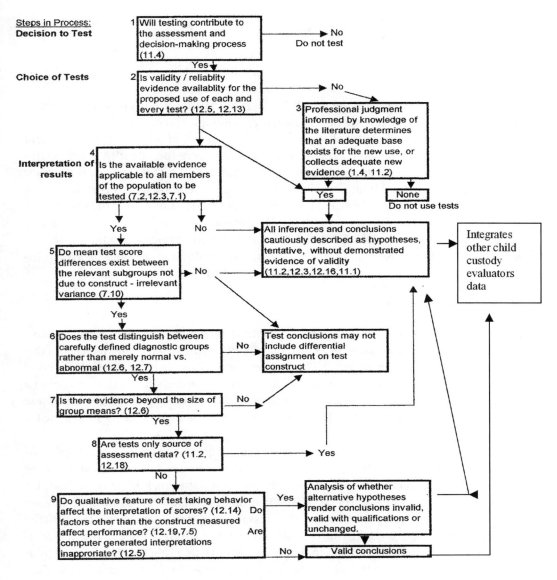

Figure 12–2. **APA standards on psychological testing applied to child custody evaluation.**

With this in mind, we propose a six-part protocol for the use of the Rorschach in a CCPPE:

1. Protecting the RIM.
2. Threshold for use of the RIM.
3. Hypothesis generation.
4. Administration and scoring of the RIM.

5. Interpretation of the RIM.
6. Integration of the RIM.

Protecting the RIM

At the outset of the evaluation, the CCPPE as part of their informed consent agreement addresses the issue of the release of test data, if psychological testing is done. A balance must be struck between the ethical provisions for disclosure of all test data to the client and contractual obligations to test manufacturers to preserve the integrity of the instruments against efforts to teach people how to "beat the test." Neither the parties nor their attorneys have any such obligations. There is a growing literature on attorney misuse of testing (Wetter & Corrigan, 1995) and Internet sites devoted to sabotaging the tests (Ruiz, Drake, Glass, Marcotte, & van Gorp, 2002). Our response has been to make a protective order part of the protocol of the CCPPE.[5] The test data will be released to the parties' attorneys for use in their case, but its re-release is strictly prohibited and after the case is litigated or settled the materials are returned to the CCPPE.[6]

Threshold Determination

There are two questions that have to be asked for determining whether or not the Rorschach is an appropriate measure in a particular CCPPE: Are the "facts in dispute" in this case ones that the RIM can address? The sources for the facts in dispute are the overlap between a state's applicable case law and statutes that determine what a court can or must consider, the model of CCPPE that directs the evaluator to the factors they should assess as part of an ethical, competent CCPPE, and the issues presented by the parties as the focus of their unique dispute.

If the answer to this question is yes, then the second question concerns whether sufficient information will be gathered from sources other than psychological testing in the CCPPE to meet its objective of convergent validity (Committee on Ethical Guidelines for Forensic Psychologists, 1991; Halikias, 1994) If this alternate source information does not exist, is not produced by the litigants, or is less reliable or valid than the RIM, then the use of the RIM is appropriate (Schutz, forthcoming). We strongly believe that the decision to use the RIM must rest on whether or not its results are probative for the particular case and further discourage the automatic use of any method without sufficient basis.

Hypotheses Generation

Hypothesis generation flows seamlessly from the threshold questions in the initial interviews with the parties. Their assertions about themselves, the other parent, and their chil-

---

[5]A copy of a sample Protective Order for Psychological Testing is available from Dr. Benjamin Schutz. Thanks to attorneys Dan Dannenbaum and Bob Eustice for permission to reprint their sample protective order.

[6]Some states have more restrictive requirements. For example, Maryland law does not allow for direct release of raw psychological test data to attorneys, but requires instead that a psychologist or psychiatrist with training in the tests administered be designated through the court to provide interpretation to the attorneys.

dren are elicited and fully elaborated. Each parent is given an opportunity to respond to the other parents' contentions. These findings are translated into psychological constructs generated by state law and the GA model of the CCPPEs profession. Then the parties are asked to provide relevant third parties who can corroborate their points of view.

The interview data provides the initial statement of the parties' description of the psychological functioning of its members. As such, it generates at least two fully articulated hypotheses that the CCPPE is meant to test. These perceptions constitute a "lay" assessment of personality by the parents that is often at the heart of their dispute (Madden-Derdich & Leonard, 2002; Pearson & Theoness, 1993; Wolchik, Fenaughty, & Braver, 1996). The RIM becomes a way to seek corroboration of their respective points of view. Because it is administered by another psychologist who is independent and blind to the parents' assertions, the RIM provides an objective and unbiased description of their personalities. The pattern of accuracy/distortion both in regard to aspects of themselves and to the others in the family can be very helpful in describing the "interpersonal dance" of action and reaction generated by what are usually complexly interacting misperceptions of themselves and the other person. The CCPPE at this point may have developed their own hypotheses to test. Ideally, in our protocol, the interviews with the parties and children, as well as relevant document review, are all completed before the RIM (and any other psychological tests) is administered. This sequence allows for the most refined and complete articulation of the hypotheses to be presented to the tester.

These hypotheses are next presented as neutrally worded questions or requests to the CCPPE's psychological test consultant. If the CCPPE is a psychiatrist or social worker, then this next step would be standard practice as they lack the training to administer the RIM. However, we recommend this protocol for psychologist CCPPEs as well. Our reasoning is that the bifurcation of interviewing and psychological testing maximizes the independence of the hypothesis generation from the hypothesis testing. Interviews of caretakers serve primarily to generate hypotheses, not to confirm them. Interviews of children serve to complete the picture from a family systems perspective of the hypotheses generated by the parents. Child interviews also provide a partial confirmation of the competing hypotheses. In turn, direct observation of parent–child interactions and psychological testing serves primarily to confirm or rule out the hypotheses generated from interview. To achieve true convergent validity, the measures should not have shared method, reporter, or interpreter variance (Campbell & Fiske, 1959; Reichardt & Coleman, 1995). We seek to achieve convergent validity in CCPPE by bifurcation of these methods. Ideally, psychological test administration and even direct observation are not only administered, scored, and interpreted by someone other than the interviewer or hypothesis generator; they are done blind, that is, without any information other than the evaluation is a CCPPE. In addition to independence from the hypothesis generator, this method removes a major source of confirmatory bias (Garb, 1998) as a possible influence on the interpretation of these data. Although we strongly believe that this model is the soundest approach from both legal and scientific perspectives, we understand that many CCPPEs do not or perhaps cannot function in this way. In such circumstances, efforts still should be made to bifurcate hypothesis generation from hypothesis testing, such as administering and scoring the Rorschach before the interviewing process, but not generating a RIM Structural Summary or computer scoring the MMPI–2 until the hypothesis testing phase of the evaluation.

Based on the idiographic psychological synthesis performed at the start of the hypothesis generation, the types of questions most commonly asked of the RIM are the following:

1. Please describe the affectivity and its regulation in the parents and the children. Include whether it is predominantly positive (e.g., warm, affectionate) or negative (depressed, anxious, guilty, irritable/hostile) and how it is expressed (e.g., avoided/constricted/poorly modulated/impulsive/ disorganizing).

2. Please describe the stress levels and coping styles/resources of both the parents and children. Include appraisals of self-efficacy, locus of control, neediness, active problem solving, passivity, avoidance and withdrawal, support-seeking, self-soothing, PTSD.

3. Please provide information consistent with the following psychopathological conditions: affective disorder (depression/bipolar), psychotic processes, including schizophrenia, substance abuse, antisocial personality disorder/psychopathy (or oppositional defiant disorder/conduct disorder in children), and anxiety disorders.

4. Please provide information on conflict styles/tactics for the parents and children. Include aggressiveness, power and control, cooperation, conflict avoidance/sensitization, rigidity, and inflexibility.

5. Please provide information on the ability of the parents and children to engage in nondefensive inspection of their own behavior. Include their attributions to others.

6. Please provide information about the interpersonal relatedness of the parents and children. Include empathy, narcissism, neediness, and boundary disturbances such as enmeshment, intrusiveness, rejection, sensitivity, and responsiveness.

These six key variable sets are based on Schutz's (in press) comprehensive, empirically grounded model for CCPPE based on his extensive review of the literature on parenting, child development, and family psychology, thus anchoring the RIM to specific variables in his CCPPE model.

Administration and Scoring of the RIM

To reiterate, our RIM protocol begins with the use of the CS, the only Rorschach system meeting the requirements for admissibility in court (McCann , Evans, chap. 3, this vol.). For specific purposes, there are other independent, soundly empirically anchored scores and scales also worth adding to the CS as well, such as the Gacono and Meloy aggressive content scores (Gacono, Bannatyne-Gacono, Meloy, & Baity, 2005), the Armstrong Trauma Content Index (Armstrong & Loewenstein, 1990), Urist's Mutuality of Autonomy Scale (Urist, 1977), the Rorschach Defense scale (Cooper & Arnow, 1985), and the Rorschach Oral Dependency scale (Bornstein, Rossner, & Hill, 1994). As stated earlier, our model calls for a psychological testing consultant working for the CCPPE to administer the Rorschach blind to the hypotheses generated by the CCPPE. When parents are evaluated, they are given instructions that they are not to give information about their case and that they provide only their name, date of birth, educational level, home address, and any previous Rorschachs taken. Because of important concerns raised by Wetter and Corrigan (1995) and Ruiz et al. (2002) regarding preparation for taking psychological tests, parents are also asked to fill out a statement describing what, if any, preparation they had had for taking the Rorschach and written informed consent is obtained.[7]

Following administration, RIM protocols not scored until both parties have taken the test and the MMPI–2 have been administered. Once both protocols have been scored and MMPI–2 scores have been received from one or both of the two nationally recognized computerized scoring services,[8] then the psychological testing consultant generates an independent interpretation of these data before receiving questions from CCPPE. Once this has been accomplished, the CCPPE presents the neutrally worded questions or requests to the CCPPEs psychological test consultant, who generates a report based solely on RIM and MMPI–2 variables.

Interpretation of the RIM

This section proposes to link RIM variables to specific key parenting concerns in CCPPE. There is little or no direct research on these RIM variables in CCPPE, although Singer et al.'s (chap. 21, this vol.) data set from a large sample of child custody litigants is an important step in providing RIM forensic reference group descriptive statistics. Consistent with Erard (2005) and Weiner (2005a), we use RIM variables that are logically connected to understanding relevant clinical and dispositional variables (see Gacono & Evans, preface, this vol.). Additionally, although we emphasize particular RIM variables, it is important to remember that CS interpretation strategy is configurational and requires looking at individual variables in the context of the entire Structural Summary (Exner, 2003). Whereas what follows is our conceptualization of variables that link RIM variables to specific key concerns, we do not claim these variables to be exclusive and hope that further research and conceptualization will be spurred as a result. Additionally, rather than using Exner's (2003) key variable Interpretative Search Strategy, we use an alternative approach similar to Erdberg's (2005) case formulation model for advanced RIM interpretation.

Affectivity and Its Regulation.   The first of the key CCPPE concerns is *affectivity and its regulation* in parents and children, particularly positive and negative emotions and how emotion is expressed. The RIM offers a number of variables that can be useful in assessing these concerns, especially regarding negative emotions of anger, resentment, anxiety, pessimism, and dysphoria. With regard to anger and resentment, CS variables to be first considered are *White Space (S)* and *Aggressive Movement (AG Special Score)*,

---

[7]A copy of the form *Client Preparation for Psychological Testing* and his informed consent statement may be obtained by contacting Dr. Barton Evans.

[8]Pope, Butcher, and Seelen (2006) clearly state that computer scoring of the MMPI–2 is the only practice acceptable for forensic evaluation, because hand scoring error rates are unacceptable and the scale availability is likely truncated.

along with Gacono and Meloy's (1994) *Aggressive Content (AgC)* score. Exner (1993) reported that research on *S* suggests excessive negativity, resentment, and/or anger, although not necessarily expressed overtly. Elevated *AG* indicated hostility toward others, verbal aggressiveness, or physical aggressiveness, although its meaning must be put into context with other variables such as affective controls, conventionality, reality testing, and stress tolerance. Because both *S* and *AG* are not necessarily direct measures of aggressive behavior, we suggest that consideration of adding the non-CS variable of *Aggressive Content (AgC)*, which has received considerable empirical support as an indication of behavioral aggressiveness (see Gacono et al., 2005). Configurally, we recommend that *S*, *AG*, and *AgC* can be used together to tap traits of anger and resentment in custody litigants, along with whether or not these traits are likely to be behaviorally expressed as aggressiveness.

Exner and Erdberg (2005) report that research suggests that anxiety and stress is best found in the configuration of *Inanimate Movement (m)* and *Diffuse Shading (SumY)*, modified by components from the *D* and *Adjusted D (AdjD)* scores. This research suggests that an elevation in *m* reflects the more general state anxiety, whereas elevated *SumY* has been found in situations where stress is uncontrollable and leads to feelings of helplessness. Exner and Erdberg suggest that minus *D* and *AdjD* scores are necessary to assess trait-like manifestations of anxiety, examining the sources of internal and external demands within the score to determine the chronic stressors. In terms of severe anxiety found in posttraumatic disorders, we further consider the use of Armstrong's Trauma Content Index (TCI) (Armstrong & Loewenstein, 1990) as an important non-CS indicator for possible past trauma and dissociation.

Weiner (2005b) suggests that dysphoria, and related negative cognitions like pessimism, can best be tapped by the configuration of *Sum of Achromatic Color (C')*, discomfort and tension from constrained emotional expression; *Color Shading Blends (Col-Shd Blds)*, confusion and ambivalent experience of both positive and negative feelings about the same thing; *Morbid Content (MOR)*, pessimism and a negative self and *Vista (V)* negative emotions and rumination caused by self-inspection. Naturally, positive findings on the *Depression Index (DEPI)* and the *Suicide Constellation (S-CON)* suggest overwhelmingly painful emotional and helplessness.

With regard to how emotions are expressed, the RIM offers important variables related to affective regulation and impulsivity. Exner and Erdberg (2005) suggest a configurational approach to this issue consisting of the *FC: CF + C Ratio*, the ability to modulate the expression affect and *Human Movement (M)*, the ability to inhibit and delay affect. To these variables we add consideration of the sum of *Pure Color (C)*, as an indication of immature or explosive expression of emotion, as well as the *Affective Ratio (afr)*, as a measure of affective engagement or avoidance; the Intellectualization Index, assessing the defense of intellectualization as a way of warding off painful emotion that could be dealt with more realistically; and, although rare, *Color Projection (CP)*, as an indication of a hysterical-like denial of unwanted emotions.

Stress and Coping.   Assessment of stress and coping styles/resources of both the parents and children on the RIM begins with the CS interpretive cluster of Control and Stress

Tolerance, reflected by the *D* score (*D*), which gives a more traitlike assessment of stress tolerance and coping capacity, modified by the degree of situational stress, found in the *Adjusted D* score (*AdjD*). Exner (1993, 2003) emphasized that this interpretative cluster must be carefully reviewed to evaluate the amount and quality of psychological resources reflected in *Experience Actual* (*EA*) in relationship to the amount and sources of need states and subjective distress measured by the *Experienced Balance* (*eb*). Exner further stressed that the finding of a positive *Coping Deficit Index* (*CDI*) raises questions about stress tolerance even in light of normal scores on *D* and *AdjD*. Problem-solving style, and its implication for coping and stress management, is further captured in this cluster by the *erlebnistypus* (*EB*).

Further modifying information from the Coping and Stress Tolerance cluster as a measure of stress and coping capacity are variables useful in tapping passive avoidance of responsibility and external locus of control, such as the *Active to Passive Ratio* ($p > a + 1$) and the *Active to Passive Human Movement Ratio* ($Mp > Ma$); dependent neediness found in elevated *Texture* responses (*T*), *Food* responses (*Fd*), and the *Rorschach Oral Dependency scale* (*ROD*) (Bornstein, 1996; Masling, Rabie, & Blandheim, 1967); and withdrawal and avoidance, such as high *Lambda* style and the *Isolation Index*, including severe dissociation, evaluated by Armstrong's TCI. Weiner (2005b) also suggested reviewing *XA%* (reality testing), *Zd* (ability to take in sufficient information before arriving at a conclusion), and *a:p* ratio (cognitive flexibility) as other indicators of coping skills in custody litigants.

Psychopathology. Although the RIM is not a diagnostic instrument per se (Exner, 2003), it can provide useful information consistent with the following psychopathological conditions with a known nexus to parenting and postdivorce adjustment of children (see Schutz, forthcoming, for a review of this literature); affective disorder (depression/bipolar); psychotic processes, including schizophrenia; antisocial personality disorder/psychopathy (or oppositional defiant disorder/conduct disorder in children); substance abuse; and anxiety disorder. With regard to affective disorders, Exner (2003) reviews the utility of the *DEPI* as a measure of both cognitive and affective components of depressive or dysthymic experience commonly underlying a wide variety of mood disorders, schizoaffective disorders, and personality disorders. Singer and Brabender (1993) found that individuals with bipolar disorder in both the depressed and manic phases showed high levels of cognitive slippage on the CS, unlike those with unipolar depression. Osher, Mandel, Shapiro, and Belmaker's (2000) study using the CS also found that children of bipolar parents show significantly increased incidence and severity of thought disorder, lower cognitively mediated affective responses, and fewer conventional responses.

Perhaps, the empirically sturdiest aspect of the RIM are variables related to the psychotic processes found in schizophrenia, schizoaffective disorder, bipolar disorder, and some personality and trauma-oriented disorders, which is substantial value in CCPPE. Exner (2003) reviews the development of the *Perceptual Thinking Index* (*PTI*) as a measure of underlying processes of disordered thinking and inaccurate perception in adults, whereas Smith, Baity, Knowles, and Hilsenroth (2001) found the *PTI* to be useful in assessing thought disorder in children and adolescents. Additionally, the *Ego Impairment Index* (Perry & Viglione, 1991; Perry, Minassian, Cadenhead, Sprock, & Braff, 2003), comprised of CS variables, can be used to establish severity of cognitive perceptual disturbance.

Beginning with the ground-breaking work of Gacono and Meloy (1994), there has been substantial research on RIM characteristics of antisocial personality disorder/ psychopathy (as well as oppositional defiant disorder/conduct disorder in children), which can be used when this diagnosis is at question in a CCPPE. Much of this research is summarized in chapters 16 through 20 of this book. Although there is less than there is for these first three psychopathological conditions, there has also been research on the RIM and substance abuse (e.g., Blatt & Berman, 1990; Cipolli & Galliani 1990; Ganellen, 1994; Verma & Misra, 2002), as well as anxiety disorders such as panic disorder with agoraphobia (de Ruiter & Cohen 1992), trauma disorders (Kaser-Boyd & Evans, chap. 13, this vol.), and obsessive style using the Obsessive Style Index (OBS) (Exner, 2003).

Conflict Styles/Tactics.   Whereas conflict styles/tactics for the parents and children is primarily an interpersonal variable, the RIM can provide valuable information regarding personality predilections toward cooperative, competitive, or avoidant strategies. The CS variable of *Cooperative Movement* (*COP*), the likelihood of expecting and enjoying cooperative and collaborative relationships with others, addresses most directly a propensity toward cooperative strategies, although Exner (2003) emphasizes the importance of configurational interpretation in which *COP* is assessed in relationship to *AG*. Additionally, the *Good Human Representational* variable (*GHR*), especially when it exceeds *Poor Human Representational* variable (*PHR*), further suggests interpersonal effectiveness. With regard to aggressiveness and power and control found in high conflict, competitive relationships, the configuration of *AG*, *S*, and *AgC* mentioned earlier in the Affectivity section assesses the individual's valence toward aggressive and conflictual strategies that can result from it, whereas rigidity and inflexibility of thinking underlying an inability to negotiate can be evaluated with *a:p*. Personality variables that can bring about conflict-avoidant relationships include *afr* (backing away from affective engagement); $p > a + 1$ (passivity or even passive aggressiveness when combined with *AG*); and significant *Isolation Index* (interpersonal withdrawal), all of which could be amplified by high *Lambda* style, low *EA*, and *CDI,* suggesting limited stress tolerance and oversimplification as a defensive strategy. Another potential RIM marker of extremely aggressive, high conflict style could be an indication of traumatic stress in the other parent and/or the children, such as an elevated *TCI* and other trauma sequelae (see Kaser-Boyd & Evans, chap. 13, this vol.)

Nondefensive Introspection of Self.   Another research-based issue in CCPPE is the ability of the parents and children to engage in *nondefensive inspection* of their own behavior as a way to manage painful conflict in divorce, including their negative attributions toward others. The presence of the CS determinant of *Form Dimension* (*FD*) suggests a capacity for self-inspection, reevaluation of the self, and introspection and occurs most frequently in nonpatients, although an elevation suggests excessive, perhaps defensive, self-preoccupation (Exner, 2003). *V* involves painful, ruminative self-inspection focusing on negative aspects of the self and is found disproportionately among dysphoric individuals and may indicate a limited ability to manage a painful view of the self common in conflictual divorce proceeding. At the most defensive end of the spectrum, reflection response (*Fr*) and elevated *Egocentricity Index (3r + [2]/R)* indicates a narcissistic preoccupation with one's own interest, which suggests impairment in the capacity to reflect accurately on the self and to contain negative attributions toward others. Additionally, fewer whole human responses (*H*) than part object (*Hd*) plus fantasy-based human representations (*[H] + [Hd]*) suggests that the parents' view of themselves is not based on an accurate representation of self and others, raising concern about the capacity to accurately reflect on their experience about themselves. Further complicating accurate self-reflection is defensive obsessive preoccupation (*OBS+*), excessive worry about interpersonal threat (*Hypervigilance Index, HVI+*), and ineffective management of information by either underincorporation or overincorporation (*Zd*).

Interpersonal Relatedness and Responsiveness.   The need for children to be buffered from the conflict and attachment threats during divorce cannot be underestimated and the assessment of interpersonal relatedness and responsiveness of the parents and children in CCPPE is a central concern. As Weiner (2005b) stated, children are at great risk psychologically when their parents are disconnected, self-absorbed, and insensitive to the needs of others and are restricted in their love, warmth, and concern for their children. Indeed, Singer et al. (chap. 21, this vol.) found a much higher proportion of such individuals in their child custody reference group sample.

Schutz (forthcoming) found four sets of relevant interpersonal variables in his review of the literature. The first variable is the continuum between empathy and narcissistic preoccupation. RIM CS variables related to empathic capacity are *T* (capacity and comfort in forming close relationships), *COP* (interest in collaboration in interpersonal relationships), and accurate *M* responses (empathic capacity). Also, Urist's well-researched (1977) *Mutuality of Autonomy scale (MOA)* is useful in demonstrating reciprocal mutuality in interpersonal relationships. On the other end of the continuum, the presence of *Fr* and elevated *3r + (2)/R* is a sign of impairment in empathic capacity and mutuality, *M–* indicates odd and distorted views of others and lack of empathic attunement, *T*-less records signify discomfort and trouble in forming intimate relationships, and no *COP* suggests problems with collaboration. Disturbance on the *MOA* indicates relationships are based more on the needs of the parents than on a relationship of parent–child mutuality and synchronicity.

Schutz's next CCPPE interpersonal variable involves boundary regulation as expressed on a continuum between differentiation and fusion/enmeshment. Again the *MOA* is an important RIM measure with a 7-point scale that addresses separation-individuation perhaps better than any current CS scale, index, or variable, in the evaluation of differentiation and enmeshment issues. Related problems of parental neediness and dependency can be assessed with CS variables of elevated *T* and *Fd* and the independent *ROD* scale. Another disturbance in differentiation arises from excessive inwardness or social remoteness of the parent, which can be measured by a low *Sum H* (interest in people) and elevated *ISOL* (social withdrawal).

An important continuum of parental responsiveness noted by Schutz is support, protection, and other focusedness versus rejection, criticalness, disdain, and contempt. One of the *MOA* 7-point scales assesses coercive control of the other, whereas the CS constellation of *OBS* (especially high numbers of *Unusual Detail*, *Dd*, and *Overelaborated Detail*, *FQ+*) is also useful in assessing criticalness and the requirement of meticulousness. Additionally, disdain and contempt are frequently aspects of narcissistic preoccupation, as measured by *Fr*, and can be more precisely measured by the Cooper and Arnow's (1985) Rorschach Defense scales, particularly the Devaluation scale.

Schutz's last interpersonal relatedness continuum is accuracy of attribution toward other people versus interpersonal distortion. CS variables of accurate *M* and *H* > *(H)* + *Hd* + *(Hd)* are also helpful in evaluating parents' ability to see others as they are. The presence of more than one *M* responses with minus form quality indicates impaired and distorted thinking about interpersonal relationships and *H* < *(H)* + *Hd* + *(Hd)* signifies object relations based primarily on part object formulations and views of the other based more on the individual's inner psychology than on realistic and accurate perception. Lastly, parents with a positive *HVI* are likely to have heightened interpersonal sensitivity, which is nonetheless strongly warped by deep interpersonal fears and insecurities, and family relationships are likely to be infused with paranoid like projections.

INTEGRATION OF THE RIM

The process of integrating the data of a CCPPE proceeds through a Content × Method matrix (Schutz, in press). All the data on each factor of the CCPPE is extracted from the record and entered in a cell for each method. There will be a matrix for each caretaker and child. The data on each factor is analyzed for convergence and contradictory findings. Contradictions must be explicitly resolved or noted.

The report on the RIM (and any other tests) is reviewed after the entire interview and records data have been collected. An interim assessment is made and prediction about how the RIMs were scored is made before it is read. After the report is read, there is a follow-up consultation to answer any questions the report raises, clarify the CCPPE's understanding of the report, and identify any noteworthy responses that were not part of the referral questions to understand their implications and what hypotheses they generate for the CCPPE. They may help organize disparate or poorly understood pieces of data in the CCPPE. The answers to the specific questions are then entered in the matrix as they refer to specific content areas or factors.

This raises an interesting issue regarding convergent validity. One way of conceptualizing this (Schutz, forthcoming) is to use the metaphor of constructing an edifice on the sea. Convergent validity is achieved when data from independent methodologies converges on the same conclusion. This assumes that the constituent measures that independently converge each have a demonstrated validity as a measure. If none of the individual measures has any demonstrated validity, then the convergence is like nailing a series of floating boards to each other. Although they converge, and will "hang together," they have no ties to the underlying sea bed and will drift off with the tide.

We believe that of the current data collection methodologies in a CCPPE, the one with the best connection to the "sea bed" is psychological testing and, rather than being only a hypotheses generator, it actually serves as the hypothesis confirmation or tether that connects the convergent data to the underlying constructs.

The RIM information becomes part of the description of the individual's contributions to the dynamics of both the interparent relationship (conflict and support) and the parent–child relationship. (See Figure 11–1.)

CONCLUSIONS

We are currently working on a way for the RIM to be used specifically as a test of clinical judgment of the CCPPE. In addition to the questions asked, the CCPPE will fill out a checklist of the way he believes each person's RIM will be scored. This is then exchanged with the testing consultant before the RIM results are released. The number of correct predictions will be a measure of the accuracy of the CCPPE's judgment of the personality functioning of the parties.

We will also give the parents a checklist derived from the RIM to assess the accuracy of their predictions regarding the test descriptions of themselves and the other parent. This method is a means of assessing the accuracy of their self and other percepts. It can serve to dramatize misperceptions as an opening to reconsidering their beliefs and the actions that flow from them.

Recent research developments in RIM variables and constellations such as the proposed Complexity Index, the Gacono–Meloy aggression scores, Urist's Mutuality of Autonomy Scale, and Armstrong's Trauma Content Index are measures that promise to expand the empirically relevant domains of the GA model that the RIM can contribute to. Hopefully, future research will also provide CCPPE with specific RIM indices that are developed with this specific forensic population to more directly assess the empirical variables in the GA model.

REFERENCES

Ackerman, M. J., & Ackerman, M. C. (1996). Child custody evaluation practices: Survey of psychologists. *Family Law Quarterly, 30*(3), 565–586.

American Academy of Child and Adolescent Psychiatry. (1997). Parameters for child custody evaluations. *Journal of the American Academy of Child and Adolescent Psychiatry, 36*(10), 58–68.

American Educational Research Association, American Psychological Association, and the National Council of Measurement in Education. (1999). *Standards for educational and psychological testing*. Washington, DC: American Psychological Association.

American Psychiatric Association. (1988). *Child custody consultation: A report of the Task Force on Clinical Assessment in Child Custody*. Washington, DC: American Psychiatric Association.

American Psychological Association (2002). Ethical principles of psychologists and code of conduct. *American Psychologist, 57*, 1060–1073.

American Psychological Association, Practice Directorate. (1994). Guidelines for child custody evaluations in divorce proceedings. *American Psychologist, 49*, 677–680.

Archer, R. P., & Newsome, C. R. (2000). Psychological test usage with adolescent clients: survey update. *Assessment, 7*, 227–235.

Armstrong, J. G., & Loewenstein, R. J. (1990). Characteristics of patients with multiple personality and dissociative disorders on psychological testing. *Journal of Nervous and Mental Disease, 178*, 445–454.

Ash, P., & Guyer, M. (1984). Court implementation of mental health professionals' recommendations in contested child custody and visitation cases. *Bulletin of American Academy of Psychiatry and Law, 12*, 137–147.

Association of Family and Conciliation Courts. (1994). *Model standards of practice of child custody evaluation.* Madison, WI: Association of Family and Conciliation Courts.

Blatt, S. J., & Berman, W. H. (1990). Differentiation of personality types among opiate addicts. *Journal of Personality Assessment, 54*, 87–104.

Board of Trustees of the Society for Personality Assessment. (2005). The status of the Rorschach in clinical and forensic practice: An official statement by the Board of Trustees of the Society for Personality Assessment. *Journal of Personality Assessment, 85*, 219–237.

Bornstein, R. F. (1996). Construct validity of the Rorschach Oral Dependency scale: 1967–1995. *Psychological Assessment, 8*, 200–205.

Bornstein, R. F., Rossner, S. C., & Hill, E. L. (1994). Retest reliability of scores on objective and projective measures of dependency: Relationship to life events and intertest interval. *Journal of Personality Assessment, 62*, 398–415.

Butcher, J. N., & Rouse, S. V. (1996). Personality: Individual differences and clinical assessment. *Annual Review of Psychology, 47*, 87–111.

Cipolli, C., & Galliani, I. (1990). Addiction time and value of *Z* indicators in Rorschachs of heroin users. *Perceptual and Motor Skills, 70*, 1105–1106.

Committee on Ethical Guidelines for Forensic Psychologists. (1991). Specialty guidelines for forensic psychologists. *Law and Human Behavior, 15*, 655–665.

Cooper, S., & Arnow, D. (1985). An object relations view of borderline defenses: A Rorschach analysis. In M. Kissen (Ed.), *Assessing object relations* (pp. 143–171). New York: International Universities Press.

Daubert V. Merrell Dow Pharmaceuticals, Inc. 509, US 579 (1993).

de Ruiter, C., & Cohen, L. (1992). Personality in panic disorder with agoraphobia: A Rorschach study. *Journal of Personality Assessment, 59*, 304–316.

DSS V. Hamlet (225 Mich. App. 505; 571 N.W. 2d 750; 1997 Mich. App. Lexis 331).

Educational Research Association, American Psychological Association, & National Counsel on Measurement in Education. (1999). *Standards for educational and psychological testing.* Washington, DC: American Educational Research Association.

Erard, R. E. (2005) What the Rorschach can contribute to child custody and parenting time evaluations. *Journal of Child Custody, 2, 119–142.*

Erdberg, P. (2005, December 2–4). *Workshop on Rorschach assessment of children and adolescents.* San Francisco: Rorschach Workshop.

Exner, J. (1993). *The Rorschach: A Comprehensive System: Basic foundations* (3rd ed.). New York: Wiley.

Exner, J. (2003). *The Rorschach: A Comprehensive System: Basic foundations* (4th ed.). New York: Wiley.

Exner, J. E., Jr., & Erdberg, P. (2005). *The Rorschach: A comprehensive system: advanced interpretation* (3rd ed.). Hoboken, NJ: Wiley.

Ford v. Ford (pseudonyms). (2000, Del. Fam. Ct Lexis 104).

Garb, H. (1998). *Studying the clinician: Judgment research and psychological assessment.* Washington, DC: American Psychological Association.

Gacono, C., Bannatyne-Gacono, L., Meloy, J. R., & Baity, M. R. (2005). The Rorschach extended aggression scores. *Rorschachiana, 27*, 164–190.

Gacono, C., & Meloy, R. (1994). *The Rorschach assessment of aggressive and psychopathic personalities.* Hillsdale, NJ: Lawrence Erlbaum Associates.

Ganellen, R. J. (1994). Attempting to conceal psychological disturbance: MMPI defensive response sets and the Rorschach. *Journal of Personality Assessment, 63*, 423–437.

Gatowski, S. I., Dobbin, S. A., Richardson, J. T., Ginsberg, G. P., Merlino, M. I., & Dahir, V. (2001). Asking the gatekeepers: A national survey of judges in judging expert evidence in a post-*Daubert* world. *Law and Human Behavior, 25*(5), 433–458.

Giannelli, P. C., & Imwinkelried, E. J. (1999). *Scientific evidence* (3rd ed.). Charlottesville, VA: Lexis Law Publishing.

Grove, W. M., Barden, R. C., Garb, H. N., & Lilienfeld, S. O. (2002). Failure of Rorschach-Comprehensive-System-based testimony to be admissible under the *Daubert-Joiner-Kumho* standard. *Psychology, Public Policy, & Law, 8*(2), 216–234.

Hagan, M. A., & Castagna, N. (2001). The real numbers: Psychological testing in custody evaluations. *Professional Psychology: Research and Practices, 32*(3), 269–271.

Halikias, W. (1994). Forensic family evaluations: A comprehensive model for professional practice . *Journal of Clinical Psychology, 50,* 951–964.

Halon, R. (1990). Child Custody evaluation: A comprehensive model. *American Journal of Forensic Psychology, 8,* 19–62.

Keilin, W. G., & Bloom, L. J. (1986). Child custody evaluation practices: A survey of experienced professionals. *Professional Psychology: Research and Practice, 17*(4), 338–346.

Lilienfeld, S. O., Wood, J. M., & Garb, H. N. (2000). The scientific status of projective techniques. *Psychological Science in the Public Interest, 1,* 27–66.

Luftman, V. H., Veltkamp, L. J., Clark J. J., Iannacone, S., & Snooks, H. (2005). Practice guidelines in child custody evaluations for licensed clinical social workers. *Clinical Social Work Journal, 33*(3), 327–357.

Madden-Derdich, D. A., & Leonard, S. A. (2002). Shared experiences, unique realities: Formerly married mothers' and fathers' perceptions of parenting and custody after divorce. *Family Relations, 51*(1), 37–45.

Masling, J., Rabie, L., & Blondheim, S. H. (1967). Obesity, level of aspiration, and Rorschach and TAT measures of oral dependence. *Journal of Consulting Psychology, 31,* 233–239.

Mayo v. Mayo (2000 ND 204; 619 N.W.2d. 631; 2000 N.D. Lexis 245).

McCann, J. T. (1998). Defending the Rorschach in court: An analysis of admissibility using legal and professional standards. *Journal of Personality Assessment, 70,* 125–144.

Meloy, J. R., Hansen, T. L., & Weiner, I. B. (1997). Authority of the Rorschach: Legal citations during the past 50 years. *Journal of Personality Assessment, 69,* 53–62.

Metzger, Bradt, & Izen Jr. v. Sebek et al. (892 S.W. 2d 20; 1994 Tex App. Lexis 2382).

Osher, Y., Mandel, B., Shapiro, E., & Belmaker, R. H. (2000). Rorschach markers in offspring of manic-depressive patients. *Journal of Affective Disorders, 59,* 231–236.

Pearson, J., & Thoeness, J. (1993). When parents complain about visitation. *Mediation Quarterly, 11*(2), 139–156.

Perry, W., Minassian, A., Cadenhead, K., Sprock, J., & Braff, D. (2003). The use of the Ego Impairment Index across the schizophrenia spectrum. *Journal of Personality Assessment, 80,* 50–57.

Perry, W., & Viglione, D. J. (1991). The Ego Impairment Index as a predictor of outcome in melancholic depressed patients treated with tricyclic antidepressants. *Journal of Personality Assessment, 56,* 487–501.

Piotrowski, C., Belter, R. W., & Keller, J. W. (1998). The impact of "managed care" on the practice of psychological testing: Preliminary findings. *Journal of Personality Assessment, 70,* 441–447.

Piotrowski, C., & Keller, J. W. (1989). Psychological testing in outpatient mental health facilities: A national study. *Professional Psychology: Research and Practice, 20,* 423–425.

Pope, K. S., Butcher, J. N., & Seelen, J. (2006). *The MMPI, MMPI–2 & MMP–A in court: A practical guide for expert witnesses and attorneys* (3rd ed.). Washington, DC: American Psychological Association.

Quinnell, F. A., & Bow, J. N. (2001). Psychological tests used in child custody evaluations. *Behavioral Sciences and the Law, 19,* 491–501.

Reichardt, C. S., & Coleman, S. C. (1995). The criteria for convergent and discriminant validity in a multitrait-multimethod matrix. *Multivariate Behavioral Research, 30*(4), 513–538.

Ruiz, M. A., Drake, E. B., Glass, A., Marcotte, D., & van Gorp, W. G. (2002). Trying to beat the system misuse of the internet to assist in avoiding detection of psychological symptom dissimulation. *Professional Psychology: Research and Practice, 33,* 294–299.

Schutz, B. M. (in press). *Honing the edge: The search for excellence in child custody evaluations.* Mahwah, NJ: Lawrence Erlbaum Associates.

Schutz, B. M., Dixon, E. B., Lindenberger, J. C., & Ruther, N. J. (1989). *Solomon's sword: A practical guide to conducting child custody evaluations.* San Francisco: Jossey-Bass.

Singer, H. K., & Brabender, V. (1993). The use of the Rorschach to differentiate unipolar and bipolar disorders. *Journal of Personality Assessment, 60,* 333–345.

Smith, S. R., Baity, M. R., Knowles, E. S., & Hilsenroth, M. J. (2001). Assessment of disordered thinking in children and adolescents: The Rorschach Perceptual-Thinking Index. *Journal of Personality Assessment, 77,* 447–463.

The people of the State of Illinois v. Tanya L. and Clayton J. (351 Ill App 3d 557; 814 N.E. 2d 618; 2004 Ill App. Lexis 951; 286 Ill Dec.630).

Urist, J. (1977). The Rorschach test and the assessment of object relations. *Journal of Personality Assessment, 41,* 3–9.

Verma, M. K., & Misra, S. (2002). Rorschach's response patterns of drug addicts. *Journal of Projective Psychology & Mental Health, 9,* 62–64.

Weiner, I. B. (2005a). Rorschach assessment in child custody cases. *Journal of Child Custody, 2,* 99–119.

Weiner, I. B. (2005). The utility of Rorschach assessment in clinical and forensic practice. *Independent Practitioner, 25,* 76–83.

Wetter, M. W., & Corrigan, S. K. (1995). Providing information to clients about psychological tests: A survey of attorneys' and law students' attitudes. *Professional Psychology: Research and Practice, 26,* 474–477.

Wolchik, S. A., Fenaughty, A. M., & Braver, S. L. (1996). Residential and non-residential parents perspectives on visitation problems. *Family Relations, 4*(2), 230–237.

Wood, J. M., Nezworski, M. T., Lilienfeld, S. O., & Garb, H. N. (2003). *What's wrong with the Rorschach?: Science confronts the controversial inkblot test.* San Francisco: Jossey-Bass.

13

RORSCHACH ASSESSMENT
OF PSYCHOLOGICAL TRAUMA

Nancy Kaser-Boyd
Geffen School of Medicine, UCLA

F. Barton Evans
Private Practice, Bozeman, MT

Psychological trauma is a profoundly destabilizing phenomenon and trauma disorders take varied, puzzling forms, depending on the nature and severity of the trauma and other variables (e.g., pre-morbid personality functioning). The symptoms of trauma so mimic and overlap other disorders that they present formidable diagnostic and treatment challenges. There is a large body of clinical literature on trauma (van der Kolk, 1987, 2003) and numerous assessment instruments have been proposed for the assessment of trauma (e.g., the Minnesota Multiphasic Personality Inventory, MMPI, and its PK scale; Keane, Malloy, & Fairbank, 1984), the Millon Clinical Multiaxial Inventory (MCMI–III), PTSD scale (Millon, Bockian, Tringone, Antoni, & Green, 1989), the Trauma Symptom Inventory (Briere, 1995), and numerous checklists and structured interviews. So the question arises: Why use the Rorschach to assess trauma? There is a surprisingly robust literature on the Rorschach and trauma (Armstrong & Kaser-Boyd, 2003; Levin & Reis, 1996) and the Rorschach has been suggested as the ideal tool to "trigger" trauma memories and feelings, a process that may be similar to traumatic reliving in nightmares (van der Kolk & Ducey, 1989). The abstract images, coupled with dark and vibrant colors, call out images of danger and harm in individuals who experienced trauma and evoke the subjective experience of the trauma. The Rorschach accesses psychological variables not tapped by self-report measures (Levin & Reis, 1997), allowing the patient to communicate trauma images in the indirect mode of the testing situation that were avoided in direct interaction with the assessor. The Rorschach"s structural data and content are useful indices to current symptoms and psychological processes (Armstrong & Kaser-Boyd, 2003) and provide important information about perceptual accuracy, coping resources, stress tolerance, modulation of affect, and hypervigilance (Kaser-Boyd, 1993).

In the forensic arena, the trauma referral may be a person, for example, who has filed a civil suit claiming emotional damages or who is seeking asylum and protection from torture (Evans, chap. 23, this vol.; Van Velsen, Gorst-Unsworth, & Turner, 1996). The clients may be on trial for a crime where Posttraumatic Stress Disorder is a crucial aspect of their mental state (Kaser-Boyd, 1999), or the forensic practitioner may be conducting an assessment of criminal mitigation (e.g., see Kaser-Boyd, chap. 10, this vol.). This chapter is written for the forensic practitioner who wishes to design a test battery that competently measures the presence and severity of trauma symptoms. We begin with an overview of trauma theory and discuss its implications for Rorschach assessment. We discuss the biological response to trauma, which pinpoints physiological roots of key psychological symptoms (e.g., hyperreactivity to traumatic triggers). We review the literature on the Rorschach and trauma in adults and then discuss Complex Posttraumatic Stress Disorder. We illustrate the use of the Rorschach in a forensic case. Finally, we outline key courtroom challenges to the Rorschach in a trauma case, as well as the defenses to these challenges.

THEORETICAL AND CLINICAL PERSPECTIVES ON TRAUMA

There are two circumstances under which traumatized people come to the attention of assessment psychologists. Some people seek treatment following an identified trauma such as a natural disaster, rape, or life threatening illness or injury. In these instances, the existence and significance of the trauma is overt. Thus, the psychologist will have been alerted to the importance of considering the test data from a trauma standpoint. The contribution of performance-based tests like the Rorschach (frequently called "projective tests") to understanding "overt trauma" presentations has been explored in some detail by assessment researchers (Briere, 1997; Carlson, 1997). The Rorschach frequently can be helpful in clarifying the myriad clinical issues that are often raised by trauma. As is discussed later, Posttraumatic Stress Disorder (PTSD) is only one of many possible trauma outcomes (van der Kolk & McFarlane, 1996). Moreover, PTSD tends to be associated with multiple co-morbidities (Kessler, Sonnega, Bromet, Hughes, & Nelson, 1995). The ability of the Rorschach and other "projective tests" to elucidate aspects of the patient's self-concept, affect regulation, relational capacities, and coping mechanisms makes these measures useful in addressing the complexities of trauma diagnosis and treatment (Parson, 1998). For example, the Rorschach can offer important information on whether the patient has the psychological resources to tolerate the stress of the first line of treatment for PTSD, exposure therapy (Foa, Keane, & Friedman, 2000).

Assessment psychologists are also likely to encounter traumatized people under circumstances that are even more diagnostically challenging, when trauma reactions are present, but are not identified as such. In cases of what we will call "covert trauma," patients may be aware of having had an experience, or experiences, that we would label "traumatic." However, they are unaware of the connection between such incidents and their present symptoms. Thus, they are unlikely to directly raise these experiences in treatment. A covert trauma presentation is especially likely in cases of chronic childhood abuse and neglect, where traumatic dissociation limits conscious access to trauma memories (Williams, 1994). However, covert trauma can be found unexpectedly in a patient simply because, by its very nature, traumatic experience is difficult to capture in words, to organize in a coherent fashion, and to report in a manner that feels safe (Dalenberg, 2000). Because it is particularly useful for gathering data on processes not readily available to self-reflection and self-report, the Rorschach may reveal the first sign of covert trauma.

Studies of the prevalence of psychological trauma in psychiatric patients show rates of trauma exposure that range from 60% to over 80% (e.g., Bryer, Nelson, Miller, & Kroll, 1987). Reviewing the epidemiological data on traumatic stress, Carlson (1997) concludes that clinicians can expect at least 15% of their adult clients to have current or past trauma symptoms. In inpatient settings, the rates are even higher (Carmen, Rieker, & Mills, 1984). Studies of at-risk populations exposed to specific traumatic incidents show the highest rates in survivors of rape, military combat, captivity, and ethnically or politically motivated internment and genocide, ranging between one third to more than one half of those exposed (APA, 2000). In view of the ubiquity of trauma in the clinical population, the possibility is that the psychological effects of trauma will be complex and covert. It is especially important that assessment psychologists utilize a range of assessment methods to increase their chances of sampling and recognizing trauma reactions and familiarize themselves with the trauma research literature on the Rorschach.

THE CLINICAL FACES OF TRAUMA

Whereas the term *trauma* is used loosely in everyday speech to signify highly unpleasant events, it is used here in the precise manner described by *DSM–IV–TR* (American Psychiatric Association, 2000). Criterion A–1 for PTSD outlines that a psychological trauma consists of experiencing or witnessing an event that involves death or serious injury to oneself, or learning about the unexpected or violent death of a loved one. Simply undergoing such an experience is not enough. As delineated in Criterion A–2, the person must also react to the experience with intense fear, helplessness, or horror or, if it is a child, with disorganized or agitated behavior. Thus, being involved in a large-scale disaster as a victim or an emergency worker, being raped, or being tortured would qualify as a Criterion A experience. Being in a minor accident, an emotionally painful relationship, or suddenly and unjustly losing a job would not ordinarily meet Criterion A requirements, no matter how personally distressing these experiences are to the individual.

The distinction between a traumatic and a noxious experience is important because trauma initiates a set of distinctive psychophysiological responses that are different from the psychophysiology of stress. For example, PTSD patients show a highly sensitized hypothalamic-pituitary-adrenal axis reflecting basic changes in management of arousal level (Yehuda & MacFarlane, 1995). Brain norepinephrine system alterations associated with memory and learning disturbance have also been found (Bremner, Davis, Southwick, Krystal, & Charney, 1994). Such physiological reactions underlie the biphasic psychological response to trauma, in which hyperarousal and emotional flooding alternate with avoidance and emotional numbing (van der Kolk, 1994). Physiological dysregulation also underlies the pervasive symptoms that characterize chronic trauma and that can mask accurate diagnosis because they resemble many other psychological disorders, such as bipolar disorder, panic disorder, and borderline personality disorder.

Common trauma symptoms include somatization, panic reactions, emotional lability, anxiety, agitation, depression, hopelessness, loss of life purpose, sleep problems, inability to self-soothe, and disturbances in thinking and reality testing. Affective disregulation can interact with cognitive confusion and avoidance, producing unbidden, intrusive reminders that plunge the person back into the time of trauma or that bleed into ongoing experience. These intrusions can be experienced on a cognitive level as hallucinatory flashbacks, on a somatic level as body pains, and on an emotional level as spurts of grief, fear, or depression (van der Kolk, 1994). Psychotic-like thinking has been observed in traumatized people who were previously clinically normal (Weisath, 1989), and cognitive decline and neurological soft signs have been found in people with chronic trauma (Gurvitz et al., 2000). Traumatic dissociation can cause problems in memory and abrupt alterations in state of awareness that impede the integration of the trauma, making it difficult for the person to talk about the event. Other defensive efforts to avoid being flooded by traumatic memories may make traumatized people appear depleted, uncooperative, and unwilling to engage with the world, further complicating clinicians' efforts to understand and connect with them. As is discussed later in this chapter, if the trauma is repetitive or occurs early in development, then the survivor may show an even more complicated symptom picture (van der Kolk, 2005).

Not all trauma survivors show these symptoms. There is no one-to-one relationship between an external trauma and the person's psychological or psychobiological response. Trauma survivors develop PTSD somewhere between 25% and 30% at the lower end (Green, 1994), and 50% at the higher end of exposure (APA, 2000). Elevated rates of major depression, panic, and substance abuse disorders are also commonly observed (Shalev et al., 1998). However, many people spontaneously resolve their trauma and, in the process, develop greater coping skills (Solomon, Mikulincer, & Avitzur, 1988). Although such individual variability may be a testament to the uniqueness of the human spirit, such findings also complicate the researcher's task.

THE NEUROBIOLOGY OF TRAUMA

As with other psychiatric/psychological disorders, biology or *neurobiology* is implicated as a cause of clinical symptoms. Emerging data on Posttraumatic Stress Disorder also suggests underlying neurobiological factors in the expression of clinical symptoms. Van der Kolk (1987) asserted that physiological changes can account for most of the posttrauma symptoms noted earlier. Reviewing studies of inescapable shock and maternal deprivation, he postulated a depletion of a variety of essential neurotransmitters results. Kolb (1988), employing classical neurobiological theory, suggested that the experience of massive threat subjects the organism to excessive neuronal overload. Subsequent research supported this hypothesis, finding both a change in brain chemistry and in brain structure in traumatized subjects.

What sets acute trauma disorders apart from other psychiatric and psychological disorders is the sudden, intense experience of fear (e.g., in traumas like rape, civilian catastrophe, or the experience of criminal assault), or the chronic experience of fear (e.g., in battering relationships or repeated child sexual abuse). Fear, or more precisely, arousal from fear, is controlled by the amygdala, which controls other emotions as well. When the amygdala has been surgically removed in experimental animals, they fail to condition to a feared object (Schacter, 1996). When the amygdala is electrically stimulated in experimental animals, they show a fear response in the absence of a frightening stimulus, and electrical stimulation of the amygdala in patients with temporal lobe epilepsy produces an intense experience of fear (Schacter, 1996). While in a condition that caused intrusive recollections, Vietnam combat veterans' PET scans showed heightened activity in the right amygdala and in the visual cortex (Rauch et al., 1996). The amygdala receives input from primary sensory areas of the brain, so that it can receive an "early warning" of danger, and it also receives input from higher cortical structures, where the fear stimuli are further processed. LeDoux (1996, 1998) calls this the two brain pathways of fear.

In most mammals, the experience of fear causes brain changes that help the organism to respond. Adrenalin is released and floods the central nervous system, leading to a chain reaction, which includes (a) changes in the noradrenergic system and in the chemical messengers known as the catecholamines (epinephrine, norepinephrine, and dopamine); and (b) changes in the hypothalamic-pituitary-adrenal axis, with a release of corticotropin-releasing factor (CRF) and then a release of glucocorticoids (cortisol). Epinephrine is associated with arousal states. When rats are experimentally injected with epinephrine, they show a fear response (Schacter, 1996) and when human subjects are injected with Yohimbine, a drug that mimics arousal states, they also show a fear response. A study with Vietnam veterans revealed an association between the intrusive symptoms of PTSD and the presence of norepinephrine and dopamine in their urine (Yehuda, Southwick, Giller, Ma, & Mason, 1992). Inescapable stress or trauma depletes norepinephrine and dopamine, presumably because use exceeds synthesis; chronic depletion of norepinephrine (NE) then renders norepinephrine receptors hypersensitive to subsequent NE stimulation (van der Kolk & Greenberg, 1988).

During highly stressful experiences, the glucocorticoids (cortisol) are also released in the brain. The glucocorticoids help to mobilize energy for "fight or flight," increase cardiovascular activity, and inhibit other physiological processes (Schacter, 1996). Flooding with glucocorticoids can seriously damage neurons. Injecting glucocorticoids in rats for several months produced a permanent loss of glucocorticoid receptors in the hippocampus, and signs of degeneration of neurons were visible after only a few weeks (Salpolsky, 1992). The hippocampus has been demonstrated to control memory (Schachter, 1996). African primates exposed to various stressors (i.e., attacks from other primates, difficulty hiding, etc.) showed abnormally elevated levels of glucocorticoids (Salpolsky, 1992) and atrophy of neurons in the hippocampus. Studies in rats and other experimentally traumatized animals showed decreased hippocampal volume (Holschneider, 2000).

Studies with traumatized children and adults have shown changes in brain structure and chemistry. Neuroimaging of adults and children with PTSD showed a reduction in hippocampal volume, and in children, smaller intracranial and intracerebral volumes (Bremner, 1999; De Bellis et al., 1999). Gurvitz et al. (1996) found a strong positive correlation between degree of Vietnam combat exposure and hippocampal volume. De Bellis, Lefter, Trickett, and Putnam, 1994), using magnetic resonance imaging, found a smaller left hippocampus, compared to controls, in women who had suffered severe sexual and physical abuse. Traumatized adults and children also have been found to have adrenergic systems that are more active than normals (Southwick et. al., 1993), dysregulated HPA systems (Yehuda & McFarlane, 1995), and abnormalities in serotonergic mechanisms (Southwick et al., 1999).

How might these brain changes tie into specific symptoms of trauma? The negative symptoms of PTSD (e.g., numbing, withdrawal, emotional constriction) are similar to those shown by animals subjected to inescapable shock and may result from the depletion of norepheniphrine (van der Kolk & Greenberg, 1988). Re-experiencing traumatic memories in response to a trigger or reminder of the trauma is akin to electrical stimulation of the amygdala, where intense fear reactions in the absence of the original stimulus appear. The biphasic symptoms of PTSD are thought to come from the combination of depletion of norepinephrine and dopamine with the associated hypersensitivity of the neurons to subsequent norepenephrine stimulation (van der Kolk, 1987). In other words, in the absence of a threat stimulus, the individual appears unemotional, flat, or perhaps depressed like other norepinephrine and dopamine-depleted patients. A perceived threat causes a surge of epinephrine (like the surge of catecholamines in the original trauma) and this activates the emotions of the original trauma—fear and other emotions. Trauma survivors appear to have a continuing physiological hyperreactivity, which is likely mediated by changes in the noradrenergic system, with noradrenergic receptor hypersensitivity.

Of all of the clinical symptoms, it is the changes in memory that have been the most controversial. Schacter (1996) gives an elegant and easily understood explanation of the underlying brain changes associated with memory deficits. The damage to glucocorticoid receptors in the hypothalamus are likely associated with impaired memory. Animals who have undergone experimental oblation of the hypothalamus, but not the amygdala, do not appear to avoid a feared stimulus (i.e., have not learned or "remembered" to avoid it), but respond with fear, when it is presented to them. Studies of rats and other animals have shown that injecting epinephrine immediately after an animal learns a task enhances subsequent memory for that task (Schacter, 1996). This helps to explain why trauma-related memories may be unavailable during the constricted phase of the disorder, but, when a new threat produces epinephrine, the patient is flooded with memories of the trauma.

Dissociation may result from the same biological mechanisms. Dissociated material often surfaces during times of new threat or when "triggers," or reminders, of the trauma occur, which is again when epinephrine would be available in the brain. The memories are more inaccessible to the patient with dissociative symptoms, but are likely simply a more extreme end of the spectrum of "forgetting" about, or constriction of the memories of trauma. Schacter (1996) points out that dissociation can be horizontal (as in repressing all memories from a part of one's life) or lateral (forgetting aspects of a portion of one's life, with otherwise intact memory). LeDoux's (1995, 1998) research on the two pathways to the brain of threat stimuli and the neurobiology of fear also suggest a biological mechanism for dissociation.

Trauma can also affect cognitive functioning. Sustained abuse can result in the development of complex relational schema or internal working models (Briere & Spinazola,

2005) involving negative self-perceptions and expectations of negative outcomes. These schemata are easily evoked by new experiences reminiscent of the earlier traumatic experience, leading to perceptions that are highly colored by trauma. We may think of this process as cognitive distortion or impairments in reality testing.

MODERATING FACTORS IN TRAUMA

The psychological effects of trauma depend on a variety of moderating factors, which influence whether or not traumatized people will be able to move on with their lives or suffer disabling, long-term psychological effects. It has been increasingly recognized by trauma researchers that trauma reactions cannot simply be conceptualized as an interaction between a normal person and an extraordinary stressor, and that a diathesis-stress model best reflects the data. Certain variables that influence the trauma response do reside in the external stressor. This includes the magnitude and the severity of trauma, as well as its unpredictability, uncontrollability, and duration (Carlson, Furby, Armstrong, & Schlaes, 1997). Research indicates that highly violent, repetitive trauma has more severe psychological effects than do single or relatively nonviolent incidents (Breslau et al., 1998). Other moderating variables reside within the person. For example, people with an earlier unresolved trauma tend to respond more maladaptively to a new trauma (Resnick, Yehuda, Pitman, & Foy, 1995). Limited coping resources and history of psychological disorder are also predisposing factors for a pathological response to trauma (McFarlane, 1989; Waysmen, Schwarzwald, & Solomon, 2001). The developmental stage during which the person is traumatized is an especially powerful internal moderating variable. Research on repetitive trauma in children indicates that such experiences are likely to have a pervasive effect on personality development (Cassidy & Mohr, 2001). Still other moderating variables reflect the interaction between the person and the trauma. Involvement in a traumatic situation caused by another person is more likely to lead to a serious psychological reaction than is experiencing an impersonal trauma such as a natural disaster (Briere, 1997). If, as in incest, the relationship between the perpetrator and the traumatized person is close and dependent, it is more likely to lead to a pervasive trauma disorder, such as Complex PTSD (Trickett & Putnam, 1993; van der Kolk, 2003, 2005) with profound damage to the self and to other-relatedness.

At any age, the quality of the person's social support system functions as a significant protective factor. Positive social support is associated with integration of the traumatic event and subsequent recovery. Conversely, such factors as neglect, family, and social disorganization, as well as simply not talking about a traumatic event with a sympathetic listener, predict chronic reactions to trauma (Briere, 1997).

IMPLICATIONS FOR RORSCHACH RESEARCH

As the previous discussion details, trauma can impact a wide variety of personality and biological functions. Rorschach researchers have worked to map the effects of trauma on reality testing, emotional control, object relations, and the process by which neutral stimuli become transformed into traumatic triggers. The sophistication of Rorschach research has grown with the increasing sophistication of the trauma field. Like the early clinical research, early Rorschach research did not control for moderating variables such as severity of the traumatic stressor, prior trauma history, and developmental level of the person at time of trauma. Researchers often failed to acknowledge the biphasic nature of PTSD in their research designs, lumping "flooded" and "avoidant" patients into one PTSD group. Researchers may not have taken into account co-morbid disorders such as substance abuse, depression, suicidality, and Axis II traits, which may represent secondary reactions to untreated trauma, rather than the central trauma response itself. Conversely, the same can be said for researchers in other clinical areas, who generally do not control for the effects of past trauma on symptomatology and response to treatment. In addition, there is little research on subtypes of trauma reactions, such as people who show only a limited trauma response and appear "stuck" in an avoidant, flooded, or hyperaroused state. These limitations apply to all research on trauma, not just Rorschach research.

RESEARCH FINDINGS

The theory that traumatized people have distinctive, intense associations to ambiguous visual stimuli has received unanticipated support in the wake of our recent national trauma, the destruction of the World Trade Center towers on September 11, 2001. Immediately following this tragedy, news and Web site media documented a widespread and hotly argued debate over whether or not photographs of a smoke cloud rising over one tower depicted the face of God, the devil, Bin Laden, a conspiracy on the part of the photographers to dupe the public, or just a cloud (Wells & Maher, 2001). One psychologist opined that, in times of stress, the human brain looks for figures in ambiguous, visual stimuli. His description of the rationale for the Rorschach in cases of trauma received support from an unexpected quarter, the president of the International Association of Arson Investigators, who noted that it was not unusual for people to see unusual images in smoke clouds (Hoffman, 2001). Done over 20 years ago, the earliest projective studies of trauma (Salley & Teiling, 1984; van der Kolk & Ducey, 1984) used the test best described as photographs of smoke clouds, the Rorschach. As is described later, these findings became central to the newly developing field of posttraumatic stress.

We have outlined the difficulties diagnosing trauma on the basis of clinical symptoms and the same caveats apply to the Rorschach. In considering the findings discussed here, the reader should keep in mind that there is no single, unique, unassailable set of trauma markers. This is especially true for Rorschach findings because the major use of such tests is the delineation of personality characteristics, not diagnosis. One would expect there to be significant variability in test findings because this would follow the very real variation of symptoms seen in trauma presentations. For example, patients who are more flooded should have different Rorschach patterns from those who are more constricted. Test takers who experienced chronic trauma should similarly show a different pattern of Rorschach response from those whose previous functioning was normal. As Briere (1997) has pointed out, the Rorschach is as susceptible to as many pitfalls for misdiagnosis of trauma as are structured tests. No Rorschach interpretive system is free from theoretical assumptions about the meaning of a response and these assumptions can either bias or illuminate what is observed. Unless the assessor is conversant with the trauma literature, many trauma reactions are likely to be misdiagnosed. Given the complexity of differential diagnosis and, in particular, the potential overlap between trauma, personality disorder, and psychotic test responses, it is essential that clinicians be familiar with all three diagnostic entities in order to make accurate differential diagnoses with the Rorschach.

The earliest studies of Rorschach and trauma involved servicepeople in wartime. The first study of the effects of traumatic stress on Rorschach responses stands as a testament to the determination of the researcher and his subjects. Shalit (1965) administered the Rorschach to 20 servicemen in the Israeli Navy while they were in the midst of a severe storm at sea. This study was the first to demonstrate the rise in *Inanimate Movement* (*m*) that has been consistently found in later trauma research. In 1984, using the newly created diagnosis of PTSD, van der Kolk and Ducey (1984) and Salley and Teiling (1984) studied Vietnam combat veterans and became the first researchers to document traumatic intrusions on the Rorschach. Levin and Reis (1996), in their review of the state of Rorschach trauma research, point out that these early studies were important to the development of the trauma field because they helped researchers recognize and establish an understanding of the biphasic trauma response.

In the discussion that follows, we combine results from studies of military personnel and civilians because studies find equivalent trauma responses for both populations. Elsewhere (Armstrong & Kaser-Boyd, 2003), we have summarized research results for traumatized children, a body of Rorschach literature that becomes crucial in evaluations where the trauma is long past, but has had permanent effects on personality functioning. Readers will note that most Rorschach research uses the Exner Comprehensive Scoring System. However, a number of researchers have used non-Exner scores to capture phenomena not otherwise easily tracked. We first organize our discussion in terms of the biphasic trauma response to enable the reader to put some theoretical organization on the variety of findings described. Given the biphasic nature of the trauma response, it is not unexpected that Rorschach researchers have documented signs of both flooding and constriction in the Rorschach protocols of traumatized samples. Van der Kolk and Ducey (1984, 1989) and Cerney (1990) reported finding two distinct response modes among their subjects: either constriction with no color determinants, or flooding with unmodulated color. In other studies, Levin (1993), Swanson, Blount, and Bruno (1990), Hartman et al. (1990), Kaser-Boyd (1993), Armstrong (1991), and Brand, Armstrong, and Loewenstein (2006) noted a biphasic trauma pattern within their subjects' protocols. These findings included emotional lability ($CF + C > FC$) alongside a low Affective Ratio (< .05). An avoidance-flooding pattern could also be seen in the combination of high *Lambda*, low *R*, and low *Afr* along with significant Traumatic Content Index, isolated *C* and *CF*, and *PTI*. The individual protocol may show signs of both flooding and constriction or, alternatively, the protocol will be either "flooded" or "constricted," based on the phase the patient is in at the time of testing.

Signs of Traumatic Avoidance

The early exploratory work of van der Kolk and Ducey (1984) described two patterns of Rorschach responses in Vietnam veterans, marked by a paucity of affective responses and low response rate, which suggested traumatic avoidance. Traumatic avoidance has been documented empirically by a number of Rorschach researchers. The low *Affective Ratio* and low *Blends* found in these studies has been understood to reflect emotional numbing (Kaser-Boyd, 1993). The low *R* and high *Lambda* (Hartman et al., 1990; Swanson et al., 1990) can be understood as markers of cognitive avoidance. These tendencies combine to produce the unusually low *EB* generally seen in traumatized populations (Levin & Reis, 1996).

The presence of dissociation is associated with some unique Exner scores. Researchers studying dissociative disordered populations have found an unusual number of super introversive subjects, and this finding is in contrast to the extratensive pattern typically seen in nondissociative trauma groups (Armstrong & Loewenstein, 1990; Scroppo, Weinberger, Drob, & Eagle, 1998). *FD*, a sign of cognitive and emotional distancing, is characteristic of dissociation (Armstrong, 1991). These findings are consistent with developmental theory, which posits that dissociation can enable the child to distance overwhelming emotion and escape into an imaginative world that is more gratifying than the real one (Armstrong, 1994; Putnam, 1997). Using a non-Exner system framework, Leavitt and Labott (1996) and Leavitt (2000) developed and researched a dissociative index that includes references to seeing forms through obscuring medium (similar to the Exner *FV*), exaggerating the distance of objects (similar to Exner *FD*) and disorientation, a unique variable in which stimuli are seen as shifting or rapidly changing. These researchers were able to correlate their scale with scores on the Dissociative Experiences Scale, suggesting a promising approach to tracking dissociation on the Rorschach (Leavitt & Labott, 1997).

Most recently, Brand et al. (2006) reported on a Rorschach sample of 100 psychiatric inpatients who were severely dissociated and found clear signs of traumatic avoidance in this population. They reported that over 40% of their sample gave *R* < 14, a very significant finding when compared to relevant comparison groups. Brand et al. viewed this pattern as an attempt to "limit and escape painful associations." Additional signs of avoidance and numbing were the high prevalence of *FD*, replicating Armstrong's (1991) finding mentioned earlier; higher frequency of introversive individuals (including nearly one third superintroversives in the sample), suggesting intellectualization and obsessive processes; a low *Afr*, representing emotional numbing; and more *M*, indicating an absorption in fantasy as a means of withdrawal.

Signs of Traumatic Flooding

Evans (chap. 23, this vol.) describes a population of torture victims who seem incapable of defending against the triggering images of the Rorschach: The "... horrific and relentless intrusive experiences of the torture ... overwhelm pervasive and extreme attempts at avoidance and numbing." Individuals whose torture experience was recent or those for whom the trauma was especially horrific will present florid Rorschachs, as if they are unable to defend against images of danger and bodily harm. Traumatic flooding has been noted in the relatively unstructured color responses ($CF + C > FC$) and extratensive *EB* of trauma populations (van der Kolk & Ducey, 1984, 1989). Painful affect is expressed by the predominance of shading responses, particularly *Y* and *V* (Levin, 1993; Salley &

Teiling, 1984; Scroppo et al., 1998). It is not surprising that all of the aforementioned researchers find a high negative D and $AdjD$ in their samples, given the damaging effects of flooding on coping. Traumatic hyperarousal has been documented by researchers in the significant *Inanimate Movement* (m) and *Hypervigilant Index*, reflecting the sense of helplessness in the face of overwhelmingly powerful forces and hypersensitivity to great danger. The psychological meaning of the significant HVI seen in trauma populations has been recently explored in a study by Levin, Lazrove, and van der Kolk (1999). Their subjects' significant HVIs changed from positive to negative following successful EMDR treatment for PTSD. Using SPECT brain scanning, these researchers were able to show that the decrease in HVI was not associated with changes in limbic system overarousal, but was associated with increased frontal lobe function. They hypothesize that, through treatment, their subjects become better able to differentiate real from imagined threats and thus became better able to control their arousal level.

Whereas dissociation is generally viewed as an avoidant process, it can also appear in the flooding phase in the form of flashbacks. Studies have sought to track flashbacks through analysis of content. Since the early Rorschach studies of war and civilian populations, researchers have noted the presence of traumatic content (Leifer, Shapiro, Martone, & Kassem, 1991; van der Kolk & Ducey, 1989). Working with a dissociative disorder sample, Armstrong (1991) developed the Traumatic Content Index consisting of the sum of the Exner contents *Sex*, *Blood*, *Anatomy*, *Morbid*, and *Aggressive Movement* responses, divided by the total number of responses (TC/R). A TC/R of .3 and above was hypothesized to suggest traumatic intrusions. Kamphuis, Kugeares, and Finn (2000) documented the ability of the TC/R to distinguish between patients with confirmed sexual abuse from those without abuse. Leavitt and Labott (1996) were able to differentiate women with sexual abuse histories from a control group using non-Exner content indicators of sexual abuse, including body damage and images of children as victims.

Brand et al.'s (2006) Rorschach sample of 100 severely dissociated psychiatric inpatients also found marked indications of traumatic intrusion in this population. Although they reported that over 40% of their sample gave $R < 14$, even these Low R records were interpretively robust without the usual signs of defensiveness, such as high *Lambda*, high $X+$, low *Blends*, and brief *Responses*. In fact, this dissociative group experienced significantly more emotional flooding than comparison groups. Brand et al. found significantly higher scores on Armstrong's Trauma Content Index with a mean above .50 for the dissociative inpatients, replicating previous studies showing the utility of this measure. Further, Brand et al. found overcomplexity in these patients' cognitive processes, indicated by high *Blends* and low *Lambda*. Also, there was more distorted and illogical thinking ($WSum6$) and distorted views of others ($M-$), signifying "traumatic thought disorder" often found in elevations on Scale 8 on the MMPI–2. Interestingly, Brand and her colleagues also found that this dissociative group displayed positive signs as well, including an interest in others (H), less alienation than other patient groups (low %$H < 2$), as well as the capacity for cooperative relationships with others (COP) and empathy (M), suggesting that long-term insight oriented psychotherapy may be a treatment of choice. Forensic evaluators should further note that Brand et al. (2006) contains extensive tables with frequencies of 36 key CS variables and CS descriptive statistics for this data set.

In order to track traumatic intrusions in traumatized Persian Gulf War veterans, Hilsenroth developed a *Combat Content (CC)* score (Sloan, Arsenault, Hilsenroth, Harvill, & Handler, 1995). The CC includes perceptions of weapons and personalized responses referring to experiences that occurred during their course of military operations. The Sloan et al. research is particularly notable for its cross-validation of the measures of flooding discussed previously. These researchers found the theoretically expected negative correlation between the MMPI–2 PTSD scale, the *PK* scale, and the Rorschach *D* and *Adjusted D* scales, and a positive correlation between the *PK* scale and their *CC* scale. To date, there exists no Rorschach trauma content scale that can be applied cross-trauma or cross-culturally. Given the range and variety of life traumas, this may be an unrealistic goal. Nonetheless, it is clear that intrusions of traumatic associations onto the Rorschach occur in subjects who may not readily volunteer such information in interview. For example, Franchi and Andronikof-Sanglade (1993) studied a group of West African immigrant women in Paris who had had clitoridectomies. Although none of these women complained of being sexually mutilated, images of intact and clitoridectomized organs, along with scores associated with emotional distress, emerged as a dominant theme in 40% of their protocols.

Finally, all trauma researchers have found a high incidence of impaired reality testing and thought disorder on the Rorschach. This includes atypical views of reality (low *X+%*, high *Xu%*), illogical combinations of ideas (*INCOMs* and *FABCOMs*), and loss of task focus (*DR*). Carlson and Armstrong (1994) argued that, for traumatized patients, ambiguous tests like the Rorschach can cease to be a test and, instead, become a traumatic trigger. Thus, the typical interpretations of the meaning of scores cannot be utilized, because the test taker no longer has the appropriate test set. Similarly, in reviewing the Rorschach trauma literature, Levin and Reis (1996) concluded that traumatic themes often supersede otherwise intact reality testing. Considering that the essence of trauma is dealing with a reality that has acted in a chaotic and illogical fashion, Armstrong (2002) has hypothesized that these scores reflect a "traumatic thought disorder."

Special Issues

One challenging task for clinicians and researchers is to untangle Rorschach indicators of chronic trauma from Axis II disorders. Readers may have already noted the parallel between the biphasic trauma response and the Rorschach research findings on patients with Borderline Personality Disorder (Herman & van der Kolk, 1987). This parallel is not unexpected because the two groups overlap, with a large subgroup of borderlines who report childhood abuse (Herman, Perry, & van der Kolk 1989). With this said, from a practical standpoint, it is clinically important to be able to distinguish between the affective and cognitive variability and malevolent perceptions of people with borderline spectrum disorders and the traumatic intrusions and flooding seen in people with PTSD. The treatment needs, strengths, and vulnerabilities of these two populations are often quite different. The constellation of dysfunctional traits that come from early or chronic severe childhood trauma can fit neatly into other Personality Disorder categories as well, such as Antisocial Personality Disorder, Narcissistic Personality Disorder, Paranoid Personality

Disorder, to name the most prevalent. Individuals subjected to early, severe, repetitive trauma like that seen in severe child abuse are diagnosed using contemporary standards as having Disorders of Extreme Stress (DESNOS), which is also called Complex Posttraumatic Stress Disorder or Personality Disorders Resulting from Extreme Stress (Herman, 1992; van der Kolk, 2005; van der Kolk, Roth, Pelcovitz, Sunday, & Spinazzola, 2005). Impairments in Complex Posttraumatic Stress Disorder are described in six domains:

1. Alterations in regulation of affect and impulses. Deficits of affect regulation are illustrated by difficulty modulating affects, including anger, self-destructive behavior, deficits of modulation of sexual involvement, and excessive risk-taking.

2. Alterations in attention or consciousness. These alterations may be transient dissociative episodes or derealization and depersonalization.

3. Alterations in self-perception. These are exemplified by a sense of having been permanently damaged, feeling shame, ineffectiveness, excessive guilt, and other indicators of an impaired sense of self.

4. Alterations in perception of others. These individuals develop distorted beliefs about others as the result of their "distorted" experiences of childhood. Experiences of others swing from idealization to devaluation. There is a pervasive inability to trust and a preoccupation with hurting those who hurt them. In their adult lives, they may be revictimized, or may victimize others (women more likely to become victims and men more likely to become perpetrators).

5. Somatization. Although they may not have chronic pain or illness, this somatic preoccupation is more common than in normal individuals. They may have compromised functioning in one domain, for example, cardiopulmonary or digestive. They often have sexual symptoms and also may have conversion symptoms. Their physical symptoms may result from their chronic stress or may be a subjective perception of vulnerability as an offshoot of feeling profoundly threatened.

6. Alterations in systems of meaning. They have difficulty sustaining hope and quickly feel helpless and despairing in crises.

Briere & Spinozola's (2005) comprehensive review of assessment measures of the different components of Complex Posttraumatic Stress Disorder is a valuable resource, starting with broad-band instruments such as the MMPI–2 and moving to more trauma-specific instruments, such as the Trauma Symptom Inventory. In chapter 10, Kaser-Boyd (this vol.) illustrates how each of these symptom clusters can be explored with Rorschach variables in preparation of mitigation evidence for death penalty hearings.

It is often the case that the current trauma is complicated by a history of previous traumas (Follette, Polusny, Bechtle, & Naugle, 1996). Examples include the victim of sexual harassment who is an incest survivor; the battered woman who saw severe domestic violence with her parents; and the victim of political persecution who is also a rape trauma survivor. Multiple traumas have what has been described as a "kindling effect" (Schumm, Stines, Hobfoll, & Jackson, 2005). The clinical effects may not be the same as DESNOS, but the response to a current trauma may be more severe. In contemporary clinical practice with traumatized patients, treatment focus also includes dealing with a high level of "self-medication" with drugs and alcohol, which further causes difficulties in the symptom picture (Acierno, Resnick, Kilpatrick, Saunders, & Best, 1999). This highlights the importance of taking a careful history and understanding how one life event connects to the next.

CASE EXAMPLE

The case of Mr. K could be considered typical of the complexity seen in forensic cases. Mr. K went to serve in the first Gulf War when he was just 19. He was a high school graduate, and the son of Asian immigrants who were hard working and successful. He wanted to serve his country, so he joined the Army and became a member of an elite unit. His brother became a police officer. Mr. K was only 5 feet 2 inches tall, but he was physically tough and he was determined to be a good soldier. After basic and advanced training, he was deployed to Saudi Arabia, where his unit went on raids across the border into Iraq. The mission of his unit was to "clear the area." Mr. K had many painful images of combat, although his service was some 10 years prior to the forensic evaluation. For example, he described the first time he saw a dead body: "Clearing the places, we would run into dead bodies. The first body, it was like in a movie. It just zoomed out at me. The body just tears up with the bullets they use. The torso was ripped in half, and you can see the muscles and the gut, and their faces. You never forget that surprised look on their face. I will never forget that first body."

Mr. K recounted how he and his Army comrades became "hardened" to seeing bodies. He said that they started to take pictures of the dead bodies and, as their numbing to the horror increased, they stood smiling next to the bodies for the photo. Mr. K said that, as time went on, he felt that a lot of innocent Iraqis were being killed. He felt personally responsible for killing innocent people. He also felt distress and shame about the treatment of Iraqi POWs. He had several experiences where he thought he might die. For example, on one occasion he was hanging onto the outside of a helicopter that almost crashed.

Mr. K finished his tour of duty and returned to his home. He was finally safe, but he did not feel safe. He had terrible nightmares of combat and death. He could hardly sleep and he felt constantly agitated. Once, his family found him with a black plastic bag over his head. He explained, to the evaluator, that he was practicing exercises learned in combat to see if he could "still measure up." He also re-enacted war scenes with toy soldiers. He said that he was playing "to see if I could make it turn out different, you know, with actual combat with the enemy, not with innocent people." He had a sense of a foreshortened future and felt like none of his values made sense now. He felt angry and alienated, like other people did not understand. He had passive fantasies of suicide. His family thought he acted like he was hearing voices, but he said he was "reliving conversations and events," that he would "go into a trance" and "think and think and talk to myself." He felt an ever-present sense of danger and began carrying a weapon, although he lived in a safe city. He felt physically unwell, too. His hair was falling out and he had skin rashes, which he feared were the result of chemical weapons.

Because of his odd and frightening behavior, Mr. K ultimately had to leave his parents' home. He began a period of homelessness, drifting from one place in the city to another. Eventually, he met other homeless people, who introduced him to the drug culture, mostly abusing methamphetamines. Mr. K found "meth" almost immediately addictive, which was not surprising because meth alleviated some of the worst symptoms of PTSD. For example, meth users say they do not dream and indeed Mr. K's terrible nightmares went away. Meth users also report a reduction of anxiety and guilt, likely due to the drug's impact on the brain's frontal lobes. They become totally goal-focused, ignoring the past and the future, an obvious relief for someone who re-experiences traumatic images. Meth also mimics the adrenaline rush of combat. He said, "I hadn't felt that high since being over there."

Methamphetamine abuse often leads to criminal activity. Meth users often stay in groups and form small criminal rings that engage in fraud or thefts or manufacture of the drug. Mr. K was ultimately arrested for identity theft. His first trial attorney had little knowledge about PTSD or about the aftereffects of the Gulf War. For example, in court, he said that his client had been exposed to Agent Orange, a chemical used in Vietnam, but not in the Persian Gulf. Mr. K ultimately was convinced to plead guilty. Because he had not filed paperwork to become a citizen when he was in the Army, he was next faced with deportation. The evaluation was conducted for his deportation hearing.

It is always a challenge to conduct an evaluation of a mental state that occurred at some point in the past (e.g., at the time of a crime several years prior, or at the time of entering a plea, several years prior). However, most mental disorders have a typical course or history. The course of PTSD is described at the beginning of this chapter. In combat veterans, we can expect that they will be flooded with images of war and threat when they return from a combat zone. Gradually, these images will recede and there will be signs of avoidance or emotional constriction. Many soldiers can achieve the avoidant stage only through the use of drugs or alcohol and the substance abuse causes further mental deterioration, worsening and changing the presentation of the disorder.

Mr. K was tested in a prison setting. He had not used Crystal Meth for several years, and he was not receiving psychotropic medications. He presented as an intelligent, polite, modest man, without evidence of psychotic symptoms or expression of strong emotion. His MMPI–2 results were valid, with no evidence of an attempt to exaggerate or malinger. He scored slightly above significance on almost all the basic clinical scales, but had pronounced elevations on Scales 7 and 6 (T of 80 and 85, respectively). His T-score on PK was 78. Although the MMPI–2 clearly documented symptoms of PTSD, the T-scores and descriptions of their meaning paled by comparison to the data from the Rorschach. The same was true for the MCMI–III. Mr. K was not elevated on the MCMI Posttraumatic Stress Scale, but he was markedly elevated on Anxiety Disorder, and on Drug Dependence, which could be argued as the manifestations of PTSD. Triggered by these abstract blots, his Rorschach most vividly illustrated his preoccupations. Mr. K was unable to inhibit frightening and deteriorated percepts on any of the 10 Rorschach cards. The red color of the Rorschach invariably called out images of bloody, damaged, vulnerable animals and people. Almost every card contained an injured or dying creature. Some examples illustrate his preoccupation with injury and death:

Card II: Maybe two rabbits that were split in half, blood coming out from his mouth and his be-hind. Blood behind his eyes. It's awful. As soon as I saw the red, it looked like blood, and smashed. And then it looked like two rabbits, their paws and the feet, laying on their side, ears, a tail, and see how the blood is coming out from their mouth and this is coming from their rear area, like they've been smashed.

Card III: It looks like two ladies, facing each other, like they are washing clothes or something, and for some reason, these remind me of getting shot, they just got shot. Blood spotches. Maybe they are ripping something apart and they are facing each other. I saw the two red parts, it looks like they got shot. Boom! And this is red coming from behind. I said ladies because it looks like they have breasts. At first it looked like they were washing clothes, but looking at it, it looks like something is being ripped apart, like they are fighting over something and tearing it apart. They have shoes, they have faces, and they are looking at each other, and this looks like blood, like they've been shot.

Card VII: This looks sort of like a face. Like the skin area around, exactly what it would look like if they peeled off the skin, except they didn't take off the nose (which would be here in the empty space) and that would be the beard. The skin of a face, peeled open. Here the ears would go and the eyes, but they just took the skin off.

Card VIII: These look like two dead wolves, and something is stuck to their neck, an apparatus, and I guess it looks like they are sucking something out and waste is coming out of this end. Actu-ally, this kind of looks like a rifle here, it's got two scopes here, and this looks like blood, or doo doo. It's like a rifle but it's connected to their neck and it looks like its sucking stuff out of the wolves. It's got the scopes, the grips, the barrel. You see the colors. It's red, but its got a little bit of yellow and it looks like guts and waste. It looks really dirty and messy, stuff you wouldn't touch. These are animals and they really look dead, and these two really look like rifles, just like the kind of scope I had. This is the flash suppressor. This has the grip, the magazine, and it's pointing right at their neck ....

[Second response, same card] Also, it could look like someone is hanging upside down and hold-ing onto something heavy, and he has a lot of weight on him, and it ll he is being tortured, maybe being ripped apart here, his backbone. All the different colors, the way it's splotchy, looks like guts and gore.

Mr. K's protocol is littered with *Morbid* and *Aggressive Content*, and he had a high Trauma Content Index. Moreover, his *WSum6* is 35, and his *X+%* is .63, indicating the cognitive dysfunction that is depicted about individuals who have experienced a world where the abnormal has become normal. Apart from formal scores, his Rorschach proto-col is a window into his experience of the Gulf War.

Forensic Issues

Perhaps one of the most important issues when assessing trauma with the Rorschach in forensic settings is whether the protocol was malingered. First and foremost, it is impor-tant to emphasize that the diagnosis of PTSD should never rest solely on Rorschach re-sults. Like any competent forensic evaluation, one must use a multimethod approach to assessment (see Erdberg, chap. 27, this vol.). There should be indicators of PTSD in the clinical interview, in the collateral descriptions of the patient from others (e.g., his family, his boss), and data from other tests, all of which converge to support the diagnosis. In the case of Mr. K, both the MMPI and the MCMI were valid, with no signs of malingering. Although each test measured his trauma symptoms in a way unique to that test, neither broad-band self-report instrument was inconsistent with a diagnosis of PTSD.

In terms of whether or not PTSD can be malingered on the Rorschach, Wood, Nezworski, Lillienfeld, and Garb (2003) made the sweeping conclusion that PTSD can be easily malingered: "Numerous studies have shown that individuals with a minimal amount of coaching can fake schizophrenia on the Rorschach. Furthermore, research indicates that patients with depression and posttraumatic stress disorder are indistinguishable on the Rorschach from individuals who are faking."

Wood et al. cite studies by Freuh and Kinder (1994) and Popper (1992) "proving" that PTSD can be faked. Citing Popper is an example of the recurring tendency of these authors to cite dissertation research, not a peer-reviewed journal, a curious decision given the sharp unpublished studies criticism they level at Exner. A review of the Freuh and Kinder study revealed the several methodological designs flaws, including inclusion of a sample whose trauma exposure was at least 17 years prior to this study. As stated earlier, other research with combat veterans and other groups indicates that PTSD is a biphasic disorder, which waxes and wanes in terms of overt trauma symptoms (e.g, the "flooded Rorschach"). The study makes no attempt to control the trauma sample for "flooded" or "avoidant" subgroups, for example, by using *Lambda* greater than or less than 1.0, as suggested elsewhere (Armstrong & Kaser-Boyd, 2003). Because the "trauma" group was so many years past trauma exposure, there was a real likelihood that they would have constricted Rorschachs, which is born out by group statistics. Thus, the conclusion that the "fakers" showed more symptoms of trauma than the "real" PTSD group may be spurious. Additionally, Wood, Nezworski, Lilienfeld, and Garb (2003) fail to acknowledge, let alone address, three well-designed research articles by Ganellen (1994, 1996; Ganellen, Wasyliw, Haywood, & Grossman 1996), which found the Rorschach to be superior to the MMPI–2 to detecting psychological state in forensic contexts (i.e., being freer from response style bias such as malingering). Why they cite a dissertation and a methodologically flawed article and fail to cite three other articles from refereed journals contradicting their assertion is not known, although the implications from the perspective of good science are troubling.

Research in psychological assessment indicates that malingerers in general commonly feign psychological disorder by an overly dramatic presentation of symptoms (e.g., Storm & Graham, 2000; Perry & Kinder 1990; Schretlen, 1988), including malingered posttraumatic stress disorder (Elhai, Gold, Sellers, & Dorfman, 2001; Gold & Frueh, 1999; Liljequist, Kinder, & Schinka, 1998). Ganellen (chap. 5, this vol.) reviews three studies of malingering that indicate malingerers respond to the Rorschach with *Dramatic Content* and he cautions that the *Dramatic Content* score is similar to the Trauma Content Index. However, he notes that the range of scores expected on *Dramatic Content* in clinical, nonclinical, and forensic samples responding honestly and in samples of simulating and actual malingers has not been established, nor has a cut score differentiating between genuine and feigned protocols been determined. Additionally, Exner (personal communication) often said that malingerers give "blood and guts" responses with good *Form Quality*, not realizing that the mentally disordered patient generates scores associated with thought disorder and poor reality testing. As clients and their lawyers become more willing to prepare for psychological testing (Wetter & Corrigan, 1995) and Internet resources are readily accessible (Ruiz, Drake, Glass, Marcotte, & van Gorp, 2002), it behooves the careful forensic psychologist to carefully examine the Rorschach along with the other tests in the battery for the possibilities of malingering.

Once the issue of malingering has been resolved, the forensic practitioner must decide how to present Rorschach data in a simple, illustrative way. It is rarely effective to dwell on a Structural Summary and the many scores it provides, simply because this overwhelms the layperson. Attorneys seem to shy away from learning the Rorschach literature. The publication of many scholarly replies to the criticisms of Wood et al. (2003), summarized in the White Paper (SPA, 2005) likely feels overwhelming to someone not educated in psychometrics and statistics, and most of the attacks appear to be *ad hominem* (e.g., attacking Exner, or making sweeping statements such as "Isn't it the case that the Rorschach is highly controversial?"). If the Rorschach variables selected for testimony are highly associated with trauma, based on the published studies reviewed in this chapter, and if there is a commonsense explanation about how personal experience is tapped by these abstract cards, even a vicious attack based on Wood et al. (2003) may be ignored by a jury. The forensic practitioner is well advised to come to the courtroom ready to do battle on the psychometric issues of reliability, validity, and utility and also to explain the Rorschach and the findings in the simplest way possible. The variables chosen previously to illustrate Mr. K's similarity to the trauma population were limited with this in mind, even though there were many other aspects of his Rorschach of interest. When we see what the traumatized person projects onto these abstract stimuli, we can truly see how trauma has infused their perception and worldview. It is the graphic illustration of what they have seen and felt, and it communicates their trauma experience better than any other psychological instrument.

ACKNOWLEDGMENTS

This chapter is, in part, an adaptation of Armstrong and Kaser-Boyd (2003), with the exception of the section on forensic issues, which remains the sole opinion of Kaser-Boyd and Evans. They are grateful to Judy Armstrong for her permission to use a portion of her earlier chapter.

REFERENCES

Acierno, R., Resnick, H. S., Kilpatrick, D. G., Saunders, B. E., & Best, C. L. (1999). Risk factors for rape, physical assault, and posttraumatic stress disorder in women: Examination of differential multivariate relationships. *Journal of Anxiety Disorders, 13*, 541–563.

American Psychiatric Association. (2000). *Diagnostic and statistical manual of mental disorders* (4th rev. ed.). Washington, DC: Author.

Armstrong, J. G. (2002). Deciphering the broken narrative of trauma: Signs of traumatic dissociation on the Rorschach . In A. Andronikof (Ed.), *Rorschachiana XXV: Yearbook of the International Rorschach Society* (pp. 11–27). Ashland, OH: Hogrefe & Huber.

Armstrong, J. G. (1991). The psychological organization of multiple personality disordered patients as revealed in psychological testing. *Psychiatric Clinics of North America, 14*, 533–546.

Armstrong, J. G. (1994). Reflections on multiple personality disorder as a developmentally complex adaptation. *The Psychoanalytic Study of the Child, 49*, 340–364.

Armstrong, J. G., & Kaser-Boyd (2003). Projective assessment of psychological trauma. In M. Hilsenroth & D. Segal (Eds.), *Objective and projective assessment of personality and psychopathology: Vol. 2. Comprehensive handbook of psychological assessment*. New York: Wiley.

Armstrong, J. G., & Loewenstein, R. J. (1990). Characteristics of patients with multiple personality and dissociative disorders on psychological testing. *Journal of Nervous and Mental Disease, 178*, 445–454.

Brand, B. L., Armstrong, J. G., & Loewenstein, R. J. (2006). Psychological assessment of patients with dissociative identity disorder . *Psychiatric Clinics of North America, 29*, 145–168.

Bremner, J. D. (1999). Alterations in brain structure and function associated with posttraumatic stress disorder. *Seminars in Clinical Neuropsychiatry, 4*, 249–255.

Bremner, J. D., Davis, M., Southwick, S. M., Krystal, J. H., & Charney, D. S. (1994). Neurology of Posttraumatic Stress Disorder. In R. J. Pynoos (Ed.), *Posttraumatic stress disorder: A clinical review* (pp. 210–268). Maryland: Sidran.

Breslau, N., Kessler, R. C., Chilcoat, H. D., Schultz, I. R., Davis, G. C., & Andreski, P. C. (1998). Trauma and posttraumatic stress disorder in the community. *American Journal of Psychiatry, 55*, 626–632.

Briere, J. (1995). *Trauma Symptom Inventory*. Odessa, FL: Psychological Assessment Resources.

Briere, J. (1997). *Psychological assessment of adult posttraumatic states*. Washington, DC: American Psychological Association.

Briere, J., & Spinazola, J. (2005). Phenomenology and psychological assessment of complex posttraumatic states. *Journal of Traumatic Stress, 18*(5), 401–412.

Bryer, J. B., Nelson, B. A., Miller, J. B., & Krol, P. A. (1987). Childhood sexual and physical abuse as factors in adult psychiatric illness. *American Journal of Psychiatry, 144*, 1426–1430.

Carlson, E. B. (1997). *Trauma assessments*. New York: Guilford.

Carlson, E. B., & Armstrong, J. G. (1994). The diagnosis and assessment of dissociative disorders. In S. J. Lynn & J. W. Rhue (Eds.), *Dissociation: Clinical and theoretical perspectives* (pp. 159–174). New York: Guilford.

Carlson, E. B., Furby, L., Armstrong, J., & Schlaes, J. (1997). A conceptual framework for the long-term psychological effects of traumatic childhood abuse. *Child Maltreatment, 2*, 272–295.

Carmen, E. H., Rieker, P. P., & Mills, T. (1984). Victims of violence and psychiatric illness. *American Journal of Psychiatry, 141*(3), 378–383.

Cassidy, J., & Mohr, J. J. (2001). Unsolvable fear, trauma, and psychopathology. *Clinical Psychology: Science and Practice, 8*, 275–298.

Cerney, M. (1990). The Rorschach and traumatic loss: Can the presence of traumatic loss be detected from the Rorschach? *Journal of Personality Assessment, 55*, 781–789.

Dalenberg, C. J. (2000). *Countertransference and the treatment of trauma*. Washington, DC: American Psychological Association.

De Bellis, M. D., Keshavan, M. S., Clark, D. B., Casey, B. J., Giedd, J. N., Boring, A. M., Rustaci, K., & Ryan, N. D. (1999). Developmental traumatology; Part K: Biological stress systems. *Biological Psychiatry, 45*, 1271–1284.

De Bellis, M. D., Lefter, L., Trickett, P. K., & Putnam, F. W. (1994). Urinary catecholamine excretion in sexually abused girls. *Journal of the American Academy of Child and Adolescent Psychiatry, 33*, 320–327.

Elhai, J. D., Gold, S. N., Sellers, A. H., & Dorfman, W. I. (2001) The detection of malingered posttraumatic stress disorder with MMPI–2 Fake Bad Indices. *Assessment, 8*(2), 221–236.

Fine, R. (1955a). Manual for a scoring scheme for verbal projective techniques (TAT, MAPS, stories and the like). *Journal of Projective Techniques, 19*, 306–309.

Foa, E. B., Keane, T. M., & Friedman, M. J. (2000). Guidelines for treatment of PTSD. *Journal of Traumatic Stress, 13*, 539–588.

Follette, V. M., Polusny, M. A., Bechtle, A. E., & Naugle, A. E. (1996). Cumulative trauma: The impact of child sexual abuse, adult sexual assault, and spouse abuse. *Journal of Traumatic Stress, 9*(1), 25–36.

Franchi, V., & Andronikof-Sanglade, H. (1993). Methodological and epistemological issues raised by the use of the Rorschach Comprehensive System in cross cultural research. *Rorschachiana, 18*, 118–133.

Freuh, B. C., & Kinder, B. N. (1994). The susceptibility of the Rorschach Inkblot Test to malingering of combat-related PTSD. *Journal of Personality Assessment, 62,* 280–298.

Friedrich, W. N., & Share, M. C. (1997). The Roberts Apperception Test for Children: An exploratory study of its use with sexually abused children. *Journal of Child Sexual Abuse, 6*(4), 83–91.

Ganellen, R. J. (1994) Attempting to conceal psychological disturbance: MMPI defensive response sets and the Rorschach. *Journal of Personality Assessment, 63*, 423–437.

Ganellen, R. J. (1996) Exploring MMPI–Rorschach relationships. *Journal of Personality Assessment, 67*, 529–542.

Ganellen, R. J., Wasyliw, O. E., Haywood, T. W., & Grossman, L. S. (1996) Can psychosis be malingered on the Rorschach? An empirical study. *Journal of Personality Assessment, 66*, 65–80.

Gold, P. B., & Frueh, C. B. (1999) Compensation-seeking and extreme exaggeration of psychopathology among combat veterans evaluated for posttraumatic stress disorder. *Journal of Nervous & Mental Disease, 187*(11), 680–684.

Green, B. (1994). Traumatic stress and disaster: Mental health effects and factors influencing adaptation. In F. Liemac & C. C. Madelson (Eds.), *International review of psychiatry* (Vol. 2, pp. 117–210). Washington, DC: American Psychiatric Press.

Gurvitz, T. V., Gilbertson, M. W., Lasko, N. B., Tarlan, A. S., Simeon, D., Macklin, M., Orr, S. P., & Pitman, R. K. (2000). Neurological soft signs in chronic posttraumatic stress disorder. *Archives of General Psychiatry, 57*, 181–186.

Gurvitz, T. V., Shenton, M. E., Hokama, H., Ohta, H., Lasko, M. B., Orr, S. P., Kikinis, R., Jolesz, A., McCarley, R. W., & Pitman, R. K. (1996). Magnetic resonance imaging study of hippocampal volume in chronic, combat-related posttraumatic stress disorder. *Biological Psychiatry, 52*, 661–666.

Hartman, W. R., Clark, M. E., Morgan, M. K., Dunn, V. K., Fine, A. D., Perry, G. G., Jr., & Winsch, D. L. (1990). Rorschach structure of a hospitalized sample of Vietnam veterans with PTSD. *Journal of Personality Assessment, 54,* 149–159.

Herman, H. L. (1992). Complex posttraumatic stress disorder: A syndrome in survivors of prolonged and repeated trauma. *Journal of Traumatic Stress, 5*(3), 377–391.

Herman, J. L., Perry, J. C., & van der Kolk, B. A. (1989). Childhood trauma in borderline personality disorder. *American Journal of Psychiatry, 146,* 490–495.

Herman, J. L., & van der Kolk, B. A. (1987). Traumatic antecedents of borderline personality disorder. In B. Van der Kolk (Ed.), *Psychologial trauma* (pp. 111–126). Washington, DC: American Psychiatric Press.

Hoffman, B. (2001, September 13). *What is that image?* Retrieved October 2, 2001, from http://Sa.mlive.com/news/index.ssf?/news/stories/20010913ssatansface.frm

Holaday, M. (1998). Rorschach protocols of children and adolescents with severe burns: A follow-up study. *Journal of Personality Assessment, 71*(3), 306–321.

Holschneider, D.P. (2000, September). *Genotype to phenotype: Challenges and opportunities in mice and men.* UCLA School of Medicine, Department of Psychiatry, Grand Rounds.

Kamphuis, J. H., Kugeares, S. L., & Finn, S. E. (2000). Rorschach correlates of sexual abuse: Trauma content and aggression indices. *Journal of Personality Assessment, 75*, 212–224.

Kaser-Boyd, N. (1999). Defending the Rorschach in court. *Newsletter of the Society for Personality Assessment.*

Kaser-Boyd, N. (1993). Post-traumatic stress disorder in children and adults. *Western State Law Review, 20*, 319–334.

Kaser-Boyd, N. (1993). Rorschachs of women who commit homicide. *Journal of Personality Assessment, 60,* 458–470.

Keane, T. M., Malloy, P. F., & Fairbank, J. A. (1984). Empirical development of an MMPI subscale for the assessment of combat-related posttraumatic stress disorder. *Journal of Consulting and Clinical Psychology, 52,* 888–891.

Kessler, R. C., Sonnega, A., Bromet, E., Hughes, M., & Nelson, C. B. (1995). Posttraumatic stress disorder in the national comorbidity study. *Archives of General Psychiatry, 52,* 1048–1060.

Kolb, L. C. (1988). A critical survey of hypotheses regarding posttraumatic stress in light of recent research findings. *Journal of Traumatic Stress, 1,* 291–304.

Leavitt, F. (2000). Texture response patterns associated with sexual trauma of childhood and adult onset: Developmental and recovered memory implications. *Child Abuse and Neglect, 4,* 251–257.

Leavitt, F., & Labott, S. M. (1996). Authenticity of recovered sexual abuse memories: A Rorschach study. *Journal of Traumatic Stress, 9,* 483–496.

Leavitt, F., & Labott, S. M. (1997). Criterion-related validity of Rorschach analogues of dissociation. *Psychological Assessment, 9,* 244–249.

LeDoux, J. (1996). *The emotional brain: The mysterious underpinnings of emotional life.* New York: Simon & Schuster.

LeDoux, J. (1998). Fear and the brain: Where have we been and where are we going? *Biological Psychiatry, 44,* 1229–1238.

Leifer, M., Shapiro, J. P., Martone, M. W., & Kassem, L. (1991). Rorschach assessment of psychological functioning in sexually abused girls. *Journal of Personality Assessment, 56,* 14–28.

Levin, P. (1993). Assessing PTSD with the Rorschach projective technique. In J. Wilson & B. Raphael (Eds.), *The international handbook of traumatic stress syndromes* (pp. 189–200). New York: Plenum.

Levin, P., Lazrove, S., & van der Kolk, B. (1999). What psychological testing and neuroimaging tell us about the treatment of posttraumatic stress disorder by eye movement desensitization and reprocessing. *Journal of Anxiety Disorders, 13,* 159–172.

Levin, P., & Reis, B. (1996). Use of the Rorschach in assessing trauma. In J. P. Wilson & T. Keane (Eds.), *Assessing psychological trauma and PTSD* (pp. 529–543). New York: Guilford.

Liljequist, L., Kinder, B. N., & Schinka, J. A. (1998) An investigation of malingering posttraumatic stress disorder on the Personality Assessment Inventory. *Journal of Personality Assessment, 71*(3), 322–336.

McFarlane, A. C. (1989). The aetiology of posttraumatic morbidity: Predisposing, precipitating and perpetuating factors. *British Journal of Psychiatry, 154,* 221–228.

Mikkelson, B., & Mikkelson, D. P. (2001). *Images of the World Trade Center fire reveal the face of Satan.* Retrieved from http://www.snopes2.com/rumors/wtcface.html

Millon, T., Bockian, N., Tringone, R., Antoni, M., & Green, C. (1989). New diagnostic efficiency statistics: Comparative sensitivity and predictive/prevalence ratio. *Journal of Personality Disorders, 3,* 163–171.

Perry, G. G., & Kinder, B. N. (1990). The susceptibility of the Rorschach to malingering: A critical review. *Journal of Personality Assessment, 54*(1–2), 47–57.

Parson, E. R. (1998). Traumatic stress personality disorder (TrSpd), Part II. Trauma assessment using the Rorschach and self-report tests. *Journal of Contemporary Psychotherapy, 28,* 45–68.

Popper, M. D. (1992). The Rorschach on trial: Attempts to simulate disability. *Dissertation Abstracts International, 53*(2), 1073B.

Putnam, F.W. (1997). *Dissociation in children and adolescents: A developmental perspective.* New York: Guilford.

Rauch, S. L., van der Kolk, B. A., Fisler, R. E., Alpert, N. M., Orr, S. P., Savage, C. R., Fischman, A. J., Jenike, M. A., & Pitman, R. K. (1996). A symptom provocation study of posttraumatic stress disorder using positron emission tomography and script-driven imagery. *Archives of General Psychiatry, 56,* 556–578.

Resnick, H. S., Yehuda, R. Pitman, R. K., & Foy, D. W. (1995). Effect of previous trauma on acute plasma cortisol level following rape. *American Journal of Psychiatry, 152,* 1675–1677.

Ruiz, M. A., Drake, E. B., Glass, A., Marcotte, D., & van Gorp, W. G. (2002).Trying to beat the system Misuse of the internet to assist in avoiding detection of psychological symptom dissimulation. *Professional Psychology: Research and Practice, 33,* 294–299.

Salley, R., & Teiling, P. (1984). Dissociated rate attacks in a Vietnam veteran: A Rorschach Study. *Journal of Personality Assessment, 48,* 98–104.

Sapolsky, R. M. (1992). *Stress, the aging brain, and the mechanisms of neuron death.* Cambridge: MIT Press.

Schachter, D. L. (1996). *Searching for memory: The brain, the mind, and the past.* New York: Basic Books.

Schretlen, D. J. (1988). The use of psychological tests to identify malingered symptoms of mental disorder. *Clinical Psychology Review, 8*(5), 451–476.

Schumm, J. A., Stines, L. R., Hobfoll, S. E., & Jackson, A. P. (2005). The double-barreled burden of child abuse and current stressful circumstances on adult women: The kindling effect of early traumatic experience. *Journal of Traumatic Stress, 18*(5), 467–476.

Scroppo, J. C., Weinberger, J. L., Drob, S. L., & Eagle, P. (1998). Identifying dissociative identity disorder: A self-report and projective study. *Journal of Abnormal Psychology, 107,* 272–284.

Shalit, B. (1965). Effects of environmental stimulation on the M, FM and m responses in the Rorschach. *Journal of Projective Techniques and Personality Assessment, 29,* 228–231.

Shalev, A. Y., Freedman, S., Peri, T., Brandes, D., Sahar, T., Orr, S. P., & Pitman, R. K. (1998). Prospective study of posttraumatic stress disorder and depression following trauma. *American Journal of Psychiatry, 155,* 630–637.

Sloan, P., Arsenault, L., Hilsenroth, M., Harvill, L., & Handler, L. (1995). Rorschach measures of posttraumatic stress in Persian Gulf War veterans. *Journal of Personality Assessment, 64,* 397–414.

Solomon, Z., Mikulincer, & Avitzur, E. (1988). Coping, locus of control, social support, and combat related posttraumatic stress disorder: A prospective study. *Journal of Personality and Social Psychology, 55,* 279–285.

Southwick, S. M., Paige, S. R., Morgan, C. A., Bremner, J. D., Krystal, J. H., & Charney, D. S. (1999). Adrenergic and serotonergic abnormalities I PTSD: Catecholamines and serotonin. *Seminars in Clinical Neuropsychiatry, 4,* 256–266.

Southwick, S. M., Krystal, J. H., Morgan, A. C., et. al. (1993). Abnormal noradrenergic function in post traumatic stress disorder. *Archives of General Psychiatry, 50,* 266–274.

Society for Personality Assessment. (2005). Status of the Rorschach in clinical and forensic practice: An official statement by the Board of Trustees of the Society for Personality Assessment. *Journal of Personality Assessment, 85*(2), 219–237.

Storm, J., & Graham, J. R. (2000). Detection of coached general malingering on the MMPI–2. *Psychological Assessment, 12,* 158–165.

Swanson, G. S., Blount, J., & Bruno, R. (1990). Comprehensive system Rorschach data on Vietnam combat veterans. *Journal of Personality Assessment, 54,* 160–169.

Trickett, P. K., & Putnam, F. W. (1993). Impact of child sexual abuse on females. *Psychological Science, 4,* 81–87.

van der Kolk, B. A. (2003). The neurobiology of childhood trauma and abuse. *Child and Adolescent Psychiatric Clinica, 12,* 293–317.

van der Kolk, B.A. (1987). *Psychological trauma.* Washington, DC: American Psychiatric Press.

van der Kolk, B. A. (1994). The body keeps score: Memory and the evolving psychobiology of posttraumatic stress. *Harvard Review of Psychiatry, 1,* 235–265.

van der Kolk, B. A., & Courtois, C. A. (2005). Editorial comments: Complex developmental trauma. *Journal of Traumatic Stress, 18*(5), 385–388.

van der Kolk, B.A., & Ducey, C. (1984). Clinical implications of the Rorschach in post-traumatic stress disorder. In B. A. van der Kolk (Ed.), *Post-traumatic stress disorder: Psychological and biological sequelae* (pp. 29–42). Washington, DC: American Psychiatric Press.

van der Kolk, B. A., & Ducey, C. (1989). The psychological processing of traumatic experience: Rorschach patterns in PTSD. *Journal of Traumatic Stress, 2,* 259–263.

van der Kolk, B. A., & Greenberg, M. S. (1987). The psychobiology of the trauma response: Hyperarousal, constriction, and addiction to traumatic reexposure. In B. A. van der Kolk (Ed.), *Psychological trauma* (pp. 63–88). Washington, DC: American Psychiatric Press.

van der Kolk, B. A., & McFarlane, A. C. (1996). The black hole of trauma. In B. A. van der Kolk, A. C. McFarlane, & L. Weisaeth (Eds.), *Traumatic stress* (pp. 3–23). New York: Guilford.

van der Kolk, B. A., Roth, S., Pelcovitz, D., Sinday, S., & Spinazzola, J. (2005). Disorders of extreme stress: The empirical foundation of a complex adaptation to trauma. *Journal of Traumatic Stress, 18*(5), 389–399.

Van Velsen, C., Gorst-Unsworth, C., & Turner, S. (1996). Survisors of torture and organized violence: Demography and diagnosis. *Journal of Traumatic Stress, 9*(2), 181–194.

Waysman, M., Schwarzwald, J., & Solomon, Z. (2001). Hardiness: An examination of its relationship with positive and negative long term changes following trauma. *Journal of Traumatic Stress, 14,* 531–548.

Weisath, L. (1989). A study of behavioral responses to an industrial disaster. *Acta Psychiatrica Scandinavica, 355* (80), 13–71.

Wells, S., & Maher, J. (2001, September 28). *AP photographer stands by his work.* Retrieved October 2, 2001, from http://9news.com/newsroom/13294.html

Wetter, M. W., & Corrigan, S. K. (1995). Providing information to clients about psychological tests: A survey of attorneys' and law students' attitudes. *Professional Psychology: Research and Practice, 26,* 474–477.

Williams, L. M. (1994). Recall of childhood trauma: A prospective study of women's memories of child sexual abuse. *Journal of Consulting and Clinical Psychology, 62,* 1167–1176.

Wood, J. M., Nezworski, M. T., Lilienfeld, S. O., & Garb, H. N. (2003). *What's wrong with the Rorschach?* San Francisco: Jossey-Bass.

Yehuda, R., & McFarlane, A. C. (1995). Conflict between current knowledge about posttraumatic stress disorder and its original conceptual basis. *American Journal of Psychiatry, 152,* 1705–1711.

Yehuda, R., & McFarlane, A. C. (1997). Psychobiology of Posttraumatic Stress Disorder: *Annals of the New York Academy of Sciences, 821,* 556–566.

Yehuda, R., Southwick, S. M., Giller, E. L., Ma, C., & Mason, J. W. (1992). Urinary catecholamine excretion and severity of PTSD symptoms in Vietnam combat veterans. *Journal of Nervous and Mental Disease, 180,* 321–325.

14

RORSCHACH ASSESSMENT IN TORT AND EMPLOYMENT LITIGATION

Bruce L. Smith
University of California, Berkley

Among the most complex and challenging areas for the forensic psychologist are personal injury—or tort—and employment litigation. According to the classic text, *Prosser and Keeton on Torts* (Keeton et al., 1984), there is no single definition of a *tort*. In general, torts may be defined as those civil wrongs that are not breaches of contract. In general, these do not violate criminal law, although there are exceptions.[1] In addition, for an act to be considered a tort, it must create *injury*, which is defined as harm to an individual's interest or property. Included among these are personal injuries resulting from motor vehicle accidents or from negligent maintenance of property, defamation, alienation of affection, and so on. The term *tort* is derived from the Latin *tortus*, which means "twisted," as well as from the medieval French "tort," meaning "wrong." Interestingly, *tortus* is also the root of the modern word "torture." Torts are a creation of common law. For the most part, our tort law derives from English common law of the 19th century (Keeton et al., 1984). Individuals are held to have a responsibility not to harm others or their interests either through malfeasance or negligence.

TYPES OF TORT LITIGATION

Today, there are many different kinds of tort claims and tort litigation. In fact, this is one of the reasons that it has been so difficult to define a single "law of torts." In many of these, however, psychological issues are frequently an important aspect. Broadly speaking, torts can be divided into two categories, *intentional* and *negligent*. Intentional torts are those such as intentional infliction of emotional harm in which the tortfeasor intends to cause harm to the defendant (Koch et al., 2006). Many—but by no means all—of these are criminal acts such as assault, battery, or false imprisonment. Others, such as willful slander, libel, "insult and indignity," or malicious practical jokes, are not criminally sanctioned, but nonetheless are classed as intentional torts (Keeton et al., 1984). Interestingly,

---

[1]In some instances, a single act may be punishable by criminal law and damages recovered under tort law. The O. J. Simpson cases are such an example.

intentional torts, and in particular those that derive from criminal behavior, are among the few kinds of tort litigation in which the defendant's state of mind is at issue and, thus, the defendant may be subject to psychological examination. In order to prove intent, it is necessary to prove that defendants knew—or should have known—the consequences of their actions and that they intended those consequences to occur.

Negligent torts arise out the defendant's duty to the plaintiff. In order to prove a negligent tort, the plaintiff must prove four elements: "a duty or obligation to protect others from foreseeable risks; a failure on the defendant's part to discharge this duty; a reasonably close causal connection between the defendant's conduct and the injury sustained by plaintiff; and actual loss or damage to the interests of the plaintiff" (Keeton et al., 1984, pp. 164–165).

In order to evaluate the first element, courts have generally applied the "reasonable person" standard; that is, would the reasonable person "standing in the defendant's shoes" have foreseen the risk. Just who constitutes a "reasonable person" depends on the nature of the alleged tort. In medical malpractice cases, for example, it would be another physician within the same specialty; in the case of a motor vehicle accident, it would be another driver.

In evaluating the third element, the courts typically rely on what is known as the "reasonably constituted person" or "reasonable person of ordinary sensibilities" (Keeton et al., 1984, p. 63). That is, the conduct must be such that it would injure an ordinary person. For example, a plaintiff who claims to suffer emotional distress because she overheard the defendant utter a mild expletive in public would not be able to recover damages, because such an event would not be expected to be harmful to an ordinary person. The exception to this is if the defendant knew in advance that the plaintiff had some particular disability that would render him peculiarly vulnerable; for example, intentionally jostling a man on crutches would likely be treated differently by the courts than doing the same to one without any visible disability.

The most common form of negligent tort is probably that arising out of an automobile accident, in which it is alleged that the negligent actions of one driver injured another driver or a pedestrian. In this instance, operators of motor vehicles are presumed to have a duty to the public to exercise reasonable caution to avoid collisions. Other forms of personal injury also give rise to tort actions, such as "slip and fall" cases, in which it is alleged that the defendant maintained an unsafe property, cases involving product liability, and defective equipment. In all of these instances, the common thread is that there was a breach in the defendant's duty to protect the plaintiff, and the latter suffered harm as a consequence.

Another common kind of negligent tort is malpractice, in which a professional offering a service falls below a "standard of care" (Diamond et al., 2000, p. 105). Although medical malpractice is by far the most common form of malpractice litigation, malpractice suits have also been brought against dentists, psychologists, attorneys, accountants, and so forth.

RELATIONSHIP OF EMPLOYMENT LITIGATION TO TORTS

Many forms of employment litigation are also torts. *Wrongful termination* or *wrongful discharge* is one of the most common torts in which psychological damages may be alleged. Wrongful discharge occurs when employees are terminated in such a way that violates their contract, public policy, or constitutes a breach of faith and fair dealing (Kerley, 2002, p. 113). Wrongful discharges based on a breach of contract occur when the termination of employment is found to be in violation of the employee's stated contract with the employer. States vary as to whether or not they allow claims for psychological harm ("mental anguish") in such claims (Kerley, 2002, p. 114). Wrongful discharge in violation of public policy occurs when the discharge is contrary to "public policy," although there is considerable disagreement among jurisdictions as to what constitutes public policy. In general, discrimination on the basis of race, gender, disability, or age is included, as are terminations for filing a workers' compensation claim (or union grievance), for "whistle-blowing" (i.e., reporting illegal activity to law enforcement), performing a civic duty such as jury service or honoring a subpoena, and refusing to perform illegal, unethical, or unsafe activities on behalf of the employer (Kerley, 2002, p. 116).[2]

A special class of wrongful discharge is *constructive discharge*, in which the employer makes working conditions so intolerable that the employee feels compelled to resign. Most jurisdictions utilize a "reasonable person" standard (i.e., would a reasonable person presented with the same conditions also resign); a minority requires the plaintiff to prove that the employer *deliberately* made the conditions intolerable (Kerley, 2002, p. 124). Among the actions that courts have found to be sufficient to justify a constructive discharge claim are demotion (*Stephens v. C.I.T. Group/Equipment Financing,* 1992), reassignment to menial work (*Wilson v. Monarch Paper*, 1991), or harassment (*Guthrie v. J.C. Penney*, 1986).

Wrongful discharge and constructive discharge actions may also include a claim for *intentional infliction of emotional distress* in which it is alleged that the discharge was carried out in a manner that was extremely abusive, degrading, or humiliating (Kerley, 2002, p. 130).[3] In order to prevail in such a claim the employee must prove both that the actions of the employer exceeded all bounds of decency and that the employee suffered genuine harm.

Example

Ms. A, a management employee for a moderate-sized retail firm had her job title reclassified from "Human Resources Director" to "Manager" on the recommendation of an outside consultant retained by the company to help them avoid going into bankruptcy. The move, like several other re-classifications, was justified on the basis of the fact that she managed only one other employee, and the consultant felt that the company was top heavy in senior management. Neither Ms. A's salary nor her job description changed as a result of this re-classification, although future salary increases would have been affected. Ms. A felt humiliated by this and, after a few months, resigned. She subsequently sued for

---

[2]Technically, some of these, such as discrimination on the basis of disability or discharge for being a whistle-blower may not be classed as torts, per se, as they are part of statutory rather than common law. Practically, however, this distinction has little bearing on the work of the forensic psychologist.

[3]Not all states recognize this cause of action, and some only provide compensation under workers' compensation statues.

constructive termination. A psychological evaluation (including the Rorschach) conducted as part of the litigation documented severe depression, characterized by loss of self-esteem, feelings of worthlessness, and a sense of profound loss. It was opined that in large measure this depression was a reaction to her reclassification and subsequent resignation. Nonetheless, her suit failed on summary judgment, because she was unable to demonstrate that a reasonable person would have found the change in her working conditions constituted a valid reason for resignation.

Discrimination and harassment in employment are closely related issues. Title VII of the 1964 Civil Rights Act prohibits discrimination in employment on the basis of race, color, religion, gender, or national origin (Kerley, 2002, pp. 53–54). The Age Discrimination in Employment Act (ADEA) added discrimination on the basis of age to the list of prohibitions in 1967 (Kerley, 2002, p. 200), and discrimination on the basis of disability was added by the Americans with Disabilities Act (ADA) of 1990. These laws prohibit "disparate treatment" on the basis of race, color, religion, sex, national origin, age or disability. Employees may bring a suit if they feel they have been subjected to such treatment on the basis of their membership in a "protected class" (i.e., one of the previous enumerated groups). Interestingly, unlike most other kinds of tort litigation, in which the burden of proof lies with the plaintiff, discrimination suits are subject to a "shifting" burden of proof in which the plaintiff first must establish a *prima facie* case of discrimination (i.e., an adverse event); the defendant must next attempt to establish a legitimate nondiscriminatory reason for the action; the burden then shifts back to the plaintiff to prove that the defendant's rationale is just a pretext (*McDonnell Douglas v. Green*, 1973).

Harassment is considered a form of discrimination and is defined as behavior that is offensive, hostile, or threatening and is based on the victim's membership in a protected class. Sexual harassment is the most commonly encountered form of harassment; Title VII recognizes three categories of sexual harassment: *quid pro quo*, in which employment decisions (e.g., hiring, promotion, etc.) are conditional on submission to unwelcome sexual advances; *hostile work environment*, in which conduct has the purpose or consequence of interfering with an employee's performance by creating a hostile or offensive work environment; or *retaliation*, in which an adverse employment decision (e.g., termination) is made in retaliation for having complained of harassment (Kerley, 2002, pp. 279–284). Employees may bring claims of harassment on bases other than sex or gender. Employees who are taunted, threatened, or otherwise abused on the basis of their race or national origin, age, disability, or "affinity orientation" (the current preferred term for sexual orientation) may have claims for harassment as well.

Example

Ms. B was a mid-level college administrator in her middle fifties. After several years on the job, a reorganization of her department left her with a supervisor 30 years her junior. The supervisor, Ms. C, was uncomfortable with Ms. B's greater level of experience and began to make disparaging remarks about her based primarily on her age. She would remark to others in the office, for example, "people over 50 just bring an office down." When the departmental Christmas party was planned, she said to Ms. B in a public place,

"You should go with X from accounting, he's the only other old fart around here." When Ms. B complained about this behavior to the departmental head, no action was taken, but soon thereafter, she was told that her job was being eliminated and that she was welcome to apply for a lesser position that would replace it. When she refused, she was terminated; shortly thereafter, a replacement was hired who performed essentially the same functions, albeit with a different title. She then sued for age discrimination, alleging harassment and retaliation. When evaluated psychologically, she was found to manifest severe anxiety and depression that could be traced to her experiences at work. Her suit was successful and she won a sizeable award, including damages for emotional distress.

This case illustrates one other important factor in harassment cases, the fact that although the harasser was the plaintiff's immediate supervisor, the employer (in this case the college) was liable under the doctrine of *respondeat superior* (literally: "the master answers"). In this situation, employers are responsible if it can be proven that they knew of the harassment (e.g., because the plaintiff complained) or should have known (if the behavior was pervasive) and failed to prevent it (*Vance v. Southern Bell,* 1989) .

PSYCHOLOGICAL ISSUES IN TORT AND EMPLOYMENT CASES

Psychological evaluations are called for in tort litigation when the plaintiff claims emotional injury as a result of the tortuous act. Koch et al. (2006, p. 25) note that most claims for psychological injury arise in negligent torts. Thus, for example, if plaintiffs claim posttraumatic stress as a result of a serious automobile accident, they have put their emotional state at issue. A psychologist may be brought in by either or both parties to evaluate the plaintiff's psychological condition and render an opinion concerning whether or not that individual is suffering emotional damage and whether or not it is due to the alleged tort.

The concept of psychological or emotional harm was not initially part of tort law as a separate cause of action, and damages for emotional injury could usually only be recovered if they were incidental to physical injury (Diamond et al., 2000, p. 162). Interestingly, Koch et al. (2006) notes that awareness of emotional or psychological injury appears to be a consequence of the advent of rail travel, as frequent railroad accidents led to symptoms that we would recognize today as posttraumatic stress disorder. At that time, they were often referred to as "railway spine," because it was presumed that jarring of the spine was responsible for the psychological symptoms. Gradually, over the years, the recognition of emotional distress as a "free-standing" damage has grown (Diamond et al., 2000, p. 162), albeit only in fits and starts. Currently, states differ as to the requirements for recovery for emotional distress in personal injury cases. Some still hold to the narrowest requirement, called the "impact rule," in which there can only be recovery for emotional distress if there is some direct physical impact, even if the impact itself does not cause injury.[4] More commonly, states have adopted one of the broader rules, typically the "zone of danger rule," in which plaintiffs can claim emotional distress if they are in

---

[4]This rule was articulated in a somewhat amusing case, *Christie Brothers Circus v. Turnage* (1928), in which a prominent businessman claimed emotional distress from the public humiliation that occurred when a circus horse had a large bowel movement in his lap during a performance. The court ruled that the contact with the feces constituted sufficient "impact."

close enough proximity to have been in danger of physical injury, or the "bystander rule," in which a witness to a serious injury can recover if they have a significant relationship to the victim (e.g., a parent witnessing the violent death of a child). Finally, a few states, notably California, have de-coupled emotional and physical distress and have substituted a "normally constituted person" standard in which emotional distress can be claimed if a normally constituted person would be unable to cope with the circumstances of the case (*Molien v. Kaiser Foundation Hospitals*, 1980).

TWO ISSUES: LIABILITY AND DAMAGES

Although, as described previously, there is a complex set of elements that need to be established in tort or employment litigation, it is convenient for the forensic psychologist to think of two broad sets of issues: *liability* and *damages*. Liability refers to those issues that determine whether or not the defendant is responsible for the injury suffered by the plaintiff. Essentially, in order to prevail, the plaintiff must prove either that the defendant engaged in willful, extreme, or outrageous conduct toward the plaintiffs (i.e., intentional tort) or breached a duty toward them (negligent tort). In the words of Prosser, "liability must be based upon conduct that is socially unreasonable" (Keeton et al., 1984, p. 6). Damages refers to the question of whether or not the plaintiff suffered loss or injury as a result of the defendant's actions as well as the appropriate monetary compensation. If no harm befell the plaintiff, then there can be no tort. For example, if a defendant runs a red light or maintains an unsafe staircase, then there is no tort if no one is injured as a result of his actions.

When retained to conduct an evaluation as part of tort or employment litigation, it is imperative that the psychologist determine in advance precisely what issues are to be addressed. Most commonly, a psychological evaluation is requested in order to address the issue of damages (i.e., was the defendant emotionally or psychologically harmed as a result of the alleged actions of the defendant). Under such circumstances, it is not necessary for the psychologist to be concerned with whether or not the defendant behaved wrongly (e.g., whether or not termination of employment was wrongful or whether or not defendant could have avoided an accident). It is, however, necessary to determine whether or not the emotional distress is a result of the accident or harassment or termination—tortuous or otherwise. Often, this can be an extremely difficult determination to make, and it is here that Rorschach testing can often be quite important.

Example

Mr. C, an openly gay man, was a driver for a large company when he was terminated while out on temporary disability for a foot injury. Mr. C long suspected that his employer had wanted to get rid of him because of his sexual orientation; this was during a time when the AIDS epidemic was peaking, and many employers were leery of gay male employees because they feared the added cost of medical and disability insurance. As a result of the loss of his job, Mr. C became despondent and his health began to suffer. Some months later, he was diagnosed with AIDS. Mr. C's termination was clearly in violation of state employment law, and he sued for damages, claiming among other things that he suffered extreme emotional distress as a consequence. The defendant's employer claimed that Mr. C's emotional distress was primarily a reaction to learning of his AIDS diagnosis, not the loss of his job. A comprehensive psychological evaluation, however, demonstrated that in this case, the loss of his job was far more traumatic than the medical diagnosis for Mr. C. In particular, the Rorschach showed that he was a primitively narcissistic man whose self-esteem was very fragile. Furthermore, he was prone to overidentify with admired powerful men (in this case, the president of the company). Being terminated from his job was a crushing blow to his self-esteem that was far more devastating than even the diagnosis of AIDS. The jury awarded him damages in the high six figures.

Sometimes, however, the psychologist may be called on to opine about some aspect of liability. In the case of psychological malpractice, for example, a psychological expert will be called on to testify to the standard of practice. A psychological evaluation of the plaintiff may even be a part of such an evaluation in rare instances.

Example

Ms. D was evaluated by Dr. E, a psychologist who gave a full battery of tests. As a result of this evaluation, it was recommended that Ms. D go off of all psychotropic medication and terminate psychotherapy. Shortly after this, Ms. D, who had previously been diagnosed with bipolar disorder, suffered a full-blown manic episode and needed to be hospitalized. Dr. E's testing was so poorly conducted that another assessment was required. This assessment clearly supported the diagnosis of bipolar disorder, and the expert opined that a competent assessment in the first place could not have failed to reveal this and that Dr. E's recommendations were totally unsupportable.

In employment cases, whereas the defendants need only prove that they did not breach a duty to the plaintiff (i.e., did not terminate the plaintiff wrongfully and did not engage in discriminatory behavior), there are times when a psychologist may be called in to evaluate the plaintiff in order to help "tell a story" to the jury, that is, to aid the jury in understanding why the plaintiff might have misperceived the defendants' actions. Although not strictly necessary from a legal standpoint, such evidence may be useful in helping a jury better understand the facts of the case from a defendant's perspective.

Example

Ms. F was a clerical employee in a medium-sized firm who sued her employer for sexual harassment, claiming that her immediate supervisor created a hostile workplace and the company refused to do anything about it. She cited the following acts on the part of her supervisor as evidence: On two occasions, when leaning over her desk to peruse a document he touched her shoulder with his abdomen, and on several occasions she overheard him referring to her and her co-workers as "girls." She acknowledged that this was the entirety of her complaint. She contended that as a result of this "harassment" she had lost all interest in sexual relations with her husband, had developed severe anxiety and insomnia, and could no longer work for that firm. Psychological assessment revealed a very brittle woman who was prone to overinterpret her environment and to misperceive the behavior of others. (Among the Rorschach data that supported these conclusions were a positive *Hypervigilance Index*, a high $X–\%$, the presence of several $M–$ responses, and a positive *Coping Deficit Index*.) These conclusions were useful in explaining to the jury both why she might be so outraged by behavior that a "reasonable woman" might find trivial and why she might claim to be traumatized by the experience. Her suit was rejected.

In assessing whether or not a plaintiff's injury was the result of the alleged tort or wrongful employment action, psychologists need to be aware of the issues involved in determining causation in a legal context. The law distinguishes between "cause in fact" (also called percipient cause) and proximate cause; the former refers to the events that precipitated the injury, whereas the latter is a legal term that refers to what actions or events are legally responsible for the loss or injury (Keeton et al., 1984, p. 263). In general, courts utilize the "but for" rule; that is, in order for the defendant to be liable for the plaintiff's injuries, it must be determined that they would not have occurred but for the actions of defendant (Keeton et al., 1984, p. 266). Of course, in the case of psychological injury, this can be an immensely difficult determination, because it is often difficult to identify a single cause of a psychological disorder.

Further complicating the picture is the concept of contributory negligence. This refers to the fact that the plaintiff's actions may have contributed to his injury (Diamond et al., 2002, p. 259). Plaintiffs, like defendants, are held to an "objective" standard (i.e., what would a reasonable person do). If, for example, driver A is speeding, and pedestrian B crosses the street against the traffic light, then A's negligence contributed to his being struck. States vary in how they treat contributory negligence. A few states use a "pure comparative negligence" standard, in which the plaintiffs can recover a percentage of their damages equal to the percentage of liability the defendant is found to have. Most use a modified comparative negligence standard. In this standard, the defendant must be found to be at least 50% at fault (or more than 50%) in order for plaintiff to recover. One state, South Dakota, bars recovery if the plaintiff is at all negligent, unless the negligence is "slight" (Diamond et al., p. 264).

In addition to the aforementioned, plaintiffs have a responsibility to mitigate or limit loss or injury. This is sometimes referred to as the "doctrine of avoidable consequences" (Diamond, 2002, p. 248). For example, if a plaintiff who suffers PTSD as a result of an injury refuses to seek treatment, the defendant will not be held liable for that portion of the loss that might have been avoided with treatment. The psychologist who performs an evaluation of the plaintiff is likely to be asked to opine about the appropriate course of treatment as well as the likely impact of such therapy.

In determining whether a plaintiff's distress is the consequence of the alleged tort or wrongful employment action, the psychologist must be especially concerned with two concepts: preexisting conditions and the "egg-shell plaintiff." As mentioned earlier, in determining if an injury is compensable, courts use the standard of the "reasonably constituted person." Emotional distress or psychological injury is only compensable if the events would have caused such injury in the reasonably constituted person or person of "average sensibilities." In addition, a psychological injury must include some measurable decrement in some aspect of psychological functioning; mere upset at having lost a job, for instance, is insufficient. It is also important to note that distress caused by the litigation itself is not recoverable, because lawsuits are entered into voluntarily. Thus, the psychologist must attempt to partial out symptoms that are occasioned by legal procedures (e.g., depositions) and those that are the result of the original events themselves.

Preexisting Conditions

The term *preexisting conditions* refers to those deficits in functioning that predated the tortuous events and can serve as an affirmative defense against damage claims. The plaintiffs are only entitled to recover for damages that are a consequence of the tortuous behavior and only sufficiently to render them "whole," that is, return them to the state of health prior to the injury. In the case of emotional damages, it is often a challenge to differentiate between a preexisting condition (e.g., chronic depression) and an exacerbation caused by the defendant's actions. It is necessary to pay careful attention to evidence—especially from collateral sources—of the plaintiff's condition at the time of the events at issue, as well as psychological test data that provide information about long-standing personality characteristics versus current mental state.

Egg-Shell Plaintiff

Whereas courts have held that adverse consequences need to be foreseeable (i.e., would harm the "reasonably constituted person"), the extent of injury need not be foreseeable. Thus, for example, if a Halloween prank that might be expected to cause some degree of distress in an average individual provokes a fatal heart attack in a victim with a serious cardiac condition, the joker would be liable for wrongful death; it is this person's bad luck for choosing the wrong victim. The term *egg-shell plaintiff* or *egg-shell skull* first made its appearance in a British case around the turn of the last century . The term refers to the idea that if a blow to the head that might cause a bruise to most victims crushes the skull of the plaintiff, then the defendant is liable for the crushed skull (*Delieu v. White*, 1901). It is based on the notion that the defendant "takes the plaintiff as he finds him" (Diamond et al., p. 221). This concept was extended to the psychological realm in *Steinhauser v. Hertz Corp* (1970), in which the court held that a teenage girl with a fragile psyche could recover when a slight automobile accident precipitated a schizophrenic break, and in *Malcom v. Broadhurst* (1970), in which the court stated that there was no difference between an egg-shell skull and an egg-shell psyche. As can be seen, differentiating between an egg-shell plaintiff and a preexisting condition can be a real challenge to the forensic psychologist. Only a very careful analysis of the plaintiff's level of functioning pre-injury as well as the particular circumstances can enable the psychologist to make such a distinction.

Example

Ms. G, an employee of a public agency, sued for sexual and racial harassment. She alleged that she was subjected to a barrage of insulting remarks about her race and her gender as well as her physical appearance. In addition, she was ostracized by the other employees and singled out for this kind of treatment. She further alleged that her supervisors did nothing to stop the harassment; rather, they responded by further isolating her by moving her workstation. She claimed severe emotional distress as a result of these events, including panic attacks, insomnia, and depression. A psychological evaluation performed on Ms. G confirmed her account of the degree of her distress and further revealed that her history left her particularly vulnerable to the experience of ostracism. When she was an early adolescent, her mother was killed in an automobile accident, and she, alone of her 9 siblings, was sent to another state to live with an aunt and her family. There she was treated as a kind of interloper, tolerated but never included. As a consequence, her experience of ostracism at the hands of her coworkers was a re-traumatization.

It should be noted in passing that it is important when reporting on the results of such evaluations—whether in a written report or testimony—to make certain to use language that respects the fact that the issue of the defendant's liability remains to be decided. Thus, phrases such as "Mr. X's termination," or "the events at XYZ Company" should be substituted for "Mr. X's wrongful termination" or "defendant's harassment of Mr. X."

USE OF THE RORSCHACH IN TORT CASES

Assessments in tort or employment cases can be very complex. Psychologists must not only determine the nature of the plaintiff's state of mind and assess any possible emotional damage, they must also be able to assess whether or not the damage is related to the alleged tortuous action. As with any forensic evaluation, multiple sources of data are necessary in tort and employment assessments. It is useful to think of evaluations as involving three distinct data sources: collateral information, clinical interview, and psychological testing. The plaintiff's statements can be checked against the documentary record or the statements of others involved in the case. In addition, inferences drawn from psychological testing can serve as a check on the impressions drawn from interviews. As with any forensic evaluation, the psychologist needs to maintain a high "index of suspicion," as the plaintiffs are motivated by financial considerations to present themselves in a particular way. As a consequence, conclusions that are drawn should be supported by multiple sources of information.

For several reasons, the Rorschach is particularly useful in these types of evaluations. Unlike self-report inventories such as the Minnesota Multiphasic Personality Inventory–2 (MMPI–2; Butcher et al., 2001), the Millon Clinical Multiaxial Inventory–III (MCMI–III; T. C. Millon et al., 1994), or the Trauma Symptom Inventory (TSI; Briere 1995), all of which are useful, it is less subject to conscious manipulation (Ganellen, 1994; Ganellen et al., 1996; Ganellen, chap. 5, this vol.) It is not uncommon to have MMPI–2 or MCMI–III protocols of questionable validity in a battery of tests administered to a plaintiff in litigation. Secondly, such inventories are "snapshots" that give a picture of the plaintiff's functioning at the time of testing—often months or even years after the events in question—and may not shed adequate light on the plaintiff's enduring personality configuration. This is especially useful when trying to differentiate between preexisting conditions and specific vulnerabilities that might predispose a plaintiff to have a particular kind of reaction to an injury (i.e., an egg-shell plaintiff). In particular, the fact that the Comprehensive System (Exner, 1993) contains both scores that are resistant to change and, thus, reflect enduring personality characteristics and those that are sensitive to current emotional state such as *Adjusted D*, *m* (*Inanimate Movement*), and *Y* (*Diffuse Shading*) renders it especially useful for evaluating possible differences between current functioning and baseline. Finally, although as Weiner (chap. 6, this vol.) points out, inferences derived from a qualitative analysis of content are typically to be avoided in forensic evaluations, a judicious use of such interpretations can bolster conclusions that are supported by other data. For example, if subjects have numerous Rorschach responses of weak, helpless, or damaged humans or animals, and this is supported by a Structural Summary that includes several *Morbid* responses, *a:p* (*Active Movement to Passive Movement*) in the passive direction and an elevated *FM+m*, there is support for the interpretation that they are experiencing helplessness and a sense of having been beaten down. This would bolster a conclusion that the subject's current distress is a result of a sense of having been unfairly treated in the work setting.

General evidentiary considerations in the use of the Rorschach in forensic settings have been amply discussed already (see McCann & Evans, chap. 3; Meloy, chap. 4; and Weiner, chap. 6, this vol.), and no purpose would be served repeating these arguments. There are, however, specific considerations in the use of the method in tort and employment cases that need to be mentioned. As with any test, the Rorschach is only appropriate—and testimony about it admissible—to the extent that it us used appropriately. Most importantly, this means that it should be used to address appropriate questions.

Example

A psychologist administered the Rorschach to a Ms. H, plaintiff who was alleging racial harassment in the workplace. Based on a very high *Lambda*, a low *R* and a positive *HVI*, he concluded that she was defensive and paranoid, that she must have misperceived events at work, and therefore her claims of harassment were unfounded. His testimony was rightly excluded. The Rorschach cannot and should not be used to opine about what may or may not have occurred at some point in the past.

In particular, psychologists who use the Rorschach in employment cases may find themselves needing to defend the specific relevance of the method. A common tactic of opposing counsel is to ask whether there are any studies addressing the use of the Rorschach in evaluating individuals who are claiming constructive termination, or harassment based on age, or some other claim specific to the case. Of course, the answer to this question is likely to be no, but this should not be relevant. Rule 702 of the Federal Rules of Evidence (FRE) holds that scientific evidence is admissible if it "will assist the trier of fact to understand the evidence or determine a fact in issue ..." (Rothstein et al., 2003, p. 633). This was further reinforced in the *Daubert* case (1993), in which the Court held that scientific testimony should "fit" *some question* to be resolved in the case . Thus, the proper answer to the previous question is: "No, I am not aware of such studies; however, I am not using the Rorschach to determine whether or not the plaintiff was harassed (or wrongly terminated, etc.); I am using it to help determine whether or not s/he is currently suffering emotional distress as well as to assess his/her pre-morbid personality structure. There is a wealth of research supporting the use of the test for these purposes."

CASE EXAMPLE

Background

The following case illustrates the complexity of forensic evaluation in employment litigation as well as the role of the Rorschach in these evaluations. Mr. J was a middle-aged project manager for a medium-sized manufacturing company who discovered what he felt were some financial irregularities in the reports of his division's performance. When he brought these to the attention of his immediate supervisor, he was told not to pursue the matter further. Fearing that important information was being withheld from the company leadership, he attempted to communicate directly with the CEO and CFO of the firm, only to be ordered not to contact any higher level employee other than his supervisor. He later learned that the company was in merger discussions with another firm. The day the merger was announced, Mr. J was terminated from his job, being told only that it was "in the best interests of all concerned." Mr. J, who had been with the firm for about 1 year and had been earning a six-figure salary, sued in federal court for wrongful discharge, alleging that he was fired in retaliation for being a "whistle-blower." In addition to claiming loss of wages and other economic damages, Mr. J claimed "mental anguish" and emotional injury as a result of having lost his job. For their part, the defendant corporation denied the allegations, maintaining instead that Mr. J was terminated for just cause.

Mr. J was evaluated by psychological and psychiatric experts retained by both defense and plaintiff. At the time of the evaluations, the case had been going on for approximately 2 years, and he had been unemployed for that entire period. At issue were the following:

1. What was Mr. J's current psychological state, and was there evidence for emotional distress?
2. Was there evidence that Mr. J's current level of functioning and any deficits were secondary to the termination of his employment?
3. Alternatively, was there a preexisting condition that might better account for any current distress or deficit?

As is often the case, this litigation produced mountains of documents that the experts needed to review. In addition to depositions of the plaintiff and key witnesses, there were medical records dating back approximately 20 years and copies of e-mails between the plaintiff and various officials within the company. In addition to reviewing the documents, the psychiatrist retained by the defendant interviewed Mr. J for approximately 7 hours. He then produced a report in excess of 60 pages. The psychologist retained by the plaintiff met with Mr. J for approximately 8 hours during which time he interviewed him and administered the Rorschach. In addition, Mr. J completed the MMPI–2.

History

This was an extremely complicated case. Mr. J had a long history of psychiatric difficulties dating back to childhood. He admitted that he had severe anxiety attacks as a child and an episode of severe depression when he was 16. This latter was severe enough that he was taken to his pediatrician for evaluation, but no further treatment eventuated. Beginning in his 20s, he began to experience anxiety and occasional panic attacks that he assumed had a physiological basis. As a consequence, he presented at emergency rooms, fearing a heart attack. It wasn't until he was in his 40s that these episodes were correctly diagnosed. Meanwhile, he reported several depressions over the years, all of which were precipitated either by the loss of a job or the break-up of a serious romantic relationship. About 2 years prior to loss of his job, he was hospitalized involuntarily for suicidal threats; this admission lasted only 2 days, and he was released into the care of his psychiatrist at the time. Mr. J also readily admitted abusing alcohol. He stated that he began heavy drinking in his late 20s and has had periods of sobriety alternating with periods of abuse ever since. He also had one brief stay in a residential program for alcohol abuse. Over the years, he had variously been diagnosed with bipolar disorder, panic disorder, posttraumatic stress disorder, major depression, and alcohol abuse and dependence.

Mr. J reported at the time of the evaluation severe depression and anxiety. He was being maintained on both anxiolytic and antidepressant medication, although both of these were being managed by his primary care physician, not a psychiatrist. He was not in psychotherapy at the time. He stated that he had lost interest in most of his favorite activities: going to movies, eating at restaurants, gardening, even walking his dog. He also reported a marked diminution of libido; prior to the termination of his employment, he and his wife had maintained an active sex life; at the time of the evaluation, they had not engaged in sexual activity in several months.

Mr. J had a very troubled early history. Both of his parents were alcoholics and, by his account, abusive. They divorced when he was 14, and his mother re-married to another abusive alcoholic. In addition to physical abuse, Mr. J was constantly told that he was worthless and a failure. There was little support for education in his family, and he began working full-time upon graduating from high school. Over the years, he managed to attain an A.A. degree from various community colleges, but never completed university. He held a series of jobs in the manufacturing sector, each more responsible than its predecessor and, although he did lose a couple of them either through reorganization or conflict with superiors, he always received excellent performance reviews. By the time he was hired by the defendant corporation, he had held several highly responsible management positions and was earning a substantial salary.

Evaluations

The defense psychiatrist diagnosed Mr. J with a rapid-cycling Bipolar II Disorder as well as an Anxiety Disorder and Alcohol Dependence. On Axis II he suggested "avoidant and passive-aggressive traits." It was his opinion that Mr. J's symptoms were probably a result of the "natural progression" of his illness, although he did not completely rule out the possibility that his termination might have exacerbated his condition. He also opined that "it was medically probable" that Mr. J was sending too many e-mails to his superiors in the days leading up to his dismissal. He further opined that Mr. J's supervisor was "medically probably" responding appropriately to Mr. J's behavior, although he never interviewed her. These latter opinions led the court to rule most of the psychiatrist's report inadmissible, as he had gone beyond the scope of his examination. This illustrates the importance of the forensic examiner being clear on the nature of the issues to which the evaluation should be addressed.

By contrast, the plaintiff's psychologist stated that although a bipolar diagnosis could not be ruled out, it seemed somewhat less likely than a diagnosis of Major Depression as there was little evidence in either Mr. J's account or the medical records of manic episodes. Furthermore, the fact that Mr. J's periods of sobriety did not precipitate mania—as is common with patients who are self-medicating a bipolar illness with alcohol—was further evidence against a primary diagnosis of bipolar disorder.

The psychological testing—especially the Rorschach—was particularly crucial in understanding this case. The results of the MMPI–2 suggested moderate to severe subjective distress. Remarkably, despite the nature of the litigation, Mr. J's profile was not elevated on any of the validity scales; rather, he produced a profile that suggested honest reporting. The clinical scales were broadly elevated, with the highest elevations on Scales 3, 6, and 8. Analysis of the Harris–Lingoes subscales as well as the Content and Supplementary scales suggested acute distress marked by dysphoria, hopelessness, and fearfulness. He tested as someone who had difficulty handling even minor stresses at present. In addition, there was evidence that his anxiety could be understood in large measure as related to traumatic stress.

Role of the Rorschach

What is the role of the Rorschach in a case such as this? This is a case of incredible psychological complexity, and a data source from which inferences can be drawn both about current functioning and enduring structure is invaluable. As can be seen from the Structural Summary (Appendix), Mr. J produced a protocol that was valid for interpretation, although the *Lambda* of .20 suggests that his defenses are currently overwhelmed. The first finding that bears on the forensic questions in this case is the *D* of –3 and *Adjusted D* of –1. These data suggest that whereas his psychological resources may in general be limited, at present he is in a state of acute overload. Furthermore, it is likely that much of this stress is situational. Despite the concerns about a possible psychotic disorder raised in the psychiatrist's report, the *PTI* is not elevated, and Mr. J's reality testing appears intact, judging from the *XA%* and *WDA%*. Furthermore, there are only 3 of the *Sum6 Special Scores*, only one of which is a Level 2. This is suggestive of some thought slippage, although it is not consistent with a pervasive thought disorder. Rather, it is more consistent with the notion that Mr. J may have occasional lapses in judgment when particular issues are triggered. Consistent with this is the fact that his only two fabulized combination responses as well as his only *FQ–* responses occur on the last two cards, suggesting that the representation of strong affect may be particularly disruptive to him, even though he did not necessarily respond to it by expressing strong emotions. A tentative interpretation of these data would be that his cognitive processes are particularly vulnerable to stress, and, although he may be able to function adequately under normal circumstances, he is easily overwhelmed by stress or strong emotional stimuli. Thus, the high level of conflict experienced around his job may have been especially disorganizing for him. On the other hand, the presence of two *M−* responses does suggest that he may have a tendency to misperceive the behavior of others. Whereas this finding might seem relevant to the issue of whether or not Mr. J misperceived the actions of his superiors in the workplace, the caution mentioned previously about not concluding from the Rorschach about actual past events points out the fallacy of such a conclusion.

As Weiner (1994) has noted, the Rorschach should not be used primarily as a diagnostic test. Nonetheless, a Rorschach protocol is likely to produce information that is consistent or inconsistent with a particular diagnosis. In this instance, there are several data points that point in a direction other than bipolar disorder. For one thing, there are no *m* responses. Frequently, bipolar patients, especially those in a more manic state, will produce many inanimate movement responses, because they are representing the experience of an "out of control" energy. Second, there are only two *Color* responses, and neither of these are pure *C*s, contraindicating affective flooding. Thirdly, although he produced six *Shading* responses, the bulk of them were scored *Y*, rather than *C'*. This is suggestive of the fact that he experiences negative affects more as anxiety than depression and that, in large measure, they may be situationally influenced. Finally, it is frequently the case that individuals with bipolar disorder produce *DR* responses, as their disordered thinking takes the form of a flight of ideas. Mr. J's protocol contained no responses scored *DR*. It should be noted that the extremely low *Lambda* is found frequently with bipolar patients, but it is also a common feature of other forms of psychological distress (e.g., PTSD) in which overwhelming turmoil is a prominent feature. It should be stressed, of course, that the absence of evidence is not the same as evidence for an absence; ruling out a bipolar disorder diagnosis on the basis of the Rorschach would be a serious interpretive error. On the other hand, it would be correct to state that the protocol does not provide any solid evidence supporting that diagnosis.

The other data that are particularly relevant to this case have to do with Mr. J's self-esteem regulation. His protocol contains two *FD* responses, a *Vista (FV)* and four *Morbid* responses. Taken together, these suggest that he is ruminates excessively over what he perceives as negative aspects of himself and that he views himself as damaged. Significantly, his first response on the Rorschach is scored for both *Vista* and *Morbid*, suggesting that this may be the most prominent aspect of his sense of self. Such a finding is consistent both with the presence of a serious depression, as well as a recent traumatic blow to his self-esteem. Although, as Weiner (chap. 6, this vol.) notes, conclusions drawn from the Rorschach in forensic cases should stress structural variables rather than content, a judicious use of some content may be relevant. In this case, it is noteworthy that all four of Mr. J's Morbid responses involve objects that have parts missing, described variously as "cut off," "stripped down," and "torn down." These images are consistent with his statements about himself, that he felt as if a vital part of himself had been taken away.

Conclusions

Based on the totality of the evidence, the plaintiff's psychologist concluded that Mr. J was suffering from severe depression and anxiety that was severely compromising his functioning at the time of the evaluation. It was also his opinion that the percipient cause of his symptoms was the loss of his job. The psychologist concluded that, for reasons that could be traced back to his childhood, Mr. J invested an inordinate amount of his self worth in his status as a successful manager and, when that status was taken from him, the result was traumatic. Although he felt that a pre-morbid diagnosis of panic disorder, recurrent major depression, and chronic PTSD was more likely than bipolar disorder, the psychologist felt that, even if the latter were accurate, it did not alter the conclusion that the exacerbation of Mr. J's symptoms was a direct result of losing his job. He also opined that intensive treatment over a substantial period of time was likely necessary to return him to his pre-morbid state of functioning.

That Mr. J was seriously troubled was never really in doubt. Both defense's and plaintiff's experts diagnosed major mental illnesses. What was at issue, however, was whether Mr. J's history of psychological disturbance constituted a preexisting condition or rendered him an "egg-shell plaintiff." The defense tried to make the case that a long-standing bipolar disorder made him the former, that his current state was the product of the "natural progression" of this disorder. By contrast, the plaintiff's psychologist concluded that, irrespective of the formal diagnosis, the fact was that Mr. J had been functioning adequately at the time of his termination and began to deteriorate only after losing his job. The degree to which he decompensated as a result of his termination was undoubtedly due to his fragile psyche, but it was nevertheless the termination itself that triggered his symptoms. In concluding this, he relied to a significant degree on the results of the Rorschach, which were far more consistent with this conclusion than with that of a chronic psychiatric condition.

Epilogue

In addition to arguing that the termination was justified and not retaliatory, the defense attempted to argue that Mr. J's distress was not the product of losing his job, but was a preexisting condition and, therefore, he was not entitled to compensation. The plaintiff, by contrast, maintained that the illegal termination of Mr. J's employment was directly responsible for his substantial psychological injuries. During the settlement conference, when the various experts' reports were presented in evidence, the defense's claim that as Mr. J suffered from a long-standing bipolar illness and had therefore not been psychologically damaged by his termination prompted the judge to reply, "Well, I suspect that would make him even more vulnerable, huh?" In the end, Mr. J won a substantial settlement, a portion of which went toward the intensive treatment that he so desperately needed.

CONCLUSIONS

Personal injury and employment litigation are among the most challenging arenas in which the forensic psychologist operates. The issues are varied and complex, but at the same time, endlessly fascinating. This chapter has attempted to highlight some of the issues of which the forensic examiner must be aware, as well as discuss the ways in which the Rorschach can be used in such examinations. It is my view that when used appropriately and with awareness of the various legal issues involved in these cases, the Rorschach can be invaluable in tort and employment litigation.

REFERENCES

Briere, J. (1995). *Trauma Symptom Inventory (TSI) professional manual.* Odessa, FL: Psychological Assessment Resources.

Butcher, J., Dahlstrom, W. D., Graham, J. R., Tellegen, A., & Kaemmer, B. (2001). *MMPI–2 manual for administration and scoring.* Minneapolis, MN: University of Minnesota Press.

Christie Brothers Circus v. Turnage, 144 S.E., Georgia Court of Appeals: 680 (1928).

Daubert v. Dow Pharmaceuticals, Inc., 509 U.S. 113, Supreme Court: 2786 (1993).

Diamond, J. L., Levine, L. C., & Madden, M. S. (2000). *Understanding torts.* New York: LexisNexis.

Dulieu v. White, 2 K.B.: 669 (1901).

Exner, J. E. (1993). *The Rorschach: A Comprehensive System: Vol. 1. Basic foundations* (3rd ed.). New York: Wiley.

Ganellen, R. J. (1994). Attempting to conceal psychological disturbance: MMPI defensive response sets and the Rorschach. *Journal of Personality Assessment, 63,* 423–437.

Ganellen, R. J., Wasyliw, O. E., Haywood, T. W., & Grossman, L. S. (1996). Can psychosis be malingered on the Rorschach? An empirical study. *Journal of Personality Assessment, 66,* 65–80.

Guthrie v. J.C. Penney Co., Inc., 803 F.2nd, 5th Circuit: 1138, 1145 (1986).

Keeton, W. P., Dobbs, D. B., Keeton, R. E., & Owen, D. G. (Eds.). (1984). *Prosser and Keaton on torts.* St. Paul, MN: West Publishing.

Kerley, P. (2002). *Employment law for the paralegal.* New York: West Legal Studies.

Koch, W. J., Douglas, K. S., Nicholls, T. L., & O'Neill, M. L. (2006). *Psychological injuries: Forensic assessment, treatment, and law.* Oxford, England: Oxford University Press.

McDonnell Douglas Corp. v. Green, 411, U.S. 792 (1973).

Millon, T., Millon, C., & Davis, R. (1994). *Millon Clinical Multiaxial Inventory–III.* Minneapolis, MN, National Computer Systems.

Molien v. Kaiser Foundation Hospital, 27 Cal. 3rd, California Supreme Court: 819 (1980).

Rothstein, P. F., Raeder, M. S., & Crump, D. (2003). *Evidence in a nutshell.* St. Paul, MN: Thomson West.

Steinhauser v. Hertz Corp., 421 F.2nd, 2nd Circuit: 1169 (1970).

Stephens v. C.I.T Group/Equipment Financing, Inc., 955 F.2d, 5th Circuit: 1023, 1027 (1992).

Vance v. Southern Bell Telephone & Telegraph Cop., 863 F.2nd, 11th Circuit: 1503, 1516 (1989).

Weiner, I. (1994). The Rorschach Inkblot Method (RIM) is not a test: Implications for theory and practice. *Journal of Personality Assessment, 62,* 498–504.

Wilson v. Monarch Paper Co., 939 Ff2d, 5th Circuit: 1138, 1145 (1991).

APPENDIX: RORSCHACH OF MR. J.

Sequence of Scores Client Information

Sequence of Scores

Card	Resp. No	Location and DQ	Loc. No.	Determinant(s) and Form Quality	(2)	Content(s)	Pop	Z Score	Special Scores
I	1	WSo	1	FVo		A	P	3.5	MOR
	2	Wo	1	FMa, FDo		A	P	1.0	DV
II	3	D+	1	FMp, FYo	2	A		3.0	
III	4	D+	1	Mpo	2	H, Id, Cg	P	3.0	GHR
IV	5	Wo	1	Fo		(A)		2.0	
V	6	Wo	1	Fo		A	P	1.0	
VI	7	W+	1	Fo		Ad, Ay	P	2.5	
	8	Wo	1	FYu		A		2.5	MOR
VII	9	W+	1	FMpo	2	A, Id		2.5	
	10	W+	1	Mpo	2	H, Ay, Cg, Id	P	2.5	GHR
VIII	11	W+	1	FMao	2	A, Bt	P	4.5	
IX	12	Do	9	FD, FY, Mp, CF−		Hd, Sx			MOR, PHR
X	13	DdS+	99	FMa, FC'	2	A, Id		6.0	
	14	D+	7	FMa, FYu	2	A, Bt		4.0	MOR
	15	Do	2	FM pu	2	A			
	16	Dd+	99	FMa−		Ge, A		4.0	FAB2
	17	D+	6	Ma−		Id		4.0	AB, FAB, PHR
	18	D+	10	CFu		Hd, Bt		4.0	AB, PHR

Summary of Approach

I: WS.W	**VI:** W.W
II: D	**VII:** W.W
III: D	**VIII:** W
IV: W	**IX:** D
V: W	**X:** DdS.D.D.Dd.D.D

RIAP™ Structural Summary Client Information

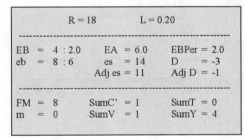

Location Features

Zf	=	16
ZSum	=	50.0
ZEst	=	52.5
W	=	9
(Wv	=	0)
D	=	7
W+D	=	16
Dd	=	2
S	=	2

DQ

		(FQ-)
+	= 11	(2)
o	= 7	(1)
v/+	= 0	(0)
v	= 0	(0)

Form Quality

	FQx	MQual	W+D
+	= 0	0	0
o	= 11	2	10
u	= 4	0	4
-	= 3	2	2
none	= 0	0	0

Determinants

Blends	Single	
FM.FD	M	= 3
FM.FY	FM	= 4
FD.FY.M.CF	m	= 0
FM.FC'	FC	= 0
FM.FY	CF	= 1
	C	= 0
	Cn	= 0
	FC'	= 0
	C'F	= 0
	C'	= 0
	FT	= 0
	TF	= 0
	T	= 0
	FV	= 1
	VF	= 0
	V	= 0
	FY	= 1
	YF	= 0
	Y	= 0
	Fr	= 0
	rF	= 0
	FD	= 0
	F	= 3
	(2)	= 8

Contents

H	=	2
(H)	=	0
Hd	=	2
(Hd)	=	0
Hx	=	0
A	=	11
(A)	=	1
Ad	=	1
(Ad)	=	0
An	=	0
Art	=	0
Ay	=	2
Bl	=	0
Bt	=	3
Cg	=	2
Cl	=	0
Ex	=	0
Fd	=	0
Fi	=	0
Ge	=	1
Hh	=	0
Ls	=	0
Na	=	0
Sc	=	0
Sx	=	1
Xy	=	0
Idio	=	5

S-Constellation

☑	FV+VF+V+FD > 2	
☑	Col-Shd Blends > 0	
☐	Ego < .31 or > .44	
☑	MOR > 3	
☐	Zd > ±3.5	
☑	es > EA	
☑	CF + C > FC	
☑	X+% < .70	
☐	S > 3	
☐	P < 3 or > 8	
☐	Pure H < 2	
☐	R < 17	
6	Total	

Special Scores

		Lvl-1	Lvl-2
DV	=	1 x1	0 x2
INC	=	0 x2	0 x4
DR	=	0 x3	0 x6
FAB	=	1 x4	1 x7
ALOG	=	0 x5	
CON	=	0 x7	

Raw Sum6	=	3
Wgtd Sum6	=	12

AB	= 2	GHR	= 2
AG	= 0	PHR	= 3
COP	= 0	MOR	= 4
CP	= 0	PER	= 0
		PSV	= 0

RATIOS, PERCENTAGES, AND DERIVATIONS

R = 18	L = 0.20

EB	= 4 : 2.0	EA	= 6.0	EBPer = 2.0
eb	= 8 : 6	es	= 14	D	= -3
		Adj es	= 11	Adj D = -1

FM	= 8	SumC'	= 1	SumT = 0
m	= 0	SumV	= 1	SumY = 4

AFFECT

FC:CF+C	= 0 : 2
Pure C	= 0
SumC' : WSumC	= 1 : 2.0
Afr	= 0.80
S	= 2
Blends:R	= 5 : 18
CP	= 0

INTERPERSONAL

COP = 0		AG = 0
GHR:PHR		= 2 : 3
a:p		= 6 : 6
Food		= 0
SumT		= 0
Human Content		= 4
Pure H		= 2
PER		= 0
Isolation Index		= 0.22

IDEATION

a:p	= 6 : 6	Sum6 = 3
Ma:Mp	= 1 : 3	Lvl-2 = 1
2AB+(Art+Ay)	= 6	WSum6 = 12
MOR	= 4	M- = 2
		M none = 0

MEDIATION

XA%	= 0.83
WDA%	= 0.88
X-%	= 0.17
S-	= 0
P	= 7
X+%	= 0.61
Xu%	= 0.22

PROCESSING

Zf	= 16
W:D:Dd	= 9:7:2
W : M	= 9 : 4
Zd	= -2.5
PSV	= 0
DQ+	= 11
DQv	= 0

SELF-PERCEPTION

3r+(2)/R	= 0.44
Fr+rF	= 0
SumV	= 1
FD	= 2
An+Xy	= 0
MOR	= 4
H:(H)+Hd+(Hd)	= 2 : 2

PTI = 1	☐ DEPI = 4	☐ CDI = 3	☐ S-CON = 6	☐ HVI = No	☐ OBS = No

Constellations Table

S-Constellation (Suicide Potential)
☐ Positive if 8 or more conditions are true:
NOTE: Applicable only for subjects over 14 years old.
☑ FV+VF+V+FD [3] > 2
☑ Col-Shd Blends [1] > 0
☐ Ego [0.44] < .31 *or* > .44
☑ MOR [4] > 3
☐ Zd [-2.5] > ±3.5
☑ es [14] > EA [6.0]
☑ CF + C [2] > FC [0]
☑ X+% [0.61] < .70
☐ S [2] > 3
☐ P [7] < 3 or > 8
☐ Pure H [2] < 2
☐ R [18] < 17
6   Total

PTI (Perceptual-Thinking Index)
☐ (XA% [0.83] < 0.70) *and* (WDA% [0.88] < 0.75)
☐ X-% [0.17] > 0.29
☐ (Sum Level 2 Special Scores [1] > 2)
and (FAB2 [1] > 0)
☐ ((R [18] < 17) *and* (WSum6 [12] > 12)) *or*
((R [18] > 16) *and* (WSum6 [12] > 17))
☑ (M- [2] > 1) *or* (X-% [0.17] > 0.40)
1   Total

DEPI (Depression Index)
☐ Positive if 5 or more conditions are true:
☑ (FV + VF + V [1] > 0) *or* (FD [2] > 2)
☑ (Col-Shd Blends [1] > 0) *or* (S [2] > 2)
☐ (3r + (2)/R [0.44] > 0.44 *and* Fr + rF [0] = 0)
or (3r + (2)/R [0.44] < 0.33)
☐ (Afr [0.80] < 0.46) *or* (Blends [5] < 4)
☐ (SumShading [6] > FM + m [8])
or (SumC' [1] > 2)
☑ (MOR [4] > 2) *or* (2xAB + Art + Ay [6] > 3)
☑ (COP [0] < 2)
or ([Bt+2xCl+Ge+Ls+2xNa]/R [0.22] > 0.24)
4   Total

CDI (Coping Deficit Index)
☐ Positive if 4 or more conditions are true:
☑ (EA [6.0] < 6) *or* (AdjD [-1] < 0)
☑ (COP [0] < 2) *and* (AG [0] < 2)
☑ (Weighted Sum C [2.0] < 2.5)
or (Afr [0.80] < 0.46)
☐ (Passive [6] > Active + 1 [7])
or (Pure H [2] < 2)
☐ (Sum T [0] > 1)
or (Isolate/R [0.22] > 0.24)
or (Food [0] > 0)
3   Total

HVI (Hypervigilance Index)
☐ Positive if condition 1 is true and at least 4 of the others are true:
☑ (1) FT + TF + T [0] = 0
☑ (2) Zf [16] > 12
☐ (3) Zd [-2.5] > +3.5
☐ (4) S [2] > 3
☐ (5) H + (H) + Hd + (Hd) [4] > 6
☐ (6) (H) + (A) + (Hd) + (Ad) [1] > 3
☐ (7) H + A : Hd + Ad [14:3] < 4 : 1
☐ (8) Cg [2] > 3

OBS (Obsessive Style Index)
☐ (1) Dd [2] > 3
☑ (2) Zf [16] > 12
☐ (3) Zd [-2.5] > +3.0
☐ (4) Populars [7] > 7
☐ (5) FQ+ [0] > 1
☐ Positive if one or more is true:
☐ Conditions 1 to 5 are all true
☐ Two or more of 1 to 4 are true *and* FQ+ [0] > 3
☐ 3 or more of 1 to 5 are true
and X+% [0.61] > 0.89
☐ FQ+ [0] > 3 *and* X+% [0.61] > 0.89

NOTE: '' indicates a cutoff that has been adjusted for age norms.*

	SCZI (Schizophrenia Index)

☐ Positive if 4 or more conditions are true:

☐ ((X+% [0.61] < 0.61) *and* (S-% [0.00] < 0.41))
or (X+% [0.61] < 0.50)

☐ X-% [0.17] > 0.29

☐ (FQ- [3] ≥ FQu [4])
or (FQ- [3] > FQo [11] + FQ+ [0])

☐ (Sum Level 2 Special Scores [1] > 1)
and (FAB2 [1] > 0)

☐ (Raw Sum of 6 Special Scores [3] > 6) *or*
(Weighted Sum of 6 Special Scores [12] > 17)

☑ (M- [2] > 1)
or (X-% [0.17] > 0.40)

1 Total

15

THE RORSCHACH IN FITNESS FOR DUTY EVALUATIONS

James F. Gormally
Private Practice, Silver Spring, MD

Fitness for duty (FFD) evaluations involve psychological assessment guided by knowledge of discrimination law. A core aspect of the law is the individualized assessment of disabled employees, taking into account how a disability like depression affects job performance, as well as strengths and weaknesses in the personality that impact the effect of the depression on functioning. This chapter posits that the Comprehensive System (CS; Exner, 2003) provides a well-differentiated description of the disabled employee. Vulnerability and resilience can be described by the CS. Case material is presented to illustrate this application of the test. When interview findings are integrated with test data from the CS, conclusions about the employee's fitness can be supported by empirical data, which is the benchmark standard for psychological opinions.

Diagnosed disorders do not define a disability. Obviously, many employees can function at work with a diagnosed disorder. Although there is a prevailing standard for disability from the Americans With Disabilities Act of 1990 (ADA), clinical judgment is integral to this assessment. In effect, the forensic psychologist needs to form an opinion about whether a diagnosed disorder impairs the employee to such a substantial degree as to disable them. Key concepts of discrimination law are explained in this chapter, followed by a model that can be used to make an assessment of an ADA disability. Defensiveness is common in FFD evaluations and data on response set is presented to clarify this problem.

THE ORGANIZATIONAL CONTEXT

Multiple parties are interested in the results of a FFD, and they frequently have competing needs and motivations, as this case demonstrates. A correctional officer (Mr. C.O.) was physically assaulted by an inmate; the officer was alone at his post at the time. The assault resulted in a cut lip and loosened teeth, which required medical attention but not hospitalization. The correctional facility supervisor put Mr. C.O. on leave for 10 weeks, after which time he returned to light duty. Mr. C.O. had been exposed to other hazards.

For example, several months prior to the current attack, he had feces and urine thrown at him. Management referred Mr. C.O. to the medical examiner (ME) for a FFD, as he did not want to leave his light duty assignment. The ME requested information from Mr. C.O.'s therapist, who believed he was not ready to return to work. The therapist diagnosed Mr. C.O. with Posttraumatic Stress Disorder (PTSD) and a depressive disorder. The ME wanted an independent assessment of Mr. C.O.'s current mental status, a diagnosis, and treatment options. There were also questions about Mr. C.O.'s fitness for work in corrections.

What follows is a discussion of underlying motivations of the various parties involved in the question of Mr. C.O.'s fitness for duties. Correctional management is under pressure to staff their facility and need Mr. C.O. off light duty and on the job. They are not medically trained and are unable to inquire knowledgeably about Mr. C.O.'s condition and prognosis. From this point of view, it is entirely understandable why they might order a FFD for Mr. C.O. It is possible that Mr. C.O. is viewed as a "below average" employee. Organizations sometimes re-assign problem employees, but those options are limited. Management may want the ME to declare an employee as completely disabled so that there is no need to deal with retaining someone on a light duty assignment.

The second party is the ME who is responsible for ensuring that accommodations in the workplace are made (e.g., ordering magnifying screens for computers for a diabetic with vision impairments). The ME's opinions would most certainly be scrutinized if a suit alleging discrimination were to be filed by Mr. C.O. Given these realities, a reasonable plan would be to confer with a mental health professional concerning whether there was a diagnosable disorder that was blocking Mr. C.O.'s ability to return to work. The ME is the client of the forensic psychologist, who provides a consultation service so that the ME can make a decision regarding Mr. C.O.'s fitness for duties.

The third party is the occupational medical department of the parent organization contracting with the ME. They are most concerned with ensuring the organization is ADA-compliant. Because the ADA regulations apply to organizations with 15 or more employees, it is important for local governments and large organizations to be well-versed with the concept of "appropriate and reasonable" accommodations in the workplace. Scheid (1999) studied organizational responses to the ADA and found a "deep pockets" phenomena. The size of the organization was a significant factor in whether the business was more or less likely to comply with ADA regulations. Businesses with more people were more likely to comply with ADA regulations.

A mental health professional is the fourth party. A therapist is treating Mr. C.O. and believes he is not ready to return to full duty, although there is reason to believe a therapist's assessment will lack objectivity. In this case, the question could be whether the professional is emphasizing vulnerability rather than resilience in the report to the medical examiner, because Mr. C.O. has said he does not want to return to work.

Foote (2000) noted that collateral reports from mental health professionals are often limited and not definitive in assessing the relationship between a mental disorder and impaired work performance. The forensic psychologist would not want to ask a treating therapist for a forensic opinion, because it creates a dual relationship between the therapist and Mr. C.O. (Greenburg & Shuman, 1997).

Finally, Mr. C.O. is required to comply with the request for a psychological FFD. Most employers or organizations have regulations for a FFD in employment contracts and refusal to comply is grounds for dismissal. He is likely to be highly threatened by the FFD, thinking that it might lead to termination. Mr. C.O. could be understandably confused about what to do; although he might not want to give up his career, he might also fear that he will be exposed to more hazards if he stays on the job.

Knowing the needs of the various parties involved in a FFD will help the psychologist avoid common pitfalls in forensic work: disputes about payment, assessing the wrong questions, using inappropriate measures, and giving the wrong level of feedback to the various parties (Weiner, 1995).

PSYCHOLEGAL ISSUES IN FFD

A quick review of the ADA Web site (at the Department of Justice, http://www.ada.gov) will show that the regulations cover a wide scope, including accessible building standards, discrimination in the workplace, and discrimination in education. The spirit behind the ADA it is to ensure that all persons are treated with fairness. Never was this clearer to me than when I was counseling a patient with dwarfism, who mentioned that some pumps are too high for her to operate. ADA has regulations about gas station design and the purpose of these regulations is not to compel society to give dwarfs extra help. In fact, the ADA is designed primarily to "level the playing field."

There are four sources of laws: the U.S. Constitution, legislation (federal and state), agency regulations (e.g., HIPPA [Health Insurance Portability and Insurance Act]), and case law. The supreme authority is the Constitution, and by extension, interpretation of the Constitution by the Supreme Court in a particular case. On the other hand, case law (from one state) may or may not guide practice in another state. A major tension in the case law was created when cases were decided based on the literal interpretation of the ADA, which states that adaptations, devices, and medications cannot be considered in determining if a person is disabled.

The Second Circuit decided in *Bartlett v. New York State Board* (1998) that learning disabilities are to be evaluated without consideration of compensatory strategies. Dr. Bartlett had a learning disability that affected her reading ability; she had documented deficits in phonological processing that impaired reading functions. She had compensated well enough to achieve an average level of reading skill. But, the average level of her reading skill did not void the protection of the ADA, which provided accommodations to her during board exams. According to the court, her compensations, and average reading level, "do not take her outside of the protective provisions of the ADA."

Thus, cases were being decided based on the language of the ADA. But these decisions appeared to be undercutting the spirit of discrimination law that ensures each person deserves to be evaluated on an individual basis. For example, evaluating a disability caused by dwarfism should include the use of compensatory strategies, like the use of a step stool to use a gas pump. Take her step stool away, and my patient will look and act like all other persons with dwarfism. When someone is assumed to be like others in a group, the individual's strengths and weaknesses are ignored. This is inherently unfair. The presumption that a disabled person is like everyone else with the same disability is what leads to discrimination in the workplace.

The confusion about whether or not to include compensations in the assessment of a disability is understandable. For example, there have been several times when parents want to know whether or not to have their child take medication when being evaluated for attention deficit hyperactivity disorder (ADHD). If a medication is used, the parent could wonder if the test scores will provide evidence of a disability. On the other hand, if the child is not medicated, the child might perform poorly on a test, which could confirm their child as disabled and therefore entitled to services. However, the cost to the child is being stereotyped ("disabled means unable"). Parents want services for their child, but they do not want their child labeled.

In 1999, the Supreme Court decided three cases that focused on the tension created by the lower court's decision making based on the literal translation of the ADA. These three opinions are important for psychologists to study, because they provide definitive guidance about who is disabled and therefore entitled to protection under ADA. (see http://www.findlaw.com). One case involved the Sutton sisters, who had been denied employment by United Airlines due to visual impairments. United Airlines had a policy that pilots for their jumbo jets could not use glasses. In *Sutton v. United Airlines* (1999), the petitioners argued that United Airlines was engaging in discriminatory hiring practices. They further asserted that they were experienced pilots, and had obtained a license to fly commercial jets, making them "qualified individuals with a disability" deserving protection under ADA. The Supreme Court decided in favor of United Airlines. This decision is quite important and, along with two other cases decided at the same time, created a standard for how an ADA disability is defined.

The other two cases both involved Department of Transportation (DOT) regulations about driving trucks. In *Murphy v. United Parcel Service* (1999), the petitioner Murphy had hypertension and was using medication to manage his blood pressure. UPS followed DOT rules specifying that truckers cannot have a "diagnosis of high blood pressure, " which could impact the ability to drive safely. In fact, at the time he was hired, Murphy's blood pressure was so high (186/124) that he was not qualified to be certified for a DOT health certificate. He started work because a certificate was given to him in error. When he was re-evaluated by the medical examiner at UPS, his blood pressure was still quite high (160/102). He was terminated because his blood pressure exceeded policy guidelines. The court found that the medical examiner evaluated Murphy when he was in a medicated state and that company policy, and not prejudice, guided the termination. He was not disabled enough by the hypertension that he could not function, and therefore he was not disabled in a basic activity of life.

In *Albertsons, Inc. v. Kirkingburg* (1999), a truck driver had monocular vision due to an uncorrectable vision condition in one eye. He also was erroneously certified by a physician as passing DOT standards. When he was re-evaluated, he received a waiver of the DOT vision standards, but his employer fired him for failing to meet vision standards. The lower court initially found that he was not qualified as a trucker without an accommodation, and he was not protected by the ADA. But the Ninth Circuit over turned this ruling and found that *Kirkingburg* was in fact disabled. This court's reasoning was that how he sees differs significantly from how most people see. The Supreme Court found that the Ninth Court made a misstep in that "seeing differently" from most people does not rise to the level of disability, as being disabled "significantly restricts" functioning.

Core Concepts of ADA

Justice O'Connor's decisions in *Sutton* and *Murphy* and Justice Souter's decision in *Kirkingburg* analyze disability law and provide clarifying definitions to language in the ADA. Those concepts that should guide FFD include: individualized approach, disability, and qualified individual with a disability.

Individualized Approach.   A disabling condition of an employee needs to be decided on a case-by-case basis. In the *Kirkingburg* decision, Justice Souter found that the Ninth Circuit did not focus sufficiently on the ADA's emphasis on an individualized approach to disability determination. Justice Souter reasoned, "Some impairments may invariably cause a substantial limitation of a major life activity, but monocularity is not one of them, for that category embraces a group whose members vary" (e.g., how restricted they are in functioning). In *Sutton*, Justice O'Connor wrote, "The (ADA) guidelines' directive that persons be judged in their uncorrected or unmitigated state runs directly counter to this individualized inquiry. The former would create a system in which persons would often be treated as members of a group having similar impairments, rather than as individuals."

Disability.   In ADA language, a disability is "a physical or mental impairment that substantially limits one or more of the major life activities of an individual." In *Sutton*, the court found that not being able to fly a jumbo jet is insufficient to meet the "substantial limits" test of a disabling condition. They went on to point out that the Sutton sisters could use their skills as a regional pilot or pilot instructor. Almost identical reasoning was used in *Murphy*. The court asserted that many jobs were open to him as a mechanic that did not involve driving a truck. Justice O'Connor wrote in *Murphy* that "to be regarded as substantially limited in the major life activity of working, one must be regarded as precluded from more than a particular job."

Temporary stress reactions (i.e., adjustment disorders) have not been considered a disability, even though the adjustment disorder can be associated with severe levels of symptoms. Goodman-Delahunty (2000) cites a case (*Hamilton v. Southwestern Bell Telephone Co.*, 1998) that involved an excessive emotional outburst at work. Expert testimony diagnosed PTSD, but found that the employee could function normally. The court concluded that the employee was impaired, but not disabled. Chronic disorders (e.g., bipolar disorder) may not qualify as a disability, particularly if the disorder is being medically managed. If the employee suffers from relapses, and the relapses substantially impact work functioning, then this fact pattern may support a disability determination.

Levine (1987) discussed a "variation-to-handicap continuum" in the context of learning problems, which has application to FFD. Variations are unusual patterns of strengths and weaknesses that are present in most of us. Dysfunctions are variations that significantly impair performance in a particular function (e.g., a dysfunction in interpersonal skill or stress tolerance, which affects functioning on the job). Dysfunctions are the kind of ordinary problems that are addressed by training and coaching on the job. Dysfunctions can be compensated for, and when the compensations are successful, a person is able to function. Sometimes, dysfunctions can lead to a disability, despite the employee's and supervisor's best efforts. Handicaps are disabilities that are uncompensated for and that compromise a critical area of performance, like working.

The presence of a *DSM–IV* diagnosis does not establish that a person is disabled. In fact, many persons function at work with a diagnosed disorder because they have found the right kind of work environment and/or developed compensations that allow them to cope. As Justice Souter wrote, "The determination of whether an individual has a disability is not necessarily based on the name or diagnosis of the impairment the person has, but rather on the effect of that impairment on the life of the individual."

Qualified Individual With a Disability.   Most FFD includes a statement about accommodations that allow a disabled person to function on the job. However, accommodations need to be reasonable, and employers are not required to re-design a job for an employee. Goodman-Delahunty (2000) describe the case of a mentally ill woman whose ability to work was found to be substantially impaired because of difficulties working with others and following directions. Even though there were periodic emotional outbursts, her job performance was rated as satisfactory. The court found her to be a QUID ("qualified individual with a disability"), who could be accommodated on the job by making duties routine and predictable, and using supportive supervision.

A MODEL FOR CONDUCTING FFD

Models vary for conducting FFD, and I imagine that most practitioners who have done more than 10 evaluations have developed one that works for them (e.g., Foote, 2000). For the purpose of this chapter, I provide a model that has evolved over 15 years of conducting FFD evaluations. The first step in the model is to gather sufficient information to ensure that a FFD will answer the referral question.

Qualify the Referral.   Many health care professionals conduct FFD. Someone who has been off work because of an injury to a knee, for example, would be sent for an evaluation by an orthopedist before being cleared to return to work. These requests for a FFD are routine. However, requests for a FFD because of behavioral or emotional issues are not routine. The kinds of problems that trigger a psychological FFD usually have history and background that needs to be obtained (e.g., mental health treatment, medical problems). Determine if something unusual happened on the job that triggered the referral (e.g., the bus driver accidentally ran over and killed a pedestrian). If the employee has been on light duty status, then find out the reasons for this placement. If the employee is on administrative leave, find out the reasons. A key question is: Who will be receiving the report? The answer to this question defines the client who will be receiving your consultation service.

The phone contact should be followed up by a letter that specifies the problems that the employee is having on the job, when the problems started, and how frequently they have been occurring. The best referral includes "good faith" efforts by management to help the employee function better, and the employee's response to those interventions (although this kind of documentation is rare). A phone conversation is insufficient to qualify the referral. It does happen that the requester may be unwilling to commit in writing to the reasons for the evaluation. When that happens, I do not accept the referral. The next step is to obtain information about what is expected from the employee at work.

Determine the Essential Duties of the Job.   A job description may be available from the Human Resource Department, but there is no substitute for behavioral descriptions of the employee's typical work day. If an employee is working in a high-stress position (e.g., as a police officer), there are typical tasks as well as duties that are infrequent but unusually demanding (e.g., an enforcement situation with a combative citizen; see P. Weiss, W. Weiss, & Gacono, chap. 25, this vol.).

Goodman-Delahunty (2000) provides a useful description of issues surrounding essential features of a job (e.g., when there is dispute between the worker and management about the essential features of the job). In addition, she discusses attendance, conduct, and on-the-job stress as it relates to whether these are essential to the job. For example, the EEOC (Equal Employment Opportunity Commission) considers attendance a policy but not an essential job function, and therefore something that may be altered as a form of an accommodation. However, violations of standards of conduct are grounds for discipline or dismissal and not protected under ADA. The examiner may choose to visit the workplace to learn about the demands of the job (e.g., ride along with police). Identifying key duties is critical in making the assessment of impairment to functioning on the job (see also Foote, 2000).

Establish a Working Relationship with the Employee.   FFD are particularly difficult to conduct because of the involuntary nature of these evaluations. The employee may have difficulty cooperating with the assessment tasks that are used. Skillful attention to the threat produced by the evaluation will create the perception that the forensic psychologist wants to conduct the assessment in a humane fashion. This will help foster a working alliance with employees and motivate them to give you the information you need to conduct the evaluation. How one deals with issues such as informed consent, requests for the report, and missed visits will further strengthen or weaken the working alliance.

It is helpful to clarify the role of the medical examiner, and to highlight who will be making the decision about returning to work. For example, during rapport building, I mention that the ME does not want someone to go back and be re-injured on the job when there is an injury. I explain that medical issues require medical evaluations, however, the ME consults with a psychologist when there is a behavioral issue. I explain the assessment process is a "psychological fit for duty evaluation." I go on to explain their role (i.e., to give me the information I need, so that I can explain their thoughts and feelings about returning to work to the medical examiner). I prepare the employee that there may be a second appointment, if psychological testing is required. I give a simply worded agreement form to sign that specifies the parameters of the relationship.

Gather Collateral Information.   Collateral information for the FFD involves, for example, performance evaluations, student ratings of teaching, arrest records (although this is rare), and mental health treatment reports. The quality level of this kind of information can vary (Foote, 2000). Personnel records are questionable because workers are reluctant to reveal a disability to management, particularly if it involves a psychiatric disorder. A more informative history would be one in which a disability was disclosed to management that was accommodated, and the results of those accommodations were described. Performance evaluations are not necessarily useful or accurate. Using telephone calls to obtain information from management is problematic, unless the informant is willing to sign an affidavit certifying that the record of the phone conversation is true and accurate. Mental health treatment reports can provide factual information (e.g., kind of medications; dates of hospitalization). However, mental health reports are not forensic reports.

Zelig's FFD model (2001) describes a wide range of collateral information, including a credit card report, statements from witnesses, and interviews with informants nominated by the employee. Fingerprints for a "personal record check" to determine if there is a criminal history are used by Zelig. Arrest records or other information that can be used to confirm self-reports are necessary when the referral background includes antisocial conduct on the job (about 12% of the FFD cases in my database included legal problems). However, a competent assessment can be performed most of the time relying on self-reports in the interview, data from the client in the letter of referral, and test data.

Use a Semistructured Interview Protocol.   The interview provides information that is not able to be obtained in any other way. This includes an assessment of the employee's development, interpersonal attitudes, mental status, and feelings about returning to work. Most notably, the employee's emphasis during the interview will reveal underlying motivation about working. For example, in response to the inquiry "Please describe your health," employees who are not ready to return to work will enumerate many problems. There are questionnaires that could be created for work history, social history, and mental health treatment history; however, the employees' thoughts and feelings about their history would not be thoroughly assessed unless they were probed during the interview. However, there are limitations to the technique in terms of lack of standardization, so I have developed an interview protocol.

I use open-ended questions, which are constructed to "open up" the employee without stimulating undue anxiety (e.g., move from easy to more difficult topics). At the beginning, I convey a curious tone and ask, "How did you wind up getting referred to the medical examiner?" Empathic responses, or head nods, build rapport when the employee is feeling distressed. Provide a listing of common life events for the employee to check-off and follow up about the personal significance of these stressors (e.g., Is a divorce a change for the better?). This allows the employee to provide important situational factors that might be affecting work (e.g., recent birth of a child with serious medical problems). Midway through the interview, confront the employees with the problems in their performance carefully noting their answers. My approach has been to write down responses, close to verbatim as possible, while noting themes when open-ended questions are used. This approach allows for actively processing the interpersonal aspect of the interview, including making behavioral observations. Use close-ended questions in the last half of the interview to assess specific content areas (e.g., last physical exam and results). Interview the employees about their familiarity with psychological testing (e.g., see the review by Ruiz et al., 2002 about websites that have tips about taking psychological tests). End with questions about their job, future plans, any requests for accommodations and thanking the employee for their cooperation.[1]

A mental status examination is a standard assessment technique in forensic psychiatry (e.g., Breger, 1997) and a recommended part of the FFD evaluation. Morrison (1995) provides a condensed and highly useful summary of the major domains of a mental status exam: appearance and behavior, mood, flow of thought, content of thought, perception, cognition, insight, and judgment. I schedule enough time after the interview to complete a form that covers these domains.

Write the Report Integrating Relevant Background With Test Data. Relevant background information should inform the interpretation of psychological test data. The employee's mental status, unique developmental experiences, work history including achievements and traumatic experiences, work demands, the employee's strengths, history of disability and mental health treatment, personal stressors, and educational background are all relevant to FFD. Houlihan and Reynolds (2001) discuss their FFD work and their descriptions of the background are excellent illustrations of what to look for. There is no current standard for how to define culture and how to integrate cultural background, so judgment is involved in how to describe cultural factors in a way that increases the precision of the assessment.

It should be emphasized that FFD is a consultation to a client. The overall goal of the assessment is to create a report that makes the employee's problems comprehensible to the client. A standard approach in the psychological report is to identify linkages between presenting problems/observations of the mental status, relevant history, and data on personality functioning. This "rule of three" is a helpful guide for writing the kind of report that effectively presents conclusions about fitness that are logical and objective.

Finally, provide the correct level of feedback to the referral source and do not provide feedback to the employee. A guideline is to give the referral the minimum information needed to make a decision about fitness for duty (fit for duty, or not; accommodations; nature of the disability). The complete report of the evaluation is kept on file. Not giving feedback to the employee prevents the potential for splitting between the referral and the forensic psychologist; it also avoids creating the perception that the relationship is helpful (which it is not).

---

[1] A copy of the interview is available by email (jfgormally@yahoo.com).

THE RORSCHACH AND FITNESS FOR DUTY EVALUATION

My FFD database includes a group of 124 employees (females, $n = 62$; males, $n = 62$) who were administered the Rorschach between 1990 and 2005. The letter of referral was coded for problems that led to the request for the evaluation. There were four groups of problems: employees who complained that they were too distressed to work, conduct problems (alcohol, anger, antisocial conduct), problems in the supervisory relationship, and dysfunctional professionals/managers. Multiple codings were made for some referrals (e.g., an employee with a drinking problem who was also distressed).

Impairment in the Distressed Employee

The most common problem (45% of referred women, 29% of men) involved employees whose distress interfered with their work. In the 6 months prior to the FFD evaluation, 19% of full sample employees (no gender differences were found) received care in a mental health unit at the hospital or went to the emergency room. The utilization of outpatient mental treatment in this sample was also high (50% women, 42% men). The following case illustrates the how the CS was used to explain how depression impaired Mr. A.'s ability to function on the job.

Mr. A., an administrator, age 47, was referred for an FFD after a prolonged absence due to a major depression. The onset of the depression was marked by a sense of paralysis at work and problems concentrating. Mr. A. lost his emotional composure managing others. He isolated himself from his wife and would retreat into the woods near his home and cry. He reported a long history of treatment for an affective disorder, starting around age 20 on an outpatient basis, and had not been hospitalized in the past, nor did he report past or current suicidal behaviors. Mr. A. had been on leave to receive treatment (both verbal therapy and medication), then tried to return to work after 1 month, but had to go back on leave. Now, after another month off, he was feeling well enough to work. The medical examiner wanted to know if part-time work was an appropriate accommodation, as well as an opinion about his fitness. Prolonged absences from work will trigger a FFD because management is usually "in the dark" about the reasons for the absence; thus it is understandable why Mr. A. was referred for a FFD.

Malingering must always be considered when evaluating distressed employees. When employees are not motivated to return to work, they often seek consultation from a mental health professional. The employee will produce a letter or form that includes a diagnosis and prognosis when the employee will be able to return to work. Ten percent of the FFD database requested that their mental health professional provide such a letter. These diagnostic opinions are rarely compelling and do not meet the standards for a forensic evaluation (Greenberg & Shuman, 1997). Although confirmation of an employee's compliance and attendance at treatment is useful, the treating professional's opinion about fitness for duties is generally not informative.

This assessment was relatively straightforward because there was no evidence of exaggeration in the interview, the symptoms that were reported were specific to depression, and the MMPI–2 F scales showed no evidence of overreporting. Indeed, his MMPI–2 validity scale profile indicated an open and cooperative test taking attitude. He was seeking return to work so there would be no reason to expect overreporting. Mr. A. produced an interpretively useful Rorschach with $R = 22$; he was obviously engaged in the task with many synthesized responses and blends. The Structural Summary showed that $DEPI = 6$ and a $CDI = 1$. These findings were interpreted as indicating a "significant and potentially disabling affective problem" marked by complaints of distress and behavioral dysfunction (Exner, 2000, p. 80). The use of the $DEPI$ and CDI can be helpful in understanding the distressed employee. It is quite common that the distress is symptomatic of coping skills that are insufficient to meet the interpersonal demands of the job (e.g., when CDI is positive and $DEPI = 5$). This pattern of scores will distinguish this kind of distress from distress caused by an affective disorder. Often, I find that employees who are malingering distress will have very low $DEPI$ scores, exaggerated MMPI–2 profiles and a positive CDI.

Mr. A. did not endorse a significant number of symptoms on the MMPI–2 depression content scale, which was consistent with the assessment made of depressive symptoms during the interview. The MMPI–2 profile was not elevated on A, anxiety content or scale 7. The profile had no clinical scales above $T = 65$. There were elevations on scales 4 ($T = 64$), 6 ($T = 64$), 2, 8 and 9. He was endorsing a clinically significant level of tension relating to others ($T = 73$ on SOD), which was related to the "phone phobia" at work and the tendency to isolate from others. The five elevations on the clinical scales suggested interpersonal problems, including irritability, argumentativeness, and a tendency to transfer blame to others.

The RIM provided an insight into this man's vulnerability to relapse, as well as strengths that might allow him to continue his recovery. His self-report in the interview and MMPI–2 did not indicate the presence of emotional distress. Problems with self-image and self-acceptance were evident ($Vista = 3$), as well as resilience that allowed him to battle his depression ($D = 0$, $AdjD = +1$, $EA = 14.5$). Whereas he struggled with self-disparagement, the record had no $Morbid$ content and an average $Egocentricity Index$.

Expanding on the theme of vulnerability to future depression, I focused on Rorschach variables that have been found to add to the predictive accuracy of self-reports of depression. Hartmann, Wang, Berg, and Saether (2003) found that $sum Y$ and $WSum6$ improved predictive accuracy of diagnosis. Mr. A.'s structural summary included $Y = 2$, and $WSum6 = 20$, with 4 level 1 $FABCOM$s. Vulnerability processing affect was noted as well, including avoidance ($Afr = .47$) as a compensation for problems with affective modulation ($FC{:}CF + C = 1{:}6$). There was unusual degree of complexity to his affective process (50% of responses containing blended determinants; 3 $Color/Shading$ blends). Mr. A.'s problems with affect were further understood by the production of 6 space responses. These problems were balanced by the finding of 4 $Cooperative Movement$ responses, no personalized responses, and the presence of a $Texture$ in the record.

The conclusion provided to the medical examiner was that the administrator met criteria for an ADA disability. The vulnerability in his personality created an ongoing risk for relapse into a major depression. The report explained that Mr. A. had a "double depression." He struggled with cycles of major depression while being "bogged down" by a chronic predisposition to dysthymia. His depression caused serious impairment in his job functioning. These functions included his ability to concentrate and administrate programs, as well as work cooperatively with others. His affect was not depressed during the interview and he was well enough to work.

Wisely, Mr. A. had sought the counsel of an attorney specializing in discrimination law. He learned that it was up to him to declare himself disabled and ask for part-time work.One might be moved by an employee's openness, but, there must be a good reason to recommend changes to duties on the job. In this case, the assessment data showed that his depression had cleared, but there was vulnerability in his personality that was not likely to change in the near future. Part-time work was a reasonable accommodation because he was early into the recovery process and vulnerable to a relapse.

Defensiveness in the Assessment of Conduct Problems

A second referral category that is frequently encountered involves inappropriate conduct. Of the 62 men who were evaluated, 32 (52%) had behavior problems, whereas 12 of 62 (19%) women had conduct issues. Problems stemming from unrecognized/untreated alcoholism were the most common conduct issue (27 of 124 or 22%, with twice as many men as women with this background). Interview methods and scales on the MMPI–2 perform an adequate assessment of the employee's awareness of a problem, however, these employees typically conceal, more than reveal, their problems on these assessment instruments.

Ganellen (1994) studied a group of male airline pilots who presumably were aware of their problems with alcohol because they were being evaluated after a period of treatment. He found high levels of defensiveness on the MMPI–2 validity scales. He also found that the Rorschach detected vulnerabilities in self-perception that might explain their defensiveness. A substantial number of pilots evidenced a fragile narcissism (*Vistas* combined with *Reflections*; Gacono, Meloy, & Heaven, 1990). The sense of self as damaged, like a cracked piece of pottery, causes pain. Yet, seeking help reinforces the sense of self as flawed in a permanent way. The defensiveness is quite understandable.

Sex offenders are difficult to interview because their conduct problems are private and, therefore, can be kept secret. Grossman, Wasyliw, Benn, and Gyoerkoe (2002) present a strong case for the Rorschach in their study of sex offenders who are defensive on the MMPI–2. One employee in the FFD database was arrested for a sex offense; he produced a valid MMPI–2 profile that was within normal limits. His Rorschach profile revealed a number of problems that made it much more clear that his offense was symptomatic of vulnerabilities in his personality (i.e., $AG = 9$, suggesting ego-dystonic aggressive tension; $Mor = 4, X-\% = 31, M- = 4, Ego = .63, a:p = 13:3$). The RIM also indicated that he may have been experiencing considerable remorse about his offense ($V = 1$).

Problems in the Supervisory Relationship

Problems with authority are acted out on the job in various ways (uncooperative attitude, sleeping on the job, unreliable attendance, misuse of sick leave). Acting out and performance problems are complex assessments because there is an interpersonal dynamic to the supervisory relationship. Issues, such as supervisory style, can be expected to impact employee morale and performance. However, it is important to keep the focus of the FFD on whether the performance problems are the result of an ADA disability.

Of the 124 referrals in the FFD RIM database, there were 31 cases (25%) that cited performance problems (no gender differences). Sick leave restrictions were being used for 20 employees of these 31 with performance issues, which obviously puts enormous stress on the supervisory relationship. Stormy and difficult supervisory–employee relationships were noted in 16 employees. Being able to work with others is a basic element of most employment. One of the four components that are used to determine impairment in functioning in workman's compensation evaluations is the capacity to work cooperatively with others (American Medical Association, 2001).

Mr. L. was a 55-year-old librarian referred because of a hostile relationship with supervision and coworkers. The background indicated that he could perform his duties well, there was no history of mental health treatment and he was perceived as an asset at other libraries. Mr. L. wrote a letter of complaint about mistreatment on the job and was unwilling or unable to take responsibility for his hostility. There was an escalating quality to the hostility, leading to a heated interchange with his supervisor. He was then placed on light duty to "cool off." He was confused about what he wanted to do after ending light duty and was considering pursuing legal action against the organization. In the FFD interview, Mr. L. was not paranoid, but he was unwilling to accept any responsibility to the unraveling of the work relationships.

The MMPI–2 showed an elevated L scale, which was not high enough to invalidate the test but did weaken the usefulness of the profile. The profile was within normal limits, indicating that he viewed his adjustment as satisfactory. Even the Work Content scale was not elevated. Mr. L. was able to complete the Rorschach without card rejections, but he gave a low number of responses ($R = 15$). The CS data indicated a positive CDI, which would be more interpretatively sound, if he had given an average number of responses. He was experiencing stress associated with the evaluation ($m=2$; $D = -1$; $AdjD = 0$), which was understandable as he was not particularly resourceful ($EA = 6$). He was prone to problems with emotional modulation ($FC:CF + C = 0:2$, and he was *Introversive*). In obvious situations he could read the cues for how to behave (*Populars* = 7) consistent with the positive and long work history. But there were three minus answers, all of which were given to the chromatic cards, further suggesting problems with emotion. This Rorschach finding was consistent with his history of an emotional "airing out" his grievances about supervision to upper administration. In both the MMPI–2 (hi L scale) and the Rorschach ($a:p = 4:8$), there was a rigid quality to his thinking and pattern of adjusting to stressors on the job. It is notable that the decline in the relationship occurred around the time when his job was being restructured, which required him to adapt.

It was quite interesting that Mr. L.'s Rorschach included three *Food* responses (including one minus response). One starts to develop the hypothesis of a hostile-dependent relationship with supervision, stemming from the librarian's personality issues. Further specifying this employee's interpersonal schema was useful to predict how Mr. L. was likely to internalize supervisory direction (*Human Content* = 4, which is average; $M- = 0$,

$COP = 1$, $AG = 1$, $GHR:PHR = 4:0$) There was strength noted in the assessment of his underlying object relations schema, despite the structure-dependent quality to his personality. After describing the findings about his personality, and integrating it with the history and collateral data, the report concluded that the employee was fit for full duty with the recommendation to use a referral to the Employee Assistance Program. The counselor might help mediate differences between the employee and the supervisor. The prediction was made that, if the supervisor could re-visit their issues in a reassuring tone, this might be calming to the employee.

Professionals/Managers Who Are Dysfunctional

The database includes a subgroup of cases evaluating professionals (dentist, physician, attorney, and psychologist), a tenured professor, ranking officers in the police department, and managers at the upper levels of administration. These referrals are relatively rare (about 10% of the entire sample). These cases can involve some problem in functioning that is highly embarrassing to the individual (e.g., a bipolar police administrator writing a bizarre note to the mayor during a period of noncompliance with his medication regimen, which has become public). Sometimes, the reasons may center on performance issues (e.g., below standard work).

Professionals are human like everyone else, and they will make mistakes. Because professionals are autonomous, they are expected to engage in self-monitoring and learn from their mistakes without supervision. If functioning slips below a standard set by codes of conduct, then the professional is expected to engage in corrective actions (e.g., seek consultation, take time off, improve skills through training, etc.). This kind of self-correction involves good judgment. The forensic psychologist must decide if the presenting problem is isolated, perhaps due to situational stress, or whether the dysfunction is symptomatic of impairment in self-monitoring and judgment. Fortunately, the Rorschach can be very helpful in the assessment of these important questions.

There is a relatively good fit between the interpretive yield of the cognitive triad cluster of variables in the CS and the kinds of questions posed by these referrals. The RIM presents a novel problem-solving task that is standardized and provides a set of normative data to assess the judgment and decision-making process. In fact, this kind of data is unique to the Rorschach, and is generally recognized as a strength to the test. There is "face validity" to the task. The responses to the test involve the same judgment and thinking that will affect work and are not unique to the test situation. The combined power of the cognitive triad that assess processing, mediation and thinking (e.g., Zd, $X-\%$, $WSum6$) is based on the ability to make predictions of thinking and judgment at work.

A relapsing alcoholic attorney, age 49, was referred for an FFD after a period of absence from work. It is notable that Mr. D. admitted to excessive drinking around the time that he was sent for an evaluation, but his awareness of a problem was low based on other data (interview responses to questions about substance abuse and alcohol use; normal score on the AAS scale of the MMPI–2).

In the review of $FQ-$ answers in a case for Mr. D., one minus response was a "squished liver" in the D9 area of Card X. Although a single Rorschach response is not sufficient in forming a conclusion, this response illustrates how unusual preoccupations can cause underlying distractions and interfere with the professional's judgment process. The sensitivity of the RIM to problems in judgment is particularly useful as Mr. D. had a personality structure that was self-protective as opposed to self-critical ($K = 60$ on the MMPI–2). His Structural Summary ($R = 34$) indicated significant problems with mediation ($X–\% = 38$, $XA\% = 62$, $WDA\% = 69$). Mr. D. also had difficulties in processing information and was likely to make hasty, underincorporative efforts at processing ($Zd = -5.5$), although he was average in his ability to synthesize information ($DQ+ = 8$). Within the ideation cluster, the special scores were elevated ($WSum6 = 14$), including one *Level 2 Special Score*. His thinking problems were fairly well compensated during the interview, but the lack of coherence to his thinking could be expected to affect decision making on the job. These liabilities on the cognitive triad were occurring in a person with an introversive style. The normal process of deliberation and delay was being influenced by distortions introduced by his problems with mediation (of the seven M responses, three had minus form quality).

The FFD evaluation requires determining what if any situational factors might be producing distress and behavioral problems. During the FFD interview, the employee is presented with a listing of 18 common life events (e.g., births, deaths, marriage, divorce) that may have happened during the previous 2 years. The employees are asked to endorse relevant events, and discuss their impact on them. Mr. D. listed major changes in the health of his mother that was not a significant source of stress. He also listed the fact that his job security was threatened, in part because he has been critical of his supervisor. Fortunately, the CS provides an empirical basis for determining the nature and severity of situationally based stress. The structural summary showed that $EA = 9.5$, $D = 0$, and $AdjD = 0$, which indicated that he was capable managing the "slings and arrows" of life.

The CS data provided clear evidence linking the history to impairments in the ability to use good judgment on the job and monitor his performance. It was unlikely that he would get treatment for his alcohol relapse, because he was not distressed and he was not aware that he had a problem with drinking. He was considered unfit for full duty pending the evaluation and treatment from the distressed attorney program.

Test Taking Attitude in FFD

APA standards for testing in forensic work specified that "a thorough knowledge of response set and its influence on test results may be needed for accurate interpretation of results" (Turner et al., 2001, p. 1110). Exaggerated responding and defensiveness are quite common in FFD, although malingered profiles are rare. The literature shows some evidence of guarded MMPI profiles that were administered as part of FFD. The Ganellen (1994) study of airline pilots who wanted to return to work after treatment for alcoholism found high scores on the K scale (average $T = 65$). Interestingly, the Rorschach was found to bypass the defensiveness of the pilots, although how that data was used to make a determination of fitness for duty was not addressed in the study. Grossman, Haywood, Ostrov, Wasyliw, and Cavanaugh (1990) studied police officers and found that motivation to work influenced MMPI validity scale data such that F

scales were elevated for officers who claimed to be disabled while those who wanted to be cleared were guarded.

Table 15–1 presents data from 135 employees who were administered the RIM as part of the FFD. The data indicates that R was in the low average range for both those who were claiming to be disabled and those who wanted to be cleared. A substantial 30% of both groups of employees produced low R records ($14 \leq R < 17$). Low R records are not to be expected, occurring in 6% of the new nonpatient norm group. These data indicate that an extra level of censoring is common for FFD. It was common that these subjects gave less than 14 answers and needed the test re-administered. This technique worked in every case but once, but almost always the second administration yielded a low R protocol. Other data in Table 15–1 (*Lambda*, *DQ+*, and *Blends*) indicate that FFD subjects avoid the demands associated with the task, tend to be less sophisticated in integrating their responses and are less complex when compared to nonpatient adults. High levels of *Populars* have been associated with defensiveness in other assessment situations (Exner & Erdberg, 2005, p. 443), but $P > 7$ was in the normative range of 18%. However, higher numbers of records with $P < 4$ were found (norm is 4%). This finding gives some insight into the perceptual problems of workers who are sent for a FFD, as these workers fail to pick up obvious cues from the workplace (e.g., not abusing sick leave), which can contribute to problems functioning. In summary, the FFD subject can be guarded and less engaged with the testing task presented by the RIM.

Meyer (1992, 1993) studied the clinical implications of R and found that the *Coping Deficit Index* (*CDI*) was significantly more likely to be positive for low R records. FFD protocols commonly include a positive *CDI*, which could explain problems functioning on the job. However, the confidence in using what we know about the CDI will be improved as research clarifies whether R confounds the interpretation of the CDI.

Table 15–2 provides MMPI–2 data from my FFD database. The elevations on F, $F(b)$, and L indicate that response set influences self-report in FFD. Not surprisingly, worker

TABLE 15–1

Rorschach Data Associated With Response Set in a FFD Sample

Rorschach Variable	Ready to Work (n = 46)	Not Ready to Work (n = 89)
R	20.2 (*SD* = 5.4)	20.7 (SD = 5.4)
14 ≤ R > 17	14 (30%)	27 (30%)
Lambda	.66 (*SD* = .47)	.71 (SD = .67)
Lambda > .99	11 (24%)	15 (17%)
Populars < 4	4 (9%)	12 (13%)
Populars > 7	7 (14%)	15 (16%)
Blends	3.5 (*SD* = 2.2)	3.9 (2.5)
DQ+	6.0 (*SD* = 2.9)	6.6 (3.6)

Note. Rate re-rate reliability for determinants = 82%; Blends = 86%; DQ = 81%; Populars = 93% based on 10 protocols that were re-scored.

TABLE 15–2

MMPI–2 Measures of Response Sets in a FFD Sample

MMPI–2 Scale	Full Sample $(n = 237)$[a]		Ready to Work $(n = 107)$		Not Ready to Work $(n = 130)$	
	M	SD	M	SD	M	SD
VRIN	50.5	10.2	48.1	10.3	52.6	9.7
TRIN	57.5	6.9	57.8	6.7	57.2	7.1
F	57.5	17.1	49.4	10.3	64.1	18.8
F(b)	58.2	20.3	50.8	12.7	64.5	23.2
L	57.0	11.1	57.9	10.3	56.2	11.7
K	51.5	11.2	54.8	11.3	48.8	10.3

Note. Differences between the Ready to Work and Not Ready to Work groups were significant ($p < .001$) except for TRIN and L.
[a]$N = 215$ for VRIN and TRIN.

attitudes about returning to work play a role in whether problems on the MMPI–2 are over or underreported. Those who do not want to return to work exaggerate self-reports; this is consistent with Rogers's (1990, 1997) work on malingering, and his interview protocol (SIRS) uses unusual symptom reporting as a marker for malingering. This response set is readily detectable in the interview using open-ended questions. Those subjects who want to be cleared are significantly more defensive on the K scale of the MMPI–2. The validity scales of the MMPI–2 also show a pervasive tendency to conceal more than reveal as a response attitude. Regardless of motivation to return to work, the average FFD subject endorses 5–6 L scale items compared to the 3–4 L scale items which is normative.

These findings have practical implications for the use of testing in FFD work. Before administering a test, use techniques to prepare the subject. Expect the RIM to threaten the subject and using calming responses to defensive verbalizations during the beginning of the test. Respond to uncooperative subjects without expressing annoyance (e.g., saying "people see more than 1 thing" at Card I in a way that communicates a challenge but not disrespect). When less than 14 responses are given, respond with calm conveying a "this happens all the time" attitude. Re-administering the MMPI–2 when K or L are highly elevated often will produce valid profiles, particularly when a supportively educational approach is used as opposed to a punitive manner. Card rejections are infrequent in FFD (about 5%). They are as unusual as excessive item omissions (>10) on the MMPI–2 (which occurs 3% in the FFD database). Ask that the cards be given to you instead of being placed on the desk. In this way, the card is not accepted until a response has been made. After single responses to the cards, use the recommended extra prompting at Card IV, saying "Would you look some more" in a slightly deferential as opposed to demanding manner. It is wise to keep in mind that the RIM is a challenging test for most persons.

In summary, motivation to return to work is easily assessed by interview and is likely to influence test taking attitude. The MMPI–2 validity scales indicate that employees who want to be cleared will underreport and those who claimed to be disabled and unable to work will overreport problems. The RIM can bypass problems with these response sets, but not always. Guarded responses to the RIM are common in FFD, so the examiner should take the time to prepare the subject and use a calm tone and facilitative verbal responses to signs of defensiveness during the test.

CONCLUSIONS

The ADA has empowered workers to expect a fair and unbiased assessment of their difficulties functioning on the job. This will invariably include an objective determination as to whether the employee is disabled by a psychological disorder (as defined by ADA and clarified by the Supreme Court). The data in the report should logically lead the reader to understand whether or not the work problems are caused by an ADA disability. The FFD also provides information about what accommodations should be made available to the employee, if the individual is qualified but unable to perform the job because of the disability. The report concludes with a statement indicating that the employee is cleared (or not) for full duty. The assessment process typically involves an interview, often requires psychological testing, and sometimes involves gathering collateral sources of data. The Comprehensive System from the RIM enables the forensic psychological evaluator to describe the employee as a person with resources and vulnerability. This assessment approach is a good fit with the individualized approach to evaluating a disability according to ADA standards.

ACKNOWLEDGMENTS

The long and rewarding association with Gawin Flynn is greatly acknowledged. William Alexy gave helpful comments; Robert Dies provided incisive comments on the entire chapter; Barton Evans and Carl Gacono provided encouragement and practical help; Lew Schlosser and James Kleiger helped on the reliability study; Clara Hill gave me invaluable help.

REFERENCES

Albertsons, Inc. v. Kirkingburg, 527 U.S. 555, 119 S. Ct. 2162 (1999).
American Medical Association. (2001). *Guides to the evaluation of permanent impairment* (5th ed.). Chicago: American Medical Association.
Americans With Disabilities Act of 1990, 42 U.S.C.A. §12101 *et seq.* (West, 1992).
Bartlett v. New York State Bd. of Law Examiners, 156 F.3d 321 (2d Cir. 1998).
Breger, S. H. (1997). *Establishing a forensic psychiatric practice.* New York: Norton.
Exner, J. E. (2000). *A primer for Rorschach interpretation.* Asheville, NC: Rorschach Workshops.
Exner, J. E. (2003). *The Rorschach: A Comprehensive System* (Vol. 1, 4th ed.). New York: Wiley.
Exner, J. E., & Erdberg, P. (2005). *The Rorschach: A Comprehensive System.* (Vol. 2, 3rd ed.). New York: Wiley.
Foote, W. E. (2000). A model for consultation in cases involving the Americans With Disabilities Act. *Professional Psychology: Research and Practice, 31,* 190–196.
Gacono, C. B., Meloy, R., & Heaven, T. (1990). A Rorschach investigation of narcissism and hysteria in antisocial personality disorder. *Journal of Personality Assessment, 55,* 270–279.

Ganellen, R. J. (1994). Attempting to conceal psychological disturbance: MMPI defensive response sets and the Rorschach. *Journal of Personality Assessment, 63,* 423–437.

Goodman-Delahunty, J. (2000). Psychological impairment under the Americans With Disabilities Act: Legal guidelines. *Professional Psychology: Research and Practice, 31,* 197–205.

Greenberg, S. A., & Shuman, D. W. (1997). Irreconcilable conflict between Therapeutic and forensic roles. *Professional Psychology: Research and Practice, 28,* 50–57.

Grossman, L. S., Haywood, T. W., Ostrov, E., Wasyliw, O., & Cavanaugh, J. L. (1990). Sensitivity of MMPI validity scales to motivational factors in psychological evaluations of police officers. *Journal of Personality Assessment, 55,* 549–561.

Grossman, L. S., Wasyliw, O. E., Benn, A. F., & Gyoerkoe, K. L. (2002). Can sex offenders who minimize on the MMPI conceal psychopathology on the Rorschach? *Journal of Personality Assessment, 78,* 484–501.

Hamilton v. Southwestern Bell Telephone Co., 136 F.3d 1047 (5th Cir. 1998).

Hartmann, E., Wang, C. E., Berg, M., & Saether, L. (2003). Depression and vulnerability as assessed by the Rorschach method. *Journal of Personality Assessment, 81,* 242–255.

Houlihan, J. P., & Reynolds, M. D. (2001). Assessment of employees with mental health disabilities for workplace accommodations: Case reports. *Professional Psychology: Research and Practice, 32,* 380–385.

Levine, M. L. (1987). *Developmental variation and learning disorders.* Cambridge, MA: Educators Publishing Service.

Meyer, G. J. (1992). Response frequency problems in the Rorschach: Clinical and research implications with suggestions for the future. *Journal of Personality Assessment, 58,* 231–244.

Meyer, G. J. (1993). The impact of response frequency on the Rorschach constellation indices and on their validity with diagnostic and MMPI–2 criteria. *Journal of Personality Assessment, 60,* 153–180.

Morrison, J. (1995). *The first interview.* New York: Guilford.

Murphy v. United Parcel Service, Inc., 527 U.S. 516, 119 S. Ct. 2133 (1999).

Rogers, R. (1990). Models of feigned mental illness. *Professional Psychology: Research and Practice, 21,* 182–188.

Rogers, R. (1997). *Clinical assessment of malingering and deception.* New York: Guilford.

Ruiz, M. A., Drake, E. B., Glass, A., Marcotte, D., & van Gorp, W. G. (2002). Trying to beat the system Misuse of the internet to assist in avoiding Detection of psychological symptom dissimulation. *Professional Psychology: Research and Practice, 33,* 294–299.

Scheid, T. L. (1999). Employment of individuals with mental disabilities: Business response to the ADA's challenge. *Behavioral Sciences and the Law, 17,* 73–91.

Sutton v. United Air Lines, Inc., 527 U.S. 471, 119 S. Ct. 2139 (1999).

Turner, S. M., DeMers, S., Fox, H. R., & Reed, G. M. (2001). APA's Guidelines for test user qualifications. *American Psychologist, 56,* 1099–1113.

Weiner, I. B. (1995). How to anticipate ethical and legal challenges in personality assessments. In J. N. Butcher (Ed.), *Clinical personality assessment: Practical approaches* (pp. 95–103). New York: Oxford University Press.

Zelig, M. (2001, August). *A forensic approach to fitness for duty evaluations.* Workshop presented for the American Psychological Association.

III

FORENSIC REFERENCE GROUPS

"In God we trust; All others must have data."

Martin Orne, M.D.

16

THE RORSCHACH AND ANTISOCIAL PERSONALITY DISORDER

Carl B. Gacono

Private Practice, Austin, TX

Lynne A. Gacono

Austin State Hospital, Austin, TX

F. Barton Evans

Private Practice, Bozeman, MT

Lindner (1943) pioneered the use of the Rorschach (Rorschach, 1942) with antisocial and psychopathic personalities. Along with others (i.e., Samuel Beck), Lindner believed that the Rorschach might prove uniquely useful in understanding these disorders. He hypothesized that at least one group of psychopaths produced recognizable, and to a degree unmistakable, Rorschach protocols, characterized by superficiality, avoidance, explosiveness, incompleteness, and egocentricity. Lindner's attempts to test his beliefs were frustrated, due primarily to difficulties assessing psychopathy and the state of Rorschach technology (in the 1940s and 1950s). Lindner's untimely death on February 27, 1956, at age 41, deprived the psychological community of a first-rate researcher and prevented him from fully testing his clinical observations.

Since Lindner's time, several advances in psychology have made a scientifically sound Rorschach study of antisocial and psychopathic personalities possible. First, the work of Hare and his colleagues (Hare, 2003) has resulted in the development of a reliable and valid method (Hare Psychopathy Checklist–Revised; PCL–R) for assessing psychopathy (Bodholdt, Richards, & Gacono, 2000; Gacono, Loving, Evans, & Jumes, 2002). Second, the development of the Comprehensive System (Exner, 1986, 2003) and advances in scoring defenses (Cooper & Arnow, 1986; Lerner & Lerner, 1980) and object relations (Kwawer, 1980) have given the researcher reliable and valid Rorschach measures. Third, the advent of computer technology has allowed the thoughtful analysis of large-sample data. Finally, developments in ego psychology and object relations theory have furthered our understanding of psychopathy by cogently conceptualizing the disorder's underlying intrapsychic and interpersonal personality organization. In particular, Kernberg's (1975) conceptualization of Antisocial Personality Disorder as a detached, pathological, aggressive, variant of Narcissistic Personality Disorder organized at a borderline level of personality has formed the theoretical basis of both theoretical and empirical work (Gacono, 1988, 1990; Meloy, 1988).

Utilizing these advances, Gacono and Meloy conducted a series of studies (Gacono, 1988, 1990; Gacono & Meloy, 1991, 1992; Gacono, Meloy, & Heaven, 1990; Meloy & Gacono, 1992), culminating in *The Rorschach Assessment of Aggressive and Psychopathic Personalities* (Gacono & Meloy, 1994), to explore the theories of Lindner and Kernberg. This work included chapters on significant Rorschach indicators for antisocial and psychopathic personality such as the Reflection response and Aggression scores, as well as Rorschach group data for Conduct Disordered children (CD; $N = 60$), CD adolescents ($N = 100$), Antisocial Personality Disordered females (ASPD; $N = 38$), ASPD males ($N = 82$), ASPD Schizophrenics ($N = 80$), psychopathic males ($N = 33$) and Sexual Homicide Perpetrators ($N = 20$). While adding empirical support to Lindner's and Kernberg's theories, the Gacono and Meloy research also provided a model for the Rorschach assessment and investigation of other personality disorders. As Erdberg (in Gacono & Meloy, 1994, p. xii) noted, "We hope that this book is the first of many in which clinical researchers use sophisticated assessment and theory to bring the sort of clarity to other syndromes." Unfortunately, to date, Gacono and Meloy's (1994) text remains the only thorough Rorschach investigation of a single personality disorder.

In all likelihood, when Meloy jokingly wrote, "Our work becomes the compulsive person's dream (JRM) or nightmare (CBG): It has just begun, or will it ever end?" (Gacono & Meloy, 1994, p. 9), he never envisioned that 10 years later, Rorschach data would continue to be added to the original forensic reference samples.[1] This chapter utilizes these expanded Rorschach data sets in providing a Rorschach understanding of Antisocial Personality Disordered and psychopathic individuals.

THE INDEPENDENT MEASURES: ANTISOCIAL PERSONALITY DISORDER AND PSYCHOPATHY

Two points are essential for understanding the use of the Rorschach in studying the *DSM* personality disorders. First, although personality disorders are currently coded as discrete categories in the *DSM–IV* (American Psychiatric Association, 1994), in reality there is considerable overlap (e.g., Gunderson & Ronningstam, 2001; Morey, 1988; Plakun, Muller, & Burkhardt, 1987). For example, paranoid persons and compulsive persons share similarities in cognitive style; narcissistic and paranoid individuals share a certain amount of grandiosity; and hysteric and narcissistic people share a need for attention. Whereas these disorders share dimensional attributes, subtle motivations underlying each personality disorder differ in important ways. Both paranoid and compulsive individuals' cognitive style includes high attention to detail, but the paranoid focuses on details to avoid anticipated interpersonal attack and the compulsive does so to avoid making mistakes, thus avoiding humiliation. This overlap must be con-

---

[1]Carl and Lynne Gacono continue to update samples.

sidered when predicting Rorschach differences between groups. For example, Gacono, Meloy, and Bridges (2000) predicted and found similar frequencies of reflections among Sexual Homicide Perpetrators, psychopaths, and Pedophiles. Rather than viewing these Rorschach variables as equivalent to a diagnosis of psychopathy, they were conceptualized as an indication of a dimensional personality trait (narcissism).

Second, each one of the personality disorder classifications includes a certain amount of heterogeneity; that is, each contains potentially identifiable subgroups. This heterogeneity is most evident when examining extremes within a given category, such as the differences between an ASPD patient with a concurrent Avoidant Personality Disorder, contrasted to an ASPD patient with a Narcissistic Personality Disorder. Consequently, the conceptually sophisticated personality disorder researcher must utilize additional *independent* measures (well beyond using the presence or absence of the disorder) when studying personality disorders. Without a doubt, the ancillary construct most relevant to studying Antisocial Personality Disorder is psychopathy.

It is important to emphasize that psychopathy is not synonymous with Antisocial Personality Disorder (Gacono & Meloy, 2002). Antisocial Personality Disorder (ASPD; *DSM–IV*; APA, 1994) evolved from a social deviancy model (Robins, 1966) and the concept of sociopathy (*DSM*; APA, 1952), with its criteria being primarily behavioral (i.e., one primary factor model). Appearing in the first *DSM* (APA, 1952), sociopathy included a variety of conditions such as sexual deviation, alcoholism, and "dissocial" and "antisocial" reactions. Whereas only the antisocial reaction was similar to psychopathy, the replacement of "Sociopathy" with ASPD in *DSM–II* (APA, 1968), and the increased focus on behavioral criteria, would widen the gap between ASPD and psychopathy.

"Psychopathy" originated from Cleckley's (1976) traditional psychiatric conceptualization that included a combination of personality traits and behaviors (two-factor model; see Table 16–1). From a *DSM–IV* perspective, psychopathy can be understood as a disorder comprised of selected behavioral and affective features of several Cluster B syndromes, including Narcissistic, Histrionic, and Borderline Personality Disorders (Gacono, Nieberding, Owen, Rubel, & Bodholdt, 2001).

Several caveats spring from psychopathy's two-factor structure versus the single factor associated with ASPD (Gacono, Loving, & Bodholdt, 2001). First, whereas one can arrive at the ASPD diagnosis by a virtually unlimited number of criteria combinations,[2] so that vastly different individuals are categorized under the umbrella of this single diagnosis, psychopathy constitutes a more homogeneous syndrome. As a result, base rates for ASPD and psychopathy are significantly different. Whereas ASPD community rates are estimated at 5.8 % of males and 1.2% of females, forensic populations will typically have rates of 50% to 80%. Psychopaths will comprise only 15% to 25% of the same forensic population. Finally, in terms of predictive validity, psychopathy assessment has important clinical and forensic implications (Gacono & Bodholdt, 2001). High PCL or PCL–R

---

[2]The possible variations in APSD diagnoses for *DSM–III* and *DSM–III–R* combined at roughly 27 trillion; the *DSM–IV* offers 3.2 million variations (Rogers, Salekin, Sewell, & Cruise, 2000). The CD (APA, 1994) diagnosis also encompasses a heterogeneous group of children and adolescents with community base rates estimated at 3% to 5% of school age children (*Male to Female Ratio* = 4:1–9:1).

TABLE 16–1

Diagnostic Criteria for DSM-IV Antisocial Personality Disorder and Psychopathy

DSM-IV Antisocial Personality Disorder

A. At least 3 of the following since age 15:

1. Arrestable Acts	4. Fights and Assaults	7. Lacks remorse
2. Lies	5. Reckless	
3. Impulsive	6. Irresponsible	

B. Current age at least 18

C. Conduct disorder, onset before 15

D. Antisocial behavior not exclusively during Schizophrenia or Manic Episode.

Psychopathic Traits and Behaviors (Hare, 1980; Hare et al., 1990)

(1) *Glibness/superficial charm

(2) *Grandiose sense of self worth

(3) Need for stimulation/proneness to boredom

(4) *Pathological lying

(5) *Conning/manipulative

(6) *Lack of remorse or guilt

(7) *Shallow affect

(8) *Callous/lack of empathy

(9) Parasitic lifestyle

(10) Poor behavioral controls

(11) Promiscuous sexual behavior

(12) Early behavioral problems

(13) Lack of realistic, long-term goals

(14) Impulsivity

(15) Irresponsibility

(16) *Failure to accept responsibility for own actions

(17) Many short-term marital relationships

(18) Juvenile delinquency

(19) Revocation of conditional release

(20) Criminal versatility

scores have been associated with higher frequency and wider variety of offenses committed (Hare, 2003); higher frequency of violent offenses (Hare, 2003); higher re-offense rates (Hare, 2003); poor treatment response (Ogloff, Wong, & Greenwood, 1990; Rice, Harris, & Cormier, 1992); and more serious and persistent institutional misbehavior (Gacono, Meloy, Sheppard, Speth, & Roske, 1995; Gacono, Meloy, Speth, & Roske,

1997; Heilbrun et al., 1998). The ASPD diagnosis is not associated with these same outcomes (Lyon & Ogloff, 2000).

Equally important for understanding the role of psychopathy in studying ASPD is the fact that it can be conceptualized both in dimensional (i.e., along a continuum of severity) and categorical terms (i.e., as a taxon or discrete syndrome). When concerned with how psychopaths nomothetically differ from nonpsychopaths, the researcher is using psychopathy as a category or taxon and should use the appropriate PCL–R cutoff (as a group, PCL–R ≥ 30 for psychopathy). Whenever possible, independent measures for the forensic samples discussed in this chapter include both a *DSM* diagnosis (Character Disorder or ASPD) and the presence or absence of a psychopathic disturbance (PCL–R ≥ 30).

Previous Rorschach Findings

In their original studies, Gacono and Meloy sought to answer several questions (Gacono & Meloy, 1994, 1997b; Meloy & Gacono, 1998):

1. Would the Rorschach empirically validate Kernberg's (1975) psychoanalytic constructs associated with psychopathy? Kernberg hypothesized that the psychopath was a detached, aggressive variant of Narcissistic Personality Disorder organized at a borderline level of personality functioning?
2. Given the behavioral differences among offenders, as noted by Lindner (1943), could the Rorschach discriminate among ASPD groups by psychopathy level?
3. Could the Rorschach also discriminate between ASPD and other Cluster B Personality Disorders?

What follows is a summary of their findings.

Borderline Personality Organization. Gacono (1988, 1990) compared the object relations and defensive operations of 14 psychopathic Antisocial Personality Disordered subjects (P–ASPD; PCL–R ≥ 30) and 19 nonpsychopathic Antisocial Personality Disordered subjects (NP–ASPD; PCL–R < 30). Although specific defenses generally failed to differentiate between the groups, this study did find that ASPDs as a group relied on devaluation, primitive denial (Lerner & Lerner, 1980), splitting, projective identification, and devaluation (Cooper & Arnow, 1986). The presence of these primitive defenses, along with the notable absence of neurotic level defenses and idealization (Lerner & Lerner, 1980), combined with a plethora of borderline object relations (Kwawer, 1980), supported the hypothesis of a common borderline level of functioning for ASPD subjects (see also Gacono & Meloy, 1992, 1997b).

Surprisingly, Kwawer's (1980) primitive (borderline) modes of interpersonal relating were produced in a proportionally greater amount ($p < .01$) by the P–ASPD group. Finding significant between group differences was "surprising" as the majority of these ASPD subjects produced PCL–R scores greater than 20. A randomly obtained prison population would be more diverse (psychopathy level), including non-ASPD subjects and low scoring PCL–R subjects. When studying offenders, expanding the range of psychopathy scores (including non-ASPD subjects) allows for the creation of more dissimi-lar groups (psychopaths, PCL–R ≥ 30, and low scorers, PCL–R < 20), thereby increasing the probability of obtaining significant between group differences.

Pathological Narcissism.   Gacono et al. (1990) examined the relationship between psychopathy, pathological narcissism (Harpur, Hare, & Hakstian, 1989; Kernberg, 1975) and hysteria (Guze, 1976; Guze, Woodruff, & Clayton, 1971). Twenty-one P–ASPD subjects were compared to 21 NP–ASPD subjects on the relevant Exner Com-prehensive System (1986) measures of *Pair* (2), *Reflection* (*rF*, *Fr*), *Personal Re-sponses* (*PER*), and *Egocentricity Index* (*3r+[2]/R*).[3] The *Impressionistic Response*[4] (*IMP*; Gacono, 1988, 1990) was used as a measure of hysterical mechanisms (Shapiro, 1965). The mean number of *Pair* and *Impressionistic Responses* did not significantly differ between the two Antisocial groups. P–ASPDs did exhibit a significantly greater mean number of *Reflections* ($p < .05$) and *Personal Responses* ($p < .05$). The *Egocen-tricity Index* scores were also significantly different ($p < .01$) with P–ASPDs producing much larger ratios (*M* = .46, *SD* = .18), along with increased *Reflections* and *Personal Responses*, than the NP–ASPDs (*M* = .30, *SD* = .14). These differences supported the hypothesis of greater pathological narcissism in P–ASPDs as compared to NP–ASPD, who demonstrated abnormally low self focus. The low *Egocentricity Ratios* produced by the NP–ASPDs suggested, "a reduced effectiveness for bolstering grandiosity and warding off the disruptive effects of internal (anxiety) and external (incarceration) threat. The internal regulating mechanisms of the severe psychopath are less tenuous" (Gacono et al., 1990, pp. 275–276).

In two related studies with adolescents, Loving and Russell (2000) found that psycho-paths were more likely to have produced a *Reflection* response than nonpsychopaths; and, although Smith, Gacono, and Kaufman (1997) failed to replicate a significant differ-ence for *PER*s and *Reflections*, they did discover that a significantly greater number of psychopathic Conduct Disordered youths (P–CDs) produced *Egocentricity Ratios* greater than .54 (P–CDs = 42%; NP–CDs = 9%). It should be noted that the Smith et al. (1997) sample contained predominately high *Lambda* subjects, which can impact the production of certain Rorschach variables such as *Reflections* (Bannatyne, Gacono, & Greene, 1999).

Attachment Deficits.   Detachment is another characteristic of psychopathy (Cleckley, 1976; Meloy, 1988). Through a comparison of Rorschach Comprehensive System variables of *Texture* (*T*, *TF*, *FT*), *Diffuse Shading* (*Y*, *YF*, *FY*), *Vista* (*V*, *VF*, *FV*),

---

[3]Meloy (1988) hypothesized that the combination of *Pairs* and *Reflections* represented an empirical measure of the grandiose self-structure in psychopaths.

[4]The *Impressionistic Response* (*IMP*; Gacono, 1988, 1990; Gacono et al., 1990), derived from Shapiro's (1965) hysterical personality's "impressionistic" cognitive style, identifies associations to the blot stimulated by color that contain abstract concepts or events (Gacono et al., 1990). It is coded by scoring achromatic (including shading) or chromatic color and an *Abstraction* (*AB*). *IMP* responses may be "sensitive indicator[s] of the degree to which cer-tain patients organized at a borderline level split off affect into rapid and diffuse symbolization" (Gacono, Meloy, & Berg, 1992, p. 45).

D scores (D) and *Adjusted D* scores (*AdjD*) between P–ASPDs ($N = 21$) and NP–ASPDs ($N = 21$), Gacono and Meloy (1991) investigated Rorschach manifestations of attachment and anxiety. *Vista* frequencies did not differ significantly between the groups. As expected, *Texture* ($p < .01$) and *Shading* ($p < .001$) frequencies were significantly less in the P–ASPDs than the NP–ASPDs. Additionally, although not reaching significance, important trends were noted with D and *AdjD*, with NP–ASPDs results suggesting more situational and chronic levels of stress, and P–ASPDs indicating that their chaotic life styles were more ego-syntonic.

The somewhat surprising presence of *Vista* in psychopaths was interpreted as representing failed grandiosity (*Fr, rF, r*) and perhaps self-pity (Gacono & Meloy, 1991), rather than representing guilt and remorse. Lower amounts of *Diffuse Shading* in the P–ASPDs, coupled with the normal D and *AdjD* score patterns suggested an absence of anxiety and helplessness, whereas the lower *Egocentricity Ratios* for NP–ASPDs pointed to the tenuous nature or vulnerability of the grandiose self structure in nonpsychopaths. A troubling implication of these findings was that the psychopaths' particular form of character pathology seemed to be effective in regulating their self-structure and narcissism, thus reducing anxiety and conflict about their antisocial behavior.

The virtual absence of T in the P–ASPD sample (5% vs. 82% in Exner's nonpatient adult normative group) empirically supported the hypothesis of profound detachment clinically observed in psychopaths (Gacono & Meloy, 1997a). Three related studies with adolescents added to these findings. Weber, Meloy, and Gacono (1992) compared inpatient CD to Dysthymic and nonpatient adolescents finding that CD subjects evidenced less attachment capacity (71%, $T = 0$), were less anxious (48%, $Y = 0$), and showed less interest in others as whole and real human objects (33%, *Pure H* = 0) than the other groups. Smith et al. (1997) found similar results supporting the Gacono and Meloy (1991) study, with P–CD adolescents (P–CD; 79%, $T = 0$; 75%, $Y = 0$). Further, Loving and Russell (2000) found that T differentiated among CD groups—psychopaths produced the lowest frequency.

Related studies with adults found that Antisocial females were less likely to produce T ($T > 1 = 29\%$) than Borderline females ($T > 1 = 100\%$; Berg, Gacono, Meloy & Peaslee, 1994) and that P–ASPDs evidenced less attachment capacity (T) and experienced less anxiety (Y) than NP–ASPDs, Narcissistic (NPD) or Borderline Personality Disordered males (BPD) (Gacono et al., 1992). In summary, there was significant evidence of attachment deficits in this population as CD and ASPD subjects rarely produce *Texture* responses, the empirically sturdy Comprehensive System (CS) variable related to attachment ($T = 0$ found in 88% of CD children, 86% of CD adolescents, 71% of ASPD females, and 91% of psychopathic males; Gacono & Meloy, 1994). Findings for Y, CS variable associated with helplessness, were equivocal ($Y > 1$, CD children = 27%; CD adolescents = 33%; ASPD females = 50%; P–ASPDs = 54%), but consistent with acting out as a defense against anxiety.

Aggression.   Aggression plays a crucial role in the development and functioning of both Conduct and Antisocial Personality Disorder and has been identified as a discriminating variable between the psychopathic and narcissistic disorders (Kernberg, 1975;

Meloy, 1988). Based on their observations, Gacono (1988) and Heaven (1988) realized the limitations of the Exner (1986) *Aggressive Movement* response (*AG*) for capturing the range and intensity of aggressive drive derivatives produced by ASPD subjects on the Rorschach. Interestingly, and counter to expectations, CD and ASPD samples uniformly produce less *AG* than nonpatients (Gacono, 1997; Gacono, Gacono, Meloy, & Baity, 2005; Smith et al., 1997), strongly suggesting the *Aggressive Movement* variable is not a reliable measure of aggressive behavior.

On closer scrutiny, despite the paucity of *AG* responses in ASPD records, other aggression imagery and aggressive manifestation were produced. The presence of other potentially scoreable aggressive imagery (see Gacono, 1988, 1990; Gacono, 1997) led to the development (Gacono, 1988) and refinement (Gacono & Meloy, 1994; Meloy & Gacono, 1992) of five additional scoring categories: *Aggressive Content* (*AgC*), *Aggressive Past* (*AgPast*), *Aggressive Potential* (*AgPot*), *Aggressive Vulnerability* (*AgV*), and *Sado-Masochism* (*SM*) (see Gacono, Bannatyne- Gacono, Meloy, & Baity, 2005; chap. 26, this vol.).

In Meloy and Gacono (1992) these experimental aggression scores, were compared between P–APSDs (*N* = 22) and NP–ASPDs (*N* = 21). Only the *SM* response appeared significantly more frequently in the psychopaths (*p* < .05), a finding that was consistent with the higher incidents of instrumental violence toward strangers associated with psychopaths (Hare, 2003). Although Meloy (1988) initially speculated about the presence of active censoring of *AG* in ASPD subjects, Gacono et al. (2005) believe that the ego-syntonic nature of the aggressive impulse and a pattern of acting out aggression for ASPDs contribute to its absence on the Rorschach. Although essential for understanding the psychology of aggressive patients, these scores warrant further study (Gacono et al., 2005).

Comparing ASPD With Other Cluster B Personality Disorders

The findings of Gacono, Meloy, and their colleagues supported Lindner's (1943) hypotheses concerning the usefulness of the Rorschach for understanding psychopathy and ASPD and were consistent with Kernberg's formulations of Antisocial Personality. Patterns emerged that were able to differentiate groups of P–ASPDs from NP–ASPDs. Although these findings were by no means conclusive, they did demonstrate the usefulness of the Rorschach in studying dimensional aspects of Antisocial and psychopathic personalities.

Gacono and Meloy next turned their attention to conducting comparative studies of ASPD with nonoffending clinical groups. Could the Rorschach elucidate the nuances that differentiate similar personality disordered groups? In order to test this hypothesis, Gacono et al. (1992) chose as comparison subjects to the P-ASPDs (N = 22). Groups of outpatient Narcissistic (*N* = 18) and Borderline (*N* = 18) Personality Disorders[5] which were similar.

Important differences and similarities between these groups emerged. Whereas both P–ASPDs and NPDs were highly narcissistic (elevated *Reflection* responses and *Egocentricity Index*), compared to P–ASPDs, NPDs were more anxious (*Y*, *YF*, *FY*), evi-

---

[5]Unfortunately, there was no sample of Histrionic Personality Disordered patients to study.

denced greater attachment capacity (*Sum T*), and produced fewer borderline object relations (Kwawer, 1980) and damaged content scores (*MOR, AgPast*). Also, BPDs were less narcissistic than P–ASPDs and NPDs, and BPDs showed equal numbers of borderline object relations scores (Kwawer, 1980) with P–ASPD subjects. BPD individuals were more anxious, produced more unsublimated aggressive (*AG*) and libidinal (*Sx*) material, and evidenced greater potential for attachment (*T*) than P–ASPDs. NP–ASPDs showed less Borderline Personality functioning than P–ASPDs or BPDs, were less narcissistic than NPD and P–ASPDs, produced less evidence of attachment capacity than the outpatient groups (although more than P–ASPDs), and were similar to BPDs in their proneness to anxiety. Consistent with Lerner's (1991) schema, the NPDs and BPDs also produced more idealization responses than the ASPDs. This difference was consistent with the outpatient subjects' capacity for forming pseudo-sublimatory channels (evident in their interpersonal attachments and a work career).

In comparing ASPD females (*N* = 38) with BPD females (*N* = 32), Berg et al. (1994) found

> both groups [to be] significantly psychopathologic when affect states, object relations, and perceptual accuracy are measured. The damage, dysphoria, and anxiety of both groups is only distinguished by the borderline females' capacity to bond (*T*) and a greater amount of affect (*CF* > BPD), positive treatment indicators that also portend a tumultuous tie to the psychotherapist. Object relations will be pre-oedipal in both groups, but much more apparent in the Borderline female. Symbiotic rather than autistic developmental themes are likely (Mahler, Pine & Bergman, 1975). Both groups will be characterologically rigid, self-absorbed, and likely to express a narcissistic sense of entitlement: the Borderline females' wish to be taken care of, the Antisocial female's wish to take. (Berg et al., 1994, pp. 18–19)

Although differences emerged in the females, none were as striking as those when comparing any of the groups to psychopathic Antisocial Personality Disordered males. In conclusion, the CS Rorschach again demonstrates a capacity for assessing subtle, highly nuanced differences in self functions, object relations, and capacity for attachment between seemingly similar, but distinct, personality disorder manifestations. As such, the Rorschach's capacity to do so can significantly add to dimensionally based psychological assessment in both clinical and forensic settings.

The Antisocial Reference Groups

In response to the dearth of normative forensic Rorschach data (CD, ASPD), two decades of Rorschach assessment and research by Gacono, Meloy, and their colleagues (Bannatyne et al., 1999; Cunliffe & Gacono, 2005; Gacono & Meloy, 1992, 1994, 1997; Smith et al., 1997) with Conduct Disordered, Antisocial, and psychopathic subjects has produced the group reference samples of such individuals similar to Exner's other patient and nonpatient groups. These samples, the first forensically oriented CS Rorschach reference data, are especially useful in presenting a cross-sectional look at the Antisocial Personality Disorder and can be considerable value to the forensic assessment psychologist.

The Rorschach forensic database discussed in this chapter is comprised of two primary groups. Group 1 includes nonrandom subjects of convenience selected from various outpatient, jail, prison, hospital, and forensic hospital populations throughout the United States who met criteria for Conduct Disorder (CD) in children and adolescents or ASPD in adults. This data set ($N = 528$) includes: 72 CD children (mostly solitary aggressive type), 179 CD adolescents, 69 ASPD females, 108 ASPD males, and 100 ASPD male Schizophrenics (mostly Paranoid Schizophrenics). These subjects were not intellectually deficient (all IQ estimates equal to or greater than 80) or diagnosed with an Axis I psychotic (with the exception of the ASPD Schizophrenics), clinically depressed, and/or organically impaired.

Group 2 ($N = 304$) includes 38 Sexual Homicide Perpetrators (SHP), 39 nonviolent Pedophiles (PED), as well as Paranoid Schizophrenic ($N = 90$), Schizoaffective ($N = 59$), Bipolar ($N = 40$), and Undifferentiated Schizophrenic ($N = 38$) Conditional Release patients (CONREP). Reliable Axis II diagnoses are unavailable for the majority of the CONREP patients (see also Bannatyne et al., 1999; Nieberding et al., 2003). The nonviolent PEDs were selected from a larger sample who met the *DSM* criteria for Pedophilia ($N = 60$; Bridges, Wilson, & Gacono, 1998). All nonviolent PEDs subjects' IQs were equal to or greater than 80, and none were psychotic, organic, diagnosed with depression, or met criteria for ASPD or psychopathy (Gacono et al., 2000; Huprich, Gacono, Schneider, & Bridges, 2003). SHPs were gathered in the same manner as Group 1 subjects. None of the SHPs were psychotic at the time of testing. In order to be included in this sample, an individual had to commit at least one sexual homicide (Gacono et al., 2000). The majority of the SHPs met the criteria for ASPD, and approximately two thirds scored ≥ 30 on the PCL–R (see Gacono et al., 2000; Huprich et al., 2003; Meloy, Gacono, & Kenney, 1994).

These 832 forensic Rorschach protocols from Groups 1 and 2 were gathered between 1982 and 2002. Geographically, protocols were obtained from Alaska, California, the District of Columbia, Florida, Illinois, Iowa, Maryland, Massachusetts, North and South Carolina, Virginia, and Wyoming. Rorschachs were administered using the Exner Comprehensive System guidelines (Exner 1991, 1993). Each Rorschach protocol was scored for Comprehensive System variables a minimum of four times each by one of several researchers. All protocols were rescored for reliability by psychologists trained in the Comprehensive System procedures. In all cases, the interjudge reliability (percentage of agreement and kappa coefficients) of our Rorschach scoring was satisfactory (see Gacono et al., 2000). Consistent with Exner's (1993) new Comprehensive System data sets, protocols with fewer than 14 responses (Exner, 1988) were excluded from all the samples (except the SHP sample). In the SHP sample, two low response protocols were deemed valid (low *Lambda*, elevated *Blends*) with less than or equal to 12 responses and were kept in the sample (both psychopaths).[6] Although we will borrow from all the data sets in our discussion, the main focus of this chapter involves samples that contain CD or

---

[6]One psychopathic response style involves a reduction in R without constricting the record. In a grandiose fashion, the psychopath may attempt to produce "perfect" W responses for all 10 cards (Gacono, 1997); or, in a paranoid manner, an increased proportion of Ws result from the need to maintain imaginary control over all perceptual aspects of the blot. This characterological construction can result in a valid < 14 response protocol (caution in interpreting the constellations).

ASPD diagnosed individuals (primarily from Group 1, also including the SHP). Group 2 subjects are discussed in chapter 20 of this volume. The following sections compare the Antisocial reference groups to the appropriate Exner (1995, 2003) Comprehensive System sample. We present our findings as group trends, and they are by no means definitive and are inadequate to capturing the many individual differences that manifest when assessing individual patients.

Conduct-Disordered Children

Core Characteristics.   The CD children (N = 72) were mostly male solitary aggressive type (Table 16–2). Their mean age was 9.7 years of age and comparisons can be reasonably made to Exner's (2003) nonpatient 10-year-old children. The CD children produced responses at a similar frequency as Exner's nonpatient (NP) 10-year-olds (CD, M = 20.35; NP, 20.97). An unusually high percentage of the CD children were *Avoidant* (CD = 63%; NP, 11%); an additional 14% were *Ambitent* (combined 77%). High *Lambdas* (CD, M = 2.16; NP, .49), an aspect of the *Avoidant* style, are consistent with cognitive constriction (Bannatyne et al., 1999) and the CD child's tendency to simplify the stimulus field by ignoring or denying its complexity and/or ambiguity (Exner, 2000). Behaviorally, the high *Lambda* highlights the CD child's limited coping strategies and propensity to act out when overwhelmed, a core characteristic of the "antisocial tendency" noted by Winnicott (1958).

Controls.   The CD child's diminished psychological resources (CD, $EA = M$ = 5.17, SD = 2.92; NP, 8.81) and reduced tolerance for stress (CD, $CDI \geq 4$ = 36%, NP, 15%) underscore their alloplastic adaptation to the environment. Acting out may result in the CD child's lowered levels of experienced stress related distress (CD, $FM + m = M$ = 3.86, $es = M$ = 5.85; NP, 6.6 & 8.45, respectively).

Affect.   Difficulty modulating affect (CD, *Pure C* = M = .57; NP) is a hallmark of Conduct Disorder. These difficulties are reflected in the imbalance of FC to CF (CD; + 2 = 1%, NP, 12%). The internal world of the CD child is characterized by dysphoria (CD, *DEPI* ≥ 5 = 25%; NP, 0%), anger (CD, $S > 2$ = 36%; NP, 12%) and malevolence (Gacono & Meloy, 1994). Affective avoidance (CD: *Aft* < .40 & 50 = 32% & 53%; NP, 2% & 13%) and emotional constriction (CD, *Blends* = 2.04; NP, 5.80) are natural, developmental reactions to an inability to deal with strong affect. This emotional constriction, avoidance, and acting out unfortunately constitutes a coping strategy that follows the CD child into adolescence and beyond.

Thinking and Processing.   CD children do not see the world as others do (CD, *PTI3* $\geq$ = 59%; NP, 0%). They tend to severely underincorporate (CD, $Zd < -.3.0$ = 24%; NP, 16%), missing important details essential to effective information processing. Their thinking contains fluidity, lacking structure and boundaries ($DQv = M$ = 1.82; $DQv > 2$ = 31%). They are prone to misperceptions (See Table 16–2: *XA, WDA, X+, Xu, X–, M–,* and

TABLE 16–2

Conduct Disordered Children (*N* = 72) Group Mean and Frequencies for Select Ratios, Percentages, and Derivations

R = 20.35 (*SD* = 4.92)		*L* = 2.16 (*SD* = 3.24)	

EB: 2.29:2.88   *EA* = 5.17 (*SD* = 2.92)

eb = 3.86 :1.99   *es* = 5.85 (*SD* = 4.00) (*FM* + m < *Sum Shading*............ 14, 19%)

D score = –0.28 (*SD* = 1.19)   *AdjD* = –0.03 (SD = .93)

EB Style

Introversive......................	8	11%
Pervasive Introversive.......	5	7%
Ambitent..........................	10	14%
Extratensive......................	9	13%
Pervasive Extratensive......	7	10%
Avoidant..........................	45	63%

EA–es Differences:D-scores

D score > 0.......................	16	22%
D score = 0.......................	33	46%
D score < 0.......................	23	32%
D score < –1.....................	10	14%
AdjD score > 0.................	18	25%
AdjD score = 0.................	38	53%
AdjD score < 0.................	16	22%
AdjD score < –1.................	4	6%

Affect

FC:CF + *C* = .60 : 2.29

Pure C = .57 (*SD* = 1.00)   (*Pure C* > 0 = 36%; *Pure C* > 1 = 13%)

FC > (*CF* + *C*) + 2.............	1	1%
FC > (*CF* + *C*) + 1.............	3	4%
(*CF* + C) > *FC* + 1...........	35	49%
(*CF* + *C*) > *FC* + 2...........	25	35%

SumC' = 1.14 (*SD* = 1.33)   *Sum V* = .35 (*SD* = .56)   *SumY* = .32 (*SD* = .85)

Afr = .49 (*SD* = .20)   (*Afr* < .40 = 23, 32%; *Afr* < .50 = 38, 53%)

S = 2.11 (*SD* = 1.51)   (*S* > 2 = 26, 36%)

Blends: R = 2.04 : 20.35

CP = .10 (*SD* = .34)

Interpersonal

COP = .67 (*SD* = .89)   (*COP* = 0 = 41, 57%; *COP* > 2 = 3, 4%)

AG = . 60 (*SD* = 1.04)   (*AG* = 0 = 49, 68%; *AG* > 2 = 5, 7%)

Food = .39 (*SD* = 1.01)

Isolate/R = .15 (*SD* = .14)

H:(H)+Hd+(Hd) = 1.82 : 3.04   (*H* = 0 = 15, 21%; *H* < 2 = 34, 47%)

(H)+(Hd):(A)+(Ad) = 1.76 :.96

H + *A:Hd* + *Ad* = 11.01 : 2.67

Sum T = .18 (*SD* = .68)   (*T* = 0 = 64, 89%; *T* > 1 = 2, 3%)

GHR = 2.17 (*SD* = 1.80)

PHR = 3.29 (*SD* = 2.21)   *GHR* > *PHR* = 24, 33%

Self-perception

    $3r + (2)/R = .25$ (*SD* = .16)   ($3r + (2)/R < .33 = 48, 67\%$; $3r + (2)/R > .44 = 6, 8\%$)

    $Fr + rF = .21$ (*SD* = .47)   ($Fr + rF > 0 = 13, 18\%$)

    $FD = .21$ (*SD* = .44)

    $An + Xy = .43$

    MOR = 1.78 (*SD* = 2.35)   (*MOR* > 2 = 15, 21%)

Ideation

    a:p = 4.24 : 1.92   ($p > a + 1 = 5,7\%$)

    Ma:Mp = 1.51 : .78   (*Mp* > *Ma* = 11, 15%)

    M = 2.29 (*SD* = 2.01)   (*M–* = .71, *SD* = 1.16; *M none* = 25%)

    FM = 2.54 (*SD* = 2.03)   *m* = 1.32 (*SD* = 1.74)

    2AB+Art+Ay = .60 (*SD* = .76)   *2AB+Art+Ay* > 5 = 0,0%

    Sum6 = 6.08 (*SD* = 3.74)   *WSum6* = 18.56 (*SD* = 13.46)

    Level 2 Sp Sc = 1.10 (*SD* = 1.86)   (*Level 2 Special scores* > 0 = 35, 49%)

Mediation

    Populars = 3.85 (*SD* = 1.81)   ($P < 4 = 34, 47\%$; $P > 7 = 2, 3\%$)

    XA% = .58 (*SD* = .14)

    WDA% = .61 (*SD* = .14)

    X+% = .37 (*SD* = .12)

    X–% = .39 (*SD* = .13)

    Xu% = .21 (*SD* = .11)

    S– = .89 (*SD* = 1.0)

XA% > .89	0	0%
XA% < .70	57	79%
WDA% < .85	70	97%
WDA% < .75	61	85%
X+% < .55	68	94%
Xu% > .20	39	54%
X–% > .20	66	92%
X–% > .30	52	72%

Processing

    Zf = 12.10 (*SD* = 4.79)

    Zd = –0.10 (*SD* = 4.19)   ($Zd > + 3.0 = 18, 25\%$; $Zd < –3.0 = 17, 24\%$)

    W:D:Dd = 10.61: 7.36: 2.38

    W:M = 10.61 : 2.29

    DQ+ = 5.14 (*SD* = 3.55)

    DQv = 1.82 (*SD* = 1.86)   (*DQv* > 2 = 22, 31%)

Constellations

PTI = 5	5	7%	*DEPI* = 7	1	1%	*CDI* = 5	3	4%
PTI = 4	19	26%	*DEPI* = 6	4	6%	*CDI* = 4	23	32%
PTI = 3	19	26%	*DEPI* = 5	13	18%		

    S-Constellation Positive 2   3%

    HVI Positive 9   13%

    OBS Positive 0   0%

S–) and unconventionality (CD, *P* < 4 = 47%; NP, 3%). Consistent with Winnicott's (1958) theory, anger disrupts the Antisocial child's developing ego by creating fears of ego-disintegration. Cognitive slippage abounds in CD children (*Level 2 Special Scores* > 0 = 49%; NP, 8%), as do other indicators of formal thought disorder (as noted in Table 16–2: *Sum6, WSum6, Level 2 Special Scores*).

Self-Perception.   Poor controls, problems managing affect, and unconventional and distorted thinking put the CD child on a collision course with others and all contribute to the child's negative evaluation of self (CD, *3r + [2]/R* < .33 = 67%; NP, 3%). Healthy self-esteem is not expected without emotional mastery. The grandiose self-structure found in the adult male psychopath (Kernberg, 1975) is not yet sufficiently functional to provide an escape from distressing feelings of being "damaged" (CD, *MOR* = M = 1.78; NP, .55).

Interpersonal.   As expected, CD children to do not experience cooperation as a natural result of interpersonal interactions (CD, *COP* = 0 = 57% & *COP* > 2 = 4%; NP, 5% & 18%). Perhaps, a combination of biological predisposition and severe disappointments (narcissistic wounding) contribute to reduced affectional relatedness (CD, *T* = 0 = 89%; NP, 12%) and a diminished interest in others (CD, *H* = 0 = 21%; NP, 3%). Certainly, low self-worth and misinterpretations of interpersonal cues further weaken the opportunity for positive interpersonal experience (Gacono & Meloy, 1997b). Aggression is beginning to serve a defensive function (i.e., Identification with the Aggressor, A. Freud; CD, *AG* = 0 = 68%; NP, 3%). As a result, CD children have poor interpersonal experiences (CD, *CDI* ≥ 4 = 36%; *GHR* > *PHR* = 33%; NP, 15% & 78%). All of these factors ultimately coalesce into an increasingly detached and exploitative view of interpersonal relations in a manner quite similar to Sullivan's (1953) concept of malevolent transformation.

Conduct-Disordered Adolescents

Core Characteristics.   These predominately male adolescents (*N* = 179) had an approximate mean age of 14.8 (see Table 16–3). PCL–R scores were not available for the entire adolescent sample; however, it is estimated that approximately 25% of the sample met the criteria for psychopathy (available PCL–R data identifies 20%). Their Rorschach *Response* production can be reasonably compared to Exner's nonpatient 15- year-olds (CD, *R* = *M* = 21.98; NP, 21.94). The CD adolescents manifest mostly dysfunctional problem-solving styles: 70% are either *Avoidant* (CD = 49%; NP, 10%; CD = *Lambda* = *M* = 1.40; NP, 65) or *Ambitent* (CD = 21%; NP, 25%). Like the CD children, their high *Lambda* styles set the stage for difficulties managing ambiguity/complexity, becoming easily overwhelmed, and adopting an alloplastic relationship to the world around them.

Controls.   The CD adolescents also have fewer available psychological resources than developmentally expected by Exner's nonpatient data (CD, *EA* = *M* = 6.18; NP,

8.82). Unlike the CD children, CD adolescents had significantly less *Sum Shading* (CD, *Sum Shading* = *M* = 2.72; NP, 4.17). Perhaps, we see some of the first clear signs of an increasingly troubled developmental trend in which the adolescent has begun to successfully ward off painful affect through acting out. Adolescent adjustment and controls were more impaired than nonpatients (CD, *CDI* ≥ 4= *37%; NP, 16%*).

Affect.   CD adolescents have difficulty modulating emotions (CD, *Pure C* > 1 = 20%; NP, 0%). Although they may still sense that something is wrong with their ability to manage their emotions (CD, *DEPI* ≥ 5 = 29%; NP, 0%), the CD adolescent is beginning to experience less of a felt sense of helplessness (CD, *Sum Y* = *M* = .43; NP, 1.30), compared to the CD child. For the adolescent with a developing antisocial lifestyle, difficulties modulating affect leads paradoxically to an alternation between a combination of avoidance of affect laden situations (CD, *Afr* < .40 = 33% & *Afr* < .50 = 54%; NP, 5% & 17%) and a diminished sense of emotional complexity (CD, *Blends* = *M* = 3.08; NP, 6.34) fluctuating with frequent and chronic experiences of anger and resentment (CD, *S* > 2 = 40%; NP, 15%) breaking through to impulsive, poorly mediated acting out.

Thinking and Processing.   As part of their strategy to simplify their increasingly chaotic world, CD adolescents, like CD children, dramatically and dysfunctionally fail to attend to the important details in their world (CD, *Zd* < −.3.0 = 30% *Underincorporation*; NP, 15%), while their thinking continues to frequently be fluid and boundariless (CD, *DQv* > 2 = 20%). Nonvolitional and distorted interpersonal ideation impairs their thinking (CD, *M*− = *M* = .76; NP, .12), while cognitive slippage (CD, *Level 2 Special Scores* > 0 = 40%; NP, 8%) and other indicators of formal thought disorder and perceptual distortion can be expected (See Table 16–3: *Sum6, WSum6, Level 2 Special Scores*). CD adolescents do not see the world as others do (CD, *PTI* ≥ 3 = 28%, *P* > 4 = 18%; NP, 1% & 3%— see Table 16–3: *XA, WDA, X+, Xu, X–*). Perhaps, *Xu%* represents a signature for the unusual thinking of character disorders. Anger (CD, *S*− = *M* = 1.21; NP, .38) plays an increasingly disruptive role in their cognitive development. All together these Rorschach findings describe well the CD adolescent's nonconsensual and anger-laden cognitive set driving him toward the accepting and "understanding" sanctuary of other troubled youth and away from societally positive interactions with normal adolescents and appropriate adult role models.

Self-Perception.   With similar emotional, cognitive, and processing deficits, many CD adolescents compare themselves quite poorly to others (CD, *3r* + *[2]/R* < .33 = 43%; NP = 6%). During adolescence, we see the beginning of a new defensive strategy, the use of self-absorption (CD, *Fr* + *rF* > 0 = 30%) as a means to ward off a painful, negative view of the self. It comes as no surprise that introspection is not prevalent among CD adolescents (CD, *FD* = *M* = .42; NP, 1.33) and that budding narcissistic defenses are increasingly used in an attempt to compensate for the deeper sense of being damaged goods (CD, *MOR* = *M* = 1.53; *MOR* > 2 = 21%; NP, .54 & 4%).

TABLE 16–3

Conduct Disordered Adolescents (N = 179) Group Mean and Frequencies for Select Ratios, Percentages, and Derivations

$R = 21.98$ ($SD = 6.98$) $\qquad$ $L = 1.40$ ($SD = 1.93$)

EB: 3.59: 2.58 $\qquad$ $EA = 6.18$ ($SD = 3.31$)

eb = 4.67: 2.72 $\qquad$ $es = 7.39$ ($SD = 4.37$) (*FM* + *m* < *Sum Shading*........... 35, 20%)

D score $= -0.37$ ($SD = 1.30$) $\qquad$ $AdjD = -0.07$ ($SD = 1.21$)

EB style

Introversive......................	39	22%
Pervasive Introversive....	28	16%
Ambitent..........................	37	21%
Extratensive....................	16	9%
Pervasive Extratensive....	10	6%
Avoidant..........................	87	49%

EA–es differences: D scores

D score > 0......................	31	17%
D score $= 0$.......................	87	49%
D score < 0.......................	61	34%
D score < -1.....................	30	17%
$AdjD$ score > 0.................	40	22%
$AdjD$ score $= 0$.................	88	49%
$AdjD$ score < 0.................	51	28%
$AdjD$ score < -1...............	16	9%

Affect

$FC{:}CF + C = .78 : 2.07$

Pure C = .26 ($SD = .62$) $\qquad$ (*Pure C* > 0 = 36, 20%; *Pure C* > 1 = 6, 3%)

$FC > (CF + C) + 2$.............. 1 $\qquad$ 1%

$FC > (CF + C) + 1$.............. 7 $\qquad$ 4%

$(CF + C) > FC + 1$............ 74 $\qquad$ 41%

$(CF + C) > FC + 2$............ 38 $\qquad$ 21%

$SumC' = 1.37$ $\quad$ ($SD = 1.76$) $\quad$ $SumV = .64$ $\quad$ ($SD = 1.01$) $\quad$ $SumY = .43$ $\quad$ ($SD = .77$)

$Afr = .51$ ($SD = .20$) $\qquad$ (*Afr* < .40 = 59, 33%; *Afr* < .50 = 96, 54%)

$S = 2.56$ ($SD = 2.16$) $\qquad$ ($S > 2 = 72$, 40%)

Blends:$R = 3.08 : 21.98$

$CP = .04$ ($SD = .19$)

Interpersonal

$COP = 1.02$ ($SD = 1.07$) $\qquad$ (*COP* = 0 = 67, 37%; *COP* > 2 = 15, 8%)

$AG = .53$ ($SD = .84$) $\qquad$ (*AG* = 0 = 116, 65%; *AG* > 2 = 5, 3%)

$Food = .31$ ($SD = .60$)

$Isolate/R = .20$ ($SD = .17$)

$H{:}(H) + Hd + (Hd) = 2.45 :$ $\qquad$ (H = 0 = 26, 15%; H < 2 = 65, 36%)
3.29

$(H) + (Hd){:}(A) + (Ad) = 1.8 : .77$

$H + A{:}Hd + Ad = 11.84 : 3.28$

$Sum\ T = .28$ ($SD = .72$) $\qquad$ (T = 0 = 148, 83%; T > 1 = 13, 7%)

$GHR = 3.00$ ($SD = 1.88$)

$PHR = 3.32$ ($SD = 2.74$) $\qquad$ $GHR > PHR = 75$, 42%

Self-perception

$3r + (2)/R = .38$ *(SD = .22)*   *(3r + (2)/R < .33 = 77, 43% 3r + (2)/R > .44 = 54, 30%)*

$Fr + rF = .62$ *(SD = 1.23)*   *(Fr + rF > 0 = 54, 30%)*

$FD = .42$ *(SD = .66)*

$An + Xy = .76$

$MOR = 1.53$ *(SD = 1.65)*   *(MOR > 2 = 38, 21%)*

Ideation

$a:p = 5.4: 2.9$ *(p > a + 1 = 15, 8%)*

$Ma:Mp = 2.26: 1.36$ *(Mp > Ma = 40, 22%)*

$M = 3.59$ *(SD = 2.51)*   *(M– = .76, SD = 1.03; M none = .02, SD = .13)*

$FM = 3.27$ *(SD = 2.32)* $m = 1.40$ *(SD = 1.45)*

$2AB+Art+Ay = 1.26$ *(SD = 1.99)* $2AB+Art+Ay > 5 = 6, 3\%$

$Sum6 = 5.04$ *(SD = 3.73)* $WSum6 = 14.60$ *(SD = 11.79)*

$Level\ 2\ Sp\ Sc = .65$ *(SD = 1.02)*   *(Level 2 Sp Sc > 0 = 72, 40%)*

Mediation

$Populars = 5.01$ *(SD = 1.73)*   *(P < 4 = 32, 18%; P > 7 = 11, 6%)*

$XA\% = .71$ *(SD = .13)*

$WDA\% = .75$ *(SD = .12)*

$X+\% = .46$ *(SD = .14)*

$X–\% = .28$ *(SD = .13)*

$Xu\% = .26$ *(SD = .11)*

$S– = 1.21$ *(SD = 1.31)*

$XA\% > .89$	10	6%
$XA\% < .70$	71	40%
$WDA\% < .85$	143	80%
$WDA\% < .75$	76	42%
$X+\% < .55$	126	70%
$Xu\% > .20$	128	72%
$X–\% > .20$	127	71%
$X–\% > .30$	65	36%

Processing

$Zf = 12.70$ *(SD = 5.17)*

$Zd = –1.00$ *(SD = 5.18)*   *(Zd > + 3.0 = 31, 17%; Zd < –3.0 = 54, 30%)*

$W:D:Dd = 10.38 : 8.70:2.90$

$W:M = 10.38 : 3.59$

$DQ + = 5.70$ (SD = 3.28)

$DQv = 1.55$ *(SD = 1.97)*   *(DQv > 2 = 35, 20%)*

Constellations

PTI = 5	2	1%	*DEPI = 7*	1	1%	*CDI = 5*	19	11%
PTI = 4	20	11%	*DEPI = 6*	12	7%	*CDI = 4*	46	26%
PTI = 3	28	16%	*DEPI = 5*	38	21%		
S-Constellation Positive	6	3%					
HVI Positive	21	12%					
OBS Positive	0	0%					

Interpersonal.   Without emotionally corrective interpersonal experiences, many CD adolescents continue to view relationships through the lens of their negative interpersonal experiences, vastly inhibiting the development of the inner representation of a mutually cooperative interpersonal world (CD, $COP = 0 = 37\%$ & $COP > 2 = 8\%$; NP, 11 & 14%). Aggression is becoming ego-syntonic, and therefore not represented as symbolic function (CD, $AG = 0 = 65\%$; NP, 25& 25%). These adolescents show a diminished interest in others (CD, $H = 0 = 15\%$; NP, 1%) and their object relations and attachments are impaired (CD, $T = 0 = 83\%$; NP, 5%). They show significant indication of social ineptness and their interpersonal functioning is problematic and ineffective (CD, $CDI > 4 = 37$ %, $GHR = M = 3.00$, $PHR = M = 3.32$; NP, 16%, 5.01 & 1.57). The CD adolescent's pervasive anger, interpersonal disconnection, and idiosyncratic and distorted conceptualizations trigger an inevitable cycle of exploitation of others and pervasive criticism and punishment by others, which further leads to an increasingly damaged interpersonal worldview. Developmentally, the CD adolescent does not learn from experience, but becomes only more defensively entrenched in detached and eccentric self-justification. These Rorschach data are remarkably consistent with psychodynamic developmental models of characterologically based defenses including identification with the aggressor, the use of grandiosity to ward off a devalued view of self, and circumvention of the experience of painful affect through avoidance and acting out.

Antisocial Personality Disordered Females

Core Characteristics.   Approximately 40% of the sample of Antisocial women ($N = 69$) produced PCL–R score ≥ 30 (Table 16–4). The females produced fewer *Responses* than expected in nonpatient adults (ASPD, $R = M = 19.84$; NP, 22.32). ASPD females are likely to be *Avoidant* (ASPD = 30%; NP, 10%) or *Ambitent* (ASPD = 36%; NP, 19%.), but not *Introversive* (ASPD = 9%; NP, 33%).

Controls.   Although ASPD women's psychological resources (*EA*) were similar to nonpatients, this finding by itself is misleading and must be interpreted in context of their dysfunctional problem-solving style and the presence of increased dysphoric affect (ASPD, $M + m < Sum\ Shading = 43\%$; NP, 15%). Combined with lessened controls (ASPD, $D < 0 = 41\%$; D score $< -1 = 23\%$; $AdjD < -1 = 12\%$; NP, 13%, 52 & 4%), their dysfunctional problem-solving style and increased dysphoria suggest that the seemingly normative *EA* for the ASPD women does not translate into adequate functioning (ASPD, $CDI \geq 4 = 32\%$; NP, $CDI > 4 = 4\%$). Instead, the average ASPD woman is socially inept, easily overwhelmed by her high level of dysphoric affect, and prone to impulsive behavior and poor decision making, even though she has what would ordinarily be quite adequate resources for problem solving. Because the ASPD woman has sufficient resources, she may be more effective in antisocial pursuits as an expression of her core psychological dysfunction, thus reinforcing this particular character adaptation.

Affect.   ASPD females have difficulty modulating emotions (ASPD, $FC = M = .86$; NP, 3.56). They experience affective flooding (ASPD, NP, 10%). Painful rumination (ASPD, $Sum\ V = M = 1.56$; NP, .28) and a sense of helplessness (ASPD, $Sum\ Y = M = 1.29$;

NP, .61) haunt the inner worlds of these women. Understandably, these women attempt to avoid emotions (ASPD, $Afr < .40 = 20\%$ & $Afr < .50 = 48\%$; NP, 3% & 11%) and have higher rates of depression (ASPD, $DEPI \geq 5 = 41\%$ & $SCON = 1\%$; NP, 5% & 0%). The chronic experience of anger and resentment is also prominent for these women (ASPD, $S > 2 = 29\%$; NP, 14%).

Thinking and Processing.   Not unlike the Conduct Disordered children and adolescents, ASPD females tended to oversimplify their inner and outer chaotic world and fail to attend to the important details (ASPD, $Zd < -3.0 = 20\%$ *Underincorporation* with thinking that is fluid and boundariless (ASP, $DQv = M = 2.57$ & $DQv > 2 = 36\%$). Female ASPDs appear to be more passive (ASPD, $p > a + 1 = 23\%$ & $Mp > Ma = 29\%$; NP, 2% & 14%) and also have more nonvolitional rumination (ASPD, $M- = M = .52$; NP, .07). Frequently, cognitive slippage and formal thought disorder impair these women's ability to think clearly (ASPD, *Level 2 Sp sc* $> 0 = 36\%$; NP, 6%—see Table 16–4: *Sum6*, *WSum6*, *Level 2 Special Scores*). Not surprisingly, ASPD females are unconventional in their thinking (ASPD, $P < 4 = 30\%$; NP, 1%). Their reality testing and perceptual accuracy are also impaired ($PTI \geq 3 = 13\%$; NP, 0%; see Table 16–4: *XA*, *WDA*, *X+*, *Xu*, *X–*). Anger and resentment disorganizes ASPD women's thinking (ASPD, $S- = M = .74$; NP, .25), which combined with their idiosyncratic thought processes makes it difficult for them to connect in positive ways with groups of normal individuals.

Self-Perception.   As would be expected, ASPD females compare themselves negatively to others (ASPD, $3r + (2)/R < .33 = 41\%$; NP, 13%) and have a damaged sense of self (ASPD, $MOR = M = 1.93$ & $MOR > 2 = 29\%$; NP, .79 & 4%). Some may attempt to overcompensate with an unrealistically high self-appraisal (ASPD, $3r + [2]/R > .44 = 36\%$; NP, 23%) and even pervasive self-absorption (ASPD, $Fr + rF > 0 = 32\%$; NP, 8%). The capacity to introspect appears to be quite limited among the ASPD females (ASPD, $FD = M = .42$; NP, 1.18).[7] Consistent with a hysterical style, somatization was common for these women (ASPD, $An + Xy = M = 1.57$; NP, .59).

Interpersonal.   ASPD women differ substantially from normal women in significant areas of interpersonal functioning. Female ASPDs do not expect cooperative interactions with others (ASPD, $COP = 0 = 36\%$ & $COP > 2 = 18\%$; NP, 17% & 36%). Anger and resentment appears to be egosyntonic (NP, $AG > 2 = 3\%$; NP, 12%). Interest in others, as opposed to viewing others as an extension of their own needs, was diminished for these women (ASPD, $H = 0 = 14\%$ & $H < 2 = 35\%$; NP, 1% & 12%), as was their capacity for attachment (ASPD, $T = 0 = 68\%$; NP, 18%). Social ineptness and problematic interper-

---

[7]Whereas high egocentricity ratios suggest inordinate self-focus, high ratios without *Reflection* indicate a sense of displeasure in doing so (Weiner, 1998). Male psychopaths (high *Reflections*, high *Egocentricity Ratio*) look at themselves exalting in self-admiration and grandiosity. In contrast, female psychopaths (high *Egocentricity Ratio* without *Reflections*) tend to experience distress with the same process. Individuals with no *Reflections*, high *Egocentricity Ratios*, and *Vistas* possess a situation-specific type of self-criticism (Weiner, 1998). Rather than remorse or guilt, the self-critical, unhappy, and dissatisfied presentation of the female psychopath can be viewed as an insidious negative self-image arising from long-standing frustration over unmet needs for attention and admiration (Cunliffe & Gacono, 2005).

TABLE 16-4

Antisocial Female ($N = 69$) Group Mean and Frequencies for Select Ratios, Percentages, and Derivations

$R = 19.84$ ($SD = 6.56$)	$L = .69$ ($SD = .46$)

EB: 3.58 : 3.84 $EA = 7.42$ ($SD = 3.96$)

eb = 4.33 : 5.38 $es = 9.71$ ($SD = 5.88$) (*FM* + *m* < *Sum Shading*............ 30, 43%)

D score = –0.38 (SD = 1.72) $AdjD = -0.35$ ($SD = 1.33$)

EB style

Introversive...........................6	9%	
Pervasive Introversive.......... 2	3%	
Ambitent..............................25	36%	
Extratensive........................ 17	25%	
Pervasive Extratensive....... 10	14%	
Avoidant..............................21	30%	

EA–es differences D scores

D score > 0............................ 7	10%
D score = 0.......................... 34	49%
D score < 0.......................... 28	41%
D score < –1........................ 16	23%
AdjD score > 0.................... 13	19%
AdjD score = 0.................... 35	51%
AdjD score < 0.................... 21	30%
AdjD score < –1.................... 8	12%

Affect

FC:CF + C = .86 : 3.11

Pure C = .59 (SD = .83)   (*Pure C* > 0 = 32, 46%; *Pure C* > 1 = 6, 9%)

FC > (CF + C) + 2................. 1   11%

FC > (CF + C) + 1................ 3   4%

(CF + C) > FC + 1.............. 41   59%

(CF + C) > FC + 2.............. 31   45%

SumC' = 2.03   (SD = 1.89)   Sum V = 1.56 (SD = 2.04)   Sum Y = 1.29   (SD = 1.43)

Afr = .54 (SD = .19)   (*Afr* < .40 = 14, 20%; *Afr* < .50 = 33, 48%)

S = 1.99 (SD = 1.56)   (*S* > 2 = 20, 29%)

Blends:R = 4.45 : 19.84

CP = .04 (SD = .21)

Interpersonal

COP = 1.20 (SD = 1.23)   (*COP* = 0 = 25, 36%; *COP* > 2 = 11, 16%)

AG = .62 (SD = .84)   (*AG* = 0 = 38, 55%; *AG* > 2 = 2, 3%)

Food = .20 (SD = .56)

Isolate/R = .23 (SD = .19)

H:(H) + Hd + (Hd) = 2.30 : 2.61   (*H* = 0 = 10, 14%; *H* < 2 = 24, 35%)

(H) + (Hd):(A) + (Ad) = 1.70 : .76

H + A:Hd + Ad = 10.14 : 2.36

Sum T = .49 (SD = .93)   (*T* = 0 = 47, 68%; *T* > 1 = 6, 9%)

GHR = 3.10 (SD = 1.91)

PHR = 2.84 (SD = 2.39)   *GHR* > *PHR* = 32, 46%

Self-perception

$3r + (2)/R = .40$ ($SD = .19$)   ($3r + (2)/R < .33 = 28$, 41%; $3r + (2)/R > .44 = 25$, 36%)

$Fr + rF = .55$ ($SD = .96$)   ($Fr + rF > 0 = 22$, 32%)

$FD = .42$ ($SD = .47$)

$An + Xy = 1.57$

$MOR = 1.93$ ($SD = 1.89$)   ($MOR > 2 = 20$, 29%)

Ideation

$a:p = 4.55 : 3.45$ ($p > a + 1 = 16$, 23%)

$Ma:Mp = 2.01: 1.62$ ($Mp > Ma = 20$, 29%)

$M = 3.58$ ($SD = 2.52$)   ($M- = .52$, $SD = .96$; M $none = .03$, $SD = .24$)

$FM = 2.84$ ($SD = 1.69$) $m = 1.49$ ($SD = 1.45$)

$2AB+Art+Ay = 2.39$ ($SD = 3.18$) $2AB+Art+Ay > 5 = 5$, 7%

$Sum6 = 6.78$ (SD $= 5.84$) $WSum6 = 20.64$ ($SD = 22.37$)

Level 2 Sp Sc $= .91$ ($SD = 2.19$) (*Level 2 Special Scores* $> 0 = 25$, 36%)

Mediation

$Populars = 4.88$ ($SD = 2.11$)   ($P < 4 = 21$, 30%; $P > 7 = 8$, 12%)

$XA\% = .78$ ($SD = .13$)

$WDA\% = .80$ ($SD = .13$)

$X+\% = .53$ ($SD = .13$)

$X-\% = .20$ ($SD = .13$)

$Xu\% = .24$ ($SD = .12$)

$S- = .74$ ($SD = 1.01$)

$XA\% > .89$............................8	12%	
$XA\% < .70$............................16	23%	
$WDA\% < .85$........................41	59%	
$WDA\% < .75$........................19	28%	
$X+\% < .55$............................35	51%	
$Xu\% > .20$............................43	62%	
$X-\% > .20$..........................28	41%	
$X-\% > .30$............................11	16%	

Processing

$Zf = 10.74$ ($SD = 3.51$)

$Zd = .05$ ($SD = 3.51$)   ($Zd > + 3.0 = 11$, 16%; $Zd < -3.0 = 14$, 20%)

$W:D:Dd = 8.88:8.96:2.00$

$W:M = 8.88: 3.58$

$DQ + = 5.39$ ($SD = 2.79$)

$DQv = 2.57$ ($SD = 2.89$)   ($DQv > 2 = 25$, 36%)

Constellations

$PTI = 5$....... 0	0%	$DEPI = 7$........ 6	9%	$CDI = 5$........ 4	6%
$PTI = 4$....... 6	9%	$DEPI = 6$...... 11	16%	$CDI = 4$...... 18	26%
$PTI = 3$....... 3	4%	$DEPI = 5$...... 11	16%		

S-Constellation Positive.... 1   1%

HVI Positive...................... 1   1%

OBS Positive..................... 0   0%

sonal relationships are also expected for ASPD women (ASPD, $CDI > 4 = 32\%$, $GHR > PHR = 46\%$; NP, 4% & 88%.

Cunliffe and Gacono (2005) summarize the Rorschach similarities and differences between male and female psychopaths:

> The male and female expressions of psychopathy differ from one another in two separate but related dimensions: interpersonal relatedness and self-perception. The female psychopath's pronounced needs for "relatedness" and adulation from others form the cornerstone of her histrionic character. Her interpersonal connections are focused on attempts to overcome her negative self-concept and dysphoric feelings that have arisen from her perceived alienation from those around her. The very dysphoria, and feelings of anger and irritation she seeks to escape have their roots in unmet needs for affiliation and desire to be "entertained" by others. The female psychopath lacks the grandiose self-structure and detachment noted in males and although she may lack the male psychopaths' desire for domination and humiliation of others, she displays a corresponding incapacity for empathy and perspective taking. The females also exhibit similar problems empathizing with others when compared to males but rather than a detached, devaluation of their victims (male psychopathy), they display a clear disregard for the welfare of others despite an outward appearance of interrelatedness. (p. 17)

Antisocial Personality Disordered Males

Core Characteristics.   Roughly 44% ($N = 47$) of the overall sample of APDS males ($N = 108$) were psychopaths ($PCL–R \geq 30$). This sample is proportionally higher than the 25% incidence found in typical prison populations. Still the majority of the males in this sample are not psychopaths and, consequently, the group data reflects the general psychological inadequacy found in ASPDs rather than the grandiosity expected from psychopaths (Gacono & Meloy, 1994). Most of the ASPD males were *Avoidant* (ASPD = 40%; NP, 10%) or *Ambitent* (22%). Fewer of these men had clearly defined problem-solving styles (ASPD *Introversive* = 18%; NP, 33%; ASPD *Extratensive* = 20%, NP, 38%). *Lambda* (M = .99) of this group was also elevated (Table 16–5).

Controls.   ASPD males had fewer psychological resources (ASPD, $EA = M = 6.36$; NP, 8.66), and more *Sum Shading* (ASPD, $FM + m < Sum\ Shading = 31\%$; NP, 15%) and they also evidenced poorer controls (ASPD, $D\ score < 0 = 0 = 31\%$ & $D\ score < –1 = 0 = 16\%$; NP, 13%). As with ASPD women, ASPD men's D and AdjD scores must always be interpreted in light of their diminished resources (affect and thinking) and other impairment, such pervasive social inadequacy (ASPD, $CDI \geq 4 = 32\%$; NP, 4%).

Affect.   As with all of the other ASPD samples, ASPD males have difficulty modulating emotions (ASPD, $FC = M = .73$; *Pure C* $> 0 = 49\%$; NP, 3.56, 10%). ASPD males were prone to painful rumination (ASPD, $Sum\ V = M = .62$) and anxiety (ASPD, $Sum\ Y = M = 1.35$), making them more susceptible to depressive experiences (ASPD, $DEPI \geq 5 = 36\%$ & $SCON = 2\%$; NP, 5% & 0%) In general, ASPD men were not comfortable with their emotions (ASPD, $Afr < .40 = 35\%$ & $Afr < .50 = 52\%$; NP, 3% & 11%), especially com-

plex emotions (*Blends*: ASPD = 3.26; NP, 5.15). As expected, ASPD men were significantly more angry and resentful than the nonpatients (ASPD, $S > 2 = 41\%$; NP, 14%).
Although these ASPD men experience painful rumination and inner distress, our clinical
observation strongly suggests that these experiences rise from their continually elevated
levels of frustration and their experience of self-pity, rather than their painful rumination
arising from remorse for their actions. Most importantly, this observation further suggests the exercise of considerable caution, when applying the usual CS interpretative
statements regarding the presence of *Shading* and particularly *Vista* with this Antisocial
and psychopathic population.

Thinking and Processing.   As with other Antisocial groups, ASPD males tend to
Underincorporate, that is, they fail to attend to the important details in their world
(ASPD, $Zd < -.3.0 = 29\%$; NP, 7%). Their thinking also evidences the characteristic
fluidness and boundary problems (ASPD, $DQv = M = 2.17$ & $DQv > 2 = 35\%$) and un-
conventionality (ASPD, $P < 4 = 27\%$ & $P > 7 = 11\%$; NP, 1% & 31%) found throughout
other Antisocial groups. ASPD men may also have profound thinking problems
(ASPD, $PTI \geq 5 = 12\%$; NP, 0%), as well as elevated levels of perceptual distortion (see
Table 16–5: *WDA*, *X+*, *Xu*, *X–*), cognitive slippage (see Table 16–5: *Sum6*, *WSum6*,
Level 2 Special Scores), and formal thought disorder (ASPD, *Level 2 sp sc* $> 0 = 39\%$;
NP, 6%). ASPD males had more nonvolitional disorganized thinking (ASPD, $M- = M =$
.59; NP, .07), and anger disorganizes their perceptual accuracy (ASPD, $S- = M = .79$;
NP, .25). Interestingly, ASPD males tend toward the abuse of fantasy (ASPD, $p > a + 1$
$= 10\%$ & $Mp > Ma = 31\%$; NP, 2% & 14%). As with other Antisocial groups, the ASPD
males evidenced significant idiosyncratic and disordered thought processes that impairs their ability to problem solve and makes it difficult for them to conform to expected social mores, and therefore, damages their ability to connect with groups of
normal individuals.

Self-Perception.   Despite sensing that they do not measure up to others (ASPD, $3r +$
$[2]/R < .33 = 49\%$; NP, 13%), ASPD males are self-absorbed (ASPD, $Fr + rF > 0 = 32\%$;
NP, 8%) and lack introspection (ASPD, $FD = M = .39$; NP, $FD = M = 1.18$). ASPDs may
somatize (ASPD, $An + Xy = M = .87$) and carry a sense of being damaged (ASPD, $MOR =$
$M = 1.79$ & $MOR > 2 = 23\%$; NP, .79 & 4%). Clearly by adulthood, the ASPD male has
now developed a brittle compensatory narcissistic stance to ward off deep feelings of inadequacy and social ineptness.

Interpersonal.   Interactions with ASPD males are based on power and control rather
than mutual cooperation (ASPD, $COP = 0 = 46\%$ & $COP > 2 = 5\%$; NP, 17% & 36%). For
many, their aggression is egosyntonic (ASPD, $AG = 0 = 68\%$; NP, 37%). They show little,
if any, interest in others (ASPD, $H = 0 = 25\%$ & $H < 2 = 42\%$; NP, 1% & 12%) and do not
experience affectional relatedness (ASPD, $T = 0 = 82\%$; NP, 18%). ASPD males suffer
from the same general social ineptness and poor interpersonal interactions (ASPD, *CDI*
$\geq 4 = 32\%$, $GHR = M = 2.41$; $GHR > PHR = 43\%$; NP, 4%, 4.93 & 88%) as do Antisocial
youth and women.

TABLE 16–5

Antisocial Male (*N* = 108) Group Means and Frequencies for Select Ratios, Percentages, and Derivations

$R = 20.87$ (*SD* = 7.62) $L = .99$ (*SD* = .75)

EB: 2.93 : 3.44	*EA* = 6.36 (*SD* = 3.13)
eb = 4.27 : 3.43	*es* = 7.69 (*SD* = 4.24) (*FM* + *m* < *Sum Shading*......... 33, 31%)
D score = –0.37 (*SD* = 1.17)	*AdjD* = 0.09 (*SD* = .88)

EB style

Introversive........................	19	18%
Pervasive Introversive......	13	12%
Ambitent............................	24	22%
Extratensive......................	22	20%
Pervasive Extratensive.....	11	10%
Avoidant............................	43	40%

EA–es differences:D scores

D score > 0..........................	14	13%
D score = 0..........................	60	56%
D score < 0..........................	34	31%
D score < –1........................	17	16%
AdjD score > 0.....................	26	24%
AdjD score = 0.....................	64	59%
AdjD score < 0.....................	18	17%
AdjD score < –1...................	4	4%

Affect

FC:CF + *C* = .73 : 2.72	
Pure C = .69 (*SD* = .92)	(*Pure C* > 0 = 53, 49%; *Pure C* > 1 = 13, 12%)
FC > (*CF* + *C*) + 2................. 0	0%
FC > (*CF* + *C*) + 1................ 3	3%
(*CF* + *C*) > *FC* + 1.............. 64	59%
(*CF* + *C*) > *FC* + 2.............. 39	36%
SumC' = 1.20 (*SD* = 1.41)	*Sum V* = .62 (*SD* = 1.00) *Sum Y* = 1.35 (*SD* = 1.92)
Afr = .50 (*SD* = .25)	(*Afr* < .40 = 38, 35%; *Afr* < .50 = 56, 52%)
S = 2.38 (*SD* = 1.80)	(*S* > 2 = 44, 41%)
Blends:R = 3.26 : 20.87	
CP = .03 (*SD* = .17)	

Interpersonal

COP = .80 (*SD* = .88)	(*COP* = 0 = 50, 46%; *COP* > 2 = 5, 5%)
AG = .50 (*SD* = .85)	(*AG* = 0 = 73, 68%; *AG* > 2 = 4, 4%)
Food = .29 (*SD* = .55)	
Isolate/R = .20 (*SD* = .14)	
H:(*H*) + *Hd* + (*Hd*) = 1.86 : 2.58	(*H* = 0 = 27, 25%; *H* < 2 = 45, 42%)
(*H*) + (*Hd*):(*A*) + (*Ad*) = 1.29 : .73	
H + *A:Hd* + *Ad* = 10.07:3.49	
Sum T = .25 (*SD* = .63)	(*T* = 0 = 89, 82%; *T* > 1 = 5, 5%)
GHR = 2.41 (*SD* = 1.62)	
PHR = 2.73 (*SD* = 2.26)	*GHR* > *PHR* = 46, 43%

Self-perception

$3r + (2)/R = .36$ (SD = .17) $(3r + (2)/R < .33 = 53,49\%$ $3r + (2)/R > .44 = 28, 26\%)$

$Fr + rF = .62$ (SD = 1.06) $(Fr + rF > 0 = 22, 32\%)$

$FD = .39$ (SD = .56)

$An + Xy = .87$

$MOR = 1.79$ (SD = 1.76) $(MOR > 2 = 25, 23\%)$

Ideation

$a{:}p = 4.68{:}\ 2.52$ $(p > a + 1 = 11, 10\%)$

$Ma{:}Mp = 1.73{:}\ 1.20$ $(Mp > Ma = 33, 31\%)$

$M = 2.93$ (SD = 2.06) $(M- = .59, SD = .85; M\ none = .02, SD = .14)$

$FM = 2.85$ (SD = 1.79) $m = 1.42$ (SD = 1.47)

$2AB+Art+Ay = 2.49$ (SD = 3.28) $2AB+Art+Ay > 5 = 13, 12\%$

$Sum6 = 5.42$ (SD = 4.00) $WSum6 = 15.48$ (SD = 12.82)

$Level\ 2\ Sp\ Sc = .62$ (SD = .97) $(Level\ 2\ Special\ Scores > 0 = 42, 39\%)$

Mediation

$Populars = 4.80$ (SD = 1.93) $(P < 4 = 29, 27\%; P > 7 = 12, 11\%)$

$XA\% = .75$ (SD = .11)

$WDA\% = .79$ (SD = .11)

$X+\% = .53$ (SD = .14)

$X-\% = .22$ (SD = .11)

$Xu\% = .23$ (SD = .11)

$S- = .76$ (SD = .99)

$XA\% > .89$............................ 8   7%

$XA\% < .70$........................... 25   23%

$WDA\% < .85$...................... 74   69%

$WDA\% < .75$...................... 32   30%

$X+\%\ < .55$........................ 60   56%

$Xu\% > .20$........................... 62   57%

$X-\%\ > .20$......................... 51   47%

$X-\%\ > .30$........................ 18   17%

Processing

$Zf = 11.36$ (SD = 4.18)

$Zd = -.88$ (SD = 3.96) $(Zd > + 3.0 = 18, 17\%; Zd < -3.0 = 31, 29\%)$

$W{:}D{:}Dd = 9.57 : 8.92 : 6.44$

$W{:}M = 9.57 : 2.93$

$DQ+ = 4.99$ (SD = 2.72)

$DQv = 2.17$ (SD = 2.18) $(DQv > 2 = 38, 35\%)$

Constellations

PTI = 5........ 3	3%	DEPI = 7........ 6	6%	CDI = 5..... 12	11%
PTI = 4........ 4	4%	DEPI = 6...... 13	12%	CDI = 4..... 23	21%
PTI = 3........ 5	5%	DEPI = 5...... 19	18%		
S-Constellation Positive...... 2	2%				
HVI Positive........................ 10	9%				
OBS Positive........................ 0	0%				

The Rorschach view of the inner relational world of the Antisocial male suggests that his long-standing, now deeply repressed needs for interpersonal attachment and appreciation from others have now undergone what Sullivan (1953) called malevolent transformation. The ASPD male pervasively devalues attachment needs in himself while the presence of such needs in others presents the ASPD male with an opportunity for exploitation and control.

Antisocial Personality Disordered Schizophrenics

The 100 Rorschach protocols of these mostly Paranoid Schizophrenic patients with a concurrent Antisocial Personality Disorder aids in understanding the relationship between an Axis I major mental disorder and Axis II character pathology (Table 16–6). Their Rorschachs clearly show characteristics of both disorders. Where meaningful, we compared our sample to Exner's (1995) Schizophrenic sample (ESCH; $N = 320$).

Core Characteristics and Controls.   ASPD Schizophrenics were cognitively constricted (SCH, *Lambda* = M = 1.14; ESCH, 1.57) and mostly *Avoidant* (SCH = 49%), with fewer *Introversives* (SCH = 22%; ESCH, 60%), although a similar number of *Extratensives* as compared to inpatient Schizophrenics (SCH = 10%; ESCH, 11%). Interestingly, ASPD Schizophrenics had even greater social ineptness than the other Schizophrenics as well as weaker controls (SCH, $EA = M = 6.97$, D score $< -1 = 0 = 11\%$; ESCH, 8.63 & 6%).

Affect.   In common with other ASPD groups, the ASPD Schizophrenics had difficulty modulating emotions (SCH, $FC = M = .60$, *Pure C* $> 1 = 15\%$; ESCH, 1.54 & 7%), but experience less inner tension, anxiety, and helplessness than other Schizophrenics (SCH, *Sum Y* = M = .61; ESCH, 2.12). They show somewhat more mood disturbance than inpatient Schizophrenics (SCH, *DEPI* $> 5 = 40\%$; ESCH, 29%), but less of a tendency toward suicide (SCH, *SCON* = 2%). This is consistent with the ASPD style where their characteristic acting out and aggression toward others substitutes for inwardly directed aggression.

Thinking and Processing.   Perhaps due to the organizing effects of the Axis II pathology, ASPD Schizophrenics tend to have lower levels of thought and perceptual disturbance, when compared to other Schizophrenics (ASPD, *PTI* $\geq 3 = 53\%$; *ESCH, SCZI* $\geq 4 = 82\%$; and Exner's (2003) high and low *Lambda* Schizophrenic groups (*PTI* $\geq 3 = 78\%$ & 74%). Their reality testing is similar (ASPD, $X - \% = M = .34$). Anger does not seem to disorganize ASPD Schizophrenic thinking as much as inpatient Schizophrenics (SCH, $S- = M = 79$; ESCH, 1.61), although ASPD Schizophrenics also appear to have even more fluid, poorly bounded thinking (SCH, $DQv = 3.22$; ESCH, 1.43). Whereas Antisocial character evidences some greater organizing effects in terms of decreasing flagrant thought disorder, ASPD Schizophrenics process information from the world in a far more vague and associational manner. This finding is perhaps the result of a profound failure to integrate their vague, poorly understood inner need states, along their grossly and unreal-

TABLE 16–6

Antisocial Schizophrenic Men ($N = 100$) Group Means and Frequencies for Select Ratios, Percentages, and Derivations

$R = 22.33$ (SD = 8.71)	$L = 1.14$ (SD = .82)	

EB: 3.72 : 3.25	EA = 6.97 (SD = 3.84)	
eb = 4.12 : 3.14	es = 7.26 (SD = 4.22) (FM + m < Sum Shading........... 30, 30%)	
D Score = –0.09 (SD = 1.33)	AdjD = 0.22 (SD = 1.36)	

EB style

Introversive........................ 22	22%	
Pervasive Introversive........ 12	12%	
Ambitent............................. 19	19%	
Extratensive........................ 10	10%	
Pervasive Extratensive......... 7	7%	
Avoidant.............................. 49	49%	

EA—es differences:D scores

D score > 0........................... 20	20%	
D score = 0.......................... 57	57%	
D score < 0........................... 23	23%	
D score < –1........................ 11	11%	
AdjD score > 0.................... 28	28%	
AdjD score = 0.................... 57	57%	
AdjD score < 0.................... 15	15%	
AdjD score < –1.................... 8	8%	

Affect

FC:CF + C = .60 : 2.63		
Pure C = .64 (SD = 1.03)	(Pure C > 0 = 41, 41%; Pure C > 1 = 15, 15%)	
FC > (CF + C) + 2................. 0	0%	
FC > (CF + C) + 1................. 2	2%	
(CF + C) > FC + 1.............. 59	59%	
(CF + C) > FC + 2.............. 47	47%	
SumC' = 1.46 (SD = 1.41)	Sum V = .62 (SD = .97) Sum Y = .61 (SD = .88)	
Afr = .47 (SD = .20)	(Afr < .40 = 41, 41%; Afr < .50 = 57, 57%)	
S = 1.93 (SD = 1.79)	(S > 2 = 30, 30%)	
Blends:R = 3.04 : 22.33		
CP = .08 (SD = .37)		

Interpersonal

COP = 1.25 (SD = 1.37)	(COP = 0 = 36, 36%; COP > 2 = 17, 17%)	
AG = .75 (SD = 1.17)	(AG = 0 = 60, 60%; AG > 2 = 10, 10%)	
Food = .43 (SD = .93)		
Isolate/R = .21 (SD = .15)		
H:(H) + Hd + (Hd) = 2.43 : 3.15	(H = 0 = 18, 18%; H < 2 = 43, 43%)	
(H) + (Hd):(A) + (Ad) = 1.81 : .60		
H + A:Hd + Ad = 11.14 : 2.86		
Sum T = .45 (SD = .99)	(T = 0 = 74, 74%; T > 1 = 10,10%)	
GHR = 2.14 (SD = 1.69)		
PHR = 4.45 (SD = 3.69)	GHR > PHR = 18, 18%	

(continued)

TABLE 16–6   *(continued)*

Self-perception

   $3r + (2)/R = .39$ $(SD = .20)$ *(3r + (2)/R < .33 = 40, 40% 3r + (2)/R > .44 = 37, 37%)*

   $Fr + rF = .60$ $(SD = 1.17)$ *(Fr + rF > 0 = 29, 29%)*

   $FD = .25$ $(SD = .50)$

   $An + Xy = 1.26$

   $MOR = 2.42$ $(SD = 2.25)$ *(MOR > 2 = 42, 42%)*

Ideation

   $a{:}p = 5.10{:} 2.75$ *(p > a + 1 = 12, 12%)*

   $Ma{:}Mp = 2.18{:} 1.55$ *(Mp > Ma = 29, 29%)*

   $M = 3.72$ $(SD = 3.17)$ *(M– = 1.49, SD = 2.09; M none = .01, SD = .10)*

   $FM = 2.54$ $(SD = 2.15)$ *m = 1.58 (SD = 1.71)*

   $2AB+Art+Ay = 2.71$ $(SD = 3.35)$ *2AB+Art+Ay > 5 = 14, 14%*

   $Sum6 = 10.49$ $(SD = 7.24)$ *WSum6 = 39.91 (SD = 31.41)*

   Level 2 Sp Sc $= 3.40$ $(SD = .3.47)$ *(Level 2 Special Scores > 0 = 76, 76%)*

Mediation

   $Populars = 4.52$ $(SD = 1.86)$ *(P < 4 = 31, 31%; P > 7 = 8, 8%)*

   $XA\% = .63$ $(SD = .17)$

   $WDA\% = .65$ $(SD = .17)$

   $X+\% = .39$ $(SD = .13)$

   $X–\% = .34$ $(SD = .17)$

   $Xu\% = .23$ $(SD = .12)$

   $S– = .79$ $(SD = 1.03)$

   $XA\% > .89$............................4   4%

   $XA\% < .70$............................66   66%

   $WDA\% < .85$.......................89   89%

   $WDA\% < .75$.......................71   71%

   $X+\% < .55$..........................86   86%

   $Xu\% > .20$...........................59   59%

   $X–\% > .20$..........................82   82%

   $X–\% > .30$..........................51   51%

Processing

   $Zf = 12.22$ $(SD = 5.23)$

   $Zd = -.93$ $(SD = 4.57)$ *(Zd > + 3.0 = 18, 18%; Zd < –3.0 = 27, 27%)*

   $W{:}D{:}Dd = 10.89{:}8.78{:}2.66$

   $W{:}M = 10.89{:} 3.72$

   $DQ+ = 5.69$ $(SD = 3.39)$

   $DQv = 3.22$ $(SD = 2.72)$ *(DQv > 2 = 49, 49%)*

Constellations

PTI = 5.......21	21%	*DEPI* = 7.......5	5%	*CDI* = 5.....14	14%
PTI = 4.......19	19%	*DEPI* = 6.....13	13%	*CDI* = 4.....19	19%
PTI = 3.......13	13%	*DEPI* = 5.....22	22%		

   S-Constellation Positive.......2   2%

   HVI Positive........................12   12%

   OBS Positive.........................0   0%

istic view of the world in which their focus on predatory opportunism and on acting out of poorly understood needs decreases the stimulus value of most other interpersonal events.

Self-Perception and Interpersonal.   A good number of ASPD Schizophrenics are self absorbed (SCH, $Fr + rF > 0 = 29\%$; NP, 13%), which might be a defense against feelings of low self worth (SCH, $MOR = M = 2.42$ & $MOR > 2 = 42\%$; ESCH, 1.47 & 22%). ASPD Schizophrenics show a markedly impaired capacity to introspect (SCH, $FD = M = .25$; ESCH, .60) and surprisingly may have even greater interpersonal deficits than inpatient schizophrenics (SCH, $CDI > 4 = 33\%$; ESCH, 25%).

Sexual Homicide Perpetrators

Core Characteristics.   We included this sample because the majority of Sexual Homicide Perpetrators (SHP) meet the criteria for ASPD and approximately two thirds of this group are psychopathic (Table 16–7). The data reveals the interplay between ASPD and sexual deviance. Unlike nonsexually offending male ASPD subjects or nonsexually offending psychopaths, the Sexual Homicide Perpetrators tended to be engaged (SHP, $R = M = 27.25$; NP, 22.32) and even pulled by the test (*Lambda M* = .71), although a subgroup had an *Avoidant* response style (SHP = 22%; NP, 10%). Fewer SHPs were *Extratensive* (SHP, *Extratensive* = 17%; NP, 30%). They often experienced dysphoric affect (SHP, $FM + m < Sum\ Shading = 28\%$; NP, 15%).

Controls.   Sexual Homicide Perpetrators had adequate psychological resources (SHP, $EA = M = 8.53$), despite less controls (SHP, $CDI \geq 4 = 38\%$, D score $< 0 = 50\%$; NP, 4% & 13%). This suggests a socially inadequate individual who has sufficient problem-solving skills, but who uses them in the service of impulse ridden needs.

Affect.   As would be expected, their Rorschachs demonstrated that SHPs have difficulty modulating affect (SHP, $Pure\ C > 0 = 44\%$, $Pure\ C > 1 = 11\%$; NP, 3.56). Perpetrators were prone to painful rumination (SHP, $Sum\ V = M = 1.36$; NP, .28) and feelings of helplessness (SHP, $Sum\ Y = 1.67$; NP, .61), making them more susceptible to depressive experiences (SHP, $DEPI \geq 5 = 42\%$ & $SCON = 8\%$; NP, 5% & 0%). They are angry and resentful (SHP, $S > 2 = 47\%$; NP, 14%), and in general were not comfortable with emotional engagement (SHP, $Afr < .40 = 31\%$ & $Afr < .50 = 44\%$; NP, 3% & 11%), which along with their social inadequacy primes them for an impulsive, hostile, dysfunctional mode of relating through sexual acting out.

Thinking and Processing.   Sexual Homicide Perpetrators show a somewhat inconsistent tendency to both fail to attend to the important details in their world through *Under-incorporation* (SHP, $Zd < -.3.0 = 36\%$; NP, 7%), while being hypervigilant (SHP, $HVI = 14\%$; NP, 3%), including having an atypical processing style of focusing on fine or unusual detail (SHP, $Dd = M = 4.17$; NP, 1.16). Their thinking evidences fluidness and boundary problems (SHP, $DQMv = 2.92$), and is unconventional (SHP, $P < 4 = 14\%$; $P > 7 = 11\%$; NP, 1% & 31%). Along with their social inadequacy, Sexual Homicide Perpetrators are more passive (SHP, $p > a + 1 = 11\%$; NP, 2%) and prone to fantasy over realistic

TABLE 16–7

Sexual Homicide Perpetrators ($N = 38$) Group Means and Frequencies for Select Ratios, Percentages, and Derivations

$R = 27.25$ $(SD = 11.67)$	$L = .71$ $(SD = .58)$
EB: $4.58 : 3.94$	$EA = 8.53$ $(SD = 3.85)$
$eb = 7.61 : 5.61$	$es = 13.22$ $(SD = 9.43)$ $(FM + m < Sum\ Shading$.......... $10, 28\%)$
D score $= -1.58$ $(SD = 2.69)$	$AdjD = -0.69$ $(SD = 1.65)$

EB style

Introversive............................ 13	36%	
Pervasive Introversive............. 6	17%	
Ambitent..................................9	25%	
Extratensive............................ 6	17%	
Pervasive Extratensive............ 3	8%	
Avoidant..................................8	22%	

EA—es differences: D scores

D score > 0............................ 4	11%
D score $= 0$.......................... 14	39%
D score < 0............................ 18	50%
D score < -1.......................... 12	33%
$AdjD$ score > 0........................ 5	14%
$AdjD$ score $= 0$...................... 19	53%
$AdjD$ score < 0...................... 12	33%
$AdjD$ score < -1..................... 10	28%

Affect

$FC:CF + C = 1.33 : 3.00$	
Pure $C = .56$ $(SD = .70)$	(Pure $C > 0 = 16, 44\%$; Pure $C > 1 = 4\ 11\%$)
$FC > (CF + C) + 2$.....................1	3%
$FC > (CF + C) + 1$.....................2	6%
$(CF + C) > FC + 1$...................19	53%
$(CF + C) > FC + 2$...................11	31%
$SumC' = 1.53$ $(SD = 1.44)$	$Sum\ V = 1.36$ $(SD = 1.96)$ $Sum\ Y = 1\ .67$ $(SD = 2.70)$
$Afr = .55$ $(SD = .23)$	$(Afr < .40 = 11, 31\%; Afr < .50 = 16, 44\%)$
$S = 3.08$ $(SD = 2.02)$	$(S > 2 = 17, 47\%)$
$Blends:R = 5.25 : 27.25$	
$CP = .14$ $(SD = .35)$	

Interpersonal

$COP = 1.31$ $(SD = 1.12)$	$(COP = 0 = 10, 28\%; COP > 2 = 6, 17\%)$
$AG = .83$ $(SD = .91)$	$(AG = 0 = 15, 42\%; AG > 2 = 3, 8\%)$
$Food = .53$ $(SD = .94)$	
$Isolate/R = .26$ $(SD = .22)$	
$H:(H) + Hd + (Hd) = 2.78 : 3.74$	$(H = 0 = 1, 3\%; H < 2 = 9, 25\%)$
$(H) + (Hd):(A) + (Ad) = 1.91 : .97$	
$H + A:Hd + Ad = 13.06 : 4.80$	
$Sum\ T = 1.06$ $(SD = 1.76)$	$(T = 0 = 20, 56\%; T > 1 = 10, 28\%)$

$GHR = 3.25\ (SD = 1.66)$

$PHR = 4.33\ (SD = 2.87)$ $GHR > PHR = 12, 33\%$

Self-perception

$3r + (2)/R = .41\ (SD = .19)$ $(3r + (2)/R < .33 = 12, 33\%; 3r + (2)/R > .44 = 13, 36\%)$

$Fr + rF = .97\ (SD = 1.56)$ $(Fr + rF > 0 = 15, 42\%)$

$FD = .42\ (SD = .69)$

$An + Xy = 1.28$

$MOR = 2.64\ (SD = 2.70)$ $(MOR > 2 = 16, 44\%)$

Ideation

$a:p = 7.50 : 4.69$ $(p > a + 1 = 4, 11\%)$

$Ma:Mp = 2.36 : 2.22$ $(Mp > Ma = 13, 36\%)$

$M = 4.58\ (SD = 2.47)$ $M– = 1.11, SD = 1.17; M\ none = .03, SD = .17$

$FM = 5.19\ (SD = 3.79)$ $m = 2.42\ (SD = 2.03)$

$2AB+Art +Ay = 2.53\ (SD = 3.03)$ $2AB + Art + Ay > 5 = 4, 11\%$

$Sum6 = 7.92\ (SD = 5.73)$ $WSum6 = 21.83\ (SD = 17.98)$

$Level\ 2\ Sp\ Sc = .72\ \ (SD = 1.14)$ $(Level\ 2\ Special\ Scores > 0 = 17, 47\%)$

Mediation

$Populars = 5.50\ (SD = 1.70)$ $(P < 4 = 5, 14\%; P > 7 = 4, 11\%)$

$XA\% = .71\ (SD = .11)$

$WDA\% = .74\ (SD = .12)$

$X+\% = .47\ (SD = .11)$

$X–\% = .27\ (SD = .11)$

$Xu\% = .24\ (SD = .10)$

$S– = 1.31\ (SD = 1.47)$

$XA\% > .89$............................ 1   3%

$XA\% < .70$........................ 17   47%

$WDA\% < .85$....................... 27   75%

$WDA\% < .75$....................... 18   50%

$X+\% < .55$.......................... 27   75%

$Xu\% > .20$........................... 21   58%

$X–\% > .20$........................ 26   72%

$X–\% > .30$........................ 11   31%

Processing

$Zf = 13.44\ (SD = 4.05)$

$Zd = -1.71\ (SD = 3.48)$ $(Zd > + 3.0 = 3, 8\%; Zd < -3.0 = 13, 36\%)$

$W:D:Dd = 9.58 : 13.50 : 4.17$

$W:M = 9.58 : 4.58$

$DQ+ = 7.31\ (SD = 3.22)$

$DQv = 2.92\ (SD = 2.50)$ $(DQv > 2 = 18, 50\%)$

Constellations

$PTI = 5$........ 0	0%	$DEPI = 7$..... 1	3%	$CDI = 5$..... 2	6%
$PTI = 4$........ 6	17%	$DEPI = 6$..... 6	17%	$CDI = 4$..... 8	22%
$PTI = 3$........ 4	11%	$DEPI = 5$..... 8	22%		

S-Constellation Positive....... 3   8%

HVI Positive........................... 5   14%

OBS Positive.......................... 0   0%

problem solving (SHP, $p > Ma = 36\%$; NP, 14%). They are given to more nonvolitional or flawed interpersonal thinking (SHP, $M- = M = 1.11$; NP, .07) and intellectualization (SHP, $2AB + ART + AY > 5 = 11\%$; NP, 2%). Sexual perpetrators do not see the world as others do (SHP, $PTI \geq 4 = 28\%$; NP, 0%) and have more perceptual distortions (XA, WDA, $X+$, Xu, $X-$), high levels of cognitive slippage (Table 16–7: $Sum6$, $WSum6$, $Level\ 2\ Special\ Scores$), and increased incidence of formal thought disorder (SHP, $Level\ 2\ sp\ sc = 47\%$; NP, 6%). Anger disorganizes their perceptual accuracy (SHP, $S- = M = 1.31$; NP, .25). These Rorschach results vividly reveal the impaired and highly unrealistic thinking, along with impaired interpersonal reasoning and proneness to fantasy, which become the dysfunctional cognitive crucible through which these sexual perpetrators hone their highly disturbed sexual fantasies.

Self-Perception. Sexual Homicide Perpetrators are pathologically self absorbed (SHP, $Fr + rF > 0 = 42\%$; NP, 8%) and are not likely to introspect (SHP, $FD = .42$; NP, 1.18), having likely developed narcissistic preoccupation as a defense against their profound inner sense of being damaged (SHP, $MOR = M = 2.64$ & $MOR > 2 = 44\%$; NP, .79 & 4%). Somatization and bodily preoccupation (SHP, $An + Xy = M = .1.28$; NP, .59) is also a much used defense against their profound personal inadequacy.

Interpersonal. These individuals tend not to anticipate interpersonal relationships as cooperative (SHP, $COP > 2 = 17\%$; NP, 36%), are less interested in others (SHP, $H < 2 = 25\%$; NP, 12%), and have not formed adequate attachments (SHP, $T = 0 = 56\%$; NP, 18%). As a result, Sexual Homicide Perpetrators are profoundly socially inadequate and have poor interpersonal interactions (SHP, $CDI \geq 4 = 28\%$, $PHR = 4.33$ & $GHR > PHR = 33\%$; NP, 4%, 1.53 & 88%).

The picture of the Sexual Homicide Perpetrator, which emerges from the Rorschach, is that of an individual who is unable to form satisfying relationships and who ambivalently feels both deep longing for, and deep resentment toward, others. The SHP's ambivalence is evident in their uncharacteristically (relative to other ASPDs or psychopaths) low *Lambda* (pulled by stimuli; *HVI*) and elevated *Blends* (pushed by stimuli). Dysphoric affect and their inability to disengage create an avenue for the expression of their deviant sexual fantasies tainted by their malevolent internal worlds. The sexual perpetrator's interpersonal confusion and fantasy-based expression of deeper attachment needs often blends his profound inner distress with impulsive emotionality, leading him to act out sexually.

CONCLUSIONS

In well-designed studies, the Rorschach continues to impress us with its usefulness and, at times, uncanny ability for understanding the complex and often impenetrable inner world of Antisocial and psychopathic personalities. Central to these disorders are difficulties dealing with complexity, a propensity to being easily overwhelmed, defensive grandiosity, affect avoidance, severe interpersonal difficulties, and highly idiosyncratic and disturbed cognitive function. Although sign approaches and making "a diagnosis" based solely on the Rorschach are likely never to be fruitful endeavors, the Rorschach data allows us to assess these crucial dimensional aspects of Antisocial Personality, which can elucidate the inner world of these highly disturbed individuals (Gacono et al., 2001; Gacono et al., 2002).

A careful evaluation of the Rorschach and psychopathy literature provides caveats for interpreting divergent findings as well as conducting future CD and ASPD research (Gacono et al., 2001). Several of these are:

1. CD and ASPD are comprised of heterogeneous groups of individuals. Whenever possible, comparative studies that treat psychopathy as a taxon must include psychopathy as an independent measure (evaluated with either the PCL–R, a "recommended" modified version of the PCL–R for adolescents or the *PCL:YV*) and use the accepted cut-off scores (PCL–R $\geq$ 30).

2. Studies need to control or discuss the limitations imposed by such variables as gender, sexual deviance, concurrent Axis I functional psychosis, age, IQ, testing setting, and legal status. These factors can also influence the production of certain Rorschach variables.

3. The influence of R (number of responses) must always be considered in Rorschach research (Meyer, 1994). With particular reference to psychopathic and Antisocial Personalities, with certain sex offender groups, increased R is predicted (Bridges et al., 1998; Gacono et al., 2000). Although R is always important related to constellations and certain variables, its interpretation is relative for others. As we expect a greater likelihood of a variable occurring when R is elevated, in studies where R is low and a low base rate variable is high (*Fr* or *T*), the interpretation that the presence of the variable represents a characterological marker of the disorder is strengthened. For example, in a group with a mean R of 14, the mean *Fr* of .50 (frequency of 50% producing at least one) provides striking evidence of self focus as a predominant trait of this group. Likewise, the absence of a variable in a high R sample similarly adds weight to its interpretation.

4. Response style must be considered when discussing the generalizability of findings across studies (Bannatyne et al., 1999). Exner (1995) has clearly demonstrated that response style (i.e., *Extratensive*, *Ambitent*, and *Introversive* styles, as well as R and high *Lambda*) can significantly impact the production of certain Rorschach variables. For example, in a high *Lambda* psychopathic ASPD group (PCL–R $\geq$ 30) with low mean IQs, a paucity of reflection responses should never be attributed with certainty to "failed replication" of previous findings with other ASPD groups. High *Lambda* and low IQ can both constrict the production of certain Rorschach variables. On the other hand, an elevation of Reflection responses in this same "constricted" group would impressively strengthen the weight of these findings. Other factors such as the presence of Schizophrenia can impact the manifestation of traits; Schizophrenic psychopathic ASPDs are not expected to produce as many *Reflection* responses as psychopathic ASPDs without psychosis (Gacono & Meloy, 1994).

Future research needed with the Rorschach and ASPD fall into two primary areas. First, well- designed studies are needed to replicate previous ones. The majority of the studies presented in the literature (mostly dissertations) are methodological flawed (see Gacono et al., 2001). Even when their methodology is sound, the researchers fail in other ways to ensure the generalizability of the samples to existing studies. A second, and perhaps the most interesting endeavor, would be to gather historical and assessment data from a large sample of carefully delineated PCL–R identified psychopaths. From this sample Rorschach and MMPI–2 data (as well as other personality methods) could aid in the important delineation of subgroups within the overall umbrella of psychopathy. Combined with attention to certain individual PCL–R item scores, these data could be used to further elucidate individual differences within the psychopathic group. Such information is essential to the research/practitioner's ongoing task of sorting out individual differences related to the institutional management and clinical treatment of offenders. The researcher in this latter area will likely demonstrate empirically what the earliest theorists' hypothesized (Karpman, 1949, 1950), that is, not all psychopaths are the same.

ACKNOWLEDGMENTS

We extend our appreciation to John Exner, Jr., and Rorschach Workshops for their assistance in analyzing the Rorschach data presented in this chapter.

REFERENCES

American Psychiatric Association. (1952). *Diagnostic and statistical manual of mental disorders.* Washington, DC: Author.

American Psychiatric Association. (1968). *Diagnostic and statistical manual of mental disorders* (2nd ed.). Washington, DC: Author.

American Psychiatric Association. (1994). *Diagnostic and statistical manual of mental disorders* (4th ed.). Washington, DC: Author.

Bannatyne, L. A., Gacono, C. B., & Greene, R. (1999). Differential patterns of responding among three groups of chronic psychotic forensic outpatients. *Journal of Clinical Psychology, 55*(12), 1553–1565.

Berg, J., Gacono, C., Meloy, J., & Peaslee, D. (1994). *A Rorschach comparison of borderline and antisocial females.* Unpublished manuscript.

Bodholdt, R., Richards, H., & Gacono, C. B. (2000). Assessing psychopathy in adults: The Psychopathy Checklists, Revised and Screening Version. In C. B. Gacono (Ed.), *The clinical and forensic assessment of psychopathy: A practitioner's guide* (pp. 55–86). Mahwah, NJ: Lawrence Erlbaum Associates.

Bridges, M., Wilson, J., & Gacono, C. B. (1998). A Rorschach investigation of defensiveness, self-perception, interpersonal relations, and affective states in incarcerated pedophiles. *Journal of Personality Assessment, 70*(2), 365–385.

Cleckley, H. (1976). *The mask of sanity* (5th ed.). St. Louis, MO: Mosby. (Original work published 1941)

Cooper, S., & Arnow, D. (1986). An object relations view of the borderline defenses: A Rorschach analysis. In M. Kissen (Ed.), *Assessing object relations phenomena* (pp. 143–171). Madison, CT: International Universities Press.

Cunliffe, T., & Gacono, C. B. (2005). A Rorschach investigation of psychopathy and hysteria in incarcerated antisocial personality disordered female offenders. *International Journal of Offender Therapy and Comparative Criminology, 49*(5), 530–546.

Exner, J. E. (1986). *The Rorschach: A Comprehensive System: Vol. 1. Basic foundations* (2nd ed.). New York: Wiley.

Exner, J. E. (1988). COP. Alumni newsletter. Asheville, ND: Rorschach Workshops.

Exner, J. (1991). *A Rorschach workbook for the Comprehensive System* (3rd ed.). Asheville, NC: Rorschach Workshops.

Exner, J. (1993). *The Rorschach: A Comprehensive System: Vol. 1. Basic foundations* (3rd ed.). New York: Wiley.

Exner, J. (1995). *A Rorschach workbook for the Comprehensive System* (4th ed.). Asheville, NC: Rorschach Workshops.

Exner, J. E. (2000). *A primer for Rorschach interpretation.* Asheville, NC: Rorschach Workshops.

Exner, J. E. (2003). *The Rorschach: A Comprehensive System* (4th ed.). Hoboken, NJ: Wiley.

Gacono, C. (1988). *A Rorschach analysis of object relations and defensive structure and their relationship to narcissism and psychopathy in a group of antisocial offenders.* Unpublished doctoral dissertation, United States International University, San Diego.

Gacono, C. (1990). An empirical study of object relations and defensive operations in antisocial personality. *Journal of Personality Assessment, 54,* 589–600.

Gacono, C. B. (1997). Is the Rorschach Aggressive Movement Response enough? *British Journal of Projective Psychology, 42*(2), 5–11.

Gacono, C. B., & Bodholdt, R. (2001). The role of the Psychopathy Checklist–Revised (PCL–R) in violence risk and threat assessment. *Journals of Threat Assessment, 1*(4), 65–79.

Gacono, C. B., Bannatyne-Gacono, L. A., Meloy, J. R., & Baity, M. (2005). The Rorschach extended Aggression scores. *Rorschachiana, 27,* 164–190.

Gacono, C. B., Loving, J. L., & Bodholdt, R. (2001). The Rorschach and psychopathy: Toward a more accurate understanding of the research findings. *Journal of Personality Assessment, 77*(1), 16–38.

Gacono, C. B., Loving, J. L., Evans, F. B., & Jumes, M. (2002). The Rorschach in forensic practice. *Journal of Forensic Psychology Practice, 2*(3), 33–53.

Gacono, C., & Meloy, R. (1991). A Rorschach investigation of attachment and anxiety in antisocial personality. *Journal of Nervous and Mental Disease, 179,* 546–552.

Gacono, C., & Meloy, R. (1992). The Rorschach and the *DSM–III–R* antisocial personality: A tribute to Robert Lindner. *Journal of Clinical Psychology, 48*(3), 393–405.

Gacono, C. B., & Meloy, J. R. (1994). *The Rorschach assessment of aggressive and psychopathic personalities.* Hillsdale, NJ: Lawrence Erlbaum Associates.

Gacono, C. B., & Meloy, J. R. (1997a). Attachment deficits in antisocial and psychopathic personalities. *British Journal of Projective Psychology, 42*(2), 47–55.

Gacono, C. B., & Meloy, J. R. (1997b). Rorschach research and the psychodiagnosis of antisocial and psychopathic personalities. *Rorschachiana, 22,* 130–145.

Gacono, C. B., & Meloy, J. R. (2002). Assessing the psychopathic personality (2nd ed.). In J. Butcher (Ed.), *Clinical personality assessment* (pp. 361–375). New York: Oxford University Press.

Gacono, C. B., Meloy, J. R., & Berg, J. (1992). Object relations, defensive operations, and affective states in narcissistic, borderline, and antisocial personality. *Journal of Personality Assessment, 59,* 32–49.

Gacono, C. B., Meloy, J. R., & Bridges, M. (2000). A Rorschach comparison of psychopaths, sexual homicide perpetrators, and nonviolent pedophiles: Where angels fear to tread. *Journal of Clinical Psychology, 56*(6), 757–777.

Gacono, C. B., Meloy, J. R., & Heaven, T. (1990). A Rorschach investigation of narcissism and hysteria in antisocial personality disorder. *Journal of Personality Assessment, 55,* 270–279.

Gacono, C. B., Meloy, J. R., Sheppard, K., Speth, E., & Roske, A. (1995). A clinical investigation of malingering and psychopathy in hospitalized insanity acquittees. *Bulletin of American Academy of Psychiatry and the Law, 23*(3), 387–397.

Gacono, C. B., Meloy, J. R., Speth, E., & Roske, A. (1997). Above the law: Escapes from a maximum security forensic hospital and psychopathy. *American Academy of Psychiatry and the Law, 25*(4), 1–4.

Gacono, C. B., Nieberding, R., Owen, A., Rubel, J., & Bodholdt, R. (2001). Treating juvenile and adult offenders with Conduct-Disorder, Antisocial, and Psychopathic Personalities. In J. Ashford, B. Sales, & W. Reid (Eds.), *Treating adult and juvenile offenders with special needs* (pp. 99–130). Washington, DC: American Psychological Association.

Gunderson, J. G., & Ronningstam, E. (2001). Differentiating narcissistic and antisocial personality disorders. *Journal of Personality Disorder, 15,* 103–109.

Guze, S. (1976). *Criminality and psychiatric disorders.* New York: Oxford University Press.

Guze, S., Woodruff, R., & Clayton, P. (1971). Hysteria and antisocial behavior: Further evidence of an association. *American Journal of Psychiatry, 127,* 957–960.

Hare, R. (2003). *Manual for the Revised–Psychopathy Checklist* (2nd ed.). Toronto: Multi-Health Systems.

Harpur, T., Hare, R., & Hakstian, R. (1989). Two-factor conceptualization of psychopathy: Construct validity and assessment implications. *Psychological Assessment: A Journal of Consulting and Clinical Psychology, 1,* 6–17.

Heaven, T. (1988). *Relationship between Hare's Psychopathy Checklist and selected Exner Rorschach variables in an inmate population.* Unpublished doctoral dissertation, United States International University, San Diego.

Heilbrun, K. et al. (1998). Inpatient and post-discharge aggression in mentally disordered offenders: The role of psychopathy. *Journal of Interpersonal Violence, 13,* 514–527.

Huprich, S. K., Gacono, C. B., Schnieder, R. B., & Bridges, M. R. (2004). Rorschach oral dependency in psychopaths, sexual homicide perpetrators, and nonviolent pedophiles. *Behavioral Sciences and the Law, 22,* 345–356.

Karpman, B. (1949). The psychopathic delinquent child. *American Journal of Orthopsychiatry, 20,* 223–265.

Karpman, B. (1950). Psychopathic behavior in infants and children: A critical survey of the existing concepts. *American Journal of Orthopsychiatry,* 223–272.

Kernberg, O. (1975). *Borderline conditions and pathological narcissism.* New York: Aronson.

Kwawer, J. (1980). Primitive interpersonal modes, borderline phenomena and Rorschach content. In J. Kwawer, A. Sugarman, P. Lerner, & H. Lerner (Eds.), *Borderline phenomena and the Rorschach test* (pp. 89–109). New York: International Universities Press.

Lerner, P. (1991). *Psychoanalytic theory and the Rorschach.* Hillsdale, NJ: Analytic Press.

Lerner, P., & Lerner, H. (1980). Rorschach assessment of primitive defenses in borderline personality structure. In J. Kwawer, A. Sugarman, P. Lerner, & H. Lerner (Eds.), *Borderline phenomena and the Rorschach test* (pp. 257–274). New York: International Universities Press.

Lindner, R. (1943, July). The Rorschach test and the diagnosis of psychopathic personality. *Journal of Criminal Psychopathology,* 69–93.

Loving, J. L., & Russell, W. (2000). Selected Rorschach variables of psychopathic juvenile offenders. *Journal of Personality Assessment, 75*(1), 126–142.

Lyon, D. R., & Ogloff, J. R. (2000). Legal and ethical issues in psychopathy assessment. In C. B. Gacono (Ed.), *The clinical and forensic assessment of psychopathy: A practitioner's guide* (pp. 139–174). Mahwah, NJ: Lawrence Erlbaum Associates.

Meloy, R. (1988). *The psychopathic mind: Origins, dynamics, and treatment.* Northvale, NJ: Aronson.

Mahler, M., Pine, F., & Bergman, A. (1975). *The psychoanalytic birth of the human infant.* New York: Basic Books.

Meloy, J. R., Gacono, C. B., & Kenney, L. (1994). A Rorschach investigation of sexual homicide. *Journal of Personality Assessment, 62,* 58–67.

Meloy, J. R., & Gacono, C. B. (1992). The aggressive response and the Rorschach. *Journal of Clinical Psychology, 48*(1), 104–114.

Meloy, J. R., & Gacono, C. B. (1998). The internal world of the psychopath: A Rorschach investigation. In T. Millon, E. Simonsen, & M. Birket-Smith (Eds.), *Psychopathy: Antisocial, criminal, and violent behaviors* (pp. 95–109). New York: Guilford.

Meyer, G. J. (1992) Response frequency problems in the Rorschach: Clinical and research implications with suggestions for the future. *Journal of Personality Assessment, 58,* 231–244.

Morey, L. C. (1988) Personality disorders in *DSM–III* and *DSM–III–R*: Convergence, coverage, and internal consistency. *American Journal of Psychiatry, 145,* 573–577.

Neiberding, R., Gacono, C., Pirie, M., Bannatyne, L., Viglione, D., Cooper, B., Bodholdt, R., & Frackowiak, M. (2003). MMPI–2 based classification of forensic psychiatric outpatients: An exploratory cluster analytic study. *Journal of Clinical Psychology, 59*(9), 907–920.

Ogloff, J., Wong, S., & Greenwood, A. (1990). Treating criminal psychopaths in a therapeutic community program. *Behavioral Sciences and the Law, 8,* 181–190.

Plakun, E. M., Muller, J. P., & Burkhardt, P. E. (1987). The significance of borderline and schizotypal overlap. *Hillside Journal of Clinical Psychiatry, 9,* 47–54.

Rice, M. E., Harris, G. T., & Cormier, C. A. (1992). An evaluation of a maximum security therapeutic community for psychopaths and other mentally disordered offenders. *Law and Human Behavior, 16,* 399–412.

Smith, A. M., Gacono, C. B., & Kaufman, L. (1997). A Rorschach comparison of psychopathic and non-psychopathic conduct disordered adolescents. *Journal of Clinical Psychology, 53,* 289–300.

Robins, L. N. (1966). *Deviant children grown up.* Baltimore, MD: Williams & Wilkins.

Rogers, R., Salekin, R. T., Sewell, K. W., & Cruise, K. R. (2000). Prototypical analysis of antisocial personality disorder: A study of inmate samples. *Criminal Justice and Behavior, 27,* 234–255.

Rorschach, H. (1942). *Psychodiagnostics.* New York: Grune & Stratton. (Original work published 1921)

Shapiro, D. (1965). *Neurotic styles.* New York: Basic Books.

Smith, A. M., Gacono, C. B., & Kaufman, L. (1997). A Rorschach comparison of psychopathic and non-psychopathic conduct-disordered adolescents. *Journal of Clinical Psychology, 53*(4), 1–12.

Sullivan, H. S. (1953). *Interpersonal theory of psychiatry.* New York: Norton.

Weber, C., Meloy, J. R., & Gacono, C. B. (1992). A Rorschach study of attachment and anxiety in inpatient conduct-disordered and dysthymic adolescents. *Journal of Personality Assessment, 58*(1), 16–26.

Weiner, I. (1998). *Principles of Rorschach interpretation.* Mahwah, NJ: Lawrence Erlbaum Associates.

Winnicott, D. (1958). *The antisocial tendency. Collected papers.* London: Tavistock.

17

A RORSCHACH UNDERSTANDING
OF ANTISOCIAL AND PSYCHOPATHIC WOMEN

Ted B. Cunliffe
California Department of Corrections and Rehabilitation, Susanville

Carl B. Gacono
Private Practice, Austin, TX

Male psychopaths are responsible for a disproportionate number of serious behavioral problems (Hare & McPherson, 1984). They are difficult to manage, even when incarcerated or maintained in forensic hospitals (Gacono, Meloy, Sheppard, Speth, & Roske, 1995; Gacono, Meloy, Speth, & Roske, 1997; Ogloff, Wong, & Greenwood, 1990; Rice, 1997; Rice, Harris, & Cormier, 1992). Although the knowledge base for female psychopaths is growing, considerably less is known about them (Hare, 2003).

Male and female psychopaths display similar behaviors and share a comparable personality organization (Borderline or psychotic), however, research suggests that the syndrome is not equivalent across genders (Cunliffe, 2002; Cunliffe & Gacono, 2005).

Findings with males have supported psychodynamics characterized by grandiosity (Gacono, 1988; Gacono & Meloy, 1991, 1994; Gacono, Meloy, & Berg, 1992; Gacono, Meloy, & Heaven, 1990), a detached (Narcissistic) interpersonal style (Kernberg, 1975; Millon & Davis, 1996), and correlations with several of the *DSM–IV* (APA, 1994) Cluster B Personality Disorders, specifically, Narcissistic (NPD), Histrionic (HPD), and Antisocial Personality Disorders (ASPD). Research with female psychopaths has suggested that Hysteria, rather than Narcissism, is their corresponding character style (Cunliffe & Gacono, 2005; Gacono & Meloy, 1994).

Millon's (Millon & Davis; 1996) conceptualization of Histrionic Personality Disorder (HPD) helps our understanding of the Hysteric's motivations and hypothesized gender differences among psychopaths. The HPD individuals' reliance on others involves an active solicitation of others in order to satisfy their pronounced needs for affiliation and attention (active/dependent style; Millon & Davis, 1996). Additionally, Hysterical

---

[1]The paucity of research with females is primarily due to the relatively low numbers of incarcerated women when compared to males (Gacono & Meloy, 1994). For example, approximately 89% of federal inmates are male (Bureau of Justice Statistics, 1999), limiting the availability of female offenders as research participants.

character has been hypothesized to defend against a consciously experienced depression and a negative self-concept (Lazare & Klerman, 1968; Pfohl, 1991; Shapiro, 1965).

This chapter uses Rorschach data as a dependent measure for understanding female Antisocial Personality Disorder and psychopathy. It provides Comprehensive System data for female psychopaths from a growing sample of Antisocial Personality Disordered Females (see chap. 16). This data may be useful to examiners evaluating similar patients. Our Rorschach study comparing the differences between psychopathic and nonpsychopathic Antisocial Personality Disordered women is also presented and discussed. Finally, conceptual and practical issues related to the assessment of the female Antisocial and psychopathic individual are explored.

FEMALE PSYCHOPATHY: THE PCL–R AND RORSCHACH

Whereas many studies have used the Psychopathy Checklists with males, there have been approximately 20 studies with female offenders.[1] Many of these included methodological problems that limit their usefulness in understanding psychopathy (Gacono & Gacono, 2006; Gacono, Loving, & Bodholdt, 2001; Gacono, Loving, Evans, & Jumes, 2002). Some researchers have utilized the PCL:SV (Hart, Cox, & Hare, 1995) to designate "psychopathy" for group comparisons (Rogers, Johansen, Chang, & Salekin, 1997; Salekin, Rogers, & Sewell, 1998), despite the fact that the PCL:SV is a screening tool and not designed to make a categorical designation of psychopathy (Bodholdt, Richards, & Gacono, 2000; Gacono et al., 2001). Other studies have lowered their PCL–R cut-off scores (PCL–R < 30; Peaslee, Fleming, Baumgardner, Silbaugh, & Thackrey, 1992) and/or had few psychopaths (PCL–R $\geq$ 30) in their samples (Vitale & Newman, 2001; Vitale, Smith, Brinkley, & Newman, 2002). Finally, some investigators have discussed ASPD and psychopathy as synonymous constructs and attempted to discuss specific items on the PCL–R as indicative of psychopathy (Shipley & Arrigo, 2004). This "psychopathic traits" approach marks a return to the days prior to the advent of the PCL–R and has been sharply criticized (Hare, 2003; Gacono, 2000b; Gacono & Gacono, 2006).

Investigators have ignored these essential issues, and even though they had few or no psychopaths in their studies (PCL–R $\geq$ 30), have presented their findings "as if" this were not the case (Peaslee et al., 1992; Salekin et al., 1998). Specifically, whereas it would be acceptable to discuss dimensionally based findings in terms of the relative differences between high and low scores within a given sample, theorizing about "psychopaths (taxon)" in the absence of PCL–R $\geq$ 30 designated subjects is unjustified (Gacono & Gacono, 2006). Concerning the Rorschach/PCL–R studies, findings with male psychopaths or female ASPDs may not be relevant to female psychopaths (Gacono et al., 2001).

COMPREHENSIVE SYSTEM RORSCHACH DATA FOR FEMALE PSYCHOPATHS (N = 27)

Our psychopathic women are taken from a larger database of Antisocial Personality Disordered females (N = 69; see chap. 16; also Gacono & Meloy, 1994). Although our sample size is small, it offers trends that may be of interest to the reader. They are by no means de-

TABLE 17–1

Female Psychopaths (*N* = 27) Group Mean and Frequencies for Select Ratios, Percentages, and Derivations

R = 19.86 (*SD* = 6.66)	*L* = .71 (*SD* = .48)

EA = 7.30 (*SD* = 4.16)

es = 10.00 (*SD* = 6.60)

FM + *m* < *Sum Shading*.... 14 (50%)

D score = –1.04 (*SD* = 2.05)   *AdjD* = –0.54 (*SD* = 1.69)

EB style

Introversive.......................... 1   4%

Ambitent............................ 11   39%

Extratensive....................... 6   21%

EA–es differences:D scores

D score > 0.......................... 3   11%

D score = 0......................... 15   54%

D score < 0......................... 10   36%

D score < –1.........................9   32%

AdjD score > 0..................... 6   21%

AdjD score = 0................... 12   43%

AdjD score < 0................... 10   36%

AdjD score < –1................... 4   14%

Affect

FC:CF + *C* = .93 : 2.96

Pure C = .46 (*SD* = .58)   (*Pure C* > 0 = 43%; *Pure C* > 1 = 4%)

FC > (*CF* + *C*) + 2............... 1   4%

FC > (*CF* + *C*) + 1................ 2   7%

(*CF* + *C*) > *FC* + 1............. 16   57%

(*CF* + *C*) > *FC* + 2............. 11   39%

SumC' = *1.89* (*SD* = 1.95)

SumV = 2.04 (*SD* = 2.56)

SumY = 1.36 (*SD* = 1.42)

Afr = .54 (*SD* = .23)   (*Afr* < .40 = 8, 29%; *Afr* < .50 = 17, 61%)

S = 2.64 (*SD* = 1.97)   (*S* > 2 = 12, 43%)

Blends:R = 4.64 : 19.86

CP = .04 (*SD* = .19)

Interpersonal

COP = 1.39 (*SD* = 1.37)   (*COP* = 0 = 11, 39%; *COP* > 2 = 5, 18%)

AG = . 57 (*SD* = .92)   (*AG* = 0 = 17, 61%; *AG* > 2 = 1, 4%)

Food = .43 (*SD* = .79)

Isolate/R = .17 (*SD* = .13)

H:(*H*) + *Hd* + (*Hd*) = 2.36 : 3.82   (*H* = 0 = 4, 14%; *H* < 2 = 9, 32%)

(*H*) + (*Hd*):(*A*) + (*Ad*) = 2.07 : .72

H + *A:Hd* + *Ad* = 9.90 : 2.79

Sum T = .75 (*SD* = 1.21)   (*T* = 0 = 16, 57%; *T* > 1 = 4, 14%)

Self-perception

$3r + (2)/R = .40$ (SD = .16) $(3r + (2)/R < .33 = 12, 43\%; 3r + (2)/R > .44 = 9, 32\%)$

$Fr + rF = .54$ (SD = 1 .04) $(Fr + rF > 0 = 8, 29\%)$ $(FrrF = 0$ and $3r + (2) \geq .44 = 5, 18.5\%)$

$FD = .18$ (SD = .39)

$An + Xy = 2.04$ (SD = 2.14

$MOR = 2.39$ (SD = 2.46) $(MOR > 2 = 11, 39\%)$

Ideation

$a:p = 4.50 : 3.25$ $(p > a + 1 = 5, 18\%)$

$Ma:Mp = 1.93 : 1.82$ $(Mp > Ma = 9, 32\%)$

$M = 3.64$ (SD = 2.44) $(M- = .71, SD = 1.27; M\ none = 25\%)$

$FM = 2.50$ (SD = 1.64) $m = 1.46$ (SD = 1.57)

$2AB+Art+Ay = 2.57$ (SD = 2.60) $2AB+Art+Ay > 5 = 3, 11\%$

$Sum6 = 7.68$ (SD = 6.04) $WSum6 = 24.0$ (SD = 20.69)

$(Level\ 2\ Sp\ Sc > 0 = 12, 43\%)$

Mediation

$Populars = 4.61$ (SD = 2.20) $(P < 4 = 9, 32\%; P > 7 = 2, 7\%)$

$XA\% = .73$ (SD = .15)

$WDA\% = .76$ (SD = .16)

$X+\% = .51$ (SD = .14)

$X-\% = .25$ (SD = .15)

$Xu\% = .22$ (SD = .11)

$S- = 1.25$ (SD = 1.17)

$XA\% > .89$.............................1   4%

$XA\% < .70$.............................9   32%

$WDA\% < .85$.......................17   61%

$WDA\% < .75$.......................11   39%

$X+\% < .55$.........................15   54%

$Xu\% > .20$...........................15   54%

$X-\% > .20$...........................14   50%

$X-\% > .30$.............................7   25%

Processing

$Zf = 10.82$ (SD = 3.70)

$Zd = .61$ (SD = 3.52) $(Zd > + 3.0 = 6, 21\%; Zd < -3.0 = 4, 14\%)$

$W:D:Dd = 8.92:8.52:2.19$

$W:M = 8.86 : 3.64$

$DQ + = 5.29$ (SD = 3.02)

$DQv = 2.64$ (SD = 2.16) $(DQv > 2 = 13, 46\%)$

Constellations

$PTI = 5$........ 0	0%	$DEPI = 7$...... 2	7%	$CDI = 5$...... 1	4%
$PTI = 4$........ 4	14%	$DEPI = 6$...... 5	18%	$CDI = 4$...... 9	32%
$PTI = 3$........ 0	0%	$DEPI = 5$...... 4	14%		

S-Constellation Positive...... 1   4%

HVI Positive........................ 0   0%

OBS Positive....................... 0   0%

finitive or adequate for capturing the many individual differences that manifest when assessing individual patients. This sample was analyzed by Rorschach Workshops using RIAP4 Plus (Exner, Weiner, & Par Staff, 2002). Understanding the Rorschach data (core characteristics, controls, stress tolerance, affect, self-perception, thinking and processing, and interpersonal) from these psychopathic women adds to our understanding of the personality functioning of these patients. When appropriate our group data is compared to Exner (2001) Nonpatient group data ($N = 600$).

Core Characteristics, Controls, and Stress Tolerance

Female psychopaths produce less than a normative number of responses ($M = 19.86$; Exner, 2001, $M = 22.32$). She's likely to be *Ambitent* (39%) or *Extratensive* (21%) rather than *Introversive* (4%). Her diminished psychological resources ($EA, M = 7.30$, Npatient, $M = 8.66$) and reduced stress tolerance ($P, CDI \geq 4 = 36\%$, D score = 0, 54%, $AdjD = 0, 43\%$; Npatient, $CDI > 4 = 4\%$, D score = 0, 70%, $AdjD = 0, 65\%$) underscore an alloplastic adaptation to the environment. These personality characteristics are conducive to acting out that reduces the female psychopath's levels of experienced stress related distress ($P, es = M = 9.96$; NP, M = 8.74). Both the psychopathic and nonpsychopathic females, while differing from nonpatients, do not differ significantly on measures of control apart from the greater proportion of *nonpsychopathic* women producing $CDI > 4$ (Table 17–1).

Affect

Difficulty modulating affect is a hallmark of Histrionic and Borderline Personality Disorders and a predominate trait for our female psychopaths ($P, FC: CF + C = .93:2.96$, *Pure C* > 0 = 43%; Npatient, $FC:CF + C = 3.56: 2.53$, *Pure C* > 0 = 10%). The internal world of the psychopathic female is characterized by dysphoria ($P, DEPI \geq 5 = 41\%$; C', $M = 1.89$, $V, M = 2.04$; Npatient, $DEPI > 5 = 5\%$; C', M = 1.49, $V, M = .28$) and anger ($P, S > 2 = 43\%$; Npatient, 14%). Affective avoidance ($Afr, M = .54$, $Afr < .40$ & $.50 = 29\%$ & 61%; Npatient, $Afr < .40$ & $.50 = 3\%$ & 11%) and emotional constriction (P, *Blends* = 4.64) are natural, developmental reactions to an inability to deal with strong affect. Emotional constriction, avoidance, and acting out are similar to what is found in male psychopaths.

Thinking and Processing

Psychopathic women do not see the world as others do ($P, PTI > 3 = 15\%$; Npatient, $PTI > 3 = 0\%$). They tend to underincorporate ($P, Zd < -.3.0 = 14\%$; Npatient, $Zd < -.3.0 = 7\%$), missing important details essential to effective information processing. Their thinking contains fluidity, lacking structure and boundaries (DQv = 2.64; DQv > 2 = 46%). They are prone to misperceptions and unconventionality (*P*, *Populars [P]*, *M* = 4.61; Npatient, *P*, *M* = 6.58). Cognitive slippage abounds in psychopathic women (*Level 2 Special Scores* > 0 = 43%; Npatient, 6%) as do other indicators of formal thought disorder.

Self-Perception

Poor controls, problems managing affect, and unconventional and distorted thinking all contribute to the female psychopath's negative evaluation of self (*P, 3r + [2]/R* < .33 = 43%; Npatient, *3r + [2]/R* < .33 = 13%). Healthy self-esteem is not expected without emotional mastery. The grandiose self-structure found in the adult male psychopath (Kernberg, 1975) is not manifested in the same way in female psychopaths. These women perceive themselves as "damaged" (*P, MOR, M* = 2.39; Npatient, *MOR, M* = .79), and although they possess a corresponding self focus to males, the female psychopath's self-perception is characterized by poor self-regard and chronic self criticism (*3r + [2]/R, < .33; P*, 43%; *Sum V, M* = 2.04. Npatient, 13%; *Sum V, M* = .28).

Interpersonal

As expected, psychopathic women do not experience cooperation as a natural result of interpersonal interactions (*P, COP* = 0 = 39%; Npatient, *COP* = 0 = 17%). Perhaps, a combination of biological predisposition and severe disappointments (narcissistic wounding) contribute to reduced affectional relatedness (*P, T* = 0 = 57%; Npatient, *T* = 0 = 18%) and a diminished interest in others (*P, H* < 2 = 32%; Npatient, *H* < 2 = 12%). Certainly, low or inflated self-worth and misinterpretations of interpersonal cues further weaken the opportunity for positive interpersonal experience (Gacono & Meloy, 1997). As a result, psychopathic women have poor interpersonal experiences (*P, CDI* ≥ 4 = 37%; GHR > PHR = 32%; Npatient, *CDI* > 4 = 4%; *GHR* > PHR = 88%). All of these factors ultimately coalesce into an increasingly detached and exploitative view of interpersonal relations in a manner quite similar to Sullivan's (1953) concept of malevolent transformation.

THE RORSCHACH STUDY: PSYCHOPATHIC AND NONPSYCHOPATHIC ANTISOCIAL PERSONALITY DISORDERED WOMEN

Our comparison samples were comprised of 40 participants from 3 women's correctional facilities and 5 subjects from Gacono and Meloy's (1994) ASPD female offender files. Twenty-three were collected from 2 low-medium security women's federal prisons in northern California (Federal Correctional Institution–Dublin [FCI–Dublin], Federal Prison Camp–Dublin [FPC–Dublin]) and 17 were collected from a larger sample of women incarcerated in a female prison in Wyoming (see Gacono & Meloy, 1994; Peaslee, 1993). Whereas the 17 subjects from the Peaslee (1993) sample and the 5 subjects from the Gacono and Meloy (1994) ASPD sample were previously presented as part of ASPD group data ($N = 38$; Gacono & Meloy, 1994), none of these 22 subjects have been previously used in comparisons of PCL–R identified psychopathic (PCL–R $\geq$ 30) and low scoring female ASPD offenders (PCL–R < 25). The combined sample consisted of two distinct groups: psychopathic (PCL–R $\geq$ 0; $n = 27$) and nonpsychopathic (PCL–R < 25; n = 18) offenders.

The ethnicity of the combined female sample was 65% Caucasian, 15% African American, 15% Hispanic, and 2% Asian. Ages ranged from 21 to 70 years ($M = 32.40$, $SD =$ 10.70), IQ estimates fell between 80 and 155 ($M = 106.12$, $SD = 14.37$), and over 50% of the women possessed a high school diploma or GED. The psychopathy group (PCL–R $\geq$ 30) contained 14 Caucasians (52%), 7 African Americans (26%), 5 Hispanics (18%), and 1 participant of unidentified racial origin (4%), whereas the nonpsychopathy group was comprised of 14 Caucasians (78%), 2 Asians (11%) and 2 Hispanics (11%).

The study participants were incarcerated for violence ($N = 16$; 35%), drugs ($N = 17$; 37%), fraud ($N = 12$; 26%), theft ($N = 7$; 15%), sex offenses ($N = 5$; 11%), and unknown (N = 6; 13%). All participants met the *DSM–IV* (APA, 1994) criteria for ASPD. Although a systematic examination of other *DSM–IV* Personality Disorders was not conducted, a high percentage of subjects also met the criteria for HPD and Borderline Personality Disorder (BPD). Participants who produced PCL–R scores greater than or equal to 30 were included in the psychopathic group (P–APSD), whereas individuals scoring less than or equal to 24 were included in a nonpsychopathic group (NP–ASPD).

The Shipley Institute of Living Scale (SILS), PCL–R, and Rorschach Inkblot Method (RIM; Rorschach, 1921) were administered to 75 incarcerated women. The measures were administered in accordance with procedures outlined for the SILS (Zachary, 1986), PCL–R (Hare, 2003; Gacono, 2000a), and Rorschach (Exner, 1993). The SILS was used to screen out participants below an IQ score of 80.

The PCL–R was used to assess each participant's level of psychopathy. Participants with PCL–R scores greater than or equal to 30 were included in the psychopathy group. PCL–R administration and scoring entails an intensive review of the participant's medical, legal, and institution files succeeded by a detailed semistructured interview and rating of the individual's personality and antisocial behaviors. Gacono's (2000b, 2005) Clinical and Forensic Interview Schedule was used to organize record and interview information. Record review produced a 100% agreement between the authors for the ASPD diagnosis.

The Rorschach protocols were scored for *Fr/rF* (self-focus), *PER* (defensiveness, aggrandizement), (2), *MOR* (sense of self-damage), *V* (painful rumination), *FD* $\geq$ 1 (psychological mindedness), *T* (affectional relatedness), *COP* (expectations of cooperative

---

[2]All of the discarded Rorschach protocols had been administered by a single examiner. It was also discovered that several had been administered per day. A review of the verbatim protocols indicated inadequate inquiry, perhaps due, in part, to the rapid administration. Although a tempting method for increasing our N, rather than picking out potentially "valid" protocols, and thereby biasing the subject selection process, we eliminated all protocols administered by the single examiner.

human interactions), *Fd* (neediness), *X–%* (reality testing), *X+%* (perceptual accuracy), and the *Human Experience Variable* (*HEV*; Perry & Viglione, 1991). The *HEV* relates to the quality of interpersonal relatedness (Burns & Viglione, 1996).

Procedure

All participants were unpaid volunteers. Half of the incarcerated population at the facilities (665 inmates) randomly received a flyer requesting their participation in the study. Exclusion criteria for selection were IQ < 80, previous diagnosis of a major mental illness, pending release from the institution (< 2 months), and/or a lack of fluency in the English language.

Potential participants were informed of the purpose, procedures, risks and benefits, and limits to confidentiality were reviewed. Of the 103 women who volunteered for the study, 20 (19.6%) were eliminated due to language problems, 2 (2%) had a history of Schizophrenia, 3 (3%) had a history of Bipolar Disorder, 1 (1%) expressed suicidal ideation and intent, 1 (1%) woman was transferred from the institution before testing could be completed, and 1 (1%) individual withdrew. Seventy-five participants completed the study procedures. Unfortunately, 48 (64%) of the original 75 subjects were excluded from the study due to inadequate Rorschach administration (Gacono, Evans, & Viglione, 2002).[2] Of the remaining 27 women, 22 were medium to maximum security inmates and 5 were low security work camp inmates. Four women were not included in our analyses because their PCL–R scores fell between 25 and 29.

Prior to being interviewed, the institutional, psychological, legal, and medical files of each inmate were reviewed. PCL–R interviews and ratings were conducted by 2 PhD level graduate students trained in the administration, scoring, and interpretation of the measure. Next, Rorschach protocols were administered following Comprehensive System guidelines (Exner, 1993) and scored by a PhD level graduate student. The sample was supplemented with 17 records selected from a database of incarcerated females collected in Wyoming (Gacono & Meloy, 1994; Peaslee et al., 1992) and another 5 protocols from the Gacono and Meloy database.

Participants scoring greater than or equal to 30 on the PCL–R (*N* = 27) were assigned to the psychopathic ASPD group (P–ASPD) and those scoring less than 25 comprised the nonpsychopathic ASPD group (NP–ASPD; *N* = 18). Upon completion of the data collection phase of the study, all Rorschach protocols were sent to an independent rater for rescoring (blind to PCL–R score) to be used in the calculation of interrater reliability. Twenty Rorschachs and PCL–Rs were chosen at random for the calculation of the interrater reliability.

Results

Of the original 75 participants, PCL–R scores for the FCI–Dublin Sample were *M* = 25.46 (*SD* = 6.38), whereas the scores for the sample of 45 participants used in this study ranged

---

[3]We note that studies of female violence have found women to be less likely to engage in predatory violence (typically found in male psychopaths; Hare & McPherson, 1984) and more liable to exhibit affectively based on reactive aggression (i.e., reacting to emotion evoked by a lesbian love triangle).

TABLE 17–2

Select Structural Variables for Psychopathic and Nonpsychopathic Incarcerated Females

Variable	Psychopaths (N = 27)			Nonpsychopaths (N = 18)			Effect Size (r)
	M	SD	Freq	M	SD	Freq	
Fr/rF	.44	.79	8	.72	1.03	7	Ns
PER			18			14	Ns
(2) > 10			5			1	.32
Ego > .44			5			2	.10
Fr/rF = 0							
MOR > 2			10			4	.11
V > 0			11			3	.11
FD > 1			4			5	.19
Interpersonal relationships							
T = 0			15			14	.26
T = 1			8			3	.26
T > 2			4			1	.27
Prt Obj T			5			0	.28
COP			27			18	.18
COP > 2			13			4	Ns
COP (spoil)			27			11	.20
COP (good)			9			8	.10
Fd			6			1	.33
HEV	−.20	1.41	7	−.24	2.09	8	.24
Reality testing							
X+% < .61	.51	.14	21	.57	.14	10	.23
X−% > .15	.24	.15	6	.16	.89	2	.29
X+% < .61 +X−% > .15			18			4	.27

from 11.60 to 39 ($M = 27.80$, $SD = 6.37$). The P–ASPD group ($N = 27$) had a mean PCL–R score of 32.69 ($SD = 2.81$), whereas the NP–ASPD group ($N = 18$) had a mean PCL–R score of 20.73 ($SD = 3.38$). PCL–R interrater reliability analyses yielded Spearman Rhos of .98 (Total scores), .93 (Factor 1), and .92 (Factor 2).

No significant differences in age or IQ were noted (P–ASPD Age: $M = 33.15$, $SD = 11.07$; NP–ASPD: $M = 31.44$, $SD = 10.62$; P IQ: $M = 103.23$, $SD = 14.35$; NP: $M = 109.94$, $SD = 13.46$, $p > .05$). The P–ASPD group contained 14 Caucasians (50%), 7 African Americans (25%), 5 Hispanics (18%), and 1 Asian (3.5%), whereas the NP–ASPD group contained 16 Caucasians (89%) and 2 African Americans (11%), with no Asian or Hispanic participants. Both groups contained significantly more Caucasians than other ethnicities (X^2 = 22.26, p < .001).

P–ASPDs were incarcerated for violence (54%), drugs (50%), sex (25%), fraud (21%), and theft (21%); NP–ASPDs were incarcerated for violence (6%), drugs (25%), sex (6%), fraud (39%), and theft (17%). The P–ASPD group contained significantly more violent offenders (X^2 = 4.79, p = .029), whereas the NP–ASPD group contained significantly more women incarcerated for fraud (X^2 = 7.68, p = .006). This is consistent with the positive correlations between psychopathy level and violence in male offender samples.[3]

Rorschach Results.   There were no significant differences in the number of Rorschach responses between the groups (P–ASPD: 14–43; M=19.86 [SD=6.66]; NP–ASPD: 14–32; M = 17.66 [SD = 4.87], p ≥ .05). An overall 88% agreement was obtained for coding. For individual Rorschach variables percent agreement was as follows: *Reflections* (100%), *Personals* (84%), *Morbid* (88%), *Pairs* (89%), *Vista* (85%), *Form Dimension* (96%), *Texture* (84%), *Cooperative Human Movement* (89%), *Food Content* (84%), and *Cognitive Special Scores* (79%) (see Table 17–2).

Self-Perception.   There were no significant differences in the proportions or frequencies of Reflection responses (P–ASPD, M = .44; NP–ASPD, M = .72, p > .05). No significant differences were found in the frequency or proportions of *PER* responses or total number of *Pair* responses (2). However, significantly more psychopaths produced 11 or more *Pairs* (P = 22%; NP = 5%; p = .001) and elevated *Egocentricity Ratios* (> .44) without a *Reflection* response (P–ASPD = 18.5%; NP–ASPD = 11%; p = < .001).

P–ASPDs also produced more protocols with > 2 *MOR*s than NP–ASPDs (P–ASPD = 37%, NP–ASPD = 22%; p = .006). The difference between mean *V*s (P–ASPD, M = 1.66, SD = 1.57; NP–ASPD, M = 2.23, SD = 2.45) was not significant; however, a significantly greater number of psychopaths produced > 1 *Vista* response (P–ASPD = 41%; NP–ASPD = 17%; X^2 = 68.08, p = < .001). Fewer psychopaths (4, 15%) produced at least 1 *FD* compared to 5 (28%) of NP–ASPDs (X^2 = 49.32, p < .001).

Interpersonal Relationships

P–ASPDs produced the following distribution of *Texture* (*T*) responses: T = 0 (N = 15, 56%), T = 1 (N = 8, 30%), and T ≥ 2 (N = 4, 15%). Fourteen (78%) NP–ASPD participants produced T = 0, 3 (17%) T = 1, and 1 (6%) T ≥ 2 (P–ASPD; M = .75; NP–ASPD; M = .28; X^2 = 23.66, < .001). P–ASPDs also produced significantly more part object *T* responses (*T* with *Ad* or *Hd* content) compared to the NP–ASPDs (high = 5, 19%; low = 0; X^2 = 28.17, p < .001). Additionally, P–ASPDs produced a significantly higher mean number of *Fd* responses (P–ASPD; M = .26; NP–ASPD; M = .11; Wilcoxon U = 199.5; p = .020) and a larger proportion of *Fd* (P–ASPD; 6 [22%] NP–ASPD; 1 [5%]; X^2 = 23.17; p < .001). Of note, 5 (83%) of the 6 *Fd* responses produced by P–ASPDs were spoiled (poor form quality; Gacono & Meloy, 1991).

The P–ASPD group produced 36 *COP* responses, whereas NP–ASPDs produced 19 ($X^2 = 16.30, p = .003$). Thirteen (48%) P–ASPDs produced *COP* ≥ 2 compared to 4 (22%) NP–ASPDs ($X^2 = 3.13, p = .08$; ns). Although not significant, a trend between psychopathy and increased *COP* production was observed. Significantly more P–ASPDs produced spoiled (poor form quality; P; 27 [75%]; NP; 11 [58%]; $X^2 = 19.56$; $p < .001$) and fewer good quality *COP* (P; 9 [25%]; NP; 8 [42%]; $X^2 = 27.96$, $p \leq .001$) responses. The P–ASPD group had a mean *Human Experience Variable* (*HEV*; Perry & Viglione, 1991) of $-.20$ ($SD = 1.41$) compared to a mean of $-.24$ ($SD = 2.09$) for the NP–ASPD group (Mann-Whitney $U = 222.00$; ns). Significantly fewer psychopaths scored in the high range of interpersonal relatedness (P–ASPD = 22%, NP–ASPD = 44%, $X^2 = 7.04$, $p = .008$).

Reality Testing.   There were no significant differences found between the mean $X+\%$ values (P–ASPD; $M = .51$; NP–ASPD; $M = .57$, $p > .05$). However, significantly more of the P–ASPDs ($N = 21, 78\%$) had $X+\%$ values below .61 (NP–ASPDs, $N = 11; 61\%; X^2 = 4.79, p = .029$). Although both groups evidenced problems with reality testing ($X-\% > .15$), P–ASPDs exhibited greater impairment (P–ASPD; $M = .24$; NP–ASPD; $M = .16$; Mann-Whitney $U = 167.5$, $p = .057$). Significantly more psychopaths produced an $X-\%$ value greater than .29 (P–ASPD = 22%; NP–ASPD = 11%; $X^2 = 20.45, p < .001$). Eighteen (67%) psychopaths had a $X+\% < .61$ and $X-\% > .15$ compared to 8 (44%) of the low psychopathy group; this difference was not significant ($p > .05$).

Discussion

The mean PCL–R score ($M = 27.80$) of our sample was greater than previously reported ($M = 23.37$; Hare, 2003; $M = 21.1$; Neary, 1990; $M = 24.49$; Strachan, 1993). Specifically, there were proportionately more psychopaths (PCL–R ≥ 30) in our sample. Two primary factors impact previously reported mean PCL–R scores. First, other researchers have included fewer female psychopaths (PCL–R ≥ 30) in their samples. Second, previous studies have included subjects from the entire inmate population. In this study, we included only those female offenders with a concurrent ASPD diagnosis; thereby, elevating the mean PCL–R scores for the sample.

Our findings suggest that female psychopaths differ from their nonpsychopathic counterparts in a number of areas. Compared to NP–ASPDs, the psychopaths experienced marked disturbances in self-perception (negative self-image), dysphoric affect, poor self-regard, limited capacity for introspection, poor interpersonal relatedness (superficial interpersonal relations), limited understanding of the motivations of others, lack of empathy, and poor reality testing (cognitive distortion and unconventionality).

---

[4]Whereas female offenders have been found to be four times as likely to produce a *Reflection* response (related to self-focus) when compared to nonpatient females (Gacono & Meloy, 1994; Peaslee, 1993), they produce fewer *Reflections* than male psychopaths. Gender differences have also been observed with adolescents, whereby males were found to produce more animal than human *Reflection* responses and females produced *Reflections* involving more scenes, mirrors, and trees (Ames, Metraux, & Walker, 1959).

The greater number of female P–ASPDs who produced elevated *Egocentricity Ratios* without a *Reflection* is noteworthy. Whereas high *Egocentricity Ratios* suggest an inordinate self-focus, high ratios without Reflection indicate a sense of displeasure in doing so (Weiner, 1998). Male psychopaths look at themselves exalting in self-admiration and grandiosity (high *Reflections*, high *Egocentricity Ratio*). In contrast, our female psychopaths appear to experience distress while engaging in the same process (high *Egocentricity Ratio* without *Reflections*). Individuals with a pattern of no *Reflections*, high *Egocentricity Ratios*, and *Vistas*, possess a situation-specific type of self-criticism not related to a true sense of remorse or guilt (Weiner, 1998). This pattern suggests chronic self-criticism and shame. Rather than remorse or guilt, the self-critical, unhappy, and dissatisfied presentation of the female psychopath may be viewed as an insidious negative self-image arising from long-standing frustration over unmet needs for attention and admiration.

The similar frequencies for *Reflection* responses in our groups argue against the presence of the grandiose self-structure operating in male psychopaths (Gacono et al., 1990; Loving & Russell, 2000; Smith, Gacono, & Kaufman, 1995; Young, Justice, Erdberg, & Gacono, 2000).[4] Rather, the female psychopath struggles with a hysterical need for attention and admiration from others (Millon & Davis, 1996) in order to mediate the effects of chronic dissatisfaction and self-criticism. Their increased *COP*, *V*, *Fd*, and *T* combined with larger proportions of spoiled *COP* and part *T* responses highlight the tenuousness of a pattern reliant on others to regulate self-esteem and mood. Compared to the independent detached interpersonal style noted in male psychopaths, the female's increased superficial need for attention and interpersonal contact renders her more dependent on the views and approval of others, resulting in a chronic, negative sense of self.

The larger numbers of female psychopaths who produced *White Space* ($S > 0$; P–ASPD $= 44\%$; NP–ASPD $= 22\%$; $X^2 = 23.17$, $p < .001$) and *Sum shading* $> FM + m$ (dysphoric affect; P–ASPD $= 48\%$; NP–ASPD $= 7\%$; $X^2 = 4.79$, $p = .029$) contrasted with the NP–ASPDs production of increased C' (P–ASPD $= 18\%$; NP–ASPD $= 33\%$; $X^2 = 13.30$, $p < .001$) suggest that, in addition to the negative self-image and limited capacity for introspection ($FD \geq 1$; P–ASPD $= 15\%$, NP–ASPD $= 28\%$, $X^2 = 7.89$, $p < .001$), female psychopaths appear to experience increased dysphoric affect and negative, oppositional feelings. Because other signs of a deeper, more consciously experienced depression evidenced by social isolation ($COP < 2$), low energy (suggested by *Blends* < 4), anhedonia and difficulties sorting out their feelings (*Color Shading Blends* > 0) while experiencing more painful internalized affect (*Sum C'* > 2) are absent, it is likely that their sadness and "depression" arise from character pathology rather than true depression. Consistent with theory (Gacono & Meloy, 1994; Lazare & Klerman, 1968), the chronic self-preoccupied, critical, and negative self-image exhibited by the female psychopaths in our study supports the assertion that their regulatory mechanisms fail to bolster self-esteem. This may represent a gender difference.

Although our psychopaths displayed greater needs for "affectional relatedness" than the nonpsychopaths, further analyses of the psychopaths' *COP, Food* content, and *T* responses suggest that their poor understanding of the motivations and desires of those around them severely compromise their ability to engage in genuine and reciprocal relations with others. Despite her heightened interest in others, the female psychopath exhibits a reduced capacity for interpersonal relatedness (increased spoiled *COP* and *Fd*, part-object *T*; fewer psychopaths scoring in the high range on the *HEV*). Our findings support the superficial, shallow, and insincere character of these women, while predicting the female psychopath's preference for more frequent, superficial interpersonal contacts.

The female psychopath's interest in others is not based on a desire for greater intimacy, but rather is motivated by a need to be the center of attention. Self-focus is sought in the interests of providing a distraction from ruminative self-criticism, a sense of insecurity, a negative sense of self, and the experience of dysphoric affect. Thus, an examiner should not confuse this increased need for "connection" with empathy or caring, but instead should interpret it as an attempt to satisfy her endless needs for attention. Additionally, the female psychopath's diminished capacity for introspection (*FD*; P–ASPD = 15%; NP–ASPD = 28%; $X^2 = 7.89$, $p < .001$) further reduces her ability to establish and maintain healthy relations with others.

Millon and Davis (1996) characterized *HPD* as an amalgam of active-dependent characteristics and sensation-seeking behavior. The Histrionic Personality was distinguished from the Dependent Personality Disorder (DPD) by the manner in which the Histrionic person actively solicits attention and admiration through seductive, entertaining, and manipulative behaviors. Although both styles exhibit dependency, the Histrionic presentation is characterized by a gregarious, extroverted attempt to garner the attention and support of the intended person or group rather than by more indirect means typically employed by DPD individuals. That is, DPD individuals will employ a passive and helpless presentation to elicit caring and attending behavior from the other person whereas the HPD person, on the other hand, will gain the desired contact and attention via entertaining, dramatic, and emotionally expressive displays. The pseudo-dependency of the female psychopath is reflected in her increased production of *Texture*, *Food* content, and *COP* responses. The female psychopath's decreased interpersonal relatedness and limited capacity for genuine intimacy is consistent with HPD theory (Chodoff & Lyons, 1958; Millon & Davis, 1996; Phohl, 1991).

Poor interpersonal judgment and the misperception of interpersonal cues are highlighted by the Rorschach findings (high degree of perceptual distortion and impairment). Investigators have previously emphasized the problems Hysterical or Histrionic individuals display with reality testing (Chodoff & Lyons, 1958; Pfohl, 1991). Our female psychopaths produced elevated scores on Rorschach indices indicating impaired reality testing (*X–%*). Two of the *DSM–IV HPD* criteria are relevant here: "7) is suggestible, i.e., easily influenced by others and circumstances; and 8) considers relationships to be more intimate than they actually are" (APA, 1994, p. 658). The Histrionic person's misinterpretation of intimacy and increased suggestibility reflect the interaction of poor reality testing (distorted thinking) and interpersonal dependency.

The current conceptualization of male psychopathy is an amalgam of a self-centered, grandiose, and Narcissistic Personality style and a criminal, Antisocial lifestyle. The female psychopath's PCL–R profile suggests a person who is less grandiose, more interested in others, and behaviorally less violent. Both genders do, however, exhibit similar degrees of conning and manipulative behavior (PCL–R Item 5), pathological lying (Item

4), and Antisocial (Items 3, 9, 10, 14, & 15) and criminal activity (Items 18–20). This female PCL–R profile suggests that although, it might first appear that she is more interested in relations with others, this interest is likely to be very superficial.

Gender differences are also reflected in the differing patterns of aggression and violence displayed by men and women. Women serving a sentence for a violent offense have been found to be two times more likely to have committed their offense against an acquaintance (Bureau of Justice Statistics, 1999). Again, this indicates the importance of others in the lives of female criminals. Heightened interpersonal dependency, poor understanding of others, and limited capacity for introspection increase the risk of the female psychopath offending against her family, friends, and acquaintances. Male psychopaths, on the other hand, exhibit a detachment from others reflected in their acts of violence against strangers (Hare & McPherson, 1984). Integration of cross-sectional findings with studies of aggression suggests that male violence is driven by narcissism. (Gacono & Meloy, 1994). That is, whereas Factor 2 (Antisocial lifestyle) PCL–R scores may decline slightly over the life span, Factor 1 scores (Narcissism) do not.

Our findings have implications for the administration, scoring, and interpretation of the PCL–R with women. As with all PCL–R administrations, it is important to gain as much record information as possible before the structured interview portion of the measure is conducted. This is a particularly pertinent factor in the PCL–R administration of female offenders given their high needs for impression management and praise from others, something not seen as frequently in male offenders, whereby their interest in being seen in a positive light is in the interests of manipulating others. The naive or inexperienced rater should not interpret dysphoric affect (as reflected in Rorschach data presented in this chapter; see Tables 17–1 and 17–2) and "depression" as guilt (Item 6) or evidence against the presence of shallow affect (Item 7). As always, accurate scoring requires a full exploration of the nature of the reported symptoms (Gacono, 2000c). A chronic negative sense of self, shame, and dissatisfaction are distinct from the experience of a true depression or remorse. These latter affective states involve a sense of guilt for past behavior and a depressive presentation characterized by low energy, problems sleeping/eating, and/or anhedonia. It is suggested that the female psychopath's affective displays are more akin to rumination and self-pity than true remorse.

Incorrect PCL–R scoring may also be compounded when the examiner discovers a history of treatment for depression or "suicide attempts" noted in medical or mental health records and mistakes these behavioral markers as indicators of actual depression or a full range of affect. A careful exploration of the history is essential to distinguish between possible cutting behavior for the purposes of escaping dysphoric affect and rumination (an aspect of Hysteria and perhaps, Borderline Personality), or feigned suicidal behavior for the purposes of secondary gain and bona fide suicide attempts, whereby the individual suffers severe depression, guilt, or remorse for past actions. That is, the examiner must take care to discriminate true depressive symptoms from the experience of inner emptiness (a chronically unhappy, dissatisfied person frustrated by failed attempts to elicit attention from others). This may consist of an intensive examination of inpatient or outpatient treatment reviews, treatment contacts, and disciplinary actions taken by security staff against the inmate relating to their contact with medical or mental health staff (i.e., lying to staff or feigning illness).

The female psychopath's increased desire for contact with others may also complicate PCL–R scoring. At first glance, it may appear that her increased interest in others or stated love for her children is evidence of a capacity for attachment or empathy for others (Item 8). However, consider if the children have been placed on the individual's visiting list, the frequency of the visits, letters received, and their behavior toward others in their social milieu (behavior in court, statements about their crime/victims, conduct in the institution, and past relationships) when making this determination. In some cases, the female psychopath may use the separation from her children as a means to garner sympathy from others and draw attention to herself. Upon more careful investigation, it may be revealed that she has little interest in her children or their activities nor has she made any significant attempts to maintain contact with them. The psychopath's increased, yet superficial and self-serving, interest in others may cause less experienced or naive clinicians to misinterpret or project their own feelings brought about by empathizing with the situation presented by the psychopath onto their assessment and thereby, overvalue the quality or depth of the female psychopath's affective life and interpersonal relationships, and consequently, overestimate the inmate's capacity for empathy.

The prototypical description of the psychopath has emerged from over 100 years of scientific study of male criminal behavior and corresponding personality structure. In contrast, the study of female psychopathy is still in it's infancy. The psychopathic interpersonal style of a Narcissistic, detached, cold, calculating, hostile, and remorseless individual has evolved from studying male psychopathy (Gacono, 2000; Hare, 2003). In many respects, the female psychopath's presentation of an interpersonally needy, gregarious, superficially friendly, and self-critical individual is at first blush, at odds with the prototypic image. The engaging style of the female psychopath may catch the inexperienced or naive rater off guard. It is essential for the examiner to carefully consider the inmate's relations with others as evidenced by her actions, behaviors, and interpersonal reactions rather than her verbal reports.

The male and female expressions of psychopathy differ from one another in two separate but related dimensions: interpersonal relatedness and self-perception. The female psychopath's pronounced needs for "relatedness" and adulation from others form the cornerstone of her Histrionic character. Her interpersonal connections are focused on attempts to overcome her negative self-concept and dysphoric feelings that have arisen from her perceived alienation from those around her. The very dysphoria and feelings of anger and irritation she seeks to escape have their roots in unmet needs for affiliation and desire to be "entertained" by others. The female psychopath lacks the grandiose self-structure and detachment noted in males, and although she may lack the male psychopaths' desire for domination and humiliation of others, she displays a corresponding incapacity for empathy and perspective taking. The females also exhibit similar problems empathizing with others when compared to males. But, rather than a detached, devaluation of their victims, they display a clear disregard for the welfare of others despite an outward appearance of interrelatedness.

Although our findings offer preliminary support for the hypothesized Histrionic character of the female psychopath (Gacono & Meloy, 1994), they also provide important clues into the interpersonal and personality functioning of the female psychopath and highlight the need for continued study of female offenders, in general, and female psychopaths, in particular.

ACKNOWLEDGMENT

This is a revised and expanded version of an article previously published in the *International Journal of Offender Therapy and Comparative Criminology, 49*(5), 530–546, 2005, and is printed by permission.

REFERENCES

American Psychiatric Association. (1994). *Diagnostic and statistical manual of mental disorders* (4th ed.). Washington, DC: Author.

Ames, L., Metraux, R., & Walker, R. (1959). *Adolescent Rorschach responses*. New York: Hoeber.

Bodholdt, R. H., Richards, H. R., & Gacono, C. B. (2000). Assessing psychopathy in adults: The psychopathy checklist-revised and screening version. In C. B. Gacono (Ed.), *The clinical and forensic assessment of psychopathy: A practitioner's guide* (pp. 55–86). Mahwah, NJ: Lawrence Erlbaum Associates.

Bureau of Justice Statistics. (1999). *Women offenders (Bureau of Justice Statistics Bulletin)*. Rockville, MD: U.S. Department of Justice.

Burns, B., & Viglione, D. J. (1996). The Rorschach human experience variable, interpersonal relatedness, and object representation in nonpatients. *Psychological Assessment, 8*(1), 92–99.

Chodoff, P., & Lyons, H. (1958). Hysteria, the hysterical personality, and "hysterical" conversion. *American Journal of Psychiatry, 114,* 734–740.

Cunliffe, T. (2002). *A Rorschach investigation of incarcerated female psychopaths*. Unpublished doctoral dissertation, Pacific Graduate School of Psychology, Palo Alto, CA.

Cunliffe, T., & Gacono, C. (2005). A Rorschach investigation of incarcerated Antisocial Personality Disordered Female Offenders. *International Journal of Offender Therapy and Comparative Criminology, 49*, 530–547.

Exner, J. E. (1993). *The Rorschach: A Comprehensive System: Vol. 2. Basic foundations* (3rd ed.). New York: Wiley.

Exner, J. E. (2001) *A Rorschach workbook for the Comprehensive System* (5th ed.). Ashville, NC: Rorschach Workshops.

Exner, J. E., Weiner, I. B., & Par Staff. (2002). *Rorschach interpretation assistance program: Version 4 plus for Windows*. Lutz, FL: Psychological Assessment Resources, Inc.

Gacono, C. (2005). *A clinical and forensic interview schedule for the Hare Psychopathy Checklist–Revised and screening version*. Mahwah, NJ: Lawrence Erlbaum Associates.

Gacono, C. B. (1988). *A Rorschach interpretation of object relations and defensive structure and their relationship to narcissism and psychopathy in a group of antisocial offenders*. Unpublished doctoral dissertation, United States International University, San Diego, CA.

Gacono, C. B. (2000a). Appendix A: PCL–R clinical and forensic interview schedule. In C. B. Gacono (Ed.), *The clinical and forensic assessment of psychopathy: A practitioner's guide* (pp. 409–421). Mahwah, NJ: Lawrence Erlbaum Associates.

Gacono, C. B. (Ed.). (2000b). *The clinical and forensic assessment of psychopathy: A practitioner's guide* (pp. 175–202). Mahwah, NJ: Lawrence Erlbaum Associates.

Gacono, C. B. (2000c). Suggestions for implementation and use of the psychopathy checklists in forensic and clinical practice. In C. B. Gacono (Ed.), *The clinical and forensic assessment of psychopathy: A practitioner's guide.* Mahwah, NJ: Lawrence Erlbaum Associates.

Gacono, C. B., Evans, B., & Viglione, D. (2002). The Rorschach in forensic practice. *Journal of Forensic Psychology Practice, 2*(3), 33–53.

Gacono, C. B., & Gacono, L. A. (2006). Some caveats for evaluating the research of psychopathy. *The Corectional Psychologist, 38*(2), 7–9.

Gacono, C. B., Loving, J., Evans, B., & Jumes, M. (2002). The Psychopathy Checklist–Revised: PCL–R testimony and forensic practice. *Journal of Forensic Psychology Practice, 2*(3), 33–53.

Gacono, C. B., Loving, J., & Bodholdt, R. (2001). The Rorschach and psychopathy: Toward a more accurate understanding of the research findings. *Journal of Personality Assessment, 77*(1), 16–38.

Gacono, C. B., Meloy, J. R., & Heaven, T. R. (1990). A Rorschach investigation of narcissism and hysteria in antisocial personality disorder. *Journal of Personality Assessment, 55,* 270–279.

Gacono, C. B., & Meloy, J. R. (1991). A Rorschach investigation of attachment and anxiety in antisocial personality. *Journal of Nervous and Mental Disease, 179,* 546–552.

Gacono, C. B., & Meloy, J. R. (1992). The Rorschach and the *DSM–III–R* antisocial personality: A tribute to Robert Lindner. *Journal of Clinical Psychology, 48*(3), 393–405.

Gacono, C. B., & Meloy, J. R. (1994). *The Rorschach assessment of aggressive and psychopathic personalities.* Hillsdale, NJ: Lawrence Erlbaum Associates.

Gacono, C. B., & Meloy, J. R. (1997). Rorschach research and the psychodiagnosis of antisocial and psychopathic personalities. *Rorschachiana, 22,* 130–145.

Gacono, C. B., Meloy, J. R., & Berg, J. (1992). Object relations, defensive operations, and affective states in narcissistic, borderline, and antisocial personality disorder. *Journal of Personality Assessment, 59,* 32–59.

Gacono, C. B., Meloy, J. R., Sheppard, K., Speth, E., & Roske, A. (1995). A clinical investigation of malingering and psychopathy in hospitalized insanity acquittees. *Bulletin of the American Academy of Psychiatry and the Law, 23*(3), 387–397.

Gacono, C. B., Meloy, J. R., Speth, E., & Roske, A. (1997). Above the law: Escapes from a maximum security forensic hospital and psychopathy. *Journal of the American Academy of Psychiatry and the Law, 25,* 547–550.

Hare, R. D. (2003). *The Hare psychopathy checklist–revised* (2nd ed.). Toronto, Canada: Multi-Health Systems.

Hare, R. D., & McPherson, L. M. (1984). Violent and aggressive behavior by criminal psychopaths. *International Journal of Law and Psychiatry, 7,* 35–50.

Hart, S. D., Cox, D. N., & Hare, R. D. (1995). *Manual for the Psychopathy Checklist: Screening Version (PCL:SV).* Toronto: Multi-Health Systems.

Kernberg, O. (1975). *Borderline conditions and pathological narcissism.* New York: Aronson.

Lazare, A., & Klerman, G. L. (1968). Hysteria and depression: The frequency and significance of hysterical personality features in hospitalized depressed women. *American Journal of Psychiatry, 124*(11), 48–56.

Loving, J., & Russell, W. (2000). Selected Rorschach variables of psychopathic juvenile offenders. *Journal of Personality Assessment, 75,* 126–142.

Millon, T., & Davis, R. (1996). *Disorders of personality:* DSM–IV *and beyond.* New York: Wiley.

Neary, A. (1990). *DSM–III and psychopathy checklist assessment of antisocial personality disorder in black and white female felons.* Unpublished doctoral dissertation, University of Missouri, St. Louis.

Ogloff, J., Wong, S., & Greenwood, A. (1990). Treating criminal psychopaths in a therapeutic community program. *Behavioral Sciences and the Law, 8,* 81–90.

Peaslee, D. (1993). *An investigation of incarcerated females: Rorschach indices and Psychopathy Checklist scores.* Unpublished doctoral dissertation, California School of Professional Psychology, Fresno, CA

Peaslee, D., Fleming, G., Baumgardner, T., Silbaugh, D., & Thackrey, M. (1992). *An explication of female psychopathy: Psychopathy Checklist scores, Rorschach manifestations, and a comparison of male and female offenders with moderate and severe psychopathy.* Unpublished manuscript.

Perry, W., & Viglione, D. J. (1991). The ego impairment index as a predictor of outcome in melancholic depressed patients treated with tricyclic antidepressants. *Journal of Personality Assessment, 56*(3), 487–501.

Pfohl, B. (1991). Histrionic personality disorder: A review of available data and recommendations for *DSM–IV*. *Journal of Personality Disorders, 5*(2), 150–166.

Rice, M. E. (1997). Violent offender research and implications for the criminal justice system. *American Psychologist, 52,* 414–423.

Rice, M. E., Harris, G., & Cormier, C. (1992). An evaluation of a maximum security therapeutic community for psychopaths and other mentally disordered offenders. *Law and Human Behavior, 16,* 399–412.

Rogers, R., Johansen, J., Chang, J. J., & Salekin, R. T. (1997). Predictors of adolescent psychopathy: Oppositional and conduct-disordered symptoms. *Journal of the American Academy of Psychiatry and the Law, 25,* 261–271.

Rorschach, H. (1942). *Psychodiagnostics.* New York: Grune & Stratton.

Salekin, R., Rogers, R., & Sewell, K. (1998). Construct validity of psychopathy in a female offender sample: A multitrait-multimethod evaluation. *Journal of Abnormal Psychology, 106,* 576–585.

Shapiro, D. (1965). *Neurotic styles.* New York: Basic Books.

Shipley, S. L., & Arrigo, B. A. (2004). *The female homicide offender: Serial murder and the case of Aileen Wuornos.* Upper Saddle River, NJ: Prentice-Hall.

Smith, A., Gacono, C. B., & Kaufman, L. (1995). A Rorschach comparison of psychopathic and nonpsychopathic conduct disordered adolescents. *Journal of Clinical Psychology, 53,* 289–300.

Strachan, C. (1993). *The assessment of psychopathy in female offenders.* Unpublished doctoral dissertation, Department of Psychology, University of British Columbia, Vancouver, Canada.

Sullivan, H. S. (1953). *The interpersonal theory of psychiatry.* New York: Norton.

Vitale, J. E., & Newman, J. P. (2001). Response perseveration in psychopathic Women. *Journal of Abnormal Psychology, 110* (4), 644–647.

Vitale, J. E., Smith, S. S., Brinkley, C. A., & Newman, J. P. (2002). The Reliability and validity of the Psychopathy Checklist–Revised in a sample of female offenders. *Criminal Justice and Behavior, 29*(2), 202–231.

Weiner, I. B. (1998). *Principles of Rorschach interpretation.* Mahwah, NJ: Lawrence Erlbaum Associates.

Young, M. H., Justice, J. V., Erdberg, P. S., & Gacono, C. B. (2000). The incarcerated psychopath in psychiatric treatment: Management of treatment? In C. B.Gacono (Ed.), *The clinical and forensic assessment of psychopathy: A practitioner's guide* (pp. 313–332). Mahwah, NJ: Lawrence Erlbaum Associates.

Zachary, R. (1986). *Shipley Institute of Living Scale: Revised manual.* Los Angeles, CA: Western Psychological Services.

18

A Rorschach Understanding of Psychopaths, Sexual Homicide Perpetrators, and Nonviolent Pedophiles

Carl B. Gacono
Private Practice, Austin, TX

J. Reid Meloy
University of California, San Diego

Michael R. Bridges
Temple University

Recent studies of sexual offenders have found that the measurable constructs of *psychopathy* and *sexual deviance* can account for most of the explainable variance in reoffense rates (Brown & Forth, 1997; Rice & Harris, 1997; Rice, Harris, & Quinsey, 1990; Rice, Quinsey, & Harris, 1991). In one recent study of 288 child molesters and rapists followed for an average of 10 years, psychopathy and sexual deviance exhibited a multiplicative interaction effect on sexual recidivism, but not violent recidivism. Data suggested that sexual deviance may be the most important factor for child molesters, whereas general criminality, lack of self-control, and psychopathy may be more important for rapists. Sexual offenders whose victims include adult women and children of both genders appear to be the most dangerous of all (Rice & Harris, 1997).

Psychopathy has typically been measured by the Psychopathy Checklist–Revised (PCL–R; Hare, 1991, 2003). The PCL–R empirically quantified Cleckley's work (1941/1976) and characterized psychopathy with 20 items comprised of two primary factors, "remorseless, callous, use of others" and an "antisocial lifestyle" (Hare, 2003). Psychopathic traits included such characteristics as glibness, grandiosity, pathological lying, manipulation, shallow affect, the lack of remorse and empathy, and failure to accept responsibility for behavior (Hare, 1991). Sexual deviance has been determined by arousal to deviant stimuli (usually children, rape cues, or nonsexual violence cues) as measured by phallometric testing.

In a preliminary Rorschach study, Meloy, Gacono, and Kenney (1994) focused on comparative differences between small samples of violent psychopaths ($N = 23$) and sexually violent-sexual homicide perpetrators ($N = 18$) to determine if the Rorschach would discriminate based on the presence or absence of a sexual deviation. Rorschach differences between the groups contributed to our initially postulating five core psychodynamic characteristics for the sexual homicide perpetrator (Gacono & Meloy, 1994), and later adding a sixth: chronic anger, entitlement and grandiosity, abnormal bonding, borderline or psychotic reality testing, formal thought disorder, and obsessional thought (see Fig. 18–1). In a separate study, Bridges, Wilson, and Gacono (1998) found similar degrees of pathological self-focus ($Fr + rF > 1$) and abnormal bonding ($T = 0$ or $T > 1$) between mixed pedophiles and other offenders. Consistent with theories of sexual offending, Rorschach variables related to anxiety, painful introspection, distorted view of others, characterological anger, and primitive dependency needs were produced significantly more frequently by the pedophiles.

Despite encouraging findings, a major limitation of the study was its failure to address the question of specificity of Rorschach variables in one sexually offending group (sexual homicide perpetrators), relative to other sexually offending groups. In fact, the question of Rorschach Comprehensive System differences among various paraphilic groups (Barbara et al, 1994; Hanson et al., 1994; Knight & Prentky, 1990; Laws & O'Donohue, 1997) has yet to be addressed.

This chapter compares select Rorschach Comprehensive System variables among these three offender groups that epitomize two factors (psychopathy and sexual deviance) that contribute substantially to violence risk. We discuss the implication of these data for understanding the personality functioning of these individuals. We also offer the reader Rorschach Comprehensive System data for three clinical reference groups: primary psychopaths without a history of sexual offending (P; $N = 32$), sexual homicide perpetrators (SHP; $N = 38$), and nonviolent pedophiles (PED; $N = 39$). Whereas these group data are not fully discussed within this chapter, it is included for the use of forensic examiners evaluating similar individuals.

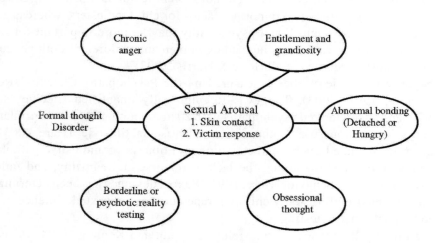

Figure 18–1.   Psychodynamics of sexual homicide.

THE RORSCHACH STUDY

Our hypotheses were developed based on a confluence of psychodynamic principles and the authors' previous research with these populations (Bridges et al., 1998; Gacono & Meloy, 1994; Meloy et al., 1994; see Figure 18–1). Psychopaths, who are prone to predatory violence (Meloy, 1988), were expected to produce less R than the sexually deviant groups. Because affective states ("internally troubled," dysphoric affect, internal press, needs, and ideational noise), in part, motivated sexually deviant behavior (Gacono & Meloy, 1994), we predicted an increased R related to these states "pressing" for expression. We predicted that psychopaths would be the most detached ($T = 0$), most affectively avoidant ($< Afr$), and least interested in others ($< COP$ & $Pure H$).

We expected higher levels of extratensiveness and less restrained hostility (S) in the SHPs and Ps due to their shared Cluster B psychopathology, specifically Antisocial Personality Disorder (ASPD; American Psychiatric Association, 1994), and consequently an associated alloplastic style of relating. On the other hand, we expected PEDs, despite their narcissism ($Fr + rF$), who at least in our sample were not psychopathic or ASPD, to evidence Cluster C traits such as rigidity, inadequacy, and overcontrol (high $Lambda$, $Introversive$, $>S$). We predicted more dysphoria and internally driven need states (V, FM, Fd, $>DEPI$) in the sexually deviant groups when compared to the psychopaths. Unlike the PEDs who manifest better overall personality controls, SHPs were expected to produce low $Lambdas$ due to their inability to distance from environmental, particularly sexually arousing stimuli. All groups were hypothesized to be self-focused ($Fr + rF$) and evidence problems with reality testing ($X-\%$) and thought disorder ($WSum6$, $SCZI$). The following summarize our hypotheses:

1. Responses; P < SH & NVP.
2. Low T, Low Afr, Low COP, Low $Pure H$ for P compared to SH & NVP.
3. More Extratensiveness & Less S in P & SHP then NVP.
4. High $Lambda$ & more Introversiveness in NVP compared to P & SHP.
5. V, FM, FD & Elevated $DEPI$; SHP & NVP > P.
6. Elevated $Reflections$ & $X-\%$ in all groups.

Method

Subjects

Subjects were comprised of three targeted sample groups: nonsexually offending psychopaths (Ps, $N = 32$), sexual homicide perpetrators (SHPs, $N = 38$), and nonviolent pedophiles (PEDs, $N = 39$). All study data were archival and taken from a computer database containing over 800 forensic Rorschach protocols. With the exception of one protocol, only protocols with ≥ 14 responses were included in the study. A single SHP produced a 13-response protocol with a $Lambda$ of .86, 4 $Reflection$ responses, 4 $Blends$, and 11 $Whole$ responses. This Rorschach pattern indicates characterological constriction (Gacono & Meloy, 1994) rather than invalidity and was included in analysis. Rorschachs were administered by advanced doctoral level clinical psychology interns or licensed clinical psychologists using Comprehensive System guidelines (Exner, 1974, 1986, 1993; Exner et al., 1995).

Psychopathy level (PCL–R score) or specific behavioral pattern (sexual offense) were our sole inclusion criteria. All other data, including demographic information, were treated as dependent variables. In treating all other data as dependent, we attempted to protect the demographic purity for individual groups. We allowed them to be representative of what is typically found in a given setting.

Psychopaths.   All psychopaths were free of mental retardation, psychosis, or neurological impairment, and were incarcerated in medium to maximum security correctional or forensic facilities when tested. Psychopathic Rorschachs (P; $N = 32$) were obtained from a larger male ASPD Rorschach sample ($N = 105$; see Gacono & Meloy, 1994; Gacono, Gacono, & Evans, chap. 16, this vol.). Forty-six of the 105 MASPD were psychopathic with PCL–R scores ≥ 30 (Hare, 1991). Of the 46, 30 subjects, although violent, had no history of sexual violence or any sex offense. Two cases (violent but not sexually violent) were randomly chosen from our female psychopathic ASPD sample ($N = 17$) and added to the male psychopaths. These 32 Rorschachs were administered between 1984 and 1996.

Sexual Homicide Perpetrators.   Sexual homicide perpetrators (SHP) were chosen from valid cases among the first two authors' sexual homicide sample ($N = 38$). All 38 Rorschachs were administered between 1986 and 1997 to individuals convicted of sexual homicide and incarcerated in various prisons and forensic hospitals in California, Florida, Illinois, Massachusetts, and the District of Columbia. Positive evidence that a sexual homicide had been committed and the production of a valid Rorschach protocol were the only inclusion criteria. Positive evidence of a sexual homicide was verified by independent record reviews by CBG and JRM and included an intentional killing and (a) physical evidence of sexual assault; (b) sexual activity in close proximity to the victim, such as masturbation; or (c) a legally admissible confession of sexual activity by the perpetrator during the homicide.

In order to accurately represent the heterogeneity of this population, individuals were not excluded due to mental retardation, mental illness, neurological impairment, or gender to accurately represent the probable heterogeneity of this population. None of the subjects, however, were mentally retarded (IQ < 70) or psychotic when tested, and although it was not formally assessed, organic impairment was not suggested from record review or clinical interviewing. Two of the 38 subjects were female.

Nonviolent Pedophiles.   Nonviolent pedophiles (PEDs; $N = 39$) were obtained randomly by MRB from a larger sample which contained violent and nonviolent subjects ($N = 60$; Bridges et al., 1998). Rorschachs were administered between 1991–1996 to subjects incarcerated in a correctional facility awaiting sex offender treatment. All subjects met the *DSM–IV* criteria (APA, 1994) for Pedophilia, as determined by agreement by two experienced clinicians (an advanced clinical psychology graduate intern or licensed psy-

chologist) from record review and interview. None of the pedophiles were mentally retarded, psychotic, neurologically impaired, or evidenced a history of interpersonal
violence. Whereas individual PCL–R scores were not available for the 39 pedophiles, a
review of their files indicated that few subjects met the criteria for ASPD and none would
meet the criteria for primary psychopathy (i.e., PCL–R ≥ 30).

Data Analysis

Available demographic data and victim data were analyzed descriptively and presented
in Tables 18–1 and 18–2, respectively. All Comprehensive System Rorschach data were
analyzed using the Rorschach Scoring Program 3–Plus (Exner & Tuttle, 1995) and other
descriptive software programs. Select Rorschach variables were compared in Table
18–3. Selection of statistical procedure depended on the variable's clinical meaning
(group proportional data or individual frequency data), and whether the variable met assumptions for parametric versus nonparametric procedures. Only those noted with an asterisk (*; see tables) were compared with parametric or nonparametric statistical
procedure (e.g., ANOVA, Kruskal–Wallis, Chi-square). Other data including Appendices A, B, and C (all descriptive Rorschach data for the three groups) were analyzed descriptively only and included for the readers perusal.

Results

Demographics

One-way ANOVAs revealed that pedophiles were significantly older ($F = 14.06$, $p <$
.000) and better educated ($F = 10.93$, $p < .005$) than psychopaths or sexual homicide perpetrators (see Table 18–1). Psychopaths and sexual homicide perpetrators were more ra-
cially diverse than the pedophiles, who were all Caucasian. There was a finding that was
not expected in nonsexually offending psychopaths (Meloy, 1988): Sexually deviant
subjects commonly reported histories of depression. Whereas psychopaths and sexual
homicide perpetrators contained male and female subjects, pedophiles were all male.
Chi-Square analysis indicated that psychopaths were more likely to be single ($p < .05$)
than the other groups. Although both psychopathic (100%) and sexual homicide groups
contained psychopaths (PC–R ≥ 30), valid PCL–R scores were only retrievable for 60%
of the sexual homicide perpetrators. Our best estimate is that from 65% to 75% of the sexual homicide perpetrators would meet criteria for psychopathy (PCL–R ≥ 30). There
were no PCL–R data for the pedophiles; however, record review indicated that few met
the criteria for ASPD and none were psychopathic.

Interrater agreement for our PCL–R scores have been reported previously for these
samples (Gacono, 1990, and Gacono, Meloy, & Heaven, 1990, Spearman Rho = .89;
Gacono & Meloy, 1992, Spearman Rho = .94; Smith, Gacono, & Kaufman, 1997,
Spearman Rho = .96; Gacono, Meloy, Sheppard, Speth, & Roske, 1995, and Gacono,
Meloy, Speth, & Roske, 1997, Spearman Rho = .98). Our interrater agreement has been
the highest reported in the PCL–R literature (R. Hare, personal communication, Novem-
ber 1995).

TABLE 18–1

Demographic Data for Nonsexually Offending Psychopaths, Sexual Homicide Perpetrators, and Nonviolent Pedophiles

Variable	Psychopaths (N = 32)	Sexual Homicide (N = 38)	Pedophiles (N = 39)	P
Age	30.3 (18–43)	32.5 (13–53)	40.5 (24–70)	$p < .000$
Education	11.4	11.8	13.7	$p < .005$
IQ	98.1 (SD = 12.3)	100.4 (SD = 18)	NA	
PCL-R Mean Total	33.1 (SD = 2.1)	30.1 (SD = 6.9)	NA	
Depression Hx[a]	NA	68%	71%	
Male	94%	95%	100%	
Female	6%	5%	0%	
White	56%	71%	100%	
Black	25%	16%	0%	
Hispanic	16%	8%	0%	
Other	0%	5%	0%	
Single[b]	75%	47%	49%	$p < .05$
Married	16%	21%	26%	
Divorced	9%	18%	23%	

[a]Verification of depression was not possible for 24% of SHPs; 38% of the SHPs with histories of depression attempted suicide. A depressive history could only be confirmed in 71% of the PEDs, however, 15% of the 71% attempted suicide. [b]The marital status was unknown for 2% of the PEDs and 13% of the SHP cases.

Victim Data

Table 18–2 illustrates victim data. Sexual homicide perpetrators were significantly more likely to target females and strangers than pedophiles. The pedophiles' instant offenses generally involved multiple events, whereas most sexual homicide perpetrators had only one sexually related homicide identified in the official record (some of the sexual homicide perpetrators committed serial murder). Pedophiles were responsible for 160 male and 77 female known victims in instant offenses alone. One hundred percent of their female victims were abused vaginally and orally. Boys were slightly less likely to be abused anally as orally (18/23). Crime scene analysis of the sexual homicide perpetrators indicated that 16 were organized, 13 disorganized, 4 mixed, and 5 undetermined (see Ressler, Burgess, & Douglas, 1988).

Rorschach Data

A limited number of Rorschach variables, related to Figure 18–1 hypotheses, were presented in Table 18–3 (only those variables designated by asterisk * were inferentially compared). Appendices A, B, and C contain all Comprehensive System data (Exner,

TABLE 18–2

Victim Data for Sexual Homicide and Nonviolent Pedophiles

Victims[a]	Sexual Homicide Perpetrators	Nonviolent Pedophiles
Male	8%	46%
Female	89%	36%
Both	3%	15%
Stranger only	63%	0%
Acquaintance only	24%	33%
Both Stranger and Acquaintance	0%	54%
Unknown	13%	13%

[a]The majority of both SHP and PED individuals had multiple prior sexual offenses and related paraphilias (e.g., 87% of PEDs were know to have previous sex offenses, and 62% were known to be compulsive masturbators).

1993) and provided more in-depth Rorschach "maps" to the core personality issues in each of these three groups.

All Rorschach protocols in our database (> 800 protocols) have been scored and re-scored by experienced raters numerous times prior to inclusion and found to be reliable (Weiner, 1991). Rorschach agreement for our computer-based archival data has also been previously reported: Gacono and Meloy (1994, p. 19), $Location = 98\%$, $DQ = 97\%$, $Determinants = 91\%$, $FQ+ = 93\%$, $Contents = 92\%$, $Z\ score = 95\%$, $Special\ Scores = 83\%$, and $Total\ Agreement = 65\%$; Smith, Gacono, and Kaufman (1997), .94 composite agreement for R, $Lambda$, $Egocentricity\ Index$, $Fr + rF$(s), Y, AG, and COP; Weber, Meloy, and Gacono (1992), $Sum\ T = 100\%$, $Sum\ Y = 100\%$, $H = 94\%$; Gacono (1998; for MASPDs), $Location = 99\%$, $Space = 100\%$, $DQ = 92\%$, $Determinants = 87\%$, $a/p = 100\%$, $FQ+ = 94\%$, $Pairs = 96\%$, $Contents = 96\%$, $Populars = 100\%$, $Z\ scores = 91\%$, and $Special\ Scores = 67\%$; Gacono and Meloy (1994, p. 293; for 19 SHPs), $Location = 99.3\%$, $DQ = 99\%$, $Determinants = 90.2\%$, $FQ+ = 99.3\%$, $Contents = 96.8\%$, $Z\ score = 98.7\%$, $Special\ Scores = 94.7\%$, and $Total\ Agreement = 85.5\%$; Bridges et al. (1998; for PEDs), $Egocentricity\ Index = 92\%$, $Reflections = 98\%$, $Sum\ V = 85\%$, $Sum\ Y = 86\%$, $m = 94\%$, $Afr = 87\%$, $S = 82\%$, $2AB + art + Ay\ (+\ 1) = 88\%$, $Fd = 96\%$, $SumT = 92\%$, $Sx = 84\%$, $M- = 90\%$, $Mp = 92\%$, $Ma = 96\%$, $H = 87\%$, $(H) = 85\%$, and $Hd = 88\%$.[1]

As predicted, the two sexually deviant groups produced significantly more responses (R; ANOVA, $F = 10.25$, $p < .001$) than the psychopaths. Although response frequency differences necessitated the need for some caution when interpreting our findings, the reader should not discount the validity of differences based on $Response$ frequency pat-

---

[1]In several studies where the general reliability of coding was checked, each response from the first rater's sequence of scores was compared to a second rater's independently coded scores. To be counted as a hit (agreement), determinants had to have achieved the same level of form domination (FC,CF,C), whereas special scores needed the same level (1 or 2); any deviation was counted as a miss (nonagreement). At times, lowered percentage of agreement for combined determinants and special scores reflect this stringent procedure (comparing response to response). In other studies, we compared and then computed % agreement for individual variables under study.

TABLE 18–3

Comparison of Select Rorschach Variables Among Nonsexually Offending Psychopaths, Sexual Homicide Perpetrators, and Nonviolent Pedophiles

Variables	Psychopaths (N = 32)			Sexual Homicide Perpetrators (N = 38)			Pedophiles (N = 39)		
	Mean	SD	Frequency	Mean	SD	Frequency	Mean	SD	Frequency
Basic personality/validity									
[a]Responses	18.9	5.17	100%	26.5	11.8	100%	29.5	11.3	100%
[a]Lambda > .99	—	—	38%	—	—	21%	—	—	51%
*Introversive	—	—	22%	—	—	39%	—	—	38%
Ambitent	—	—	47%	—	—	39%	—	—	49%
*Extratensive	—	—	31%	—	—	21%	—	—	13%
Self-perception/grandiosity									
Fr + rF	.72	.96	44%	1.11	1.62	45%	1.23	2.32	44%
Reality Testing									
X – %	22%	.12	100%	26%	.12	97%	22%	.10	100%
Thought Disorder									
WSum6	16.34	12.84	94%	23.0	19.8	92%	16.39	15.15	92%
*SCZI ≥ 4	—	—	15%	—	—	29%	—	—	20%
Obsessional thinking									
[a]FM	2.75	1.65	90%	5.08	3.76	92%	3.77	2.40	92%
Attachment/affects/interpersonal									
T = 0	—	—	100%	—	—	61%	—	—	51%
T = 1	—	—	0%	—	—	13%	—	—	28%
T > 1	—	—	0%	—	—	26%	—	—	21%
*Fd	.16	.45	12%	.53	.92	34%	.44	.68	33%
*Afr < .40	—	—	47%	—	—	34%	—	—	26%
*Afr < .50	—	—	69%	—	—	47%	—	—	44%
[a]SumV	.63	.94	44%	1.11	1.90	53%	1.77	2.03	69%
FM + m < Sum Shading	—	—	28%	—	—	24%	—	—	44%
DEPI ≥ 5	—	—	34%	—	—	37%	—	—	54%
[a]Pure H	1.66	1.31	75%	2.82	1.87	97%	2.62	2.84	87%
[a]All H	4.00	2.13	94%	6.39	3.07	100%	8.05	6.46	100%
COP > 2	—	—	0%	—	—	18%	—	—	15%
Chronic anger									
[a]Space	2.28	1.75	81%	2.92	1.99	97%	4.64	3.53	92%
Other constellations									
CDI ≥ 4	—	—	44%	—	—	27%	—	—	46%
S-CON Positive	—	—	3%	—	—	8%	—	—	18%
HVI Positive	—	—	9%	—	—	13%	—	—	28%
OBS Positive	—	—	0%	—	—	0%	—	—	3%

[a]Only those variables designated with an asterisk were compared with inferential statistics. PEDs had significantly (chi-square, $p < .05$) more high *lambda* subjects (> .99) and produced significantly more space responses (ANOVA, $p = .0006$). PEDs and SHP produced significantly more R than Ps (ANOVA, $p < .001$). SHPs produced more FM (Kruskal-Wallis, $p < .05$), whereas PEDs produced more *SumV* (Kruskal-Wallis, $p < .05$) and a trend toward more subjects who produced $V > 0$ (chi-square, $p = .10–.05$). Psychopaths produced less *T*, *Pure H* (Kruskal-Wallis, $p < .05$) and composite *H* (Kruskal-Wallis, $p < .001$) and were more likely (chi-square, $p < .05$) to produce $H = 0$.

terns that were expected and predicted. We believe that *Response* frequency differences can be understood as an artifact of each group's psychopathology. That is, it is an important dependent measure of actual group differences.

Consistent with other clinical samples, the *Ambitent* style was most frequently produced in all groups. Sexual homicide perpetrators were more likely to produce normal *Lambdas* ($X^2 = 3.84$; $p < .05$) and be *Introversive* (trend) than psychopaths, of whom a third were *Extratensive*. Pedophiles tended to produce high *Lambdas* and either *Introversive* or *Ambitent* styles. All three groups evidenced marked elevations for *Reflection* responses, suggesting abnormal self-focus or pathological narcissism, and moderate to severe levels of cognitive slippage and impaired reality testing (*WSum6*, $X - \%$). The frequency of subjects in the SHP sample who produced *Level 2 Special Scores* ($N = 19$) was slightly greater than PEDs and Ps, which each had 12 individuals.

Consistent with the sexual homicide perpetrators' and pedophiles' higher frequencies of marriage and/or divorce (see Table 18–1), they evidenced greater frequencies of *T* (SHPs: $T > 0$, 39%; PEDs: $T > 0$, 49%) than the psychopaths ($T = 0$, 100%)—although the overwhelming majority of all subjects evidenced abnormal attachment patterns ($T = 0$ or $T > 1$). The psychopaths appeared the least interested in human objects in any form, whether whole and real or part and mythical, and evidenced significantly more subjects who produced $H = 0$ ($X^2 = 3.84$, $p = .05$; 25%). Psychopaths produced a trend toward being the most affectively avoidant (*Afr*), and were significantly less likely (Kruskal-Wallis, $p < .05$) to be troubled by internal distractions such as painful rumination (*V*), nonvolitional ideation in response to physiological need (*FM*), or dependency yearnings (*Fd*).Pedophiles produced significantly more *S* responses (ANOVA, $F = 8.05, p < .0006$), a measure of passive opposition, relative to the other groups. Both sexually deviant groups experienced an elevated internal press (high *R*); however, combined with external pull (low *Lambdas*), the cognitively impaired (*WSum6*) sexual homicide perpetrators evidenced the greatest amount of nonvolitional ideation (FM, $p < .05$), or, as we previously hypothesized (Gacono & Meloy, 1994), obsessional thoughts—factors that likely provide clues to the motivation for their deviant sexual behavior (Gacono, 1997; Gacono & Meloy, 1988). Sexual homicide perpetrators also were more frequently elevated on the *SCZI* (29%), which would be consistent with the bizarre and primitive nature of their offenses. Fifty-four percent of the pedophiles elevated on *DEPI*, a finding that indicates greater dysphoria and would be consistent with less psychopathy.

CONCLUSIONS

Psychopathy and sexual deviance are personality traits and deeply conditioned arousal patterns, respectively, that contribute significantly to sexual reoffense rates (Rice et al., 1990; Rice et al., 1991; Rice & Harris, 1997). They are enduring, resilient, and highly resistant to change. Their combination is particularly malignant and lethal when expressed through sexual homicide.

In order to better understand this relationship (violence and sexual deviance), we chose *psychopathy level* (PCL–R score) or a specific *behavioral pattern* (sexual deviance) as our sole independent measures. All other variables were treated as dependent measures with the intention of using any differences to aid in understanding the unique "personality" of each group. Groups were allowed to represent "what is typically found" in a given setting.

Differences in age, ethnicity, and presence or absence of ASPD and psychopathy mirrored profiles from similar offender samples (i.e., psychopaths in a maximum security setting, sexual homicide perpetrators, nonviolent pedophiles in a federal facility). Rather than confounds, these differences acted as a measure of concurrent validity for the representativeness of our samples. For example, consistent with the largest published sexual homicide sample (Ressler et al., 1988; $N = 36$), our sexual homicide sample ($N = 38$) is predominately White and male. The presence or absence of ASPD and/or psychopathy in individual groups was consistent with related studies that have found sexual deviance to be the most influential "motivator" in nonviolent pedophiles (low ASPD & psychopathy), whereas psychopathy exerts a prominent contributing factor in rapists (more ASPD & psychopathy expected; Rice et al., 1990; Rice et al., 1991; Rice & Harris, 1997). Subsequently, differences in ethnicity and finding of less ASPD and psychopathy are less sources of concern when couched in the context of these previous findings.

Similarly, differences in *Response* frequency were expected and predicted, and were best understood as "true findings," which related to one aspect that distinguishes between sexual deviance and "psychopathic or predatory violence." Predatory violence has been described as planned and purposeful (Meloy, 1988). One would not expect elevated R in group Rorschach data of psychopathic subjects where planned and purposeful rather than affective violence is the norm (Hare & McPherson, 1984). Rather, elevated R would be expected in our sexual offending subjects where internal press (affect) motivates the behavior (Brittain, 1970; Hudson et al., 1993). It is likely that the sexual deviance contributes to elevated R in both the nonviolent pedophiles and sexual homicide perpetrators. *Response* frequency differences necessitate the need for some caution when interpreting our findings, and particularly the meaning of a sole variable or specific ratio isolated from the entire corresponding Comprehensive System description (see Appendices A, B, and C). The reader should remember that differences in R were expected and predicted.

Convergence between each group's Rorschach data and the related theoretical understanding of each disorder, as well as the congruence of specific Rorschach data with real-world behavior (i.e., less T in psychopathy—most psychopaths were single), provided additional concurrent validity. With only minor reservations, we posit the between-group differences to represent "true findings" that aid in understanding differences among the groups. Certainly safer interpretative grounds were achieved for those Rorschach variables with low base rates for which psychopaths (less R) produced greater or equal means or frequencies, or for those Rorschach variables that are not necessarily impacted by R. Additionally, less caution is warranted for questioning the validity of Rorschach variables when real-world behaviors support the group differences. This former caveat occurred with *Reflection* responses, and despite differences in R, *Reflection* frequencies were similar for all three groups. The latter also applies to the *Texture* response, where its virtual absence in the psychopaths was consistent with their real-world histories of attachment pathology.

So it is with only a minor caution that we assert that the Rorschach patterns and differences among these groups add to our understanding of both psychopathy and sexual deviance. The rigidity and simplicity (high *Lambda*) of the pedophiles' cognitive style facilitates repetition of their deviant sexual conditioning. Their high *Lambda*s support the frequent assertion by child molesters that others or situational factors are to be blamed for their behaviors (Marshall, 1997). High levels of dysphoric affect (*V, DEPI*) and primitive need states (*FM, Fd, T*) may drive their sexual acting out (Hudson et al., 1993; Pithers et al., 1989). They are interested in others (*H*), but their conception of others is based more on imagination than reality (*H < [Hd] + Hd + [Hd]*) and is contaminated by formal thought disorder (*WSum6*), borderline reality testing (*X–%*), and pathological narcissism. The pedophile feels entitled to gratify his sexualized desires for human connection through the part-object of a child. The preponderance of cartoon, science fiction, and fairy-tale figures comprising the human contents of pedophiles may reflect a narcissistic identification with children and characters associated with childhood (Bridges et al., 1998).

Introversiveness and a tendency toward dysphoric rumination distinguish the pedophiles from the nonsexually offending psychopaths with the latter group characterized more by a relatively conflict-free, remorseless dynamic state—a contribution to the absence of violence in the former and its presence in the latter group. Pedophiles, however, are significantly more characterologically angry (*S*) than the other two groups. This anger may be caused by inadequacy, less antisocial avenues for acting out, and the pedophiles' introversive inability to gratify their needs. Almost half of each group produced *Reflection* responses. Pedophiles, however, were previously found to be susceptible to negative affect or a damaged sense of self (*V > 0, Y > 1, m > 1*, or *MOR > 1*) in the context of their failed narcissistic defenses (Bridges et al., 1998). Failed narcissism may partially account for the pedophiles reliance on children for sexual gratification. At a preconscious level, nonpsychopathic pedophiles are aware that their grandiosity is a sham; feelings of damage and ineptness contribute to their inability to withstand or negotiate complexities inherent to the development and maintenance of intimate adult relationships.

Psychopaths are the least internally troubled of the three groups (less *FM, T, Fd, V, S*). They are less interested in others (*T = 0, H*), have little expectation of interpersonal cooperation (*COP*), and use people in a self-serving manner (*Fr + rF*). They are unfettered by remorse, guilt (*V*), or sustained Reflection (*FD; Introversion*). In common with pedophiles, psychopaths' perceptual and cognitive distortions (*WSum6, X–%*) add to their poor interpersonal judgment, and when combined with self-centeredness (*Fr + rF*), may contribute to a pervasive sense of entitlement. Psychopaths avoid genuine affective involvement, and although many in this group might be characterized as moving toward hypersocial sensation-seeking activities (a third are *Extratensive*), pleasure in others is experienced when others serve as an adequate mirror.

For our sexual homicide perpetrators, of which two thirds are likely psychopaths, their sexual deviance appears to emotionally disrupt their narcissistic (psychopathic) equilibrium. Unlike nonsexually offending psychopaths, sexual homicide perpetrators are internally troubled. High levels of internal dysphoria, yearning, obsession, and dependency needs (V, T, FM, Fd) push behaviors, while at the same time there is a certain loss of distance or inability to disengage from the environment and revel (*Lambda*, R). Stimuli that resonate with their sexual deviance are particularly appealing and literally irresistible. The intensity of this push–pull effect is exacerbated by less than optimal controls ($D = -1.45$, $AdjD = -0.58$; R, see Appendix B). High levels of ideational noise or, as we previously hypothesized (Gacono & Meloy, 1994), obsessional thought (*FM*), differentiate sexual homicide perpetrators from the psychopath. Like pedophiles, they are interested and perhaps drawn to others; however, their interest is contaminated by the self-centeredness ($Fr + rF$) and severe perceptual ($X-\%$) and cognitive distortions (*WSum6*), which characterize all three groups (Gacono & Meloy, 1988). Isolation is also a common defense utilized by these groups (SHP = 31.6% > .33; PED = 28.2% > .33; P = 25% > .33).

Psychopaths without concurrent sexual deviation tend to produce T-less protocols. In contrast, among sexual homicide perpetrators there was little relationship between psychopathy level and T. Psychopathic sexual homicide perpetrators were just as likely to produce one or more Ts as their nonpsychopathic counterparts. Exner (1986) and others (Klopfer, 1938; Schachtel, 1966) interpreted the *Texture* response as a measure of interpersonal closeness or affectional relatedness. Schachtel (1966) additionally theorized that, in some cases, *Texture* responses indicated ambivalence surrounding attachment and perhaps a fear of unpleasant skin contact—described elsewhere as a "negated T" response (Gacono & Meloy, 1991, 1994). *Texture* may actually constitute an intrapsychic irritant that, when coupled with sexual deviance and a propensity for violence, in part "energizes" the interpersonal behavior of these sexual murderers. Their affectional hunger surfaces in the need for direct skin contact with the victim; subsequently, ritualistic elements in the crime scene provide a canvass for the expression of their internal and stable psychosexual fantasies (Meloy, 2000).

Our findings for the three groups are also consistent with recent theories relating disturbed attachment styles to sexual offending and psychopathy (Marshall, 1997). The psychopath corresponds to Bowlby's "affectionless" style in that the individual whose capacity for attachment has been so disrupted that any basic capacity for bonding and empathy has been obliterated ($T = 0$, $H < 2$). The pedophiles appear more "anxious/ambivalent" or "preoccupied" ($T > 1$, Fd, Y, V, m), whereas the sexual homicide perpetrators seem to experience high levels of cognitive slippage, poor reality testing, and dyscontrol in the context of interpersonal relationships (*WSum6*, $X-\%$, $M-$), corresponding to what has recently been called the "disorganized/disoriented" attachment style.

The present findings expand and clarify the differences between the nonsexually offending psychopaths and sexual homicide perpetrators. Nonsexually offending psychopaths are not interested in others, evidence a complete absence of attachment capacity, lack the channeled sexual arousal to extreme violence, and are not aggressively motivated by dysphoria, obsession, or affectional hunger. Pedophiles, although angrier, display the sexual arousal integral to their offenses, but lack the emotional detachment noted in the psychopaths and evidence better controls than the sexual homicide perpetrators.

The psychological operations of all three groups—as measured by the Rorschach—show similarities and differences.[2] Two of the groups are sexually deviant (PED, SHP) and two are criminally inclined (SHP, P). The construct of psychopathy or pathological narcissism helps to understand the antisocial behavior, abnormal bonding, pathological narcissism, and cognitive problems of all the subjects, but within each group there are notable differences. Sexual deviance, however, adds to the mix. Although we did not measure sexual arousal directly, it appears to further disorganize all pathologies, the most sexually aggressive and dangerous group being the sexual homicide perpetrators. Although we may be intimidated by the psychopath, and repulsed by the pedophile, it is the sexual homicide perpetrator who truly frightens and perplexes us.

ACKNOWLEDGMENTS

The original study, *A Rorschach Comparison of Psychopaths, Sexual Homicide Perpetrators, and Nonviolent Pedophiles: Where Angles Fear to Tread*, was published in 2000 in the *Journal of Clinical Psychology, 56*(6), 757–777. The authors wish to thank Robert Bodholdt for suggestions and Philip Erdberg for his help with data analysis in that study. The authors also wish to thank Reneau Kennedy, Lynne Kenney, Greg Meyer, Bruce Smith, Anita Boss, Maureen Christianson, Paul Fautek, and Ron Ganellen for contributing protocols to the SHP sample.

REFERENCES

American Psychiatric Association. (1994). *Diagnostic and statistical manual of mental disorders* (4th ed.). Washington, DC: Author.

Barbara, H. E., Set, M. C., Serin, R. C., Amos, N. L., & Presto, D. L. (1994). Comparison between sexual and nonsexual rapist subtypes. *Criminal Justice and Behavior, 21*, 95–114.

Bridges, M., Wilson, J., & Gacono, C. B. (1998). A Rorschach investigation of defensiveness, self-perception, interpersonal relations, and affective states in incarcerated pedophiles. *Journal of Personality Assessment, 70*(2), 365–385.

Brittain, R. (1970). The sadistic murderer. *Medicine, Science, and the Law, 10*, 198–207.

Brown, S., & Forth, A. (1997). Psychopathy and sexual assault: Static risk factors, emotional precursors, and rapist subtypes. *Journal of Consulting and Clinical Psychology, 65*(5), 848–857.

Cleckley, H. (1976). *The mask of sanity* (5th ed.). St. Luis, MO: Mosby. (Original work published 1941)

Exner, J. E. (1974). *The Rorschach: A Comprehensive System* (Vol. 1). New York: Wiley.

Exner, J. E. (1986). *The Rorschach: A Comprehensive System: Vol. 1. Basic foundations* (2nd ed.). New York: Wiley.

Exner, J. E. (1993). *The Rorschach: A Comprehensive System: Vol. 1. Basic foundations* (3rd ed.). New York: Wiley.

Exner, J. E., Colligan, S. C., Hillman, L. B., Ritzler, B. A., Sciara, A. D., & Viglione, D. J. (1995). *A Rorschach workbook for the Comprehensive System* (4th ed.). Asheville, NC: Rorschach Workshops.

---

[2]Whereas these group differences are clinically useful and consistent with the literature on sexual deviance and psychopathy in accurately portraying the major personality constructs and traits associated with each of the groups (Gacono & Meloy, 1994; Marshall, 1997), and therefore describe the typical group member, we are not suggesting that the emergent Rorschach profiles distinguish all psychopaths, pedophiles, or sexual homicide perpetrators.

Exner, J., & Tuttle, K. (1995). *Rorschach scoring program–version 3-plus*. Psychological Assessment Resources, Inc.

Gacono, C. B. (1990). An empirical study of object relations and defensive operations in Antisocial Personality Disorder. *Journal of Personality Assessment, 54*, 589–600.

Gacono, C. B. (1997). Borderline personality organization, psychopathology, and sexual homicide: The case of Brinkley. In J. R. Meloy, M. W. Acklin, C. B. Gacono, J. F. Murray, & C. A. Peterson (Eds.), *Contemporary Rorschach interpretation* (pp. 217–238). Mahwah, NJ: Lawrence Erlbaum Associates.

Gacono, C. B. (1998). The use of the Psychopathy Checklist–Revised (PCL–R) and Rorschach in treatment planning with antisocial personality disordered patients. *International Journal of Offender Therapy and Comparative Criminology, 42*(1), 49–64.

Gacono, C. B., & Meloy, J. R. (1988). The relationship between cognitive style and defensive process in the psychopath. *Criminal Justice and Behavior, 15*(4), 472–483.

Gacono, C. B., & Meloy, J. R. (1991). A Rorschach investigation of attachment and anxiety in antisocial personality. *Journal of Nervous and Mental Disease, 179*, 546–552.

Gacono, C. B., & Meloy, J. R. (1992). The Rorschach and the *DSM–III–R* antisocial personality: A tribute to Robert Lindner. *Journal of Clinical Psychology, 48*(3), 393–405.

Gacono, C. B., & Meloy, J. R. (1994). *The Rorschach assessment of aggressive and psychopathic personalities*. Hillsdale, NJ: Lawrence Erlbaum Associates.

Gacono, C. B., Meloy, J. R., & Bridges, M. (2000). A Rorschach comparison of psychopaths, sexual homicide perpetrators, and nonviolent pedophiles: Where angels fear to tread. *Journal of Clinical Psychology, 56*(6), 757–777.

Gacono, C. B., Meloy, J. R., & Heaven, T. (1990). A Rorschach investigation of narcissism and hysteria in antisocial personality disorder. *Journal of Personality Assessment, 55*, 270–279.

Gacono, C. B., Meloy, J. R., Sheppard, K., Speth, E., & Roske, A. (1995). A clinical investigation of malingering and psychopathy in hospitalized insanity acquittees. *Bulletin of the American Academy of Psychiatry and the Law, 23*(3), 387–397.

Gacono, C. B., Meloy, J. R., Speth, E., & Roske, A. (1997). Above the law: Escapes from a maximum security forensic hospital and psychopathy. *Journal of the American Academy of Psychiatry and the Law, 25*(4), 547–550.

Hanson, R. K., Gizzarelli, R., & Scott, H. (1994). The attitudes of incest offenders: Sexual entitlement and acceptance of sex with children. *Criminal Justice and Behavior, 21*, 187–202.

Hare, R. D. (2003). *The Hare Psychopathy Checklist–Revised (PCL–R) manual* (2nd ed.). Toronto: Multi-Health Systems, Inc.

Hare, R. D., & McPherson, L. (1984). Violent and aggressive behavior by criminal psychopaths. *International Journal of Law and Psychiatry, 7*, 35–50.

Hudson, S. M., Marshall, W. L., Wales, D., McDonald, E., Bakker, L. W., & McLean, A. (1993). Emotional recognition skills of sex offenders. *Annals of Sex Research, 6*, 199–211.

Klopfer, B. (1938). The shading responses. *Rorschach Research Exchange, 2*, 76–79.

Knight, R. A., & Prentky, R. A.(1990). Classifying sexual offenders: The development and corroboration of taxonomic models. In W. L. Marshall & H. E. Barbara (Eds.), *Handbook of sexual assault: Issues, theories, and treatment of the offender* (pp. 23–52). New York: Plenum.

Laws, D. R., & O'Donohue, W. (Eds.). (1997). *Sexual deviance: Theory, assessment and treatment*. New York: Guilford.

Marshall, W. L. (1997). Pedophilia: Psychopathology and theory. In D. R. Laws & W. O'Donohue (Eds.), *Sexual deviance: Theory, assessment, and treatment* (pp. 152–174). New York: Guilford.

Meloy, J. R. (1988). *The psychopathic mind: Origins, dynamics and treatment*. Northvale, NJ: Aronson.

Meloy, J. R. (2000). The nature and dynamics of sexual homicide: An integrative review. *Aggression and Violent Behavior, 5*, 1–22.

Meloy, J. R., Gacono, C. B., & Kenney, L. (1994). A Rorschach investigation of sexual homicide. *Journal of Personality Assessment, 62*(1), 58–67.

Pithers, W. D., Kashima, K., Cumming, G. F., & Bueil, M. M. (1988). Relapse prevention: A method of enhancing maintenance of change in sex differences. In A. C. Slater (Ed.), *Treating child sex offenders and victims* (pp. 131–170). Newbury, CA: Sage.

Ressler, R., Burgess, A., & Douglas, J. (1988). *Sexual homicide: Patterns and motives.* Lexington, MA: Lexington Books.

Rice, M., & Harris, G. (1997). Cross-validation and extension of the violence risk appraisal guide for child molesters and rapists. *Law and Human Behavior, 21*, 231–241.

Rice, M., Harris, G., & Quinsey, V. (1990). A follow-up of rapists assessed in a maximum-security psychiatric institution. *Journal of Interpersonal Violence, 5*, 435–448.

Rice, M., Quinsey, V., & Harris, G. (1991). Sexual recidivism among child molesters released from a maximum security psychiatric institution. *Journal of Consulting and Clinical Psychology, 59*, 381–386.

Schachtel, E. (1966). *Experiential foundations of Rorschach's test.* New York: Basic Books.

Smith, A., Gacono, C. B., & Kaufman, L. (1995). A Rorschach comparison of psychopathic and non-psychopathic conduct disordered adolescents. *Journal of Clinical Psychology, 53*(4), 289–300.

Weber, C., Meloy, J. R., & Gacono, C. B. (1992). A Rorschach study of attachment and anxiety in inpatient conduct-disordered and dysthymic adolescents. *Journal of Personality Assessment, 58*(1), 16–26.

Weiner, I. B. (1991). Editor's note: Interscorer agreement in Rorschach research. *Journal of Personality Assessment, 56*, 1.

Descriptive statistics for Nonviolent Pedophiles ($N = 39$)

VARIABLE	MEAN	SD	MIN	MAX	FREQ	MEDIAN	MODE	SK	KU
AGE	40.54	10.18	24.00	70.00	39	39.00	27.00	0.72	0.59
R	29.46	11.31	14.00	61.00	39	27.00	20.00	1.05	0.74
W	10.69	6.96	2.00	40.00	39	10.00	7.00	2.05	7.16
D	13.31	9.06	0.00	36.00	38	13.00	4.00	0.45	−0.44
Dd	5.46	4.53	0.00	21.00	36	5.00	6.00	1.22	2.10
SPACE	4.64	3.53	0.00	19.00	36	4.00	2.00	1.82	5.93
DQ+	8.31	7.38	1.00	39.00	39	7.00	7.00	2.93	9.99
DQo	16.82	8.00	3.00	35.00	39	15.00	12.00	0.52	−0.24
DQv	2.54	2.22	0.00	8.00	33	2.00	1.00	0.89	−0.18
DQv/+	1.79	2.21	0.00	9.00	25	1.00	0.00	1.71	2.92
FQx/+	0.51	1.41	0.00	8.00	9	0.00	0.00	4.32	21.52
FQxo	14.08	5.43	5.00	26.00	39	14.00	11.00	0.39	−0.53
FQxu	7.82	3.91	1.00	16.00	39	7.00	7.00	0.42	−0.52
FQx−	6.80	5.31	1.00	29.00	39	6.00	6.00	2.39	7.57
FQxNone	0.26	0.44	0.00	1.00	10	0.00	0.00	1.16	−0.69
MQ+	0.20	0.69	0.00	4.00	5	0.00	0.00	4.66	24.35
MQo	2.28	1.81	0.00	7.00	33	2.00	1.00	0.71	−0.11
MQu	1.05	1.30	0.00	6.00	23	1.00	0.00	1.88	4.69
MQ−	1.51	3.29	0.00	20.00	22	1.00	0.00	4.95	27.55
MQNone	0.05	0.22	0.00	1.00	2	0.00	0.00	4.23	16.78
SQual−	1.90	2.20	0.00	12.00	31	1.00	1.00	2.82	11.07
M	5.10	5.59	1.00	34.00	39	4.00	2.00	3.96	19.21
FM	3.77	2.40	0.00	12.00	36	4.00	4.00	1.02	2.57
m	1.85	1.68	0.00	5.00	29	1.00	0.00	0.64	−0.81
FM+m	5.61	3.43	1.00	17.00	39	5.00	5.00	0.89	1.75
FC	1.36	2.02	0.00	11.00	23	1.00	0.00	3.16	13.32
CF	2.59	2.44	0.00	9.00	29	2.00	0.00	0.89	0.16
C	0.36	0.74	0.00	4.00	11	0.00	0.00	3.36	14.74
CN	0.00	0.00	0.00	0.00	0	0.00	0.00	0.00	0.00
Sum Color	4.31	4.01	0.00	19.00	34	4.00	4.00	1.80	4.39
WSumC	3.81	3.45	0.00	16.00	34	3.50	3.50	1.73	4.00
SumC'	1.23	1.56	0.00	8.00	25	1.00	0.00	2.47	8.45
Sum T	0.92	1.37	0.00	6.00	19	0.00	0.00	2.05	4.59
Sum V	1.77	2.03	0.00	8.00	27	1.00	0.00	1.50	1.84
Sum Y	1.23	1.33	0.00	5.00	24	1.00	0.00	1.05	0.58
Sum Shading	5.15	3.98	0.00	16.00	37	4.00	3.00	1.08	0.48
Fr + rF	1.23	2.32	0.00	13.00	17	0.00	0.00	3.66	17.28
FD	0.77	0.84	0.00	3.00	21	1.00	0.00	0.75	−0.36
F	13.49	6.68	2.00	30.00	39	14.00	8.00	0.46	0.12
(2)	8.15	6.07	1.00	32.00	39	7.00	3.00	1.72	4.93
3r+(2)/R	0.40	0.21	0.04	0.92	39	0.36	0.36	0.58	−0.04

VARIABLE	MEAN	SD	MIN	MAX	FREQ	MEDIAN	MODE	SK	KU
Lambda	1.02	0.65	0.11	2.67	39	1.00	1.00	0.93	0.70
EA	8.91	8.30	2.00	47.50	39	6.50	4.00	3.34	13.12
es	10.77	6.74	2.00	33.00	39	9.00	7.00	1.20	1.61
D Score	−0.51	2.72	−6.00	10.00	39	−1.00	0.00	1.54	5.68
AdjD	0.08	2.68	−4.00	11.00	39	0.00	0.00	2.72	9.42
a (active)	6.41	4.08	0.00	20.00	38	6.00	3.00	1.13	1.78
p (passive)	4.31	5.14	0.00	29.00	34	3.00	1.00	3.24	13.86
Ma	2.54	2.21	0.00	10.00	34	2.00	1.00	1.35	2.17
Mp	2.56	4.11	0.00	24.00	30	2.00	1.00	4.11	20.04
Intellect	4.44	4.58	0.00	21.00	34	3.00	3.00	1.72	3.49
Zf	15.92	8.73	6.00	50.00	39	15.00	15.00	2.51	7.95
Zd	0.82	7.37	−12.00	26.00	36	0.00	3.00	1.32	3.53
Blends	4.92	5.26	0.00	29.00	37	3.00	1.00	2.77	10.87
Blends/R	0.17	0.14	0.00	0.57	37	0.14	0.03	1.31	1.58
Col-Shd Blends	0.95	1.12	0.00	4.00	22	1.00	0.00	1.28	1.18
Afr	0.57	0.23	0.20	1.11	39	0.59	0.60	0.33	−0.49
Populars	5.36	1.81	2.00	9.00	39	5.00	5.00	−0.09	−0.37
X+%	0.51	0.12	0.30	0.81	39	0.50	0.50	0.49	0.11
F+%	0.49	0.19	0.00	0.83	37	0.50	0.50	−0.68	0.70
X−%	0.22	0.10	0.05	0.48	39	0.21	0.13	0.47	−0.14
Xu%	0.27	0.10	0.04	0.50	39	0.27	0.25	−0.09	0.70
S−%	0.26	0.20	0.00	0.71	31	0.25	0.00	0.36	−0.66
Isolate/R	0.24	0.17	0.00	0.79	—	—	—	—	—
H	2.62	2.84	0.00	15.00	34	2.00	1.00	2.56	8.77
(H)	1.77	1.97	0.00	8.00	29	1.00	1.00	1.57	2.23
HD	2.56	2.69	0.00	11.00	31	2.00	1.00	1.57	2.34
(Hd)	1.10	1.33	0.00	5.00	21	1.00	0.00	1.14	0.60
Hx	0.00	0.00	0.00	0.00	0	0.00	0.00	0.00	0.00
H+(H)+Hd+(Hd)	8.05	6.46	2.00	39.00	39	6.00	5.00	3.20	13.63
A	8.92	4.18	3.00	20.00	39	8.00	8.00	1.20	1.18
(A)	0.90	1.12	0.00	5.00	22	1.00	0.00	1.75	3.77
Ad	3.20	2.25	0.00	8.00	34	3.00	4.00	0.33	−0.63
(Ad)	0.20	0.47	0.00	2.00	7	0.00	0.00	2.29	4.92
An	1.56	1.59	0.00	6.00	28	1.00	1.00	1.32	1.65
Art	1.31	1.95	0.00	8.00	20	1.00	0.00	1.99	3.98
Ay	1.74	1.85	0.00	8.00	30	1.00	1.00	1.85	3.75
Bl	0.15	0.43	0.00	2.00	5	0.00	0.00	2.96	8.91
Bt	1.51	1.59	0.00	5.00	24	1.00	0.00	0.75	−0.59
Cg	2.56	3.00	0.00	15.00	33	2.00	1.00	2.57	8.07
Cl	0.33	0.66	0.00	3.00	10	0.00	0.00	2.38	6.40
Ex	0.26	0.50	0.00	2.00	9	0.00	0.00	1.81	2.65
Fi	0.82	0.97	0.00	4.00	21	1.00	0.00	1.29	1.78

(continued)

APPENDIX A   Descriptive statistics for Nonviolent Pedophiles ($N = 39$)

VARIABLE	MEAN	SD	MIN	MAX	FREQ	MEDIAN	MODE	SK	KU
Food	0.44	0.68	0.00	2.00	13	0.00	0.00	1.30	0.46
Ge	0.38	0.67	0.00	2.00	11	0.00	0.00	1.53	1.07
Hh	0.56	0.94	0.00	4.00	14	0.00	0.00	2.01	4.25
Ls	1.08	1.38	0.00	5.00	20	1.00	0.00	1.24	0.67
Na	1.51	1.89	0.00	8.00	23	1.00	0.00	1.57	2.63
Sc	1.72	2.15	0.00	11.00	27	1.00	0.00	2.58	8.83
Sx	0.85	1.39	0.00	6.00	16	0.00	0.00	2.04	4.28
Xy	0.05	0.22	0.00	1.00	2	0.00	0.00	4.23	16.78
Idiographic	0.90	1.21	0.00	5.00	18	0.00	0.00	1.43	2.02
DV	0.82	0.94	0.00	3.00	21	1.00	0.00	0.97	0.09
INCOM	1.05	1.23	0.00	5.00	24	1.00	0.00	1.76	3.71
DR	1.31	1.67	0.00	6.00	20	1.00	0.00	1.19	0.50
FABCOM	1.10	1.27	0.00	4.00	23	1.00	0.00	1.17	0.53
DV2	0.00	0.00	0.00	0.00	0	0.00	0.00	0.00	0.00
INC2	0.18	0.39	0.00	1.00	7	0.00	0.00	1.74	1.07
DR2	0.18	0.51	0.00	2.00	5	0.00	0.00	2.89	7.70
FAB2	0.13	0.41	0.00	2.00	4	0.00	0.00	3.43	12.18
ALOG	0.49	1.02	0.00	4.00	9	0.00	0.00	2.14	3.78
CONTAM	0.00	0.00	0.00	0.00	0	0.00	0.00	0.00	0.00
Sum 6 Sp Sc	5.26	4.44	0.00	15.00	36	3.00	3.00	0.90	−0.35
Lvl 2 Sp Sc	0.49	0.82	0.00	3.00	12	0.00	0.00	1.53	1.31
WSum6	16.39	15.15	0.00	56.00	36	11.00	0.00	1.11	0.29
AB	0.69	1.49	0.00	7.00	11	0.00	0.00	2.78	8.41
AG	0.38	0.78	0.00	3.00	9	0.00	0.00	1.97	2.95
CONFAB	0.08	0.35	0.00	2.00	2	0.00	0.00	4.92	24.93
COP	1.18	1.25	0.00	4.00	26	1.00	1.00	1.16	0.51
CP	0.00	0.00	0.00	0.00	0	0.00	0.00	0.00	0.00
MOR	1.28	1.79	0.00	8.00	22	1.00	0.00	2.13	5.13
PER	2.15	2.11	0.00	7.00	28	1.00	0.00	0.73	−0.63
PSV	0.36	0.74	0.00	4.00	11	0.00	0.00	3.36	14.74

APPENDIX B   Descriptive statistics for Psychopaths (*N* = 32)

VARIABLE	MEAN	SD	MIN	MAX	FREQ	MEDIAN	MODE	SK	KU
AGE	30.03	6.38	18.00	43.00	32	30.00	30.00	0.02	−0.43
R	18.88	5.17	14.00	39.00	32	17.50	15.00	2.17	6.42
W	9.63	3.71	5.00	22.00	32	9.00	9.00	1.29	2.79
D	6.94	4.68	0.00	24.00	31	6.00	3.00	1.66	4.44
Dd	2.31	2.22	0.00	9.00	27	2.00	1.00	1.56	2.35
SPACE	2.28	1.75	0.00	7.00	26	2.00	2.00	0.59	0.17
DQ+	4.84	2.45	0.00	12.00	30	5.00	5.00	0.53	1.83
DQo	11.19	5.41	6.00	34.00	32	9.50	8.00	2.84	9.94
DQv	1.94	1.68	0.00	6.00	26	2.00	1.00	1.06	0.68
DQv/+	0.91	1.23	0.00	5.00	15	0.00	0.00	1.53	2.54
FQx/+	0.03	0.18	0.00	1.00	1	0.00	0.00	5.66	32.00
FQxo	9.47	3.07	3.00	17.00	32	9.50	10.00	0.17	0.46
FQxu	4.44	2.70	1.00	11.00	32	4.00	4.00	0.82	0.32
FQx−	4.34	3.38	1.00	18.00	32	3.50	3.00	2.34	7.72
FQxNone	0.59	0.95	0.00	4.00	13	0.00	0.00	2.15	5.24
MQ+	0.03	0.18	0.00	1.00	1	0.00	0.00	5.66	32.00
MQo	1.47	1.32	0.00	4.00	22	1.50	2.00	0.57	−0.50
MQu	0.47	0.88	0.00	3.00	9	0.00	0.00	1.92	2.88
MQ−	0.59	0.67	0.00	3.00	17	1.00	1.00	1.39	3.85
MQNone	0.00	0.00	0.00	0.00	0	0.00	0.00	0.00	0.00
SQual−	0.59	0.80	0.00	2.00	13	0.00	0.00	0.89	−0.80
M	2.56	1.85	0.00	7.00	28	2.00	2.00	0.56	−0.32
FM	2.75	1.65	0.00	7.00	29	3.00	2.00	0.47	0.44
m	1.50	1.92	0.00	10.00	20	1.00	0.00	2.88	12.05
FM+m	4.25	2.84	0.00	13.00	31	4.00	2.00	0.96	1.36
FC	0.41	0.67	0.00	2.00	10	0.00	0.00	1.42	0.85
CF	1.66	1.31	0.00	5.00	26	1.50	1.00	0.78	0.26
C	0.75	0.95	0.00	4.00	17	1.00	0.00	1.74	3.73
CN	0.00	0.00	0.00	0.00	0	0.00	0.00	0.00	0.00
Sum Color	2.81	1.71	0.00	7.00	29	2.50	2.00	0.39	−0.05
WSumC	2.98	1.84	0.00	7.00	29	2.75	2.00	0.42	−0.10
SumC'	1.47	1.48	0.00	6.00	23	1.00	1.00	1.34	1.96
Sum T	0.00	0.00	0.00	0.00	0	0.00	0.00	0.00	0.00
Sum V	0.63	0.94	0.00	4.00	14	0.00	0.00	2.09	5.05
Sum Y	1.13	1.54	0.00	5.00	16	0.50	0.00	1.36	0.83
Sum Shading	3.22	2.59	0.00	9.00	26	3.00	0.00	0.73	0.01
Fr + rF	0.72	0.96	0.00	3.00	14	0.00	0.00	1.08	0.05
FD	0.38	0.66	0.00	2.00	9	0.00	0.00	1.57	1.29
F	8.56	4.43	3.00	25.00	32	7.00	7.00	1.95	5.32
(2)	4.91	2.58	2.00	15.00	32	4.50	4.00	1.92	6.42
3r+(2)/R	0.38	0.14	0.14	0.67	32	0.38	0.44	0.59	−0.17

(continued)

VARIABLE	MEAN	SD	MIN	MAX	FREQ	MEDIAN	MODE	SK	KU
Lambda	0.97	0.64	0.18	2.50	32	0.76	0.50	1.11	0.40
EA	5.55	2.82	1.00	12.00	32	4.75	4.00	0.82	0.04
es	7.47	4.22	1.00	22.00	32	8.00	8.00	1.12	3.15
D Score	−0.47	1.39	−4.00	2.00	32	0.00	0.00	−0.61	0.39
AdjD	0.00	1.08	−3.00	3.00	32	0.00	0.00	0.00	2.61
a (active)	4.22	2.90	0.00	13.00	31	4.00	2.00	1.40	2.58
p (passive)	2.59	1.85	0.00	6.00	28	2.50	1.00	0.25	−1.11
Ma	1.16	1.27	0.00	5.00	22	1.00	1.00	1.59	2.36
Mp	1.41	1.19	0.00	4.00	24	1.00	1.00	0.61	−0.38
Intellect	2.94	4.60	0.00	25.00	25	1.50	1.00	3.79	17.54
Zf	11.31	3.57	4.00	21.00	32	11.50	12.00	0.44	1.54
Zd	−0.63	3.40	−7.50	4.00	30	−0.50	3.00	−0.63	−0.41
Blends	3.00	2.14	0.00	9.00	31	3.00	1.00	0.93	0.53
Blends/R	0.16	0.12	0.00	0.45	31	0.14	0.07	0.89	0.40
Col-Shd Blends	0.66	1.13	0.00	5.00	12	0.00	0.00	2.34	6.47
Afr	0.43	0.17	0.19	1.00	32	0.42	0.47	1.26	2.93
Populars	4.63	2.18	1.00	9.00	32	4.50	3.00	0.12	−0.73
X+%	0.51	0.15	0.20	0.79	32	0.53	0.47	−0.25	−0.36
F+%	0.55	0.24	0.00	1.00	31	0.60	0.67	−0.13	−0.15
X−%	0.22	0.12	0.05	0.60	32	0.20	0.27	1.05	1.70
Xu%	0.23	0.13	0.06	0.55	32	0.20	0.07	0.64	−0.32
S−%	0.12	0.17	0.00	0.67	13	0.00	0.00	1.54	2.05
Isolate/R	0.21	0.15	0.00	0.56	—	—	—	—	—
H	1.66	1.31	0.00	5.00	24	2.00	2.00	0.42	−0.18
(H)	1.03	1.23	0.00	5.00	19	1.00	0.00	1.60	2.83
HD	1.03	1.36	0.00	6.00	18	1.00	0.00	2.01	5.06
(Hd)	0.28	0.58	0.00	2.00	7	0.00	0.00	2.01	3.19
Hx	0.00	0.00	0.00	0.00	0	0.00	0.00	0.00	0.00
H+(H)+Hd+(Hd)	4.00	2.13	0.00	11.00	30	4.00	3.00	1.01	2.92
A	7.22	3.20	3.00	16.00	32	7.00	7.00	1.33	1.63
(A)	0.78	0.98	0.00	3.00	15	0.00	0.00	0.92	−0.37
Ad	1.81	1.71	0.00	8.00	28	1.00	1.00	2.04	5.14
(Ad)	0.09	0.30	0.00	1.00	3	0.00	0.00	2.93	7.00
An	1.13	1.13	0.00	4.00	20	1.00	MODE	0.75	−0.21
Art	1.06	1.41	0.00	5.00	18	1.00	0.00	1.71	2.48
Ay	0.56	0.76	0.00	3.00	14	0.00	0.00	1.43	2.11
Bl	0.28	0.58	0.00	2.00	7	0.00	0.00	2.01	3.19
Bt	0.97	1.00	0.00	3.00	20	1.00	1.00	0.89	−0.09
Cg	0.75	0.92	0.00	3.00	16	0.50	0.00	1.08	0.37
Cl	0.41	0.67	0.00	3.00	11	0.00	0.00	2.12	6.10
Ex	0.22	0.49	0.00	2.00	6	0.00	0.00	2.26	4.77
Fi	0.28	0.46	0.00	1.00	9	0.00	0.00	1.02	−1.02

VARIABLE	MEAN	SD	MIN	MAX	FREQ	MEDIAN	MODE	SK	KU
Food	0.16	0.45	0.00	2.00	4	0.00	0.00	3.05	9.43
Ge	0.00	0.00	0.00	0.00	0	0.00	0.00	0.00	0.00
Hh	0.56	0.72	0.00	3.00	15	0.00	0.00	1.46	2.92
Ls	0.75	0.98	0.00	3.00	15	0.00	0.00	1.19	0.43
Na	0.69	0.93	0.00	3.00	14	0.00	0.00	1.20	0.50
Sc	0.91	1.12	0.00	5.00	18	1.00	0.00	1.82	4.64
Sx	0.56	0.67	0.00	2.00	15	0.00	0.00	0.79	−0.39
Xy	0.09	0.30	0.00	1.00	3	0.00	0.00	2.93	7.00
Idiographic	1.16	1.11	0.00	4.00	22	1.00	1.00	1.03	0.90
DV	1.03	1.31	0.00	5.00	16	0.50	0.00	1.23	1.12
INCOM	1.13	1.26	0.00	6.00	22	1.00	1.00	2.21	6.71
DR	1.97	2.52	0.00	12.00	21	1.50	0.00	2.38	7.46
FABCOM	0.44	0.80	0.00	4.00	11	0.00	0.00	3.03	12.20
DV2	0.00	0.00	0.00	0.00	0	0.00	0.00	0.00	0.00
INC2	0.19	0.54	0.00	2.00	4	0.00	0.00	2.87	7.43
DR2	0.09	0.30	0.00	1.00	3	0.00	0.00	2.93	7.00
FAB2	0.34	0.75	0.00	3.00	7	0.00	0.00	2.32	5.05
ALOG	0.03	0.18	0.00	1.00	1	0.00	0.00	5.66	32.00
CONTAM	0.22	0.49	0.00	2.00	6	0.00	0.00	2.26	4.77
Sum 6 Sp Sc	5.44	3.91	0.00	14.00	30	6.00	2.00	0.50	−0.63
Lvl 2 Sp Sc	0.63	1.01	0.00	4.00	12	0.00	0.00	1.85	3.34
WSum6	16.34	12.84	0.00	42.00	30	13.50	0.00	0.56	−0.83
AB	0.66	1.83	0.00	10.00	9	0.00	0.00	4.63	23.66
AG	0.53	0.84	0.00	3.00	11	0.00	0.00	1.45	1.19
CONFAB	0.00	0.00	0.00	0.00	0	0.00	0.00	0.00	0.00
COP	0.56	0.76	0.00	2.00	13	0.00	0.00	0.95	−0.54
CP	0.03	0.18	0.00	1.00	1	0.00	0.00	5.66	32.00
MOR	1.50	1.59	0.00	5.00	21	1.00	0.00	1.01	0.16
PER	2.56	2.39	0.00	8.00	24	2.00	0.00	0.72	−0.50
PSV	0.47	0.67	0.00	2.00	12	0.00	0.00	1.14	0.19

APPENDIX C   Descriptive Statistics for Sexual Homicide Perpetrators ($N = 38$)

VARIABLE	MEAN	SD	MIN	MAX	FREQ	MEDIAN	MODE	SK	KU
AGE	32.34	8.96	13.00	53.00	38	31.00	27.00	0.16	−0.34
R	26.50	11.80	13.00	54.00	38	23.00	19.00	0.96	−0.25
W	9.58	3.62	2.00	19.00	38	10.00	10.00	0.19	0.14
D	12.97	9.47	0.00	37.00	37	9.50	5.00	1.01	0.22
Dd	3.95	4.63	0.00	17.00	25	2.00	0.00	1.27	0.91
SPACE	2.92	1.99	0.00	7.00	37	2.00	1.00	0.57	−1.10
DQ+	7.29	3.19	1.00	16.00	38	7.00	4.00	0.41	0.38
DQo	15.53	9.62	4.00	41.00	38	13.00	4.00	1.01	0.40
DQv	2.76	2.52	0.00	9.00	30	2.00	0.00	0.99	0.44
DQv/+	0.92	1.36	0.00	6.00	19	0.50	0.00	2.11	4.85
FQx/+	0.10	0.51	0.00	3.00	2	0.00	0.00	5.40	30.35
FQxo	12.16	6.04	4.00	30.00	38	10.00	12.00	1.24	1.10
FQxu	7.13	5.22	2.00	19.00	38	5.00	4.00	1.15	0.06
FQx−	6.55	3.45	0.00	16.00	37	6.50	4.00	0.25	0.28
FQxNone	0.55	1.00	0.00	5.00	13	0.00	0.00	2.71	9.54
MQ+	0.08	0.36	0.00	2.00	2	0.00	0.00	4.85	24.25
MQo	2.05	1.41	0.00	5.00	32	2.00	3.00	0.20	−0.70
MQu	1.29	1.16	0.00	5.00	27	1.00	1.00	0.93	1.25
MQ−	1.05	1.16	0.00	4.00	22	1.00	1.00	0.88	−0.27
MQNone	0.03	0.16	0.00	1.00	1	0.00	0.00	6.16	38.00
SQual−	1.24	1.46	0.00	6.00	22	1.00	0.00	1.32	1.70
M	4.50	2.42	0.00	10.00	37	4.00	3.00	0.58	0.00
FM	5.08	3.76	0.00	16.00	35	4.50	3.00	0.81	0.56
m	2.32	2.03	0.00	7.00	30	2.00	0.00	0.75	−0.35
FM+m	7.39	4.84	0.00	22.00	36	7.00	5.00	0.77	0.91
FC	1.29	1.52	0.00	5.00	26	1.00	1.00	1.51	1.26
CF	2.42	2.02	0.00	9.00	32	2.00	2.00	1.23	1.87
C	0.58	0.72	0.00	2.00	17	0.00	0.00	0.85	−0.55
CN	0.03	0.16	0.00	1.00	1	0.00	0.00	6.16	38.00
Sum Color	4.32	2.99	0.00	13.00	37	3.00	3.00	1.19	1.17
WSumC	3.93	2.69	0.00	11.50	37	3.50	3.00	1.10	1.30
SumC'	1.42	1.29	0.00	5.00	27	1.00	0.00	0.83	0.42
Sum T	0.95	1.71	0.00	9.00	15	0.00	0.00	3.11	12.82
Sum V	1.11	1.90	0.00	10.00	20	1.00	0.00	3.23	12.87
Sum Y	1.68	2.80	0.00	12.00	21	1.00	0.00	2.56	6.83
Sum Shading	5.16	5.66	0.00	28.00	36	3.00	2.00	2.34	6.53
Fr + rF	1.11	1.62	0.00	8.00	17	0.00	0.00	2.30	7.68
FD	0.42	0.68	0.00	3.00	13	0.00	0.00	1.91	4.40
F	9.68	6.55	0.00	25.00	37	7.50	5.00	0.84	0.07
(2)	7.76	4.80	0.00	26.00	37	7.50	11.00	1.40	4.28
3r+(2)/R	0.45	0.24	0.05	1.15	38	0.44	0.44	1.05	1.48

400

VARIABLE	MEAN	SD	MIN	MAX	FREQ	MEDIAN	MODE	SK	KU
Lambda	0.70	0.57	0.00	2.17	37	0.54	0.15	1.16	0.70
EA	8.43	3.79	1.00	17.00	38	7.75	6.50	0.51	0.05
es	12.55	9.30	1.00	41.00	38	11.00	6.00	1.49	2.19
D Score	−1.45	2.66	−11.00	1.00	38	0.00	0.00	−1.88	3.91
AdjD	−0.58	1.65	−6.00	2.00	38	0.00	0.00	−1.55	2.78
a (active)	7.29	3.75	1.00	18.00	38	7.00	6.00	0.55	0.56
p (passive)	4.61	3.73	0.00	14.00	36	4.00	4.00	1.13	0.60
Ma	2.34	1.53	0.00	5.00	35	2.00	1.00	0.20	−1.26
Mp	2.16	1.73	0.00	6.00	31	2.00	2.00	0.80	0.14
Intellect	2.61	3.05	0.00	15.00	30	2.00	1.00	2.25	6.54
Zf	13.32	3.99	6.00	26.00	38	13.00	10.00	0.73	1.64
Zd	−1.61	3.67	−8.50	4.50	34	−1.00	−6.00	−0.27	−0.89
Blends	5.08	3.83	0.00	17.00	36	4.00	4.00	1.14	1.53
Blends/R	0.20	0.13	0.00	0.46	36	0.20	0.21	0.37	−0.61
Col-Shd Blends	1.03	1.30	0.00	5.00	20	1.00	0.00	1.34	1.26
Afr	0.53	0.23	0.19	1.09	38	0.50	0.36	0.82	0.04
Populars	5.32	1.77	2.00	9.00	38	5.00	6.00	0.14	−0.38
X+%	0.47	0.12	0.21	0.77	38	0.47	0.50	0.10	−0.12
F+%	0.47	0.25	0.00	1.00	35	0.47	1.00	0.39	0.66
X−%	0.26	0.12	0.00	0.47	37	0.26	0.30	−0.20	−0.52
Xu%	0.25	0.09	0.09	0.47	38	0.25	0.20	0.33	−0.24
S−%	0.17	0.19	0.00	0.67	22	0.14	0.00	0.98	0.22
Isolate/R	0.28	0.24	0.00	0.92	—	—	—	—	—
H	2.82	1.78	0.00	7.00	37	2.50	2.00	1.02	0.60
(H)	0.92	1.00	0.00	4.00	22	1.00	0.00	1.03	0.96
HD	1.74	1.78	0.00	6.00	26	1.00	0.00	0.97	0.10
(Hd)	0.92	1.36	0.00	5.00	17	0.00	0.00	1.57	1.62
Hx	0.29	0.61	0.00	2.00	8	0.00	0.00	2.01	2.93
H+(H)+Hd+(Hd)	6.39	3.09	2.00	13.00	38	6.50	4.00	0.39	−0.70
A	10.00	5.26	3.00	22.00	38	9.00	6.00	0.94	0.30
(A)	0.68	0.93	0.00	3.00	16	0.00	0.00	1.11	0.11
Ad	2.89	3.09	0.00	14.00	30	2.00	3.00	1.80	3.81
(Ad)	0.32	0.52	0.00	2.00	11	0.00	0.00	1.40	1.13
An	1.16	1.40	0.00	4.00	21	1.00	0.00	1.00	−0.41
ART	0.92	1.24	0.00	5.00	19	0.50	0.00	1.60	2.47
AY	0.89	1.06	0.00	4.00	21	1.00	0.00	1.23	0.99
Bl	0.50	0.76	0.00	3.00	14	0.00	0.00	1.55	2.05
Bt	1.11	1.50	0.00	6.00	19	0.50	0.00	1.48	1.78
Cg	1.29	1.41	0.00	5.00	24	1.00	0.00	1.15	0.80
Cl	0.68	0.96	0.00	4.00	17	0.00	0.00	1.66	2.93
Ex	0.24	0.43	0.00	1.00	9	0.00	0.00	1.29	−0.36
Fi	0.58	1.00	0.00	5.00	14	0.00	0.00	2.65	9.32

(continued)

APPENDIX C   Descriptive Statistics for Sexual Homicide Perpetrators ($N = 38$)   *(continued)*

VARIABLE	MEAN	SD	MIN	MAX	FREQ	MEDIAN	MODE	SK	KU
Food	0.53	0.92	0.00	4.00	13	0.00	0.00	2.21	5.30
Ge	0.10	0.31	0.00	1.00	4	0.00	0.00	2.68	5.46
Hh	0.55	0.83	0.00	3.00	15	0.00	0.00	1.63	2.35
Ls	1.13	1.77	0.00	7.00	19	0.50	0.00	2.15	4.35
Na	1.89	2.49	0.00	12.00	25	1.00	0.00	2.32	6.85
Sc	1.29	1.50	0.00	6.00	24	1.00	0.00	1.48	1.99
Sx	0.61	1.00	0.00	3.00	13	0.00	0.00	1.57	1.26
Xy	0.05	0.23	0.00	1.00	2	0.00	0.00	4.17	16.27
Idiographic	1.03	1.44	0.00	7.00	20	1.00	0.00	2.29	7.08
DV	1.89	2.02	0.00	8.00	26	1.00	0.00	1.14	0.87
INCOM	1.47	1.55	0.00	7.00	26	1.00	0.00	1.60	3.44
DR	2.32	2.74	0.00	12.00	24	1.50	0.00	1.55	2.94
FABCOM	1.16	1.48	0.00	6.00	21	1.00	0.00	1.51	2.05
DV2	0.00	0.00	0.00	0.00	0	0.00	0.00	0.00	0.00
INC2	0.26	0.55	0.00	2.00	8	0.00	0.00	2.07	3.51
DR2	0.42	1.35	0.00	8.00	8	0.00	0.00	5.10	28.55
FAB2	0.32	0.74	0.00	4.00	9	0.00	0.00	3.65	16.59
ALOG	0.16	0.37	0.00	1.00	6	0.00	0.00	1.95	1.92
CONTAM	0.00	0.00	0.00	0.00	0	0.00	0.00	0.00	0.00
Sum 6 Sp Sc	8.00	5.64	0.00	18.00	35	6.00	6.00	0.59	−0.79
Lvl 2 Sp Sc	1.00	1.87	0.00	10.00	19	0.50	0.00	3.64	15.31
WSum6	23.00	19.08	0.00	71.00	35	16.50	0.00	1.01	0.19
AB	0.40	0.89	0.00	4.00	9	0.00	0.00	2.79	8.23
AG	0.79	0.90	0.00	3.00	21	1.00	0.00	1.13	0.75
CONFAB	0.00	0.00	0.00	0.00	0	0.00	0.00	0.00	0.00
COP	1.37	1.13	0.00	4.00	28	1.00	1.00	0.41	−0.74
CP	0.16	0.37	0.00	1.00	6	0.00	0.00	1.95	1.92
MOR	2.63	2.62	0.00	12.00	30	2.00	0.00	1.82	4.37
PER	2.42	3.12	0.00	13.00	25	2.00	0.00	1.98	3.91
PSV	0.29	0.56	0.00	2.00	9	0.00	0.00	1.87	2.70

19

Inmates in Prison Psychiatric Treatment: A Multimethod Description

Myla H. Young
Private Practice, Walnut Creek, CA

Philip S. Erdberg
Private Practice, Corte Madera, CA

Jerald Justice
Private Practice, Walnut Creek, CA

As state mental hospitals have been closed throughout the United States, an increasing number of mentally ill persons have been incarcerated in adult correctional facilities. One survey described this trend, reporting that from 1988 to 2000 the number of mentally ill persons receiving treatment in state mental hospitals decreased by 56% while the number of mentally ill persons in adult correctional facilities increased by 114.5% (Manderscheid, Gravesande, & Goldstrom, 2004). Correctional systems have responded to this trend by endeavoring to provide psychiatric treatment within the prisons. From 1988 to 2000, the number of prisons providing mental health services increased by 56%, with 1,097 facilities providing mental health services in 2000 (U.S. Department of Justice, 2001). Mental health services included 24-hour mental health care, counseling or therapy, psychotrophic medication management, and testing or assessment. Of particular relevance to the information presented in this chapter, psychotherapy and counseling were provided by 84% of prisons providing services to mentally ill inmates and testing/assessment was provided in 78.8% (U.S. Department of Justice, 2002). Although information for 2006 was not available at the time this chapter was written, there is no reason to believe that the number of mentally ill inmates or the number of prisons providing services to mentally ill inmates has decreased since 2000 and there is substantial reason to believe that the numbers will continue to increase.

As the number of mentally ill persons in prisons grows, the necessity of describing inmates who require psychiatric treatment in prison becomes increasingly clear. The purpose of this chapter is to provide a description of one group of mentally ill inmates who were receiving psychiatric treatment while in prison and to provide a description of Rorschach findings for this group of inmates. We also provide Comprehensive System data for inmates with ≤ 13 and > 14 responses. Our hope is that this data may be useful as a comparison point for examiners that conduct psychological evaluations with this population. Additionally, our group data provides a window into the psychology of these offenders and how they differ from other forensic samples (Cunliffe & Gacono, chap.17, this vol.; Gacono, Gacono, & Evans, chap. 16, this vol.; Gacono, Meloy, & Bridges, chap. 18, this vol.; Gacono & Gacono, chap. 20, this vol.; Singer et al., chap. 21, this vol.).

PSYCHIATRIC TREATMENT PROGRAM

Participants were inmates who were referred and admitted to a specialized psychiatric treatment program located inside a large state prison. The program evaluates and treats any male inmate in the state correctional system thought to be experiencing a mental disorder and/or presenting risk of self-harm. Referrals are made by mental health professionals throughout the correctional system. The primary reasons for referrals are self-harm concerns (61%) or psychosis (24%). Only 5% of referrals identify depression as a major problem. About 5% cite danger to others as the reason for recommending hospitalization, and 5% list other reasons, mostly for diagnostic clarification. Evaluation and treatment is carried out by interdisciplinary treatment teams comprised of psychiatrists, psychologists, psychiatric social workers, rehabilitation therapists, and nursing personnel. The goals are to conduct comprehensive psychiatric evaluations, implement treatment programs to reduce the acuteness of the disorders, and to facilitate discharge to appropriate levels of care or treatment. Bed allocation is limited and the treatment period is necessarily short term, with utilization reviews on admission, at 10 days, and at 30 days.

The continuum of psychopathology in this population ranges from no mental disorder or personality disorders not warranting inpatient psychiatric treatment to acute psychosis. Thirty-six percent of the population is found to either have a psychiatric condition not requiring inpatient treatment or no mental illness at all. At the other end of the spectrum, a similar percentage of the patients are so compromised as to require longer term hospitalization and are referred to a state forensic hospital. Treatment modalities include pharmacotherapy, group therapy, and individual therapy. The treatment program is based on a cognitive behavioral model, emphasizing psychoeducational groups to increase understanding of relevant aspects of mental health, and skill-building groups to develop and refine coping abilities. Those patients whose conditions are stabilized within length of stay parameters are returned to the prison system for placement at a level of follow-up treatment or case management in accordance with their individual needs. A few patients parole or are released from prison directly from the program and in those cases follow-up care is provided by community resources.

METHOD

Data were collected from 1997 through 2005. Participants were 259 male inmates who were receiving psychiatric treatment in the previously described prison psychiatric treatment program located within the confines of a state prison. Each month the program's medical records department provided names of inmates who had been admitted for treatment. Inmates were randomly selected from this list and invited to participate. Signed informed consent was provided by all inmates prior to initiating procedures.

Participation in the study was voluntary and participants were not compensated for their participation. This research project was approved and annually reviewed by the Department of Mental Health and Department of Corrections Human Research Boards. Procedures included a comprehensive review of records and interdisciplinary treatment team (IDT) progress notes, a semistructured interview, neuropsychological testing, Rorschach, and Psychopathy Checklist–Revised (PCL–R; Hare, 1991, 2003).

Record Review

Correctional (Central File), medical, and psychiatric treatment records were reviewed. Offense, prison adjustment, medical, psychiatric, developmental, educational, and work histories were obtained from those reviews.

Semistructured Interview

The semistructured interview included description of the inmate's criminal offenses and prison adjustment, as well as psychiatric, drug use, developmental, relationship, medical, social, school, and work histories.

Neuropsychological Functioning

Neuropsychological testing included tests from the Halstead–Reitan Neuropsychological Battery (Finger Tapping Test, Trail Making A and B, Seashore Rhythm, Speech Perception, Tactual Performance Test, Category Test), as well as additional independent neuropsychological instruments (Wide Range Achievement Test and Wisconsin Card Sorting Test).

Psychological Functioning

Evaluation of psychological functioning included the Rorschach and the Psychopathy Checklist–Revised (PCL–R).

Rorschach.   The Rorschach was administered and coded using Comprehensive System guidelines (Exner, 2001). To establish intercoder agreement 15 Rorschach protocols were scored by two independent scorers. Agreement findings were based on Cohen's (1960) kappa, a chance-corrected agreement statistic. Landis and Koch (1977) suggested the following guidelines for describing levels of agreement as characterized by kappa: .01 to .20, slight agreement; .21 to .40, fair agreement; .40 to .60, moderate agreement; .61 to .80, substantial agreement; and .81 to 1.00, nearly perfect agreement. Intercoder agreement for this sample ranged from .75 to 1.00.

Psychopathy Checklist–Revised (PCL–R).   The PCL–R was administered by two of the authors of this chapter. Both individuals were certified in administration of the PCL–R (Hare PCL–R Training Program). The PCL–R was administered without knowledge of psychological and/or neuropsychological testing results. Using the criteria of agreement within two total points, there was 88% intercoder agreement for 10% of PCL–R interviews. For the entire sample, using the criteria of agreement within three total points, there was 100% interrater agreement, with significant correlation between raters for PCL–R Total Score ($r = .95, p = .01$).

RESULTS

Demographics

Ages ranged from 18 to 65, with a mean age of 35.53 ($SD = 8.08$), and with the majority of inmates in their 30s. There was a wide range of educational experience. Although the average and most frequent educational level was 10th grade, education ranged from 3rd grade to college graduate degree (3 years to 18 years of education). Twelve percent of inmates completed elementary school (1st–6th grades); 23% of inmates completed Junior High School (7th–9th grades); and 58% of inmates completed high school (10th–12th grades). Seven percent of inmates completed at least 1 year of college. Twenty percent of inmates completed a GED while in prison.

Caucasians not of Hispanic origin and African Americans were the largest racial groups, followed by Latino. (Caucasian = 36%; African American = 37%; Latino = 21%). Inmates from other races (Asian, Indian, Philippino, Arabian, etc.) comprised only 6% of the research sample.

Drug Use Histories

Drug abuse was pervasive. Eighty-eight percent of inmates reported drug abuse that met *DSM–R* criterion for abuse and/or dependence. Of those with drug abuse histories, 76% reported poly-substance abuse. Alcohol and/or marijuana were the drug most frequently used first (76%). The average age of first drug use was 12 years ($M = 12.46, SD = 2.75$). Age range for first alcohol use, however, ranged from 2 years to 21 years, with 3% of inmates reporting that they were given alcohol by their "caretakers" when they were as young as 2 years old. Although alcohol and/or marijuana were the first and most used drugs, drugs other than alcohol and/or marijuana (cocaine, amphetamine, heroin, etc.) were most frequently the drug of choice (52%).

Offense History

Offense history was obtained from a review of the inmate's Central File. Recognizing that the number and severity of offenses obtained from this review likely underestimate actual offenses, a conservative approach of reporting only those offenses for which the inmate was convicted was used for research purposes. Each offense was ranked on a

7-point scale ranging from nonviolent (1) to extreme violence (7). Using the offense that represented the most severe violence, 25% of inmates were incarcerated for offenses that did not involve physical harm to the victim (1 through 4). The majority (75%), however, were incarcerated for an offense that did result in serious physical harm to the victim. Nineteen percent of inmates were serving a life sentence. Forty-three percent had previously been incarcerated as juveniles.

Neuropsychological Functioning

Composite scores for each neuropsychological function (Attention, Memory, Psychomotor, Language, and Executive Functioning) were used to determine levels of functioning and impairment (Mild, Moderate, Severe).

Intellectual Functioning.   The average Intellectual Quotient (*IQ*) was 82.55 (*SD* = 14.02). There was, however, a wide range and a broadly skewed distribution of *IQ* scores. *IQ* scores ranged from Extremely Low (*IQ* = 50) to Very Superior (*IQ* = 134). Distribution of *IQ* scores is described in Figure 19–1.

Overall Neuropsychological Functioning.   Overall neuropsychological functioning was determined by using the Halstead–Reitan Impairment Index (Finger Tapping-Dominant; Seashore Rhythm Test; Speech Perception Test; Tactual Performance Test, TPT;

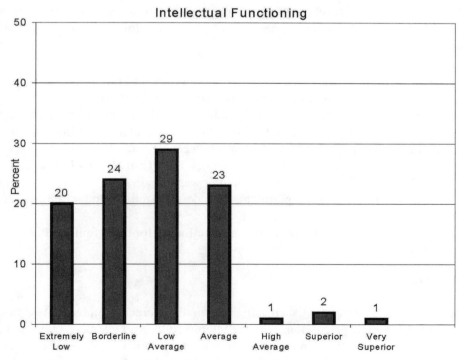

Figure 19–1.   Intellectual functioning.

Memory and Location; and Category Test) (Reitan & Wolfson, 1985). Using age and adjusted T-scores (Heaton, Grant, & Matthews, 1991), 81% of inmates had neuropsychological functioning in the impaired range ($T \leq 40$). Of those inmates demonstrating impairment, 57% experienced Mild Impairment, 15% experienced Moderate impairment, and 9% experienced Severe Impairment

Motor Functioning. Motor functioning was evaluated using the Finger Tapping Test (Dominant and Nondominant). Forty four percent demonstrated Mild Impairment; 24% demonstrated Moderate Impairment, and 13% demonstrated Severe Impairment of motor functioning.

Attention and Concentration. Attention and concentration were evaluated using the Seashore Rhythm Test, Speech Perception Test, and Trail Making A. Using a composite score, 28% of inmates were Mildly Impaired, 22% were Moderately Impaired, and 5% were Severely Impaired.

Memory. Memory was evaluated using TPT–Memory and TPT–Location scores. Sixty-eight percent (68%) of inmates demonstrated memory impairment, with 15% experiencing Mild Impairment, 38% experiencing Moderate Impairment, and 15% experiencing Severe Impairment).

Visual-Perceptual-Motor. Visual-Perceptual-Motor functioning was evaluated using the TPT–Total Time. An exceptionally high number of inmates demonstrated impairment of this function (Mild Impairment = 39%, Moderate Impairment = 25%, Severe Impairment = 9%).

Executive Functioning. Executive functioning is an umbrella construct that describes processes responsible for guiding, directing, and managing cognitive, emotional, and behavioral functions. Mature executive functioning allows the individual to engage in purposeful, goal-directed, and problem-solving actions and includes impulse control, abilities to initiate, attend, inhibit, shift, monitor, organize, and control behaviors. Executive Functioning was evaluated using the Category Test, Trail Making B Test, and Wisconsin Card Sorting Test. Executive functioning was impaired for 70% of the inmates, with 37% demonstrating Mild Impairment, 29% demonstrating Moderate Impairment, and 4% demonstrating Severe Impairment.

Further description of neuropsychological functioning for these inmates is described in Table 19–1.

Psychiatric Diagnosis

Psychiatric diagnosis was established using information gained from record reviews, interview with the inmate, discussions with the Interdisciplinary Treatment Team, and psychological and neuropsychological testing. Interrater reliability for Axis I diagnosis was established by comparing Structured Clinical Interview for *DSM–III–R* Patient Edition

TABLE 19–1

Neuropsychological Functioning of Inmates in Prison Psychiatric Treatment

Function	n	M	SD
Intellectual	259	82.55	14.02
Overall Impairment[a]	259	35.75	9.97
Motor			
Finger Tap—Dom	259	34.67	13.02
Finger Tap—Non-Dom	259	37.14	12.74
Attention			
Trails A	259	35.82	11.54
Speech Perception	201	38.27	9.59
Seashore Rhythm	259	40.82	13.44
Memory			
TPT[b]—Memory	242	40.32	11.63
TPT—Location	242	40.47	10.80
Psychomotor			
TPT—Total Time	242	35.38	11.42
Executive			
Category	259	37.01	11.69
Trails—B	259	36.83	12.23
Wisconsin[c]	155	31.45	2.12

Note.   Except for Intellectual, all scores are age and education adjusted *T* scores. *T* scores ≥ 40 are considered to be impaired.
[a]Overall Impairment is Halstead Reitan Impairment Index. [b]TPT is Tactual Performance Test. [c]Wisconsin is Wisconsin Card Sort Perseverative Responses.

(SCID–P) (Spitzer, Williams, Gibbon, & First, 1990) to diagnosis classification used in this research. The SCID–P was administered by an investigator who was blind to diagnosis based on all other information. There was 79% agreement between SCID–P diagnosis and psychiatric diagnosis used in this study.

Many participants had received psychiatric treatment prior to prison (55%) and the majority of inmates were diagnosed with an Axis I Clinical Disorder (64%). Using the primary Axis I diagnosis, Psychotic disorders (Schizophrenia, Psychosis NOS, Psychosis Due to Medical Disorder) accounted for 26% of the sample; Mood disorders (Major Depression, Bipolar Disorder, Depression NOS) accounted for 21% of the sample; disorders with both Psychotic and Mood features (Schizoaffective Disorder; Depression with Psychotic Features; Bipolar Disorder with Psychotic Features) accounted for 12%; and "Organic" disorders (Dementia) accounted for 5% of those diagnosed with a major mental disorder. Although inmates were participating in psychiatric treatment for severely mentally ill inmates in prison, 36% were not diagnosed with a severe mental disorder.

Cognitive Disorder NOS was the primary diagnosis for 9% of these inmates. Twenty-seven percent of inmates had No Diagnosis as the primary Axis I diagnosis.

Axis II Personality Disorders primarily were among *DSM–R* Cluster B (Antisocial, Borderline, Narcissistic, Paranoid) diagnoses. Of those diagnosed with a Cluster B disorder, 60% were diagnosed with Antisocial Personality Disorder, 18% with Borderline Personality Disorder, and 17% with Narcissistic Disorder. Of note, for 34% of inmates, Axis II Personality Disorder, without Axis I Clinical Disorder, was the primary diagnosis.

Psychopathy.   Psychopathy was identified as PCL–R total score $\geq$ 30and those moderate in psychopathic traits were identified by a PCL–R score of 20–29. Using these classifications, 26% were identified as psychopathic and 38% were in the moderate ranges.

Neurological Status

Neurological injury/disorder was defined as head trauma resulting in loss of consciousness, seizure disorder, loss of consciousness for reasons other than seizure, and\or medical disorder resulting in documented brain damage. A remarkably high incidence of neurological injury was identified for this sample (63%). The number of injuries ranged from 1 to 5, the most frequent number of injuries was 1, and the Mean number of injuries was 2. Age at first neurological injury ranged from 1 year old to 59 years old.

Rorschach Findings

Rorschach data was available for 249 inmates. Of these, 38 inmates gave records with fewer than 14 responses, even after repetition of the test (Exner, 2001). Descriptive statistics for the 211 inmates who gave records of 14 or more responses are presented in Table 19–2 and data for the 38 inmates with records of fewer than 14 answers are presented in Table 19–3.

We compared findings for *Lambda*, *X–%*, and *WSum6* for the 211 inmates with 14 or more responses against those for the 38 men who had given fewer than 14 answers. Interestingly, there were no significant differences for the *X–%* or for *WSum6*, and *Lambda* was significantly lower for the low *R* group ($M = 1.05$, $SD = 1.09$) than for the higher *R* group ($M = 2.0$, $SD = 2.8$, $t(247) = 2.04$, $p = .04$ (two-tailed). Neuropsychological comparisons between the two groups indicated that inmates with fewer than 14 Rorschach responses had significantly lower IQ scores and significantly greater impairment on tests of executive functioning.

CONCLUSIONS

This chapter has provided a multimethod description of 259 randomly selected male inmates who were admitted for psychiatric treatment while in prison. Demographic, drug use, offense, intellectual, neuropsychological, Rorschach, psychiatric diagnosis, and Psychopathy ratings were described. Rorschach protocols for inmates providing fewer than 14 responses and those with at least 14 responses were described separately.

TABLE 19–2

Rorschach Data for Inmates in Prison Psychiatric Treatment (*R* > 13)

MARITAL STATUS			AGE			RACE		
Single 116	55%		18–25 36	17%		White 89	42%	
Lives w/S.O. 0	0%		26–35 98	46%		Black 68	32%	
Married 17	8%		36–45 65	31%		Hispanic .. 45	21%	
Separated 6	3%		46–55 9	4%		Asian 1	0%	
Divorced 21	10%		56–65 3	1%		Other 4	2%	
Widowed 2	1%		Over 65 0	0%				

EDUCATION

SEX			Under 12 119	56%
Male 211	100%		12 Years 31	15%
Female 0	0%		13–15 Yrs 10	5%
			16+ Yrs 2	1%

RATIOS, PERCENTAGES AND SPECIAL INDICES

STYLES

			FORM QUALITY		
Introversive 28	13%		*XA% > .89* 16	8%	
Pervasive Introversive 20	9%		*XA% < .70* 121	57%	
Ambitent 37	18%		*WDA% < .85* 175	83%	
Extratensive 23	11%		*WDA% < .75* 123	58%	
Pervasive Extratensive 16	8%		*X+% < .55* 183	87%	
Avoidant 123	58%		*Xu% > .20* 135	64%	
			X–% > .20 158	75%	
			X–% > .30 113	54%	

D SCORES

D score > 0 30	14%
D score = 0 109	52%
D score < 0 72	34%
D score < –1 34	16%

		FC:CF + C RATIO		
Adj D score > 0 38	18%	*FC > (CF + C) + 2* 20	9%
Adj D score = 0 119	56%	*FC > (CF + C) + 1* 37	18%
Adj D score < 0 54	26%	*(CF + C) > FC + 1* 48	23%
Adj D score < –1 17	8%	*(CF + C) > FC + 2* 34	16%

Zd > +3.0 (Overincorp) 35	17%	*S-Constellation Positive* 10	5%			
Zd < –3.0 (Underincorp) 74	35%	*HVI Positive* 24	11%			
		OBS Positive 0	0%			

PTI = 5 25	12%	*DEPI* = 7 5	2%	*CDI* = 5 26	12%
PTI = 4 21	10%	*DEPI* = 6 14	7%	*CDI* = 4 70	33%
PTI = 3 44	21%	*DEPI* = 5 29	14%		

(continued)

TABLE 19–2 *(continued)*

R < 17	63	30%	*(2AB + Art + Ay)* > 5	14	7%
R > 27	34	16%	*Populars* < 4	69	33%
DQv > 2	23	11%	*Populars* > 7	15	7%
S > 2	58	27%	*COP* = 0	101	48%
Sum T = 0	172	82%	*COP* > 2	23	11%
Sum T > 1	14	7%	*AG* = 0	143	68%
3r + (2)/R < .33	93	44%	*AG* > 2	6	3%
3r + (2)/R > .44	69	33%	*MOR* > 2	39	18%
Fr + rF > 0	30	14%	*Level 2 Sp Sc* > 0	97	46%
Pure C > 0	55	26%	*GHR* > *PHR*	70	33%
Pure C > 1	18	9%	*Pure H* < 2	98	46%
Afr < .40	75	36%	*Pure H* = 0	43	20%
Afr < .50	115	55%	*p* > *a* + 1	30	14%
(FM + m) < *Sum Shading*	51	24%	*Mp* > *Ma*	56	27%

VARIABLE	MEAN	SD	MIN	MAX	FREQ	MEDIAN	MODE	SK	KU
AGE	33.17	7.91	18.00	65.00	211	32.00	26.00	0.69	0.88
R	21.17	7.88	14.00	59.00	211	19.00	17.00	1.94	4.35
W	8.84	5.06	0.00	34.00	210	8.00	5.00	1.45	4.70
D	8.49	5.89	0.00	32.00	207	7.00	5.00	1.17	1.53
Dd	3.83	[4.51]	0.00	43.00	184	3.00	2.00	4.51	31.45
S	1.99	[2.98]	0.00	34.00	149	1.00	0.00	6.32	63.23
DQ+	4.76	3.21	0.00	21.00	199	4.00	4.00	1.12	2.67
DQo	15.34	7.30	3.00	52.00	211	13.00	12.00	1.86	5.52
DQv	1.03	[1.59]	0.00	10.00	102	0.00	0.00	2.47	7.90
DQv/+	0.03	[0.19]	0.00	2.00	5	0.00	0.00	7.56	62.78
FQx+	0.02	0.34	0.00	5.00	1	0.00	0.00	14.52	211.00
FQxo	7.67	3.56	0.00	19.00	210	7.00	7.00	0.64	0.55
FQxu	5.58	3.47	0.00	22.00	208	5.00	5.00	1.45	3.62
FQx–	7.46	5.86	0.00	50.00	205	6.00	6.00	2.84	14.84
FQxNone	0.43	[1.08]	0.00	7.00	50	0.00	0.00	3.95	18.46
MQ+	0.01	0.07	0.00	1.00	1	0.00	0.00	14.52	211.00
MQo	1.01	1.05	0.00	5.00	129	1.00	0.00	1.00	0.69
MQu	0.67	1.00	0.00	4.00	83	0.00	0.00	1.49	1.52
MQ–	0.91	[1.24]	0.00	6.00	104	0.00	0.00	1.68	2.85
MQNone	0.02	[0.17]	0.00	2.00	3	0.00	0.00	9.80	103.19
SQual–	0.98	[2.43]	0.00	31.00	92	0.00	0.00	9.31	112.23
M	2.61	2.10	0.00	13.00	180	2.00	1.00	1.13	2.27
FM	2.58	2.30	0.00	16.00	177	2.00	2.00	1.93	6.63
m	1.29	1.41	0.00	6.00	131	1.00	0.00	1.10	0.62
FC	1.23	1.55	0.00	7.00	122	1.00	0.00	1.61	2.43
CF	1.01	1.38	0.00	6.00	104	0.00	0.00	1.57	2.07
C	0.41	[0.88]	0.00	5.00	55	0.00	0.00	2.91	9.87
Cn	0.01	[0.14]	0.00	2.00	1	0.00	0.00	14.52	211.00

VARIABLE	MEAN	SD	MIN	MAX	FREQ	MEDIAN	MODE	SK	KU
Sum Color	2.66	2.26	0.00	10.00	172	2.00	2.00	0.78	−0.10
WSumC	2.25	2.05	0.00	11.00	172	2.00	0.00	1.09	1.29
Sum C'	1.57	[1.79]	0.00	10.00	134	1.00	0.00	1.48	2.78
Sum T	0.28	[0.67]	0.00	3.00	39	0.00	0.00	2.66	6.79
Sum V	0.15	[0.56]	0.00	6.00	21	0.00	0.00	6.51	57.68
Sum Y	0.64	[1.18]	0.00	8.00	70	0.00	0.00	2.62	8.96
Sum Shading	2.64	2.92	0.00	15.00	152	2.00	0.00	1.60	3.12
Fr + rF	0.26	[0.74]	0.00	4.00	30	0.00	0.00	3.22	10.24
FD	0.39	[0.74]	0.00	4.00	58	0.00	0.00	2.31	6.09
F	11.56	6.50	1.00	54.00	211	11.00	9.00	2.06	9.21
(2)	6.98	4.65	0.00	33.00	202	6.00	5.00	1.56	5.12
3r+(2)/R	0.37	0.20	0.00	1.07	202	0.35	0.50	0.46	0.48
Lambda	2.01	2.82	0.07	18.00	211	1.25	1.00	3.80	16.17
FM+m	3.87	2.95	0.00	19.00	191	3.00	3.00	1.48	3.93
EA	4.86	3.05	0.00	16.00	205	4.50	3.00	0.83	0.85
es	6.51	4.88	0.00	30.00	201	5.00	4.00	1.58	4.11
D Score	−0.51	1.52	−9.00	3.00	102	0.00	0.00	−2.12	8.27
AdjD	−0.20	1.24	−7.00	3.00	92	0.00	0.00	−2.08	9.98
a (active)	3.72	2.78	0.00	14.00	189	3.00	3.00	0.97	1.05
p (passive)	2.79	2.10	0.00	12.00	184	3.00	1.00	0.99	1.86
Ma	1.51	1.53	0.00	8.00	149	1.00	1.00	1.41	2.73
Mp	1.11	1.23	0.00	5.00	127	1.00	0.00	1.09	0.62
Intellect	1.66	2.32	0.00	19.00	136	1.00	0.00	3.20	16.34
Zf	11.44	5.31	2.00	37.00	211	11.00	9.00	1.62	5.32
Zd	−1.28	5.24	−15.50	34.50	206	−1.00	−3.50	1.26	9.50
Blends	2.32	2.39	0.00	11.00	155	2.00	0.00	1.23	1.10
Blends/R	0.12	0.12	0.00	0.60	155	0.07	0.00	1.31	1.52
Col-Shd Blends	0.40	[0.80]	0.00	4.00	56	0.00	0.00	2.45	6.73
Afr	0.49	0.21	0.17	1.43	211	0.45	0.50	1.34	3.01
Populars	4.47	2.04	0.00	11.00	206	5.00	5.00	0.28	0.28
XA%	0.64	0.18	0.12	1.00	211	0.66	0.60	−0.31	−0.32
WDA%	0.68	0.18	0.11	1.00	211	0.71	0.71	−0.44	−0.03
X + %	0.37	0.15	0.00	0.74	210	0.37	0.50	−0.01	−0.47
X – %	0.34	0.18	0.00	0.87	205	0.33	0.07	0.28	−0.39
Xu%	0.26	0.13	0.00	0.59	208	0.26	0.33	0.19	−0.55
Isolate/R	0.17	0.14	0.00	0.66	179	0.14	0.00	1.09	1.19
H	1.97	1.80	0.00	10.00	168	2.00	1.00	1.56	3.56
(H)	0.98	0.99	0.00	4.00	131	1.00	0.00	0.93	0.39
HD	1.47	1.93	0.00	18.00	141	1.00	0.00	3.88	26.15
(Hd)	0.52	0.86	0.00	4.00	70	0.00	0.00	1.78	2.81
Hx	0.33	[0.71]	0.00	3.00	45	0.00	0.00	2.23	4.33
H+(H)+Hd+(Hd)	4.93	3.18	0.00	24.00	208	4.00	3.00	1.97	7.52
A	9.18	4.39	1.00	27.00	211	8.00	8.00	0.98	1.48
(A)	0.46	[0.79]	0.00	5.00	69	0.00	0.00	2.26	6.84

(continued)

413

TABLE 19–2 *(continued)*

VARIABLE	MEAN	SD	MIN	MAX	FREQ	MEDIAN	MODE	SK	KU
Ad	1.45	[1.58]	0.00	10.00	140	1.00	0.00	1.76	5.13
(Ad)	0.12	[0.35]	0.00	2.00	23	0.00	0.00	3.01	9.00
An	0.87	[1.17]	0.00	5.00	103	0.00	0.00	1.50	1.98
Art	0.76	1.45	0.00	14.00	87	0.00	0.00	4.66	34.41
Ay	0.48	[0.86]	0.00	6.00	66	0.00	0.00	2.42	8.63
Bl	0.35	[0.78]	0.00	5.00	46	0.00	0.00	2.89	10.13
Bt	1.11	1.50	0.00	7.00	111	1.00	0.00	1.73	3.05
Cg	1.12	1.37	0.00	8.00	122	1.00	0.00	1.70	3.74
Cl	0.23	[0.58]	0.00	3.00	36	0.00	0.00	2.81	8.28
Ex	0.13	[0.43]	0.00	3.00	22	0.00	0.00	3.72	15.52
Fi	0.34	[0.70]	0.00	4.00	49	0.00	0.00	2.36	5.88
Food	0.37	[0.73]	0.00	4.00	57	0.00	0.00	2.64	8.48
Ge	0.08	[0.31]	0.00	2.00	15	0.00	0.00	4.06	17.39
Hh	0.74	1.35	0.00	12.00	100	0.00	0.00	5.19	37.64
Ls	0.62	0.92	0.00	4.00	83	0.00	0.00	1.49	1.62
Na	0.71	[1.19]	0.00	8.00	83	0.00	0.00	2.54	8.88
Sc	0.82	[1.17]	0.00	6.00	97	0.00	0.00	1.81	3.66
Sx	0.40	[1.15]	0.00	14.00	54	0.00	0.00	8.27	92.81
Xy	0.14	[0.46]	0.00	3.00	23	0.00	0.00	3.88	17.18
Idiographic	1.32	1.68	0.00	12.00	129	1.00	0.00	2.58	10.92
DV	1.40	[1.68]	0.00	8.00	129	1.00	0.00	1.63	2.91
INCOM	1.11	[1.20]	0.00	5.00	132	1.00	0.00	1.17	0.97
DR	1.03	[1.64]	0.00	8.00	90	0.00	0.00	2.11	4.92
FABCOM	0.49	[0.79]	0.00	4.00	74	0.00	0.00	1.88	3.95
DV2	0.22	[0.84]	0.00	7.00	25	0.00	0.00	5.91	41.41
INC2	0.29	[0.73]	0.00	4.00	39	0.00	0.00	2.97	9.28
DR2	0.37	[1.06]	0.00	7.00	34	0.00	0.00	3.74	16.35
FAB2	0.49	[0.99]	0.00	6.00	56	0.00	0.00	2.52	7.35
ALOG	0.12	[0.34]	0.00	2.00	24	0.00	0.00	2.74	6.85
CONTAM	0.02	0.15	0.00	1.00	5	0.00	0.00	6.30	38.15
Sum 6 Sp Sc	5.55	4.35	0.00	24.00	199	5.00	3.00	1.24	1.84
Lvl 2 Sp Sc	1.38	[2.22]	0.00	12.00	97	0.00	0.00	2.20	5.39
WSum6	16.71	15.47	0.00	71.00	199	12.00	0.00	1.29	1.19
AB	0.21	[0.66]	0.00	5.00	27	0.00	0.00	4.21	21.16
AG	0.48	0.82	0.00	5.00	68	0.00	0.00	2.01	4.96
COP	0.96	1.22	0.00	6.00	110	1.00	0.00	1.47	2.26
CP	0.06	[0.34]	0.00	4.00	10	0.00	0.00	8.41	88.31
GOODHR	2.25	1.65	0.00	9.00	183	2.00	1.00	0.80	0.93
POORHR	3.38	2.93	0.00	22.00	188	3.00	3.00	2.16	8.69
MOR	1.25	[1.57]	0.00	8.00	122	1.00	0.00	1.68	3.24
PER	0.92	1.48	0.00	9.00	91	0.00	0.00	2.39	7.90
PSV	0.35	[0.78]	0.00	7.00	53	0.00	0.00	4.23	27.42

TABLE 19–3

Rorschach Data for Inmates in Prison Psychiatric Treatment ($R < 14$)

MARITAL STATUS			AGE			RACE		
Single 23	61%		18–25 5	13%		White 11	29%	
Lives w/S.O. 0	0%		26–35 18	47%		Black 16	42%	
Married 3	8%		36–45 8	21%		Hispanic 10	26%	
Separated 0	0%		46–55 5	13%		Asian 0	0%	
Divorced 5	13%		56–65 2	5%		Other 0	0%	
Widowed 0	0%		Over 65 0	0%		Unlisted xx	xx%	
Unlisted 0	0%							

EDUCATION

SEX

			EDUCATION		
Male 38	100%		Under 12 21	55%	
Female 0	0%		12 Years 10	26%	
			13–15 Yrs 0	0%	
			16+ Yrs 0	0%	

RATIOS, PERCENTAGES AND SPECIAL INDICES

STYLES			FORM QUALITY DEVIATIONS		
Introversive 9	24%		*XA% > .89* 3	8%	
Pervasive Introversive 7	18%		*XA% < .70* 23	61%	
Ambient 16	42%		*WDA% < .85* 33	87%	
Extratensive 0	0%		*WDA% < .75* 25	66%	
Pervasive Extratensive 0	0%		*X + % < .55* 29	76%	
Avoidant 13	34%		*Xu% > .20* 17	45%	
			X – % > .20 31	82%	
D-SCORES			*X – % > .30* 19	50%	
D score > 0 10	26%				
D score = 0 18	47%		*FC:CF + C* RATIO		
D score < 0 10	26%		*FC > (CF + C) + 2* 0	0%	
D score < –1 3	8%		*FC > (CF + C) + 1* 4	11%	
			(CF + C) > FC + 1 10	26%	
Adj D score > 0 11	29%		*(CF + C) > FC + 2* 5	13%	
Adj D score = 0 20	53%				
Adj D score < 0 7	18%				
Adj D score < –1 1	3%				
			S-Constellation Positive ... 2	5%	
Zd > +3.0 (Overincorp) 8	21%		*HVI Positive* 0	0%	
Zd < –3.0 (Underincorp) 6	16%		*OBS Positive* 0	0%	

PTI			DEPI			CDI		
PTI = 5 4	11%		*DEPI* = 7 0	0%		*CDI* = 5 8	21%	
PTI = 4 6	16%		*DEPI* = 6 2	5%		*CDI* = 4 14	37%	
PTI = 3 7	18%		*DEPI* = 5 5	13%				

TABLE 19-3 *(continued)*

MISCELLANEOUS VARIABLES

R < 17 38	100%	(2AB + Art + Ay) > 5 0	0%
R > 27 0	0%	Populars < 4 19	50%
DQv > 2 3	8%	Populars > 7 1	3%
S > 2 4	11%	COP = 0 18	47%
Sum T = 0 33	87%	COP > 2 2	5%
Sum T > 1 0	0%	AG = 0 29	76%
3r + (2)/R < .33 13	34%	AG > 2 1	3%
3r + (2)/R > .44 21	55%	MOR > 2 7	18%
Fr + rF > 0 9	24%	Level 2 Sp Sc > 0 17	45%
Pure C > 0 9	24%	GHR > PHR 15	39%
Pure C > 1 2	5%	Pure H < 2 18	47%
Afr < .40 25	66%	Pure H = 0 6	16%
Afr < .50 32	84%	p > a + 1 7	18%
(FM + m) < Sum Shading 7	18%	Mp > Ma 12	32%

VARIABLE	MEAN	SD	MIN	MAX	FREQ	MEDIAN	MODE	SK	KU
AGE	36.05	9.97	21.00	60.00	38	34.00	31.00	0.84	0.20
R	12.18	0.98	10.00	13.00	38	13.00	13.00	−0.75	−0.80
W	7.13	2.85	1.00	13.00	38	7.00	10.00	−0.27	−0.33
D	3.82	3.05	0.00	10.00	32	3.00	0.00	0.55	−0.59
Dd	1.24	[1.19]	0.00	4.00	26	1.00	1.00	0.91	0.24
S	0.79	[0.96]	0.00	3.00	20	1.00	0.00	1.21	0.69
DQ+	4.45	2.65	0.00	10.00	36	5.00	5.00	0.10	−0.78
DQo	6.97	2.73	2.00	13.00	38	7.00	5.00	0.41	−0.35
DQv	0.74	[1.13]	0.00	5.00	16	0.00	0.00	1.97	4.49
DQv/+	0.03	[0.16]	0.00	1.00	1	0.00	0.00	6.16	38.00
FQx+	0.00	0.00	0.00	0.00	0	0.00	0.00	—	—
FQxo	5.21	2.24	1.00	10.00	38	5.00	7.00	−0.23	−0.60
FQxu	2.45	1.27	0.00	5.00	37	2.00	2.00	0.25	−0.77
FQx−	4.18	2.15	1.00	10.00	38	3.50	3.00	0.75	0.29
FQxNone	0.34	[0.74]	0.00	3.00	8	0.00	0.00	2.23	4.34
MQ+	0.00	0.00	0.00	0.00	0	0.00	0.00	—	—
MQo	1.08	0.82	0.00	3.00	29	1.00	1.00	0.47	−0.05
MQu	0.61	0.82	0.00	3.00	16	0.00	0.00	1.17	0.55
MQ−	1.10	[1.62]	0.00	7.00	17	0.00	0.00	1.81	3.76
MQNone	0.00	[0.00]	0.00	0.00	0	0.00	0.00	—	—
SQual−	0.32	[0.70]	0.00	3.00	8	0.00	0.00	2.44	5.85
M	2.79	2.09	0.00	9.00	35	2.50	1.00	0.79	0.41
FM	1.95	1.63	0.00	6.00	32	1.00	1.00	0.92	0.31
m	1.00	1.38	0.00	5.00	18	0.00	0.00	1.51	1.94
FC	0.58	0.83	0.00	3.00	15	0.00	0.00	1.25	0.67
CF	1.05	1.18	0.00	4.00	22	1.00	0.00	1.02	0.27

(continued)

VARIABLE	MEAN	SD	MIN	MAX	FREQ	MEDIAN	MODE	SK	KU
C	0.29	[0.57]	0.00	2.00	9	0.00	0.00	1.86	2.70
Cn	0.00	[0.00]	0.00	0.00	0	0.00	0.00	—	—
Sum Color	1.92	1.51	0.00	5.00	30	2.00	1.00	0.38	−0.86
WSumC	1.78	1.42	0.00	5.00	30	1.50	0.00	0.56	−0.43
Sum C'	1.13	[1.86]	0.00	7.00	16	0.00	0.00	1.83	2.59
Sum T	0.13	[0.34]	0.00	1.00	5	0.00	0.00	2.27	3.33
Sum V	0.03	[0.16]	0.00	1.00	1	0.00	0.00	6.16	38.00
Sum Y	0.32	[0.74]	0.00	3.00	7	0.00	0.00	2.37	4.95
Sum Shading	1.60	2.41	0.00	9.00	20	1.00	0.00	1.81	2.55
Fr + rF	0.42	[0.86]	0.00	3.00	9	0.00	0.00	2.01	3.09
FD	0.37	[0.68]	0.00	3.00	11	0.00	0.00	2.18	5.48
F	5.24	2.68	1.00	11.00	38	5.00	4.00	0.25	−0.55
(2)	4.21	1.99	0.00	8.00	37	4.50	6.00	−0.11	−0.72
3r + (2)/R	0.45	0.25	0.00	1.09	37	0.46	0.46	0.59	0.16
Lambda	1.05	1.09	0.08	5.50	38	0.83	0.83	2.35	6.82
FM + m	2.95	2.22	0.00	9.00	35	3.00	1.00	0.96	0.57
EA	4.57	3.00	1.00	12.00	38	3.75	1.00	0.83	−0.09
es	4.55	3.52	0.00	13.00	36	4.00	4.00	0.94	0.18
D Score	−0.05	1.04	−3.00	2.00	20	0.00	0.00	−0.50	0.98
AdjD	0.18	1.06	−3.00	3.00	18	0.00	0.00	0.04	2.07
a (active)	3.68	2.03	0.00	9.00	35	3.50	2.00	0.23	−0.03
p (passive)	2.16	1.97	0.00	8.00	29	2.00	2.00	1.09	1.23
Ma	1.60	1.24	0.00	4.00	30	1.00	1.00	0.37	−0.85
Mp	1.29	1.63	0.00	7.00	22	1.00	0.00	1.65	3.09
Intellect	1.21	1.45	0.00	5.00	21	1.00	0.00	1.16	0.66
Zf	8.40	2.88	2.00	13.00	38	9.00	9.00	−0.64	0.07
Zd	0.54	3.61	−7.50	9.00	38	0.50	0.50	0.03	0.24
Blends	2.37	2.50	0.00	8.00	28	1.00	0.00	0.95	−0.45
Blends/R	0.20	0.21	0.00	0.70	28	0.09	0.00	1.03	−0.14
Col-Shd Blends	0.26	[0.45]	0.00	1.00	10	0.00	0.00	1.12	−0.79
Afr	0.40	0.14	0.22	0.86	38	0.38	0.30	1.72	2.88
Populars	3.53	1.78	0.00	8.00	37	3.50	4.00	0.43	0.29
XA%	0.63	0.20	0.18	0.92	38	0.68	0.77	−0.60	−0.41
WDA%	0.64	0.19	0.20	0.91	38	0.70	0.73	−0.60	−0.50
X + %	0.43	0.17	0.08	0.77	38	0.46	0.54	−0.41	−0.51
X − %	0.35	0.19	0.08	0.82	38	0.29	0.23	0.78	0.03
Xu%	0.20	0.10	0.00	0.40	37	0.18	0.15	0.23	−0.90
Isolate/R	0.23	0.21	0.00	0.82	29	0.17	0.00	1.03	0.91
H	1.97	1.67	0.00	8.00	32	2.00	1.00	1.40	3.22
(H)	0.76	0.97	0.00	4.00	19	0.50	0.00	1.44	2.22
HD	0.55	0.86	0.00	4.00	15	0.00	0.00	2.11	5.84
(Hd)	0.32	0.47	0.00	1.00	12	0.00	0.00	0.82	−1.40
Hx	0.18	[0.46]	0.00	2.00	6	0.00	0.00	2.54	6.35
H+(H)+Hd+(Hd)	3.61	2.15	0.00	8.00	37	4.00	4.00	0.49	−0.46
A	5.60	2.56	1.00	13.00	38	5.00	4.00	1.00	0.81

TABLE 19–3   *(continued)*

VARIABLE	MEAN	SD	MIN	MAX	FREQ	MEDIAN	MODE	SK	KU
(A)	0.24	[0.49]	0.00	2.00	8	0.00	0.00	1.99	3.45
Ad	0.76	[0.88]	0.00	4.00	22	1.00	1.00	1.73	4.31
(Ad)	0.05	[0.32]	0.00	2.00	1	0.00	0.00	6.16	38.00
An	0.47	[0.69]	0.00	2.00	14	0.00	0.00	1.15	0.12
Art	0.63	0.97	0.00	3.00	14	0.00	0.00	1.38	0.77
Ay	0.32	[0.57]	0.00	2.00	10	0.00	0.00	1.69	2.03
Bl	0.53	[0.89]	0.00	3.00	13	0.00	0.00	1.84	2.72
Bt	0.45	1.00	0.00	5.00	10	0.00	0.00	3.18	11.67
Cg	0.95	1.25	0.00	6.00	21	1.00	0.00	2.11	6.13
Cl	0.16	[0.37]	0.00	1.00	6	0.00	0.00	1.95	1.92
Ex	0.08	[0.27]	0.00	1.00	3	0.00	0.00	3.25	9.06
Fi	0.21	[0.47]	0.00	2.00	7	0.00	0.00	2.24	4.70
Food	0.42	[1.06]	0.00	4.00	7	0.00	0.00	2.69	6.45
Ge	0.03	[0.16]	0.00	1.00	1	0.00	0.00	6.16	38.00
Hh	0.45	0.65	0.00	2.00	14	0.00	0.00	1.16	0.31
Ls	0.50	0.86	0.00	3.00	12	0.00	0.00	1.73	2.23
Na	0.74	[1.13]	0.00	4.00	17	0.00	0.00	1.97	3.56
Sc	0.45	[0.69]	0.00	2.00	13	0.00	0.00	1.26	0.35
Sx	0.24	[0.49]	0.00	2.00	8	0.00	0.00	1.99	3.45
Xy	0.08	[0.36]	0.00	2.00	2	0.00	0.00	4.85	24.25
Idiographic	1.29	1.29	0.00	5.00	27	1.00	1.00	1.40	2.14
DV	1.08	[1.40]	0.00	6.00	21	1.00	0.00	1.71	3.20
INCOM	0.97	[1.28]	0.00	6.00	23	1.00	1.00	2.23	5.94
DR	0.92	[1.94]	0.00	10.00	14	0.00	0.00	3.44	13.70
FABCOM	0.42	[0.83]	0.00	4.00	11	0.00	0.00	2.69	8.90
DV2	0.18	[0.46]	0.00	2.00	6	0.00	0.00	2.54	6.35
INC2	0.40	[1.10]	0.00	5.00	6	0.00	0.00	3.20	10.30
DR2	0.55	[1.22]	0.00	4.00	8	0.00	0.00	2.16	3.42
FAB2	0.45	[0.76]	0.00	3.00	12	0.00	0.00	1.74	2.61
ALOG	0.13	[0.41]	0.00	2.00	4	0.00	0.00	3.38	11.78
CONTAM	0.00	0.00	0.00	0.00	0	0.00	0.00	—	—
Sum 6 Sp Sc	5.10	4.88	0.00	20.00	33	4.00	3.00	1.39	1.84
Lvl 2 Sp Sc	1.58	[2.30]	0.00	7.00	17	0.00	0.00	1.35	0.62
WSum6	16.53	17.22	0.00	62.00	33	10.50	0.00	1.23	0.58
AB	0.13	[0.48]	0.00	2.00	3	0.00	0.00	3.63	12.35
AG	0.37	0.75	0.00	3.00	9	0.00	0.00	2.09	3.81
COP	0.82	1.11	0.00	5.00	20	1.00	0.00	2.12	5.60
CP	0.03	[0.16]	0.00	1.00	1	0.00	0.00	6.16	38.00
GOODHR	1.82	1.20	0.00	4.00	33	2.00	1.00	0.27	−0.78
POORHR	2.10	1.94	0.00	7.00	28	2.00	0.00	0.75	−0.17
MOR	1.13	[1.45]	0.00	5.00	19	0.50	0.00	1.14	0.27
PER	0.79	1.28	0.00	4.00	14	0.00	0.00	1.56	1.31
PSV	0.13	[0.41]	0.00	2.00	4	0.00	0.00	3.38	11.78

This multimethod description produced a picture of an exceptionally compromised group of men. Intellectual functioning was quite negatively skewed, with almost three quarters (73%) demonstrating intellectual functioning below the Average range.

Neuropsychological functioning was also negatively skewed, with 81% of inmates demonstrating overall impairment indicative of diffuse brain dysfunction. Seventy percent had impaired executive function. Executive function is an umbrella construct that describes the ability for guiding and managing cognitive, emotional, and behavioral functions. It is associated with brain impairment predominantly in the frontal cortex and is responsible for thinking, reasoning, problem solving, planning ahead, anticipating consequences of actions, and changing actions based on information that is obtained from the environment. Although there are multiple reasons for brain dysfunction in these psychiatrically hospitalized inmates, some contributing reasons are likely their histories of drug abuse, neurological injuries, and experiences of severe psychiatric disorder.

Drug abuse was pervasive (88%) and predominantly characterized by poly-substance abuse (76%). Alcohol and/or marijuana were most frequently used first and most, but drugs other than alcohol and/or marijuana were the drugs of choice. Neurological injury also was predominant with 63% of inmates experiencing a significant neurological injury and/or disorder. Fifty-nine percent of inmates experienced severe psychiatric disorders with known associations with brain impairment and 5% experienced frank dementia. Although all inmates were receiving psychiatric treatment while in prison, approximately one third (36%) were not diagnosed with an Axis I Clinical Disorder, but were primarily diagnosed with an Axis II Personality Disorder. Twenty-six percent were severely Psychopathic (PCL–R Total Score $\geq$ 30).

As is often the case in psychiatric treatment programs, almost 19% of inmates in this research provided Rorschach protocols with a low number of responses ($R < 14$). Although psychologists are advised to consider low response Rorschach records with extreme caution as being of questionable usefulness and likely to produce misleading results (Exner, 1991, pp. 119, 122), a response style suggestive of withdrawal from the assessment process did not differentially characterize the inmates who gave shorter records. This finding suggests that, at least for this group of psychiatrically hospitalized inmates, Rorschach records with $R < 14$ can be useful for clinical interpretation, a finding also suggested by Gacono and Gacono (chap. 20, this vol.). It is also noteworthy that inmates with low response Rorschach records were significantly more likely to demonstrate low intellectual functioning ($p = .001$) and impaired executive functioning ($p = .01$).

ACKNOWLEDGMENT

Information presented and/or opinions expressed in this chapter reflect the opinions of the authors only and do not reflect the opinions of any state agency.

REFERENCES

Cohen, J. (1960). A coefficient of agreement for nominal scales. *Educational and Psychological Measurement, 20*, 37–47.

Exner, J. E. (1991). *The Rorschach: A comprehensive system interpretation* (2nd ed.). New York: Wiley.

Exner, J. E. (2001). *A Rorschach workbook for the comprehensive system* (5th ed). Asheville, NC: Rorschach Workshops.

Hare, R. (2001). *Hare Psychopathy Checklist–Revised technical manual*. New York: Multi-Health Systems.

Hare, R. (2003). *Hare Psychopathy Checklist–Revised technical manual* (2nd ed.). New York: Multi-Health Systems.

Heaton, R., Grant, I., & Matthews, C. (1991). *Comprehensive norms for an expanded Halstead–Reitan battery: Demographic corrections, research findings, and clinical applications*. Odessa, FL: Psychological Assessment Resources.

Landis, J. R., & Koch, G. G. (1977). The measurement o observer agreement for categorical data. *Biometrics, 33*, 159–174.

Manderscheid, R., Gravesande, A., & Goldsrom, I. (2004). *Growth of mental health services in state adult correctional facilities 1988 to 2000*. Retrieved May 31, 2006, from http://www.namiscc.org

Reitan, R., & Wolfson, D. (1985). *The Halstead–Reitan neuropsychological test battery: Theory and clinical interpretation*. Tucson, AZ: Neuropsychology Press.

Spitzer, R., Williams, J., Gibbon, M., & First, M. (1990). *Structured clinical interview for* DSM–III–R *patient edition*. Washington, DC: American Psychiatric Press.

U.S. Department of Justice. (2001). *Provision of mental health care in prisons* (Publication No. J1C0–110). Washington, DC: Author.

U.S. Department of Justice. (2002). *Mental health treatment in state prisons, 2000* (Publication No. NCJ188215). Washington, DC: Author.

20

SOME CONSIDERATIONS FOR THE RORSCHACH ASSESSMENT OF FORENSIC PSYCHIATRIC OUTPATIENTS

Lynne A. Gacono
Austin State Hospital, Austin, TX

Carl B. Gacono
Private Practice, Austin, TX

The manner in which mental illness and the forensic setting impact psychological test findings is unique in forensic psychiatric outpatients (Bannatyne, 1996). Both are influential in shaping the patient's approach to the evaluation process (response style). In fact, after addressing the issue of malingering, the forensic examiner's understanding of response style is the first step in interpreting assessment findings (Melton, Petrila, Poythress, & Solbogin, 1998). Constricted protocols should never be immediately attributed to "resistance." Elevated validity indices should not be routinely disregarded as invalid. Irregularities in the testing data may be accurate measurements of personality functioning of these patients (Bannatyne, Gacono, & Greene, 1999).

Consequently, before dismissing data, the examiner must first determine if irregularities in the findings are an accurate reflection of the patient's psychopathology. This often involves assessing the extent to which guardedness, defensiveness, and/or denial contribute to a constricted protocol (Bannatyne, 1996). Other factors such as social desirability (Bagby, Rogers, & Buis, 1994; Grossman & Wasyliw, 1988; Roman, Tuley, Villanueva, & Mitchell, 1990; Wasyliw, Grossman, Haywood, & Cavanaugh, 1988), the use of primitive defensives (Coyle & Heap, 1965; Fjordbak, 1985; Gacono & Meloy, 1994; Weiner, 1966), illness chronicity (stabilization on psychotropic medications), cognitive and emotional impoverishment, and/or concurrent character pathology (Bannatyne, 1996; Bannatyne et al., 1999; Gacono & Meloy, 1994) influence the response style of these patients. Determining the extent to which these factors are operating in an individual evaluation helps the examiner to more fully understand the patient while also allowing for a determination regarding the validity of the assessment findings. Assessment protocols that initially appear invalid frequently turn out to be accurate portrayals of the patient's psychology (Bannatyne et al., 1999).

Although response style is best assessed across multiple methods, in this chapter we focus primarily on the Rorschach. We begin with a discussion of the forensic outpatient groups we studied and their associated response style. An understanding of the response style provides a template for interpreting the Comprehensive System data that is presented. The reader may find the comparative data discussed in the latter part of this chapter for Paranoid Schizophrenic ($N = 90$), Undifferentiated/Disorganized Schizophrenic ($N = 38$), Schizoaffective ($N = 59$), and Bipolar ($N = 40$) useful in their evaluation of similar patients.

FORENSIC PSYCHIATRIC OUTPATIENTS (FPOs)

All of our participants were patients in the California Conditional Release Program (CONREP). CONREP is the California Department of Mental Health's statewide system of community-based services for specified forensic patients. Participants attend mental health treatment as a condition of community parole (Meloy, Haroun, & Schiller, 1990). The goal of CONREP is to ensure greater public protection and safety via an effective outpatient treatment system, which allows for greater supervision and support (California Forensic Services, 2001).

Thorough assessment and screening ensures treatment matching and increases the likelihood that patients will benefit from the program. *Successful patients* are those who are compliant with and benefit from outpatient mental health parole. Whereas these patients may overlap somewhat with the inpatient forensic patients discussed in chapter 19, they are less likely to include large numbers of mentally ill offenders with concurrent psychopathy.

ASSESSMENT METHODS

In addition to screening procedures, the MMPI–2 and Rorschach are routinely administered to every CONREP patient that is in the program for a time less than or equal to 18 months. MMPI–2s are administered in the presence of a licensed psychologist and scored using the NCS computerized scoring system. MMPI–2s whose *TRIN*, *VRIN*, or *L* scale was greater than or equal to 91 (Roger Greene, personal communication, 1995) were excluded from our samples.

Rorschach tests were administered and scored by licensed psychologists well versed in the Rorschach Comprehensive System guidelines (Exner, 1991). Each Rorschach protocol has been scored for Comprehensive System variables a minimum of four times by one of several researchers, including being rescored independently by a licensed psychologist. A minimum of 80% agreement for all Rorschach variables is assured for all protocols (Exner et al., 1995a; Weiner, 1991, 1995). Any and all discrepancies between the scorers were resolved by an independent scorer. In all cases, the interjudge reliability (percentage of agreement and kappa coefficients) of Rorschach scoring was satisfactory (see Gacono, Meloy, & Bridges, 2000). Protocols with fewer than 14 responses were excluded from all our samples (Exner, 1995b).

FPOs for whom a valid Rorschach were available, who met the *DSM–IV* (APA, 1994) criteria for Paranoid Schizophrenia, Undifferentiated/Disorganized Schizophrenia,

Schizoaffective Disorder, and Bipolar I Disorder, and were prescribed neuroleptic medications were included (N = 227). Psychiatric diagnoses were determined by consensus between several evaluators (licensed psychologists and psychiatrists). Charts were examined by the senior author to confirm and record demographics, history of the diagnosis, and Rorschach data. High levels of agreement (> 90%) were obtained between consensus derived primary diagnoses and subsequent record review. Reliable Axis II diagnoses were unavailable for the majority of the CONREP patients (Bannatyne et al., 1999; Nieberding et al., 2003).

RESPONSE STYLE IN FORENSIC PYSCHIATRIC OUTPATIENTS

In considering the impact of response style on FPOs, Bannatyne et al., (1999) studied a group of CONREP patients (N = 180) that included Paranoid Schizophrenics (N = 89), Schizoaffective Disorders (N = 53), and Undifferentiated/Disorganized Schizophrenics (N = 38). These patients had been found to be not guilty by reason of insanity (85%), incompetent to stand trial, or a mentally disordered offender. Fifty-six percent of the sample were Caucasian, 36% African American, 5% Hispanic, 2% Asian, and .05% Native American. The majority were male (87%), with a mean age at testing of 48 years. All patients were in outpatient treatment and on neuroleptic medication at the time of psychological testing.

Response Style

FPOs tended to answer the MMPI–2 in an unsophisticated and naive manner (L scale, M = 59.61). Interpreting ego-strength as adequate (K scale = M = 53.79) would be inconsistent with the documented histories of these patients. Rather, what is suggested is that these patients see themselves as having adequate ego strength. *Response frequency* (Rf) and *Lambda* for this forensic psychiatric sample (Rf = M = 21.03, SD = 6.37; $Lambda$ = M = 1.40, SD = 2.16) were similar to Exner's (1995b) inpatient Schizophrenic sample (Rf = M = 23.44, SD = 8.66; $Lambda$ = M = 1.57, SD = 3.47).

When the groups were divided by high L, there was also a significant but small positive correlational relationship (r = .18, p = .02) between L and $F\%$. When R and $F\%$ were used as the independent variables and L was the dependent variable, significant mean differences occurred for $F\%$; L increased when $F\%$ increased; however, L and R did not exhibit a similar relationship.

These findings suggest that when examining FPOs, the forensic examiner should always determine if rather than measuring defensiveness or denial, the presence of high L and $F\%$ are accurately reflecting a simplistic problem-solving style, reduced engagement in the testing process, lack of cognitive and emotional complexity, and a lack of attending to the self (Bannatynne et al., 1999).

Reporting of Psychotic Symptomatology

The overuse of *Pure Form* ($F\%$) by FPOs raises concerns about the usefulness of Rorschach structural variables for identifying psychosis and magnifies the problems with using sign approaches when interpreting the Rorschach. This is particularly true for FPOs with MMPI–2s that include elevated L scales. Although these patients endorsed moderate levels of unusual and bizarre symptomatology ($Sc8 = M = 64.39$), they did not acknowledge outright psychotic symptomatology ($BIZ = M = 56.61$). Patients with high L did not evidence as much psychotic symptomatology (BIZ, $Sc8$, F, $SCZI$) as those patients with lower L scores . High L patients produced Rorschachs with high $F\%$, and reported less psychotic symptomatology on both scales (BIZ, $Sc8$) than did the low L patients. As L elevated, K elevated, and F, $F - K$, $8(Sc)$, and BIZ decreased.

Regarding psychotic symptomatology on the Rorschach, no significant differences were found between high and low L scorers and the $SCZI$. This may be a result of the overall low mean $SCZI$ score ($M = 2.47$) for the FPOs (note that 82% of Exner's, 1995b, sample was positive on $SCZI \geq 4$). For the whole sample, a small, but significant positive correlation was found between BIZ and $SCZI$ ($r = .19$, $p = .01$). $SCZI \geq 4$ identified psychosis in less than 36% of each FPO sample compared to Exner et al's. (1995b) 82% for inpatient Schizophrenics.

Although this study was done prior to the PTI, this poor showing, although perhaps not unexpected, warrants an explanation. Exner (1991) stated that "pharmacological intervention, especially when the subject has been stabilized reasonably well on the medication, has relatively little impact on most Rorschach variables" (p. 121), and "that the Schizophrenic organization does not alter substantially, especially during brief intervals, even though intervention by pharmacological and other therapeutic tactics aids the newly hospitalized subject to reenter his her social environment" (Exner, 1986, p. 461). Our findings, however, suggested the need for re-evaluating this hypothesis and re-exploring older ones concerning psychometric differences between acute versus chronic psychosis (Weiner, 1966), and the need for considering the impact of the presence or absence of neuroleptic medication on responding. The $SCZI$ may not have been the best Rorschach index of psychosis, particularly for chronic FPOs. The PTI may prove otherwise.

Differences between the MMPI–2 and Rorschach in identifying psychotic symptomatology may in part be explained by more filtering on the MMPI–2. The Rorschach reality testing index ($X-\% \geq .20$) was elevated for the majority of patients, but the MMPI–2 psychosis scales were not. The MMPI–2 was, however, more accurate in identifying psychotic symptomatology for those patients producing lower L scores in that they produced significantly higher BIZ, F and $Sc8$. Although volition may contribute to the total number of Rorschach responses produced, it is less likely to contribute to Rorschach perceptual accuracy and reality testing measures.

Diagnosis and Response Style

Schizoaffective patients were less constricted and scored significantly lower than the Undifferentiated/ Disorganized Schizophrenic patients on L ($M = 57$ vs. $M = 65$) and $F\%$ ($M = .41$ vs $.51$). Paranoid Schizophrenics fell between the other groups ($L = M = 59$, $F\% = M = .48$). The three groups did not differ on R. The Undifferentiated/Disorganized and Paranoid Schizophrenic groups each differed significantly from the Schizoaffective group on $F\%$ with the latter having a lower mean $F\%$. Patients with a concomitant mood disorder

(Schizoaffective) were not as constricted as Schizophrenics without a mood disorder (Undifferentiated/Disorganized and Paranoid) and were more likely to elevate on the *DEPI* (Table 20–1).

Consistent with diagnostic criteria, Undifferentiated/Disorganized Schizophrenics were particularly dysfunctional in terms of impaired perceptual accuracy, reality testing problems, cognitive slippage, and elevations on both *SCZI* and *CDI* when compared to other groups. Because chronic, psychotic forensic patients, as a group, tend to be inadequate and unsophisticated, with less than normal psychological resources (elevated *CDI*s, low *EA*; Gacono & Meloy, 1994), *K* scale scores of these patients were not significantly elevated, despite the constriction across testing instruments. Actually, the *L* scale scores were more useful for examining response style.

If *Lambda* and *F%* measure cognitive and emotional complexity, then it follows that Schizophrenics with a concomitant mood disorder would be more emotionally complicated than Schizophrenics without mood problems (e.g., *PureC* ≥ 1 = Schizoaffective = 52%, Undifferentiated/Disorganized = 15%, Paranoid = 25%) and have less *Pure Form* in their Rorschach protocols. Testing constriction in the Undifferentiated/Disorganized

TABLE 20–1

Comparison of MMPI-2 and Rorschach Variables for Psychotic Subgroups

Variables	Undifferentiated (N = 38)			Schizoaffective (N = 53)			Paranoid (N = 89)			Inpatient Schizophrenics (N = 320)		
	Mean	*SD*	*Freq.*	*Mean*	*SD*	*Freq.*	*Mean*	*SD*	*Freq.*	*Mean*	*SD*	*Freq.*
MMPI-2												
L Scale	65a	13	100%	57b	12	100%	59b	11	100%	—	—	—
RORSCHACH												
Cognitive & Perceptual												
X–% ≥ 20	—	—	78%	—	—	70%	—	—	69%	—	—	90%
X–% ≥ 30	—	—	45%	—	—	37%	—	—	39%	—	—	69%
X+% ≤ 50	—	—	67%	—	—	60%	—	—	57%	—	—	73%
F+% ≥ 50	—	—	58%	—	—	49%	—	—	47%	—	—	—
F%	51a	.21	—	.41b	.17	—	.48a	.19	—	—	—	—
WSum6 ≥ 20	—	—	15%	—	—	33%	—	—	17%	—	—	—
WSum6 ≤ 10	—	—	60%	—	—	54%	—	—	56%	—	—	—
Constellations												
+SCZI ≥ 4	...	...	36%	...	...	21%	—	—	26%	—	—	82%
+DEPI ≥ 5	—	—	21%	—	—	40%	—	—	30%	—	—	29%
+CDI ≥ 4	—	—	52%	—	—	32%	—	—	32%	—	—	25%
+Suicide ≥ 8	...	—	0%	—	—	11%	—	—	3%	—	—	6%
+HVI	—	—	18%	—	—	19%	—	—	7%	—	—	18%

Note.   Means and standard deviations were rounded to whole numbers. Means with subscripts were statistically significant (*p* < .05). Inpatient schizophrenic data are from Exner et al. (1995b).

group likely resulted from the high levels of general cognitive and emotional impoverishment observed in these patients (high $F\%$ and L), whereas elevated scores in Paranoid Schizophrenics might have occurred due to affective avoidance ($Afr < .50 = 60\%$), impaired tolerance for emotions, and a need to be in control. In adjudicated forensic Schizophrenic populations, high L and $F\%$ may be measuring a defensive response style; however, it is just as likely an accurate depiction of a defended, unsophisticated, uninsightful, emotionally and cognitively impoverished person who lacks the cognitive and emotional resources to contend with the self and the world effectively, and perhaps also needs to see themselves in a virtuous, ideal, and emotionally healthy light or both (MMPI–2 L scale $T \geq 65$), an apt depiction of the Undifferentiated/Disorganized Schizophrenic forensic patient (Bannatyne, et al., 1999).

Although many psychotic forensic patients may intentionally underreport their psychopathology on the MMPI–2, Schizophrenic offenders with *lower L* scores as well as Schizoaffective patients appeared to more accurately report their psychopathology. Although unlikely, another explanation for self-reporting psychopathology may be that these patients wanted to appear mentally ill. For this sample of CONREP patients, this latter hypothesis would mean that patients wanted to stay in the program for secondary gain or unconscious fear of being without the program's support. Clinical experience suggests that this usually was not the case. Significantly lower scores on L and $F\%$ for the Schizoaffective patients, might relate to better treatment prognosis for those patients and patients with nondefensive (lower L and reasonable $F\%$) MMPI–2 and Rorschach protocols. Their *openness* to the task and their own affect, however, may or may not correlate with specific treatment interventions.

COMPREHENSIVE SYSTEM RORSCHACH DATA FOR FPOS

In order to compile Comprehensive System data for the FPOs, we increased the sample sizes of the individual groups and added a fourth, Bipolar I Disorder FPOs. The FPOs we discuss include: Paranoid Schizophrenic ($N = 90$), Undifferentiated/Disorganized Schizophrenic ($N = 38$), Schizoaffective ($N = 59$), and Bipolar ($N = 40$) patients. These samples were analyzed in 2002 by Exner's Rorschach Workshops using RIAP 4. Understanding the Rorschach data (core characteristics, controls, stress tolerance, affect, self-perception, thinking and processing, and interpersonal) from the FPOs adds to our understanding of the personality functioning of these patients. The following sections compare the FPO groups to the appropriate Exner (1995b, 2001) Comprehensive System sample. We present our findings as group trends, and they are by no means definitive or adequate for capturing the many individual differences that manifest when assessing individual patients.

Forensic Paranoid Schizophrenic Outpatients (PS; $N = 90$): Core Characteristics, Controls, and Stress Tolerance

Although they produced a normative number of responses ($R = M = 21.67$) our Paranoid Schizophrenics (PS) were cognitively constricted (*Lambda* $= M = 1.22$). Consistent with a paranoid style, they were mostly *Avoidant* (38%) and *Introversive* (24%), rather than *Extratensive* (10%). Like other patient groups, a significant proportion of the PS were *Ambitent* (28%).

PS were socially inept (*CDI* ≥ 4 = 34%). When compared to the Exner (1995b) inpatient Schizophrenic sample (*N* = 320; *EA* = *M* = 8.63), the PS group evidenced fewer psychological resources (*EA* = *M* = 6.54), as well as weaker controls (PS = *D* score <0 = 39%, *AdjD* < 0 = 30%; Exner, 1995b; *D* score <0 = 22%, *AdjD* <0 = 11%). (See Table 20–5.)

Affect. PS were emotionally constricted *(WSumC =, M* = 2.88), compared to nonpatient adults (*WsumC =, M* = 4.36; Exner, 2001). They had more difficulty modulating emotions (PS = *Pure C* > 1 = 12%, *[CF + C]* > *FC* + *1* = 43%) than inpatient Schizophrenics (*Pure C* > 1 = 7%, *[CF + C]* > *FC* + *1* = 25%; Exner, 1995b), and consequently, they tended to avoid emotional engagement (PS = *Afr* < .50 = 54%). When compared to Exner's (1995b) inpatient Schizophrenics, the PS experienced similar levels of dysphoric affect (PS = *Sum Shading M* = 4.28; Exner group *M* = 4.68) and painful rumination (PS = *Sum V* = *M* = 1.00; Exner group, *Sum V* = *M* = .60). The PS, however, were more likely to elevate on *DEPI* (PS, *DEPI* ≥ 5 = 39%; Exner, *DEPI* ≥ 5 = 19%). However, anxiety (PS, *Sum Y* = *M* = .87) was less likely to be contributing to their depression than expected in inpatient Schizophrenics (*Sum Y* = *M* = 2.12; Exner, 1995b).

Like inpatient Schizophrenics (*S* = *M* = . 2.77 & *S* > 2 = 43%; Exner, 1995), PS patients are prone to anger and resentment (*S* = *M* = 2.27 & *S* > 2 = 34%). However, like other forensic groups (Gacono & Meloy, 1994), their aggression may be more egosyntonic (PS, *AG* = 0 = 64% & *AG* > 2 = 4%). Aggression toward others is expected rather than aggression toward self (*SCON* + = 0%). These Rorschach findings are consistent with an alloplastic style where acting out is used to avoid and discharge anxiety and aggression.

Self-Perception. PS patients produce reflections (*Fr* + *rF* > 0 = 13%) and *Egocentricity Index* (> .44 = 41%; < .33 = 32%) at a similar rate to inpatient Schizophrenics (*Fr* + *rF* > 0 = 13%; 35% & 36%; Exner, 1995b), but exceed findings for nonpatient adults (*Fr* + *rF* > 0 = 8%; 13% & 23%; Exner, 2001). They experience a sense of being damaged (*MOR* = *M* = 1.34, *MOR* > 2 = 17%), and evidence a preoccupation with somatic features of self image (*An* + *Xy* = 1.10). These patients demonstrate impairment in their ability to introspect (*FD* = *M* = .27) when compared to inpatient Schizophrenics (*FD* = *M* = .60; Exner, 1995b). They are also prone to painful rumination (*Sum V/M* = 1.0; nonpatients, *Sum V* = *M* = .28; Exner, 2001). It does not come as a surprise that PS patients are considered to have serious adjustment problems (*Pure H* < 2 = 29%).

Information Processing. PS patients evidenced normative processing effort and organizational activity (*Zf* = *M* = 11.93; Exner's, 2001; Nonpatients = 11.84). However, their efficiency is marred by the tendency to miss important information (*Zd* = *M* = –1.62, Exner's, 2001; Nonpatients = .57). The impact of their psychosis likely reversed the expected ratio of *Underincorporators* (36%) to *Overincorporators* (13%) in these paranoid individuals. PS patients process information in a vague and associational manner, and their thinking is fluid and poorly bounded (*DQv* = *M* = 2.19). They may also have more

TABLE 20–2

Paranoid Schizophrenic Patient ($N = 90$) Group Mean and Frequencies for Select Ratios, Percentages, and Derivations

$R = 21.67$ ($SD = 6.31$)	$L = 1.22$ ($SD = 1.37$)

EB: 3.67:2.88	$EA = 6.54$ ($SD = 3.62$)	
$eb = 4.30$:4.28	$es = 8.58$ ($SD = 5.47$) ($FM + m < Sum\ Shading$......... 35, 39%)	
D Score $= -0.62$ ($SD = 1.59$)	$AdjD = -0.31$ ($SD = 1.35$)	
EB style		
Introversive........................ 22		24%
Pervasive Introversive........14		16%
Ambitent............................. 25		28%
Extratensive........................ 9		10%
Pervasive Extratensive........ 5		6%
Avoidant............................. 34		38%
EA–es differences:D scores		
D score > 0........................ 12		13%
D score $= 0$........................ 43		48%
D score < 0........................ 35		39%
D score < -1....................... 19		21%
AdjD score > 0.................... 15		17%
AdjD score $= 0$.................... 48		53%
AdjD score < 0.................... 27		30%
AdjD score < -1................. 14		16%
Affect		
FC:CF + C = .86 : 2.20		
Pure C = .50 (*SD*. = [1.04])	(*Pure C* $> 0 = 26$; 29%; *Pure C* $> 1 = 11$; 12%)	
FC > (CF + C) + 2.............. 2	2%	
FC > (CF + C) + 1.............. 5	6%	
(CF + C) > FC + 1............ 39	43%	
(CF + C) > FC + 2............ 25	28%	
SumC' = 1.83 (*SD* = 2.49)		
SumT = .58 (*SD* = .90)		
SumV = 1.00 (*SD* = 1.24)		
SumY = .87 (*SD* = 1.14)		
Afr = .52 (*SD* = .19)	(*Afr* $< .40 = 18$, 20%; *Afr* $< .50 = 49$, 54%)	
S = 2.27 (*SD* = 2.63)	(*S* $> 2 = 31$, 34%)	
Blends:R = 2.04 : 21.67		
CP = .11 (*SD* = .41)		
Interpersonal		
COP = 1.28 (*SD* = 1.25)	(*COP* $= 0 = 31$, 34%; *COP* $> 2 = 15$, 17%)	
AG = .54 (*SD* = .96)	(*AG* $= 0 = 58$, 64%; *AG* $> 2 = 4$, 4%)	
Food = .57 (*SD* = 1.01)		
Isolate/R = .18 (*SD* = .13)		
H:(H)+Hd+(Hd) = 2.63 : 2.96	(*Pure H* $= 0 = 11$, 12%; *Pure H* $< 2 = 26$, 29%)	
(H)+(Hd):(A)+(Ad) = 1.47 : .69		
H+A:Hd+Ad = 11.10 : 3.42		

Sum T = .58 (SD = .90)　　　　　　　(Sum T = 0 = 55, 61%; Sum T > 1 = 10, 11%)
GHR = 3.10 (SD = 2.07)
PHR = 3.17 (SD = 2.50)　　　　　　　(GHR > PHR = 38, 42%)

Self-perception
3r +(2)/R = .39 (SD = .17)　　　　　(3r+(2)/R < .33 = 29, 32%; 3r+(2)/R > .44 = 37, 41%)
Fr + rF = .17 (SD = .46)　　　　　　(Fr+rF > 0 = 12, 13%)
FD = .27 (SD = .52)
An+Xy = 1.10
MOR = 1.34 (SD = 1.66)　　　　　　(MOR > 2 = 15, 17%)

Ideation
a:p = 4.81 : 3.19　　　　　　　　　(p > a+1 = 14,16%)
Ma:Mp = 2.29 : 1.40　　　　　　　　(Mp > Ma = 17, 19%)
M = 3.67 (SD = 2.50)　　　　　　　(MQ– = .83, SD = 1.10; MQ None = .02, SD = 0.15)
FM = 2.91 (SD = 2.43)　　　　　　　m = 1.39 (SD = 1.45)
2AB+Art+Ay = 1.70　　　　　　　　2AB+Art+Ay > 5 = 3.3%
Sum 6 Sp Sc = 6.16　(SD = 4.33)
WSum6 = 19.94 (SD = 16.40)
Level 2 Sp Sc = .87　(SD = 1.33)　(Level 2 Special Scores > 0 = 38, 42%)

Mediation
Populars = 5.56　(SD = 1.98)　　　(P < 4 = 12,13%; P > 7 = 14, 16%)
XA% = .70 (SD = .14)
WDA% = .75 (SD = .13)
X + % = .46 (SD = .15)
X – % = .28 (SD = .13)
Xu% = .23 (SD = .09)
S– = 1.08 (SD = 1.72)
XA% > .89............................ 4　　　　　　　　4%
XA% < .70.......................... 42　　　　　　　47%
WDA% < .85...................... 65　　　　　　　72%
WDA% < .75...................... 38　　　　　　　42%
X + % < .55......................... 61　　　　　　　68%
Xu% > .20........................... 53　　　　　　　59%
X – % > .20......................... 61　　　　　　　68%
X – % > .30......................... 34　　　　　　　38%

Processing
Zf = 11.93 (SD = 4.82)
Zd = –1.62 (SD = 4.80)　　　　　　(Zd > + 3.0 = 12, 13%; Zd < –3.0 = 32, 36%)
W:D:Dd = 9.07:9.46:3.14
W:M = 9.07: 3.67
DQ+ = 5.93 (SD = 3.69)
DQv = 2.19 (SD = 2.25)　　　　　　(DQv > 2 = 32, 36%)

Constellations

PTI = 5............ 7	8%	DEPI = 7.......... 9	10%	CDI = 5....... 12	13%		
PTI = 4............ 6	7%	DEPI = 6.......... 8	9%	CDI = 4....... 19	21%		
PTI = 3.......... 10	11%	DEPI = 5........ 18	20%				
S-Constellation Positive....... 0	0%						
HVI Positive.......................... 8	9%						
OBS Positive......................... 0	0%						

difficulty shifting attention ($PSV = M = .40$; Exner's, 2001, Nonpatients = .04). Added to these deficits, their grandiosity ($W:M$ = 9:3) may further weaken an already inefficient processing effort and strategy ($W:D:Dd$ = 9:9.5:3; Exner's, 2001; Nonpatients = 8.28:12.88:1.16) resulting in the patients overextending themselves (poor judgment) and adding to their stress.

Mediation and Ideation.   Inappropriate use of form ($XA\% > .89 = 4\%$ & $WDA\% < .85 = 72\%$) and impaired reality testing ($X-\% = M = .28$; $X-\% > .20 = 68\%$, $WSum6$ $M = 19.94$; Lvl $2 = M = .87$; $M- = .83$) are consistent with the diagnosis of these patients, although these variables appear less pathological than those for the inpatient Schizophrenics ($X-\% = M = .37$; $X-\% > .20 = 90\%$, Exner, 1995b). Anger impacts the already disordered thinking of these patients ($S- = M = 1.08$). PS patients are prone to unconventional thinking ($Popular = M = 5.56$ & $Xu\% = M = .23$). Both PS patients and inpatient Schizophrenics produce some evidence of abusing fantasy (PS = $Mp > Ma = 19\%$; Exner, 1995b, 35%). Taken together, PS patients tend to have significantly lower levels of overall perceptual thought disturbance ($PTI \geq 3 = 26\%$), as measured by the Rorschach, when compared to Exner's (1995b) inpatient Schizophrenics ($SCZI \geq 4 = 82\%$), Exner's (2001) high $Lambda$ Schizophrenics ($PTI \geq 3 = 72\%$), and his low $Lambda$ Schizophrenics ($PTI \geq 3 = 74\%$).

Interpersonal.   PS patients may have even greater interpersonal deficits than nonforensic inpatient Schizophrenics (PS, $CDI \geq 4 = 34\%$; Exner, 1995b, $CDI \geq 4 = 25\%$,). Their attachment capacity (Sum $T = 0$, 61%) is impaired and similar to inpatient Schizophrenics (Sum $T = 0$. 70%, Exner, 1995b). Consistent with Schizophrenia, interest in others is diminished ($Pure$ $H = 0$, 12%; $Pure$ $H < 2$, 29%), but when present may be imbued with more primitive need states ($Fd = M = .57$). As expected, they are likely to miss important interpersonal cues ($Underincorporators = 36\%$; $Popular = M = 5.56$).

PS patients produce more $COPs$ ($COP = 0$, 34%; $COP > 2$, 17%) than inpatient Schizophrenics ($COP = 0$, 51%; $COP > 2$, 7%; Exner, 1995b). However, interpreting this finding as meaning greater expectations of mutually cooperative relationships would be premature without a careful analysis of their quality. Impaired interpersonal relationships are further supported by low levels of GHR ($M = 3.10$; $GHR > PHR = 42\%$).

Forensic Undifferentiated/Disorganized Schizophrenic Outpatients (UND; *N* = 38): Core Characteristics, Controls, and Stress Tolerance

Although they produced a normative number of responses ($R = M = 20.60$), the Undifferentiated/Disorganized Schizophrenics (UND), not surprisingly, were the most cognitively constricted ($Lambda = M = 1.33$) forensic group. Consistent with a Schizophrenic style, they were mostly *Avoidant* (45%) and split almost evenly between *Ambient* (24%) and *Introversive* (21%). Few were *Extratensive* (11%). As one would expect, the UND were the most socially inept ($CDI \geq 4 = 48\%$) out of all four groups. When compared to the Exner (1995b) inpatient Schizophrenic sample ($N = 320$; $EA = M = 8.63$) the UND group had dramatically fewer psychological resources ($EA = M = 5.58$), as well as weaker controls (D score $< 0 = 53\%$, $AdjD < 0 = 37\%$; Exner's D score $< 0 = 22\%$, $AdjD < 0 = 11\%$) and were the lowest scorers in our forensic sample (Table 20–3).

Affect. The UND patients were emotionally constricted ($WSumC = M = 2.58$), and had difficulty modulating emotions (*Pure C* $> 1 = 11\%$, *[CF + C]* $> FC + 1 = 29\%$) much like inpatient and high *Lambda* Schizophrenics (*Pure C* $> 1 = 7\%$, *[CF+C]* $> FC + 1 = 25\%$, Exner, 1995b; *Pure C* $> 1 = 8\%$, *[CF + C]* $> FC + 1 = 17\%$, Exner, 2001). Difficulties modulating emotions contributes to their tendency to avoid emotional engagement (*Afr* $< .50 = 63\%$).

Compared to Exner's (1995b) inpatient Schizophrenics, UND patients experienced similar levels of dysphoric affect (*Sum Shading* $= M = 4.39$; Exner group, $M = 4.68$), but much more than his (2001) inpatient Schizophrenic *Lambda* $> .99$ (*Sum Shading* $= M = 1.88$). This pattern was also observed for painful rumination (UND $=$ *Sum V* $= M = .82$; Exner, 1995b, *Sum V* $= M = .60$; Exner, 2001, *Sum V* $= M = .16$). These patients, however, were more likely to elevate on *DEPI* (*DEPI* $\geq 5 = 42\%$; Exner, 1995b, *DEPI* $\geq 5 = 19\%$; *Exner, 2001, DEPI* $\geq 5 = 22\%$). *But like their forensic counterparts and the Exner (2001) high Lambda* group, the quality of their dysphoria was less likely to be due to anxiety (*Sum Y* $= M = 1.32$)—unlike inpatient Schizophrenics (*Sum Y* $= M = 2.12$, Exner, 1995b).

Like other inpatient and forensic groups, these patients have difficulty with anger and hostility ($S = M = 2.53$ & $S > 2 = 42\%$). *Egosyntonic Aggression* ($AG = 0 = 63\%$) is directed toward others rather than directed toward self (*SCON* $+ = 3\%$).

Self-Perception. UND patients produce reflections ($Fr + Rf > 0 = 13\%$) and *Egocentricity Index* ($> .44 = 45\%$; $< .33 = 32\%$) at a similar rate to the (1995b) inpatient Schizophrenics ($Fr + rF > 0 = 13\%$; 35% & 36%), but unlike the (2001) high *Lambda* Schizophrenics ($Fr + rF > 0 = 3\%$; 25% & 55%). They also experience a similar sense of being damaged (*MOR* $= M = 1.68$, *MOR* $> 2 = 18\%$) as the (1995b) inpatient group (*MOR* $= M = 1.47$, *MOR* $> 2 = 22\%$), but again, more so then the (2001) high *Lambda* (*MOR* $= M = .81$, *MOR* $> 2 = 8\%$). Like other Schizophrenic groups they are more preoccupied with somatic features of self-image ($An + Xy = 1.18$). They demonstrated a marked impairment in their ability to introspect ($FD = M = .21$), when compared to the (1995b) inpatient Schizophrenics ($FD = M = .60$), but not when compared to the (2001) high *Lambdas* ($FD = M = .17$), and the same pattern is seen for painful rumination (UND $=$ *Sum V* $= M = .82$; (1995), *Sum V* $= M = .60$; (2001), *Sum V* $= M = .82$). These patients demonstrate serious adjustment problems (*Pure H* $< 2 = 42\%$) when compared to the (1995b) inpatient group and the other forensic groups.

Information Processing. UND patients demonstrated normative processing effort and organizational activity ($Zf = M = 11.55$; Exner's, 2001, Nonpatients $= 11.84$). However, their approach to scanning the environment misses important information ($Zd = M = -.61$). Their disorganization is evident in the ratio of *Underincorporators* (26%) to *Over-*

TABLE 20–3

Undifferentiated Schizophrenic Patient (N = 38) Group Mean and Frequencies for Select Ratios, Percentages, and Derivations

R = 20.60 (SD = 6.00)	L = 1.31 (SD = 1.46)

EB: 3.00:2.58	EA = 5.58 (SD = 3.87)
eb = 4.16 :4.39	es = 8.55 (SD = 5.43) (*FM* + *m* < *Sum Shading*........ 16, 42%)
D Score = –0.90 (SD = 1.39)	$AdjD$ = –0.42 (SD = 1.20)

EB style

Introversive...................... 8		21%
Pervasive Introversive...... 6		16%
Ambitent........................... 9		24%
Extratensive...................... 4		11%
Pervasive Extratensive..... 3		8%
Avoidant.......................... 17		45%

EA–es differences:D scores

D score > 0........................ 3	8%
D score = 0...................... 15	39%
D score < 0...................... 20	53%
D score < –1.................... 12	32%
AdjD score > 0.................. 4	11%
AdjD score = 0................ 20	53%
AdjD score < 0................ 14	37%
AdjD score < –1................ 7	18%

Affect

FC:CF + *C* = .97 : 1.87	
Pure C = .45 (SD = 1.03)	(*Pure C* > 0 = 9 ; 24%; *Pure C* > 1 = 4 ;11%)
FC > (*CF* + *C*) + 2............ 2	5%
FC > (*CF* + *C*) + 1........... 3	8%
(*CF* + *C*) > *FC* + 1.......... 11	29%
(*CF* +*C*) > *FC* + 2........... 8	21%
SumC' = 1.97 (SD = 2.19)	
SumT = .29 (SD = .77)	
SumV = .82 (SD = 1.04)	
SumY = 1.32 (SD = 1.43)	
Afr = .45 (SD = .13)	(*Afr* < .40 = 14, 37%; *Afr* < .50 = 24, 63%)
S = 2.53 (SD = 2.51)	(*S* > 2 = 16, 42%)
Blends:R = 2.97 : 20.60	
CP = .08 (SD = .27)	

Interpersonal

COP = 1.08 (SD = 1.26)	(*COP* = 0 = 15, 39%; *COP* > 2 = 4, 11%)
AG = .74 (SD = 1.13)	(*AG* = 0 = 24, 63%; *AG* > 2 = 4, 11%)
Food = .53 (SD = .83)	
Isolate/R = .19 (SD = .18)	
H:(H)+Hd+(Hd) = 2.40 : 2.71	(*Pure H* = 0 = 5, 13%; *Pure H* < 2 = 16, 42%)
(H)+(Hd):(A)+(Ad) = 1.03 :.37	
H+A:Hd+Ad = 11.61 : 3.71	
Sum T = .29 (SD = .77)	(*Sum T* = 0 = 32, 84%; *Sum T* > 1 = 3, 8%)

GHR = 2.24 (*SD* = 1.85)

PHR = 3.63 (*SD* = 3.02)   *GHR* > *PHR* = 14, 37%

Self-perception

   3r+(2)/R = .43 (*SD* = .26)   (*3r+(2)/R* < .33 = 12, 32%; *3r+(2)/R* > .44 = 17, 45%)

   Fr + rF = .40 (*SD* = 1.24)   (*Fr + rF* > 0 = 5, 13%)

   FD = .21 (*SD* = .41)

   An+Xy = 1.18

   MOR = 1.68 (*SD* = 1.80)   (*MOR* > 2 = 7, 18%)

Ideation

   a:p = 4.00 : 3.21   (*p* > *a*+1 = 11, 29%)

   Ma:Mp = 1.74 : 1.29   (*Mp* > *Ma* = 14, 37%)

   M = 3.00 (*SD* = 2.54)   (*MQ-* = .84, *SD* = 1.20; *MQNone* = 0.00)

   FM = 3.03 (*SD* = 2.94)   *m* = 1.13 (*SD* = 1.32)

   2AB+Art+Ay = 1.32   *2AB+Art+Ay* > 5 = 1, 3%

   Sum 6 Sp Sc = 6.26 (*SD* = 4.66)

   WSum6 = 20.24 (*SD* = 20.21)

   Level 2 Sp Sc = 1.18 (*SD* = 2.29) (*Level 2 Special Scores* > 0 = 16, 42%)

Mediation

   Populars = 4.79 (*SD* = 2.41)   (*P* < 4 = 10, 26%; *P* > 7 = 5, 13%)

   XA% = .66 (*SD* = .16)

   WDA% = .70 (SD = .16)

   X+% = .40 (*SD* = .16)

   X–% = .32 (*SD* = .16)

   Xu% = .26 (*SD* = .11)

   S– = 1.42 (*SD* = 1.67)

   XA% > .89............ 4   11%

   XA% < .70............ 23   61%

   WDA% < .85...................... 30   79%

   WDA% < .75...................... 22   58%

   X+% < .55.......................... 30   79%

   Xu% > .20.......................... 29   76%

   X–% > .20.......................... *31*   82%

   X–% > .30......................... *22*   58%

Processing

   Zf = 11.55 (*SD* = 5.23)

   Zd = –.61 (*SD* = 4.80)   (*Zd* > +3.0 = 6, 16%; *Zd* < –3.0 = 10, 26%)

   W:D:Dd = 8.34:8.37:3.90

   W:M = 8.34: 3.00

   DQ+ = 5.32 (*SD* = 3.77)

   DQv = 1.71 (*SD* = 2.15)   (*DQv* > 2 = 10, 26%)

Constellations

PTI = 5............ 1	3%		*DEPI* = 7........... 0	0%		*CDI* = 5........... 6	16%
PTI = 4............ 5	13%		*DEPI* = 6........... 7	18%		*CDI* = 4.......... 12	32%
PTI = 3.......... 10	26%		*DEPI* = 5........... 9	24%			
S-Constellation Positive....... 1	3%						
HVI Positive.......................... 6	16%						
OBS Positive....................... 0	0%						

incorporators (16%). The UND patients also process information in a vague and associational manner, and their thinking is fluid and poorly bounded ($DQv = M = 1.71$). The UND appear to have more difficulty shifting attention ($PSV = M = .76$) than any of the other forensic or Exner (1995b, 2001) inpatient Schizophrenic and Schizophrenic high *Lambda* groups. Consistent with this, their *Economy Index* ($W:D:Dd = 8:8:4$) suggests that their processing effort and strategy during problem-solving or decision-making tends to be less efficient. Similar to the high *Lambda* Schizophrenic group (Exner, 2001, $W:M = 7:2$), there is also a trend toward grandiosity ($W:M = 8:3$).

   Mediation and Ideation.   Inappropriate use of form ($XA\% > .89 = 11\%$ & $WDA\% < .85 = 79\%$) and impaired reality testing ($X-\% = M = .32$; $X-\% > .20 = 82\%$, $WSum6 = M = 20.24$, $Lvl\,2 = M = 1.18$, $M- = .84$) are consistent with the diagnosis of these patients. Although these variables appear less pathological than Exner's (1995b) inpatient Schizophrenics ($X-\% = M = .37$; $X-\% > .20 = 90\%$), they are more similar to his (2001) high *Lambda* Schizophrenics ($XA\% > .89 = 0\%$ & $WDA\% < .85 = 89\%$, $X-\% = M = .38$; $X-\% > .20 = 89\%$, $WSum6 = M = 26.31$, $Lvl\,2 = M = 3.19$, $M- = .95$). As we know from the other forensic groups, anger impacts the already disordered thinking of the UND patients ($S- = M = 1.42$), they are prone to unconventional thinking (*Popular* $= M = 4.79$ & $Xu\% = M = .26$), and they produce some evidence of abusing fantasy ($Mp > Ma = 37\%$). Taken together, UND tend to have significantly lower levels of overall perceptual thought disturbance ($PTI \geq 3 = 42\%$) when compared to Exner's (1995b) inpatient Schizophrenics ($SCZI \geq 4 = 8\,2\%$), Exner's (2001) high *Lambda* Schizophrenics ($PTI \geq 3 = 72\%$), and his low *Lambda* Schizophrenics ($PTI \geq 3 = 74\%$).

   Interpersonal.   UND patients may have even greater interpersonal deficits than nonforensic inpatient Schizophrenics (UND, $CDI \geq 4 = 48\%$; Exner, 1995b, $CDI \geq 4 = 25\%$), but are more similar to Exner's (2001) High *Lambda* group ($CDI \geq 4 = 55\%$). Their attachment capacity ($Sum\,T = 0 = 84\%$) is greatly impaired and similar to inpatient and high *Lambda* Schizophrenic groups (Exner, 1995b, $Sum\,T = 0 = 70\%$; High *Lambda* Exner, 2001, $Sum\,T = 0 = 94\%$). Out of all our forensic psychiatric patient groups, the UND patients had the most diminished interest in others (*Pure H* $= 0$, 13%; *Pure H* < 2, 42%), but similarly to them, their interest may be imbued with primitive need states ($Fd = M = .53$).

   UND patients produce more *COP*s ($COP > 2 = 11\%$) than inpatient and high *Lambda* Schizophrenics ($COP > 2 = 7\%$, Exner, 1995b; $COP > 2 = 2\%$; Exner, 2001). Impaired interpersonal relationships are supported by low levels of *GHR* ($M = 2.24$; $GHR > PHR = 37\%$). Like other groups, they are likely to miss important interpersonal cues (*Underincorporators* $= 26\%$; *Popular* $= M = 4.79$).

Forensic Schizoaffective Outpatients (SAF; N = 59): Core Characteristics, Controls, and Stress Tolerance

The forensic Schizoaffective patients (SAF) produced a normative number of responses ($R = M = 19.87$) and were less cognitively constricted (*Lambda* $= M = .80$) when compared to our Paranoid Schizophrenics (*Lambda* = *M* = 1.22). Most were either *Avoidant* (36%) or *Extratensive* (32%, *Pervasive* 27%), and few *Ambitent* (7%). Many were socially inept (*CDI* ≥ 4 = 32%) and evidenced reduced psychological resources (*EA* = *M* = 7.32), as well as weakened controls (*D* score < 0 = 44%, *AdjD* < 0 = 44%) (Table 20–4).

Affect. As one might expect with an affective disorder, the SAF patients were less emotionally constricted (*WSumC* = *M* = 4.05). They had more difficulty modulating emotions (*Pure C* > 1 = 49%, *[CF + C]* > *FC* + 1 = 42%) than inpatient Schizophrenics (Exner, 1995b) or the forensic Paranoid Schizophrenics. Perhaps, as a defense, they tended to avoid emotional engagement (*Afr* < .50 = 22%). Dysphoric affect (*Sum Shading* = *M* = 5.76) and painful rumination (*Sum V* = *M* = 1.17) were consistent with elevated *DEPI*s (*DEPI* ≥ 5 = 44%). The SAF patients did not appear as angry (*S* > 2 = 25%) as Exner's (1995b) inpatient Schizophrenics (*S* > 2 = 43%), and unlike other forensic groups (Gacono & Meloy, 1994), their aggression causes them problems (*AG* > 2 = 58%). It impacts their thinking and behavior, and in some cases, is being directed toward self (*SCON* + = 32%).

Self-Perception. If self-absorption is considered a defense against core feelings of worthlessness, then it is understandable that forensic patients with an affective disorder produce more reflections (*Fr* + *rF* > 0 = 31%) and have an *Egocentricity Index* (> .44 = 49%; < .33 = 14%) higher than Exner's (1995b) inpatient Schizophrenics (*Fr* + *rF* > 0 = 13%; *Ego Index* > .44 = 35%, < .33 = 36%). SAF patients also experience a sense of being damaged (*MOR* = *M* = 1.83). This may be a byproduct of their cognitive impoverishment, grandiosity, and marked impairment in their ability to introspect (*FD* = *M* = .39). They are prone to painful rumination (*Sum V* = *M* = 1.17), and appear to be preoccupied with somatic features of self image (*An* + *Xy* = 1.16). Their serious affective dysregulation is likely reflected in their adjustment problems (*Pure H* < 2 = *61%*) and possibly feeling vulnerable (*HVI* = 25%).

Information Processing. The SAF patients evidenced normative processing efforts and organizational activity (*Zf* = *M* = 12.42). However, their processing inefficiency is similar to the other forensic groups (*Zd* = *M* = –03; *Underincorporators*, 22% & *Overincorporators*, 14%). They process information in a vague and associational manner, their thinking is fluid and poorly bounded (*DQv* = *M* = 1.90), and they may also have more difficulty shifting attention (*PSV* = *M* = .49). Their *Economy Index* suggests inefficiency (*W:D:Dd* = 10.61:6.83:2.34). Despite these deficits, grandiosity is reflected in their aspirations that exceed their real-world abilities (*W:M* = 10.61: 3.27).

Mediation and Ideation. As expected in a patient group where mood disturbance co-exists with thought disorder, SAF patients evidence elevated levels of impaired reality testing (*X–%* > .20 = 76%; *XA%* > .89 = 19% & *WDA%* < .75 = 76%), similar to that of Exner's (1995b) inpatient Schizophrenics (*X–%* > .20 = 90%). However, unlike that sample, their levels of cognitive slippage (*WSum6* = *M* = 24.56, *Lvl 2 M* = 1.34, *M–* = .63), as

TABLE 20–4

Schizoaffective Patient (*N* = 59) Group Mean and Frequencies for Select Ratios, Percentages, and Derivations

R = 19.78 (*SD* = 6.65)	*L* = .80 (*SD* = .78)

EB: 3.27:4.05   *EA* = 7.32 (*SD* = 4.28)

    eb = 4.25 : 5.76   *es* = 10.02 (*SD* = 6.12) (*FM + m < Sum Shading* 12, 20%)

    D Score = –0.85 (*SD* = 1.57)   *AdjD* = –0.36 (*SD* = 1.30)

EB style

    Introversive 13   22%

    Pervasive Introversive 7   12%

    Ambitent 4   7%

    Extratensive 19   32%

    Pervasive Extratensive 16   27%

    Avoidant 21   36%

EA–es differences:D scores

    D score > 0 12   20%

    D score = 0 6   10%

    D score < 0 26   44%

    D score < –1 27   46%

    AdjD score > 0 15   25%

    AdjD score = 0 9   15%

    AdjD score < 0 29   49%

    AdjD score < –1 21   36%

Affect

    FC:CF + C = 1.22 : 3.00

    Pure C = .88 (*SD* = 1.16)   (*Pure C* > 0 = 8; 14%; *Pure C* > 1 = 29, 49%)

    FC > (*CF* + *C*) + 2 6   10%

    FC > (*CF* + *C*) + 1 1   2%

    (*CF* + *C*) > *FC* + 1 25   42%

    (*CF* + *C*) > *FC* + 2 31   53%

    SumC' = 2.58 (*SD* = 2.41)

    SumT = .64 (*SD* = .89)

    SumV = 1.17 (*SD* = 1.38)

    SumY = 1.37 (*SD* = 1.68)

    Afr = .50 (*SD* = .22)   (Afr < .40 = 33, 56%; Afr < .50 = 13, 22%)

    S = 2.17 (*SD* = 2.08)   (*S* > 2 = 15, 25%)

    Blends:R = 4.54 : 19.78

    CP = .03 (*SD* = .18)

Interpersonal

    COP = 1.69 (*SD* = 1.46)   (*COP* = 0 = 5, 8%; *COP* > 2 = 15, 25%)

    AG = .68 (*SD* = 1.02)   (*AG* = 0 = 7, 12%; *AG* > 2 = 34, 58%)

    Food = .68 (*SD* = .97)

    Isolate/R = .20 (*SD* = .16)

    H:(H)+Hd+(Hd) = 2.17 : 3.20   (*Pure H* = 0 = 25, 42%; *Pure H* < 2 = 36, 61%)

    (H)+(Hd):(A)+(Ad) = 2.01 : .48

    H+A:Hd+Ad = 9.24 : 3.19

    Sum T = .64 (*SD* = .89)   (*Sum T* = 0 = 8, 14%; *Sum T* > 1 = 33, 56%)

$GHR = 2.73\ (SD = 2.12)$

$PHR = 3.41\ (SD = 2.30)$ $GHR > PHR = 17, 29\%$

Self-perception

$3r + (2)/R = .38\ (SD = .21)$ $(3r + (2)/R < .33 = 8, 14\%; 3r + (2)/R > .44 = 29, 49\%)$

$Fr + rF = .37\ (SD = 1.16)$ $(Fr + rF > 0 = 18, 31\%)$

$FD = .39\ (SD = .59)$

$An+Xy = 1.16$

$MOR = 1.83\ (SD = 2.08)$ $(MOR > 2 = 2, 3\%)$

Ideation

$a{:}p = 4.69 : 2.83$ $(p > a + 1 = 26, 44\%)$

$Ma{:}Mp = 1.98 : 1.29$ $(Mp > Ma = 8, 14\%)$

$M = 3.27\ (SD = 2.51)$ $(MQ- = .63, SD = 1.03; MQNone = 0.00)$

$FM = 2.78\ (SD = 2.35)$ $m = 1.47\ (SD = 1.75)$

$2AB+Art+Ay = 2.14$ $2AB+Art+Ay > 5 = 18, 31\%$

$Sum\ 6\ Sp\ Sc = 7.27\ (SD = 5.31)$

$WSum6 = 24.56\ (SD = 21.42\ )$

$Level\ 2\ Sp\ Sc = 1.34\ \ (SD = 2.55)$ $(Level\ 2\ Special\ Scores > \ 0 = 17, 29\%)$

Mediation

$Populars = 5.25\ (SD = 1.76)$ $(P < 4 = 4, 7\%; P > 7 = 8, 14\%)$

$XA\% = .69\ (SD = .15)$

$WDA\% = .72\ (SD = .16)$

$X+\% = .42\ (SD = .13\ )$

$X-\% = .25\ (SD = .15\ )$

$Xu\% = .27\ (SD = .12)$

$S- = 1.20\ (SD = 1.42)$

$XA\% > .89$.......................... 11 19%

$XA\% < .70$.......................... 4 7%

$WDA\% < .85$...................... 29 49%

$WDA\% < .75$...................... 45 76%

$X+\% < .55$.......................... 36 61%

$Xu\% > .20$.......................... 50 85%

$X-\% > .20$.......................... 45 76%

$X-\% > .30$.......................... 36 61%

Processing

$Zf = 12.42\ (SD = 5.71)$

$Zd = -.03\ (SD = 4.26)$ $(Zd > + 3.0 = 8, 14\%; Zd < -3.0 = 13, 22\%)$

$W{:}D{:}Dd = 10.61{:}6.83{:}2.34$

$W{:}M = 10.61{:} 3.27$

$DQ+ = 5.80\ (SD = 3.81)$

$DQv = 1.90\ (SD = 2.32)$ $(DQv > 2 = 5, 8\%)$

Constellations

$PTI = 5$........... 1	2%		$DEPI = 7$.......... 11	19%		$CDI = 5$.......... 15	25%
$PTI = 4$........... 0	0%		$DEPI = 6$............ 2	3%		$CDI = 4$............ 4	7%
$PTI = 3$......... 10	17%		$DEPI = 5$.......... 13	22%			
S-Constellation Positive..... 19	32%						
HVI Positive........................ 15	25%						
OBS Positive...................... 50	85%						

measured by the Rorschach, are considerably less than inpatient Schizophrenics (*WSum6* = *M* = 44.69, *M–* = *M* = 2.42, Exner, 1995b). Like the other forensic groups, anger further impacts their already disordered thinking (*S–* = *M* = 1.20) and they are prone to unconventional thinking (*Popular* = *M* = 5.25 & *Xu%* = *M* = .27). A small percentage may abuse fantasy (*Mp* > *Ma* = 14%), and they tend to have lower levels of overall perceptual thought disturbance (*PTI* ≥ 3 = 19%), as compared to Exner's (1995b) inpatient and both high and low *Lambda* Schizophrenics (*SCZI* ≥ 4 = 82%, Exner, 1995b; High *Lambda*, *PTI* ≥ 3 = 72%, low *Lambda PTI* ≥ 3 = 74%, Exner, 2001).

Interpersonal.   SAF patients may have even greater interpersonal deficits than nonforensic inpatient Schizophrenics (SAF, *CDI* ≥ 4 = 32%; Exner, 1995b, *CDI* ≥ 4 = 25%). Whereas their attachment capacity appears (*Sum T* = 0 = 14%) greater than the forensic Paranoid Schizophrenics (*Sum T* = 0 = 61%) or inpatient Schizophrenics (*Sum T* = 0 = 70%, Exner, 1995b), their interest in others (*Pure H* = 0 = 42% & *Pure H* < 2 = 61%) is also greater. However, it is imbued with primitive need states (*Fd* = *M* = .68) and influenced by their psychosis. Additionally, they are likely to miss important interpersonal cues and are prone to unconventional thinking (*Underincorporators* = 22% & *Popular* = *M* = 5.25).

SAF patients produce more *COP*s (*COP* = 0 = 8% & *COP* > 2 = 25%) than Exner's (1995) inpatient Schizophrenics (*COP* = 0 = 51% & *COP* > 2 = 7%) and forensic Paranoid Schizophrenics (*COP* = 0 = 34% & *COP* > 2 = 17%). Impaired interpersonal relationships are supported by low levels of *GHR* (*M* = 2.73 & *GHR* > *PHR* = 29%). Whereas affect may fuel their desire for interpersonal relatedness, other Rorschach identified deficits make relationships difficult.

Forensic Bipolar Outpatients (BP, *N* = 40): Core Characteristics, Controls, and Stress Tolerance

The Bipolar Patients (BP) produced a normative number of responses (*R* = *M* = 19.28). Their *Lambdas* (*M* = .73) were more similar to the Schizoaffective group (M = .80) than the Paranoid Schizophrenics (M = 1.22). Interestingly, few were *Avoidant* (18%), but they were evenly divided among *Extratensives* (28%), *Introversives* (28%), and *Ambitents* (28%). More were socially inept (*CDI* ≥ 4 = 40%) than the other forensic groups. They tended to evidence few psychological resources (*EA* = *M* = 6.88) and weakened controls (*D* score < 0 = 43% & *AdjD* < 0 = 3 5%) (Table 20–5).

Affect.   Like our other affective group (SAF), these patients were not emotionally constricted (*WSumC* = *M* = 3.38). However, they tended to avoid emotional engagement (*Afr* < .50 = 58%) much more so than our Schizoaffective group. BP patients experienced dysphoric affect (*Sum Shading* = *M* = 4.57), painful rumination (*Sum V* = *M* = 1.02), and were more likely to elevate on *DEPI* (*DEPI* ≥ 5 = 48%) than inpatient Schizophrenics (*DEPI* ≥ 5 = 19%, Exner, 1995b), but less than inpatient Depressives with *Lambda* less than 1.0 (*DEPI* ≥ 5 = 71%; Exner, 2001). These patients did not appear as

TABLE 20–5

Bipolar Patient (*N* = 40) Group Mean and Frequencies for Select Ratios, Percentages, and Derivations

R = 19.28 (*SD* = 5.09)	*L* = .73 (*SD* = .62)

EB: 3.50:3.38	*EA* = 6.88 (*SD* = 2.94)
eb = 4.75 :4.57	*es* = 9.33 (*SD* = 5.39) (*FM* + *m* < *Sum Shading*....... 18, 45%)
D score = –0.78 (*SD* = 1.86)	*AdjD* = –0.40 (*SD* = 1.41)

EB style

Introversive.......................... 11	28%
Pervasive Introversive.......... 6	15%
Ambitent............................... 11	28%
Extratensive........................ 11	28%
Pervasive Extratensive......... 8	20%
Avoidant............................... 7	18%

EA–es differences:D scores

D score > 0............................. 5	13%
D score = 0.......................... 18	45%
D score < 0.......................... 17	43%
D score < –1.......................... 9	23%
AdjD score > 0...................... 6	15%
AdjD score = 0.................... 20	50%
AdjD score < 0.................... 14	35%
AdjD score < –1.................... 8	20%

Affect

FC:CF + *C* = 1.13 : 2.60	
Pure C = .43 (*SD* = .75)	(*Pure C* > 0 = 12; 30%; *Pure C* > 1 = 4; 10%)
FC > (*CF* + *C*) + 2............... 1	3%
FC > (*CF* + *C*) + 1............... 2	5%
(*CF* + *C*) > *FC* + *1*............. 15	38%
(*CF* + *C*) > *FC* + 2............. 13	33%
SumC′ = 1.65 (*SD* = 1.59)	
SumT = .83 (*SD* = 1.17)	
SumV = 1.02 (*SD* = 1.14)	
SumY = 1.07 (*SD* = 1.33)	
Afr = .48 (*SD* = .23)	(*Afr* < .40 = 16, 40%; *Afr* < .50 = 23, 58%)
S = 1.88 (*SD* = 2.00)	(*S* > 2 = 11, 28%)
Blends:R = 4.57 : 19.28	
CP = .08 (*SD* = .27)	

Interpersonal

COP = 1.38 (*SD* = 1.15)	(*COP* = 0 = 9, 23%; *COP* > 2 = 5, 13%)
AG = .68 (*SD* = 1.09)	(*AG* = 0 = 25, 63%; *AG* > 2 = 2, 5%)
Food = .60 (*SD* = 1.17)	
Isolate/R = .23 (*SD* = .19)	
H:(H)+Hd+(Hd) = 2.38 : 2.53	(*Pure H* = 0 = 5, 13%; *Pure H* < 2 = 16, 40%)
(*H*)+(*Hd*):(*A*)+(*Ad*) = 1.68 : .65	
H+A:Hd+Ad = 10.33 : 2.60	
Sum T = .83 (*SD* = 1.17)	(*Sum T* = 0 = 21, 52%; *Sum T* > 1 = 8, 20%)

(continued)

TABLE 20–5 *(continued)*

GHR = 3.03 (*SD* = 1.76)

PHR = 2.73 (*SD* = 2.73)   *GHR > PHR* = 21, 52%

Self-perception

   3r + (2)/R = .48 (*SD* = .23)   (*3r + (2)/R < .33* = 11, 28%; *3r + (2)/R > .44* = 20, 50%)

   Fr + rF = .78 (*SD* = 2.17)   (*Fr + rF > 0* = 10, 25%)

   FD = .40 (*SD* = .59)

   An+Xy = 1.03

   MOR = 1.97 (*SD* = 1.97)   (*MOR > 2* = 11, 28%)

Ideation

   a:p = 5.15 : 3.15   (*p > a+1* = 4, 10%)

   Ma:Mp = 2.33 : 1.20   (*Mp > Ma* = 12, 30%)

   M = 3.50 (*SD* = 2.43)   (*MQ–* = .80, *SD* = 1.56; *MQ None* = 0.00)

   FM = 3.15 (*SD* = 1.82)   m = 1.60 (*SD* = 1.48)

   2AB+Art+Ay = 1.97   2AB+Art+Ay > 5 = 4, 10%

   Sum 6 Sp Sc = 6.65 (*SD* = 4.36)

   WSum6 = 23.23 (*SD* = 18.45)

   Level 2 Sp Sc = 1.33 (*SD* = 1.75) (*Level 2 Special Scores > 0* = 25, 63%)

Mediation

   Populars = 5.65 (*SD* = 2.26)   (*P < 4* = 5, 13%; *P > 7* = 6, 15%)

   XA% = .73 (*SD* = .16)

   WDA% = .75 (*SD* = .16)

   X+% = .53 (*SD* = .17)

   X–% = .26 (*SD* = .15)

   Xu% = .20 (*SD* = .10)

   S– = .75 (*SD* = .90)

   XA% > .89.......................... 4   10%

   XA% < .70....................... 14   35%

   WDA% < .85.................... 28   70%

   WDA% < .75................... 17   43%

   X+% < .55......................... 22   55%

   Xu% > .20........................ 18   45%

   X–% > .20........................ 22   55%

   X–% > .30........................ 14   35%

Processing

   Zf = 12.70 (*SD* = 5.08)

   Zd = –1.34 (*SD* = 4.74)   (*Zd > +3.0* = 10, 25%; *Zd < –3.0* = 17, 43%)

   W:D:Dd = 11:6.62:1.65

   W:M = 11: 3.50

   DQ+ = 5.95 (*SD* = 3.12)

   DQv = 1.52 (*SD* = 2.04)   (*DQv > 2* = 8, 20%)

Constellations

PTI = 5........... 1	3%	DEPI = 7........... 2	5%	CDI = 5......... 6	15%
PTI = 4........... 3	8%	DEPI = 6........... 8	20%	CDI = 4....... 10	25%
PTI = 3........... 7	18%	DEPI = 5........... 9	23%		

   S-Constellation Positive.... 3   8%

   HVI Positive...................... 6   15%

   OBS Positive.................... 0   0%

angry ($S > 2 = 28\%$) as Exner's (1995) inpatient Schizophrenics ($S > 2 = 43\%$) or (2001) inpatient Depressives ($S > 2 = 37\%$). Their aggression does not seem to be directed toward self ($SCON + = 8\%$).

Self-Perception.   The Bipolar patients produced reflections ($Fr + rF > 0 = 25\%$) at a higher frequency than the Paranoid and Undifferentiated/Disorganized groups and inpatient Schizophrenics ($Fr + rF > 0 = 13\%$, Exner, 1995b), but lower than the Schizoaffective group (31%). Their inflated *Egocentricity Ratios* ($> .44 = 50\%$ & $< .33 = 28\%$) coexisted with a sense of being damaged ($MOR = M = 1.97$). These patients have a marked impairment in their ability to introspect ($FD = M = .40$), are prone to painful rumination ($Sum\ V = M = 1.02$), and appear to be preoccupied with somatic features of self image ($An + Xy = 1.03$). Although not as impaired as the SAF group, their serious affective dysregulation is likely reflected in their adjustment problems ($Pure\ H < 2 = 40\%$).

Information Processing.   Like our other forensic outpatient psychiatric groups, the BP patients evidenced normative processing efforts and organizational activity ($Zf = 12.70$), concurrent to inefficiency ($Zd = -1.34$ & *Underincorporators* 43% & *Overincorporators* 25%). These patients process information in a vague and associational manner, their thinking is fluid and poorly bounded ($DQv = 1.52$), they may also have more difficulty shifting attention ($PSV = .43$), and their *Economy Index* suggests that processing effort and strategy during problem solving or decision making tends to be inefficient ($W{:}D{:}Dd = 11{:}6.62{:}1.65$). Despite these deficits, grandiosity is an aspect of their personality ($W{:}M = 11{:}\ 3.5$).

Mediation and Ideation.   Although not as impaired as the SAF patients, BP patients evidence elevated levels of impaired reality testing ($X-\% > .20 = 55\%$; $XA\% > .89 = 10\%$ & $WDA\% < .85 = 70\%$), similar to that of inpatient Schizophrenics ($X-\% > .20 = 90\%$, Exner, 1995b). Their levels of cognitive slippage ($WSum6 = M = 23.23$, $Lvl\ 2 = M = 1.33$, $M- = M = .80$) are considerably less than inpatient Schizophrenics ($WSum6 = M = 44.69$, $M- = M = 2.42$, Exner, 1995b). Decreased levels of *Special Scores* do not suggest the absence of a thought disorder. Anger further impacts their already disordered thinking ($S = M = 1.88$). BP patients are prone to unconventional thinking ($Popular = M = 5.65$ & $Xu\% = M = .20$), may abuse fantasy ($Mp > Ma = 30\%$), and tend to have significantly lower levels of overall perceptual thought disturbance ($PTI \geq 3 = 29\%$) when compared to inpatient Schizophrenics ($SCZI \geq 4 = 82\%$, Exner, 1995b) and both high and low *Lambda* Schizophrenics ($PTI \geq 3 = 72\%$, $PTI \geq 3 = 74\%$, Exner, 2001).

Interpersonal.   BP patients exhibit interpersonal deficits ($CDI \geq 4 = 40\%$) similar to UND patients ($+CDI = 48\%$), but greater than inpatient Schizophrenics ($+CDI = 25\%$, Exner, 1995b). Their attachment capacity ($Sum\ T = 0 = 52\%$) is somewhat greater than the PS and UND groups, but less than inpatient Schizophrenics ($Sum\ T = 0 = 70\%$, Exner, 1995b). Although interested in others ($Pure\ H = 0 = 13\%$ & $Pure\ H < 2 = 40\%$), the interest is imbued with primitive need states ($Fd = M = .60$) and grandiosity. Additionally, they are likely to miss important interpersonal cues and are prone to unconventional thinking (*Underincorporators* = 43% & *Popular* = *M* = 5.65). BP patients produce few *COPs* (*COP* = 0 = 23% & *COP* > 2 = 13%), and impaired interpersonal relationships are further supported by a lower than normative *GHR* (*M* = 3 & *GHR* > *PHR* = 52%).

CONCLUSIONS

Rorschach findings highlight what these four outpatient forensic psychiatric groups share in common. They exhibit limited or reduced psychological resources (*EA*), difficulties managing complexity (elevated *Lambda*), vulnerabilities to disorganization, reality testing problems, and interpersonal and social deficits. The data also is consistent with important clinical differences. The Paranoid Schizophrenic and Bipolar Patients were the most grandiose, as suggested by *W:M*. The Schizoaffective patients tended to be *Avoidant, Extratensive* and less emotionally avoidant. The Undifferentiated/Disorganized Schizophrenics tended to be *Avoidant, Introversive* (like the Paranoid patients), perseverative, with the lowest psychological resources and the most severe cognitive and emotional impoverishment. All of the forensic patients process information in a vague and associational manner, likely the result of a profound failure to integrate their vague, poorly understood inner need states, along their distorted, grossly unrealistic view of the world in which predatory opportunism and acting out decreases the stimulus value of most other interpersonal events.

These Rorschach patterns are helpful in guiding treatment recommendations and understanding treatment response. Deficient psychological resources and limited coping skills must always be considered when assessing treatment progress and need for continued treatment. Frequently, behavioral stability during treatment (adequate *D* and *AdjD*) is dependent on the structure of the CONREP program and not due to in depth personality change. Consequently, despite positive behavioral change, these patients continue to need the ongoing program structure, despite producing flat MMPI–2 profiles. When considering the financial, personal, and humanitarian costs of managing these patients on an outpatient basis versus hospitalization or incarceration, the CONREP structure becomes very cost-effective.

During treatment, coping style (emotional avoidance) is also important when aiding the patient in preventing relapse. In higher functioning patient groups, defenses are more likely to be challenged. For the high *Lambda* Paranoid and Undifferentiated/Disorganized Schizophrenics, the assessment data suggests that the best strategy is to bolster defenses while attempting small steps to increased comfort with affect. This approach can be contrasted to more emotional groups, where the goal of treatment—to utilize Rorschach language—may actually be to increase their *Lambda*, that is, to help them to avoid affect and gain better distance from it. The Rorschach can aid the clinician in determining the degree to which emotional avoidance represents an important coping strategy for all these outpatients. Acting out can be precipitated by emotional flooding, which leads to increased reality testing difficulties. Emotional flooding can be exacerbated by affectively oriented therapies, changes in therapeutic structure (including therapist characteristics), and interpersonal interactions. Based on Rorschach data and history, these disruptions are frequently predictable.

For these forensic outpatients aggression is problematic. Although it tends to be primarily egosyntonic, aggression toward self must always be monitored (a third of the SAF patients produce Rorschachs similar to individuals at risk for suicide). For most of these patients the data is consistent with an alloplastic style, where acting out is used to avoid and discharge distress and aggression. It appears that out of all the groups, the Schizoaffective patients may demonstrate the most motivation to engage with their therapists. Even so, the impact of cognitive impairment, processing issues, grandiosity, and primitive object relations should be kept in mind when formulating treatment goals and assessing treatment progress. Interpreting Rorschach data concretely (as meaning greater expectations of attachment capacity and mutually cooperative relationships) will likely lead to inaccurate formulations. A better understanding of object relations can be gleaned from a careful analysis of the quality of their *T* and *COP* responses. The meaning of these variables rests on an analysis of their quality—whether they are good or spoiled—and must be always be considered within the context of their real-world relationships. For some offenders, *COP*s have been interpreted as reflecting superficial charm rather than an expectation of interpersonal cooperation (Gacono & Meloy, 1994).

Our study of forensic psychiatric outpatients highlights the need for interpreting assessment data within the context of patient's response style (Melton et al., 1998). Atypical patterns of constriction are common and frequently represent accurate portrayals of the patient's psychology. For example, the higher rate of positive *SCZI*, *PTI*, and *Level 2 Special Scores* among Schizophrenic groups (with exception of the high *Lambda* inpatient Schizophrenic group, Exner, 2001) compared to our outpatient forensic groups does not indicate a lack of psychotic process among these patients. It also does not, necessarily, suggest resistance to the testing process. Rather, this finding must be interpreted in light of the patient's chronicity and their cognitive and emotional impoverishment. Rorschach constriction or expansion must always be explained within the context of the entire assessment battery and the patient's psychosocial history.

ACKNOWLEDGMENT

Portions of this chapter were published in 1999 in the Journal of Clinical Psychology, and have been reprinted here with permission.

REFERENCES

American Psychiatric Association. (1994). *Diagnostic and statistical manual of mental disorders* (4th ed.). Washington, DC: Author.

Bagby, R. M., Rogers, R., & Buis, T. (1994). Detecting malingered and defensive responding on the MMPI–2 in a forensic inpatient sample. *Journal of Personality Assessment, 62,* 191–203.

Bannatyne, L. A. (1996). *The effects of defensiveness on select MMPI–2 and Rorschach variables in schizophrenic forensic patients.* Unpublished doctoral dissertation, Pacific Graduate School of Psychology, California.

Bannatyne, L. A., Gacono, C., & Greene, R. (1999). Differential patterns of responding among 3 groups of chronic psychotic forensic outpatients. *Journal of Clinical Psychology, 55*(12), 1553–1565.

California Forensic Services. (2001). *State of California, Special Programs—The CONREP Program* (Publication No. 18). Sacramento: Author

Coyle, F. A., Jr., & Heap, R. F. (1965). Interpreting the MMPI *L* scale. *Psychological Reports, 17,* 722.

Exner, J. E., Jr. (1986). Some Rorschach data comparing schizophrenics with borderline and schizotypal personality disorder. *Journal of Personality Assessment, 50,* 455–471.

Exner, J. E., Jr. (1991). *The Rorschach: A Comprehensive System* (Vol. 2, 2nd ed.). New York: Wiley.

Exner, J. E., Jr. (Ed.). (1995a). *Issues and methods in Rorschach research.* Hillsdale, NJ: Lawrence Erlbaum Associates.

Exner, J. E., Jr. (1995b). *A Rorschach workbook for the Comprehensive System* (4th ed.). Asheville, NC: Rorschach Workshops.

Exner, J. E., Jr. (2001). *A Rorschach workbook for the Comprehensive System* (5th ed.). Asheville, NC: Rorschach Workshops.

Fjordbak, T. (1985). Clinical correlates of high lie scale elevations among forensic patients. *Journal of Personality Assessment, 49,* 253–255.

Gacono, C. B., & Meloy, J. R. (1994). *The Rorschach assessment of aggressive and psychopathic personalities.* Hillsdale, NJ: Lawrence Erlbaum Associates.

Gacono, C. B., & Meloy, J. R., & Bridges, M. (2000). A Rorschach comparison of psychopaths, sexual homicide perpetrators, and nonviolent pedophiles: Where angels fear to tread. *Journal of Clinical Psychology, 55*(6), 757–777.

Grossman, L. S., & Wasyliw, O. E. (1988). A psychometric study of stereotypes: Assessment of malingering in a criminal forensic group. *Journal of Personality Assessment, 52,* 549–563.

Meloy, R., Hanoun, A., & Schiller, E. (1990). *Clinical guidelines for involuntary outpatient treatment.* Sarasota, FL: Professional Resource Exchange.

Melton, G., Petrila, J., Poythress, N., & Solbogin, C. (1998). *Psychological evaluations for the courts: A handbook for mental health professionals and lawyers.* New York: Guilford.

Nieberding, R., Gacono, C. B., Pirie, M., Bannatyne, L., Viglione, D., Cooper, B., Bodholt, R., & Frackowiak, M. (2003). MMPI–2 classification of forensic psychiatric outpatients: An exploratory cluster analytic study. *Journal of Clinical Psychology, 59*(9), 907–920.

Roman, D. D., Tuley, M. R., Villanueva, M. R., & Mitchell, W. E. (1990). Evaluating MMPI validity in a forensic psychiatric population. *Criminal Justice and Behavior, 17,* 186–198.

Wasyliw, O. E., Grossman, L. S., Haywood, T. W., & Cavanaugh, J. L., Jr. (1988). The detection of malingering in criminal forensic groups: MMPI validity scales. *Journal of Personality Assessment, 52,* 321–333.

Weiner, I. B. (1966). *Psychodiagnosis in schizophrenia.* New York: Wiley.

Weiner, I. B. (1991). Editor's note: Interscorer agreement in Rorschach research. *Journal of Personality Assessment, 56,* 1.

Weiner, I. B. (1995a). Methodological considerations in Rorschach research. *Psychological Assessment, 7,* 330–337.

Weiner, I. B. (1995b). Variable selection in Rorschach research. In J. E. Exner, Jr. (Ed.), *Issues and methods in Rorschach research* (pp. 73–98). Hillsdale, NJ: Lawrence Erlbaum Associates.

21

CHILD CUSTODY LITIGANTS: RORSCHACH DATA FROM A LARGE SAMPLE

Jacqueline Singer
Private Practice, Sonoma, CA

Carl F. Hoppe
Private Practice, Beverly Hills, CA

S. Margaret Lee
Private Practice, Greenbrae, CA

Nancy W. Olesen and Marjorie G. Walters
Private Practice, San Rafael, CA

Over 50% of all marriages end in divorce and approximately one million children per year experience the divorce of their parents. Of all children born in 1990, from 50% to 60% will live in a single parent family. Of these divorces, 10% are high conflict (Glick, 1988). An even smaller percentage require a child custody evaluation to resolve custody disputes (Hoppe & Kenney, 1994).

Whereas there have been few studies to date using the Rorschach to examine the personality characteristics of parents involved in custody disputes (Bonieskie, 2000; Hoppe & Kenney, 1994; Lee, 1996; Singer, 2001), much has been written clinically about this population. But, are divorcing couples who must litigate custody fundamentally different from the nonpatient population on the Rorschach?

Wallerstein and Kelly's seminal work, *Surviving the Break-up* (1980), described the intense anger that was exhibited in a group of parents who could not resolve custody issues, with residual anger occurring in four fifths of their sample. Wallerstein and Kelly (1980) noted that the anger experienced by these parents was so intense that "no amount of reasoning could deter them from their goals" (Ellis, 2000 p. 238). The anger seemed to serve two purposes: to ward off a devastating depression and to organize themselves, that is, to create a sense of equilibrium where none existed. These parents exhibited behavior that had previously been uncharacteristic of them, including behavior that could be perceived as paranoid (e.g., spying on the other parent, making excessive phone contact, being assaultive, and attempting to get the children to align with them).

Johnston and Campbell's study of 80 divorced couples was summarized in their work *Impasses of Divorce* (1988). They delineated external, interactional, and internal components of a divorce impasse. The internal components, that is, the psychological state of each of the parents, is most conducive to examination with personality measures. They note that it is the preexisting psychological vulnerabilities of these parents, when coupled with the stress of the divorce that "provoke regression and produce more rigid defensive styles that *look like* [italics added] or exacerbate personality disorders" (Johnston & Roseby, 1997, p. 16). Johnston and Roseby (1997) described the characterological difficulties in these parents: "Compared to the norm, these individuals lack a firm approach to problem solving, are more likely to perceive inaccurately, reason idiosyncratically, and cognitively simplify their world. Moreover, they are hypersensitive to criticism and inordinately concerned about their own needs and perspectives" (p. 16).

Johnston and Roseby (1997) noted that 64% of their sample had personality disorder diagnoses and an additional 27% were found to have personality disorder traits. Men received diagnoses of compulsive, paranoid, avoidant, schizoid, and passive–aggressive disorders, whereas women were diagnosed as dependent, histrionic, or borderline. Fifteen percent of these parents had a diagnosis of an intermittent explosive disorder and 25% had a substance abuse problem (Johnston & Campbell, 1988). Johnston, Campbell, and Tall (1985) described the need for these borderline parents to keep things stirred up, and the obsessive parents as agonizing over small decisions or details; they were rigid, inflexible, and would not consider alternatives. The deficits of both of these sets of parents often led to custody disputes. Despite all of these difficulties, these authors found that prior to the current dispute, these parents were functioning quite well, a factor that did not seem to fit the personality disorder diagnosis. Johnston and Campbell (1988) believed that the custody litigation group was psychologically vulnerable: that is, the postdivorce dispute reawakened unresolved problems and traumas from the parents' pasts.

A narcissistic vulnerability was at the core of these divorcing couples' problems. These parents showed difficulty in maintaining a positive self-image or clear sense of identity. They seemed to utilize the "other" to maintain an inflated sense of self, and to regulate their self-esteem (Johnston & Campbell, 1988). The narcissistic vulnerability ranged from mild (45%) to moderate (36%) to severe (18%). In the mild group, parents felt betrayed and cheated. They showed their anger through their barrage of complaints; they held onto exaggerated views and made demands that far outweighed the reality of the situation. In the moderate group, parents had a grandiose sense of self and feelings of entitlement. Their negative view of their ex-spouse was a projection of their own inadequacy and protected them from seeing themselves as flawed in any way. Requests by the other parent to cooperate were perceived as an irritation. The severe group (18%) formed a paranoid delusion about their ex-spouse, forcing each image of the marriage into their now extremely narrow and toxic view of the other. A reactivation of early traumas, unresolved losses, and the failure to separate and individuate was hypothesized to account for the difficulties that these parents have in resolving the postdivorce custody disputes (Johnston & Campbell, 1988). In her book *Divorce Wars*, Ellis (2000) notes that the most prominent feature of these parents is their use of projection, splitting, and their lack of introspection.

Hoppe and Kenney's (1994) previously unpublished Rorschach data of 180 child custody litigants shows "cognitive simplicity," poor impulse control, and poor problem-solving skills in this group. These parents were needy and demanding, and had unrealistic expectations from their ex-spouses. They reacted to emotionally charged situations with denial, projection of blame, and defensiveness. This group was characterized as utilizing pathological narcissism to defend against intense feelings of inadequacy.

Child custody litigants are prone to distortion on self-report measures such as the MMPI (Bagby, Nicholson, Buis, Radovanovic, & Fidler, 1999; Bathurst, Gottfried, & Gottfried, 1997; Medhoff, 1999; Posthuma & Harper, 1998; Strong, Greene, Hoppe, Johnston, & Olesen, 1999). Given the positive response bias of this group of litigants, significant psychopathology is often absent. However, within normal limit MMPI–2 profiles can be misleading (Graham, 2000). Caldwell (2005) notes that MMPI–2 profiles of both male and female child custody litigants are more deliberately and consciously defensive (*Mp* and *Sd* elevations). He states these litigants are "more repressed and denying; relatively lacking in awareness of how they upset others; more emotionally restrained and constricted; prone to hold resentments and perhaps exceptionally slow to forgive; responsible and self-controlled; high needs (sic) to be in control of everyone's decisions; and prone to role-play an exaggerated amount of virtue as a parent" (p. 109).

As Erard (2005) points out, although other sources of data including clinical interviews and questionnaires are treated in child custody evaluations as "multiple sources," these are, in fact, "monomethod approaches" in that they are all based on self-report. In clinical interviews, these litigant parents may also be prone to positive response bias, as they attempt to minimize or deny problematic components of their history or deny behaviors of which they are accused by their ex-spouse. The Rorschach is uniquely suited to the evaluation of personality characteristics of these litigants because it is less impacted by conscious distortion. Many (e.g., Archer & Krishnamuthry, 1993; Blais, Hilsenroth, Castelbury, Fowler, & Baity, 2001; Ganellen, 1996; Weiner, 1999) have discussed the incremental validity when the MMPI and Rorschach are used jointly and how, when used in conjunction with the MMPI–2, the Rorschach can significantly add data about the psychological functioning of these litigants.

Additionally, the Rorschach is frequently used in custody evaluations (Ackerman & Ackerman, 1997; Bow & Quinnell, 2001). Nearly 44% to 48% of custody evaluators use the Rorschach as part of a multimodal approach to data gathering. It should be noted, however, that the Rorschach is not a test of parenting ability, and it cannot provide information about what parenting time arrangement is in the child's best interest. Personality testing can, however, provide much information about how the personality dynamics of these litigant parents have resulted in their inability to resolve child custody issues without the intervention of the court system.

This chapter utilizes Rorschach data to determine if the personality characteristics described in the literature are valid. Do these parents show character pathology and narcissistic vulnerability or show characteristics that would make resolving postdivorce disputes over custody more challenging? Finally, we believe that readers will find this data to be useful for comparison in forensic practice. Erard (2005) has suggested that comparison of a child custody litigant to a reference sample may shed some light on what is or is not usual for Rorschach protocols administered under such circumstances.

OUR SAMPLE

The sample consists of 728 child custody litigants (CCL). This California sample represents the Los Angeles and San Francisco Bay areas. Ninety-seven percent of our sample is in the 26–55 year old age range. This is an educated group, with at least 38% of the sample having some college or graduate level education. The majority of the sample is Caucasian (60%) and is divided near equally between men and women.

The data were collected through the course of conducting child custody evaluations for the courts over approximately a decade in the 1990s. The protocols were scored utilizing the Rorschach Interpretative Assistance Program–3 (Exner, Weiner, & Par Staff, 1995). Eighty one protocols (10%) were independently recoded. These raters, who were blind to the original scoring, were graduate students supervised by Donald Viglione at his laboratory at Alliant International University, San Diego. An overall 99% agreement was obtained for coding. Data were also analyzed by each data sample to insure consistency among the three data sets. For multicategory coding, percentage of agreement was as follows: *Location* (98%), *Developmental Quality—DQ* (97%), *Human Movement—M* (98%), *Animal Movement—FM* (99%), *Inanimate Movement—m* (98%), *Color* (99%), *Achromatic Color—C'* (100%), *Texture—T* (100%), *Vista—V* (99%), *Shading—Y* (99%), *Reflections* (100%), *Form Quality* (95%), *Z Score* (96%), and *Cognitive Special Scores* (99%). Iota (Janson & Olsson, 2001, 2004; Viglione & Meyer, chap. 2, this vol.) was calculated for all scoring categories. For the four scoring segments (*Location*, *Determinants*, *Contents*, and *Special Scores*), iota ranged from .89 for *Special Scores* to .97 for *Location*. Data were also analyzed, and iota calculated, for each data set to insure that scoring was consistent throughout the three data sets and there were no significant discrepancies between the data sets and the overall sample.

FINDINGS

The following areas are discussed regarding these litigants: Core Characteristics; Problem Solving; Affect, Stress Tolerance, and Control; Self- and Interpersonal Perception, and Cognitive Style, Ideation, Mediation, and Processing. The data that follows shows trends in this sample and future research will be required in order to tie specific variables to case specific questions.

Core Characteristics

Our CCL sample produced a number of responses (R) consistent with the nonpatient (NP) data (Exner & Erdberg, 2005), although our range was slightly greater than the nonpatient group (CCL M = 22.84, SD = 9.07; NP M = 23.36, SD = 5.68). We have used the $F\%$ to look at constriction (Viglione, Meyer, & Exner, 2001), given the skew of Lambda. Some of our sample is rather rigid and constricted (CCL L M = 1.07, SD = 1.31, $F\%$ = .43) in comparison to the nonpatients (NP L M = .58 and SD = .37; $F\%$ = .33). It is the elevated $F\%$ (*Lambda*) that has contributed to a CDI of 4 or 5 in 37% of the CCL sample. Weiner (2003) notes that elevated CDI in conjunction with adequate coping resources suggests difficulties, not so much in psychological competence across many aspects of the individual's life, but rather is indicative of marked deficits in managing interpersonal relationships (CCL, EA M = 6.62; NP, M = 9.37). (See Table 21–1.)

It may also be that the inability of CCLs to permit, process, or work through complex emotions has resulted in their elevated *Lambdas*. The failure of these parents to adequately mourn the loss of the marital relationship and their role as a parent has resulted in their limited capacity to experience affect in a modulated manner and, thus, they must constrict it. Noteworthy is that the difference in the nonpatient EA and the CCL sample EA is almost solely accounted for by the lack of *Sum C* in the CCL protocols as compared to the NP group (CCL *Sum C M* = 3.70 NP *Sum C M* = 5.95). This finding seems to support the notion that it is in the realm of the interpersonal/relational aspects of the divorce that these individuals show impairment. It is not so much a pervasive impairment in coping that results in a large proportion of the CCLs having positive *CDI*, rather, it is the lower R and high *Lambda* variables that contribute to elevated *CDIs*.

Problem-Solving Style

The Rorschach scores of these litigants are clearly reflective of the problem-solving deficits that have been noted for these parents. Only 10% of our sample had an adaptive problem-solving style, as compared to 69% of nonpatients (Exner, 2005). The remaining 90% are *Ambitents* (CCL = 48%; NP = 18%), *Superintroversives* (CCL = 28%; NP = 6%), or *Superextratensives* (CCL = 14%; NP = 4%). What might this mean in terms of the ability of this group to negotiate custody issues? For the 48% of our sample who are *Ambitents*, the problem-solving style is one of maladaptive inconsistency. "I thought we had an agreement, but we do not," or "I have changed my mind." These individuals have inconsistent coping efforts, unpredictable behavior, and an uncertain self-image. They have difficulty making decisions, and use varying but inconsistent problem-solving methods. They can be highly unpredictable and variable in their approach to even similar circumstances.

The *Superintroversives* (CCL = 28%) have an excessive and maladaptive preference for dealing with experience primarily through ideation. They fail to give their emotions their due. And whereas M is adaptive when it is active, of good form quality, and represents whole human figures, this is not the case in our group. Twenty-four percent of our sample also had $Mp > Ma$, suggesting that they use fantasy versus constructive problem solving. They do not think through what they should or should not do, but imagine instead how others, or external events, will solve problems for them. This *Superintroversive* sample is ruminative and seldom takes feelings and intuition into consideration. They do

TABLE 21–1

Child Custody Litigant Sample (*N* = 728) Group Mean and Frequencies for Select Ratios,
Percentages, and Derivations

R = 22.78 (*SD* = 9.15)	*L* = 1.06 (*SD* = 1.31)

EB: 3.69: 2.93   *EA* = 6.62 (*SD* = 3.81)

   eb = 4.98: 2.47   *es* = 8.71 (*SD* = 5.41) (*FM+ m < Sum Shading*............... 214   29%)

   D Score = –0.63 (*SD* = 1.48)   *AdjD* = –0.15 (*SD* = 1.17)

EB style

   Introversive........................ 43   6%

   Pervasive Introversive..... 200   28%

   Ambitent........................... 349   48%

   Extratensive...................... 28   4%

   Pervasive Extratensive.... 108   15%

   Avoidant........................... 266   37%

EA–es differences:D scores

   D score > 0......................... 91   13%

   D score = 0....................... 347   48%

   D score < 0...................... 290   40%

   D score < –1.................... 150   21%

   AdjD score > 0................. 140   19%

   AdjD score = 0................. 401   55%

   AdjD score < 0................. 187   26%

   AdjD score < –1................. 72   10%

Affect

   FC:CF + C = 1.86 : 1.84   (*Pure C > 0* = 136, 19%; *Pure C > 1* = 56, 8%)

   Pure C = .37 (*SD* = .72)

   FC > (CF + C) + 2.............. 0   0%

   FC > (CF + C) + 1......... 178   25%

   (CF + C) > FC + 1........... 78   11%

   (CF + C) > FC + 2........... 94   13%

   SumC' = .91 (*SD* = 1.15)   *SumV* = .31 (*SD* = .67)   *SumY* = .80 (*SD* = 1.14)

   Afr = .51 (*SD* = .21)   (*Afr < .40* = 215, 30%; *Afr < .50* = 378, 52%)

   S = 2.25 (*SD* = 2.19)   (*S > 2* = 262, 36%)

   Blends:R = 3.71 : 22.78

   CP = .03 (*SD* = .18)

Interpersonal

   COP = 1.18 (*SD* = 1.33)   (*COP* = 0 = 278, 38%; *COP > 2* = 113, 16%)

   AG = .33 (*SD* = .72)   (*AG* = 0 = 563, 77%; *AG > 2* = 17, 2%)

   Food = .43 (*SD* = .73)

   Isolate/R = .18 (*SD* = .14)

   H:(H)+Hd+(Hd) = 2.56 : 2.95   (*H* = 0 = 82, 11%; *H < 2* = 162, 22%)

   (H)+(Hd):(A)+(Ad) = 1.59 : .63

   H+A:Hd+Ad = 11.25:3.45

   Sum T = .44 (*SD* = .64)   (*T* = 0 = 373, 51%; *T > 1* = 134, 18%)

   GHR = 3.16 (*SD* = 2.01)

   PHR = 3.19 (*SD* = 2.97)   GHR > PHR = 343, 47%

Self-perception

$3r+(2)/R = .30\ (SD = .13)$ $(3r+(2)/R < .33 = 302, 42\%;\ 3r+(2)/R > .44 = 222, 31\%)$

$Fr + rF = .55\ (SD = 1.06)$ $(Fr + rF > 0 = 226, 31\%)$

$FD = .61\ (SD = .92)$

$An+Xy = 1.54$

$MOR = .84\ (SD = 1.29)$ $(MOR > 2 = 69, 10\%)$

Ideation

$a:p = 6.83: 2.89$ $(p > a+1 = 94, 13\%)$

$Ma:Mp = 2.49: 1.23$ $(Mp > Ma = 169, 23\%)$

$M = 3.69\ (SD = 2.72)$ $(M- = .91\ SD = 1.37;\ M\ none = .03, SD = .23)$

$FM = 3.31\ (SD = 2.51)$ $m = 1.67\ (SD = 1.65)$

$2AB+Art+Ay = 2.18\ (SD = 2.80)$ $2AB+Art+Ay > 5 = 28, 4\%$

$Sum6 = 4.32\ (SD = 4.06)$ $WSum6 = 14.69\ (SD = 16.70)$

$Level\ 2\ Sp\ Sc = .88\ (SD = 1.54)$ $(Level\ 2\ Special\ Scores > 0 = 291, 40\%)$

Mediation

$Populars = 4.93\ (SD = 1.78)$ $(P < 4 = 151, 21\%;\ P > 7 = 56, 8\%)$

$XA\% = .73\ (SD = .13)$

$WDA\% = .77\ (SD = .12)$

$X+\% = .51\ (SD = .13)$

$X-\% = .26\ (SD = .12)$

$Xu\% = .21\ (SD = .10)$

$S- = .16\ (SD = .21)$

$XA\% > .89$	2	.3%	
$XA\% < .70$	668	92%	$(X+\% < .61 = 572, 79\%)$
$WDA\% < .85$	506	70%	$(X+\% < .50 = 319, 44\%)$
$WDA\% < .75$	298	41%	
$X+\% < .50$	319	44%	
$Xu\% > .20$	375	52%	
$X-\% > .20$	469	64%	
$X-\% > .30$	238	33%	

Processing

$Zf = 12.25\ (SD = 5.14)$

$Zd = -2.06\ (SD = 5.07)$ $(Zd > +3.0 = 105, 14\%;\ Zd < -3.0 = 279, 38\%)$

$W:D:Dd = 9.73:9.88:3.15$ $(Dd > 3 = 232, 32\%)$

$W:M = 9.73: 3.69$

$DQ+ = 5.82\ (SD = 3.86)$

$DQv = 1.54\ (SD = 1.85)$ $(DQv > 2 = 202, 28\%)$

Constellations

$PTI = 5$	22	3%	$DEPI = 7$	14	2%	$CDI = 5$	73	10%
$PTI = 4$	48	7%	$DEPI = 6$	62	9%	$CDI = 4$	201	28%
$PTI = 3$	107	15%	$DEPI = 5$	122	17%			

$SCZI = 6$	33	5%
$SCZI = 5$	48	7%
$SCZI = 4$	120	17%

S-Constellation Positive...... 5 1%

HVI Positive.................... 181 25%

OBS Positive........................ 2 0%

not take steps toward resolution, have difficulty dealing with emotionally arousing situations, and become overwhelmed and disorganized when confronted with intensely emotional issues.

The *Superextratensives* (CCL = 14%) are highly expressive and action oriented. They rarely contemplate their decisions. They solve problems in a trial-and-error method, make decisions based on instinct and intuition, and may have difficulty with delay between feelings and actions. Chances are that, in any given custody dispute, we have two parents who both have maladaptive styles of solving problems.

Additionally, these parents have more PERs (CCL $M = 1.90$, $SD = 2.24$; NP $M = .99$, $SD = 1.10$) and more PSV than the nonpatient group (CCL $M = .51$, $SD = .92$ vs. NP $M = .12$, $SD = .22$). This only adds to the already rigid and defensive approach that these parents take toward each other.

Weiner (2003) has differentiated between three kinds of PER responses: Self-Justifying, also labeled Inadequate (Gacono & Meloy, 1994; Gacono, Meloy, & Heaven, 1990); Self-Aggrandizing, also identified as Omnipotent (Gacono & Meloy, 1994; Gacono et al., 1990); and Self-Revealing. Although we have not done a formal analysis of the entire sample in this regard, it does appear that the PER of our group are primarily the former two types. The Self-Justifying PER is primarily defensive. These individuals are trying to minimize the report of an inaccurate impression or appear to lack a good reason for having reported it. The group that gives these kinds of PER responses is insecure, lacks confidence in their capacity and judgment, and defends against the anxiety of their uncertainty by letting others know the basis of their actions and opinions. The second kind of PER, most likely occurring in the narcissistic subset of this sample, is the Self-Aggrandizing PER. This response is given by those that are trying to impress others but have an overpowering, self-focused, know-it-all attitude that may make it impossible for others to hear them. In the CCL group, these individuals have a "not invented here" attitude. If they did not think of it themselves, then it must not be a good idea, making compromise or solutions offered by the other parent nearly impossible to accept. The third kind of PER, the self-revealing, has the most positive implications for treatment and relationships. These individuals have a genuine interest in sharing. Unfortunately few, if any, of our sample showed this kind of response.

Affect, Stress Tolerance, and Self-Control

The psychological resources available to the CCL group are limited by their somewhat constricted and possibly defensive protocols. Both in their capacity to think through problems and in their ability to engage others in effective problem solving, the CCL group has less to draw from than nonpatients (CCL M $M = 3.74$; $SD = 2.79$; NP $M = 4.83$; $SD = 2.18$) (CCL *WsumC* – $M = 2.97$; $SD = 2.52$; NP $M = 4.54$; $SD = 1.98$). Additionally, CCLs appear to be under stress both situationally and chronically. Almost 40% of our sample has a D score < 0; and 25% of the sample have *AdjD* scores < 0. Compare this to nonpatients with D score $< 0 = 17\%$ and $AdjD < 0 = 10\%$. The D scores suggest difficulties with frustration tolerance and impulse control in some of our sample. The D score may indicate a mild degree of distress that is likely to be experienced more intensely in unstructured settings. It may be that this group is unable to negotiate the necessary changes to the postdivorce family due to their somewhat limited resources, their inability to acknowledge painful affect and their intense, yet unmodulated, experience of emotion. The CCL group seems, however, to have difficulty in experiencing their own distress, preferring instead to deny or project it. The negative D score also seems to identify a susceptibility to episodic losses of self-control. Twenty-five percent of our sample may have long-standing difficulties in adjustment ($AdjD$), which may preclude resolution at any stage short of a trial. Although we have a constricted sample ($L > .99 = 37\%$), we also find that the $FC: CF + C$ is closer to 1:1 vs. 2:1 found in nonpatients (Exner & Erdberg, 2005). Additionally, almost 19% of the CCLs had one $Pure\ C$ and 8% had more than 1 $Pure\ C$. Thus, when these parents do express affect, they do so in an immature, overly intense, and impulsive manner. Despite all the apparent affect, these parents do not want to process their feelings (CCL $Afr < .50$ in 52%). But, it is also likely that the combination of strong feelings, coupled with an inability or unwillingness to express them, contributes to difficulties these parents have in communicating with each other. When problems tolerating and integrating affect are coupled with impaired problem-solving skills, communication and negotiation is nearly impossible.

Self-Perception and Object Relationships

Seventy-two percent of our sample are either self-absorbed or compare themselves negatively to others. The self-absorption seen in this group takes the form of a rather self-centered, selfish, and self-serving stance. Nearly one third (31%) of these parents have one or more reflection responses (CCL $Fr + rF > 0$, 31%; NP $Fr + rF > 0$, 12%). Their own needs come before the needs of others. Unable to be accountable for their own behavior, they externalize responsibility for failure, deny shortcomings in themselves, and blame problems on other's actions or events that are outside of their control. They feel superior and entitled. Weiner (2003) also distinguishes between the nice versus the nasty narcissists. Those described as nasty are angry and avoidant, lack a genuine interest in others, do not have close attachments, and prefer emotional distance. They are competitive versus collaborative, often manipulating others to get their own needs met. Thirty-one percent of the CCL have $EgoC > .44$ and may be described like those who have one or more $Reflection$ responses. However, those with a high $EgoC$ and no $Reflection$ responses seem to have an underlying depressive component. That is, they may pay a lot of attention to themselves, but do not really like what they see or enjoy it much. The underbelly of this elevation in $EgoC$ may also be a sense of inadequacy and devaluation of their sense of self that is then projected into the ex-spouse. Forty-two percent of the CCLs have a low estimate of their personal worth, comparing themselves negatively to others (CCL $EgoC < .33 = 42\%$; NP $EgoC < .33 = 20\%$). This may be most severely felt in the 27% of CCLs who have a positive $DEPI$ and is consistent with the depressive characteristics observed in this group (Wallerstein & Kelly, 1980).

Finally, *FD* is lacking in the CCLs (CCL *M* = .61; NP *M* = 1.43). It appears that the inability of child custody litigants to reflect on their behavior is one aspect of the problem in resolution of these conflicts. It may also reflect the parents' inability to understand how to meet their own needs while at the same time being sensitive to the impact of their behavior on others.

In the area of object relations and perception, CCLs show a poor capacity to utilize the resources that they have for thinking through problems. Not only is there distortion in their capacity for empathy (CCL, *M* – = .91; NP *M* –= .23), but also difficulty in effective problem solving (*Mp* > *Ma* in 23%). Additionally, they show problematic object relations. A limited capacity for engagement may result in the deficits in effectively resolving conflicts with the ex-spouse, and stems from the kinds of difficulties with identification Weiner (2003) describes or is consistent with Johnston and Campbell's (1988) notion of this sample showing a reactivation to early trauma. In considering the human responses, 22% had *H* < 2 with 11% having no *H* responses in their protocols (NP *H* < 2 = 12%; *H* = 0 1%). Their *H: (H) + Hd + (Hd)* (2.56: 2.95) may reflect an unstable sense of self and the use of splitting.

The CCL group has less *COP* and *AG* than nonpatients (CCL, *COP M* = 1.18; *AG M* = .33; NP, *COP M* = 2.07; *Ag M* = .89). This appears consistent with difficulties working collaboratively with others. It may also suggest an inability to symbolically work through their aggression, thus needing to bring it into their relationships. Almost 40% of CCLs (NP = 11%) had no *COP*. Certainly this describes one of the core difficulties of this sample. *COP* responses suggest an interest in engaging with other collaboratively (Weiner, 2003). As Weiner (2003) notes, "The absence of COP, by contrast, identifies a maladaptive deficiency in the capacity to anticipate and engage in collaborative activities with others" (p. 169). Additionally, the low mean *AG* scores are not inconsistent with other more antisocial groups (Gacono & Meloy, 1994) and may suggest for the 77% of the CCLs who have no *AG*, an inability to channel, contain, or sublimate their aggression within the context of the custody dispute. When taken in combination, the lack of *AG* and the limited number of *COP* responses is consistent with the inability of this group to cooperatively work out difficulties.

Whereas *T* = 0 is present in 50% of our sample, we are not certain what this means, or if it effects the 24% of the parents that have a positive *HVI*. Despite the questions that have been raised about how normative *T* = 0 is (Exner & Erdberg, 2005; Erdberg & Shaffer, 1999; Shaffer, Erdberg, & Haroian, 1999), it is our clinical impression, along with that of other researchers, that some of these litigants are quite vigilant. Additionally, a slight elevation in Scale 6 on the MMPI–2 has been noted in this group (Bagby et al., 1999; Bathurst et al., 1997). Whereas half of the child custody sample has *T* = 0, 18% of the group has *T* > 1, suggesting either a situationally related dependency or individuals who feel chronically interpersonally deprived.

Is the positive *HVI* situational or a chronic state that describes an individual who perceives potential danger or threat in their environment? This can only be determined by a thorough review of the history and other test data. It is our clinical experience, however, that profound issues of trust often fuel the intractable custody disputes.

Cognitive Style, Ideation, Mediation, and Processing

Although few in the CCL group showed any kind of serious psychiatric disorder, 24% of the sample has a *PTI* $\geq$ 3 (*SCZI* $\geq$ 4, 26%) and 10% has a PTI $\geq$ 5 (*SCZI* $\geq$ 5, 12%). This seems to reflect the impaired reality testing, distortions in perceptions of others, and the introceptive/extroceptive or affectively charged boundary problems in this group. The mean *X–%* of our sample is .26. This is higher than all nonpatient (Exner & Erdberg, 2005) and international samples (Erdberg & Shaffer, 1999) and occurs in 64% of the CCLs. Additionally, 32% of CCLs have an *X–%* > .30.

Although 39% of the sample has *Level 2 special scores*, this seems to consist primarily of *INCOM2* and *DR2*. The child custody litigant group also has an elevated number of *ALOGS*. These kinds of boundary and thinking deficits suggest affectively charged, illogical thinking in these parents. The Level 2 *INCOM*s are, however, the more worrisome finding. Meloy and Singer (1991) noted that the merging of two components into one object may be a more pathological finding than two objects inappropriately combined (*FABCOM*). Our group has a lower mean number of *INCOM2*s than Exner's character disordered sample, but our mean *WSum6* is 14.93, two times higher than other nonpatients (NP, *WSum6 M* = 7.12). The elevated *DR* in our sample suggests a misattribution of affective states and is consistent with the projection that often occurs in this group of litigants (CCL *DR2 M* = .35;NP *DR2 M* = .03).

Male and Female Samples

There was a slight difference in demographic data of the male (*N* = 360) and female (*N* = 368) samples (Males: Age *M* = 40.62, Education *M* = 16.14 years; Females: Age *M* = 37.51 Education = *M* 14.76 years), and some Rorschach variables differed as well (see Tables 21–2 and 21–3). However, in comparison to other samples in which male and female populations are compared (Gacono & Meloy, 1994), the differences are minimal.

Male litigants appear to experience more situational and long-term stress (Male *D* < 0 43%, *AdjD* < 0 28%; Female *D* < 0 37%, *AdjD* < 0 23%). Men seem to jump to conclusions without considering all sources of data more frequently than women (Male *Zd* < –3.0 = 42%, Female *Zd* < –3.0 = 35%). One measure of capacity for relatedness also seems to differ with men showing more of a constricted approach to interpersonal relationships and women showing more intense desire for connectedness (Male *T* = 0 54%; *T* >1 14%; Women *T* = 0 48%, *T* > 1 22%); however, women may appear more anxious and less need driven (Male *FM* + *m* < *Sum Shading* 25%, *FM* + *m* => *Sum Shading* 75%; Female *FM* + *m* < *Sum Shading* 34%, *FM* + *m* => *Sum Shading* 66%). Finally, men appear more passive in their ideation, whereas women are more likely to be active when they do attempt to solve problems through their own internal process (Male *Mp* > *Ma* 26% and *Mp* <= *Ma* 74%; Women *Mp* > *Ma* 20% and *Mp* <= *Ma* 80%).

In evaluating the conflict between parents in any specific case, it is important to examine the dynamic interplay between the personality characteristics of each pair of parents in order to determine what results in their inability to resolve divorce-related impasses.

TABLE 21–2

Male Child Custody Litigant Sample (*N* = 360) Group Mean and Frequencies for Select Ratios, Percentages, and Derivations

R = 23.34 (*SD* = 9.80)	*L* = 1.10 (*SD* = 1.42)

EB: 3.60: 2.85   *EA* = 6.45 (*SD* = 3.98)

   eb = 5.23: 2.35   *es* = 8.77 (*SD* = 5.47) (*FM+m* < *Sum Shading*........... 214   29%)

   D Score = –0.70 (*SD* = 1.41)   *AdjD* = –0.21 (*SD* = 1.15)

EB Style

   Introversive........................ 22   6%

   Pervasive Introversive....... 99   28%

   Ambitent........................... 170   47%

   Extratensive....................... 13   4%

   Pervasive Extratensive...... 56   16%

   Avoidant........................... 134   37%

EA–es differences:D scores

   D score > 0.......................... 42   12%

   D score = 0........................ 163   45%

   D score < 0....................... 155   43%

   D score < –1....................... 87   24%

   AdjD score > 0................... 64   18%

   AdjD score = 0................. 195   54%

   AdjD score < 0................. 101   28%

   AdjD score < –1................. 44   12%

Affect

   FC:CF + C = 1.86 : 1.75   (*Pure C* > 0 = 62 17%; *Pure C* > 1 = 33, 9%)

   Pure C = .38 (*SD* = .72)

   FC > (*CF* + *C*) + 1............ 89   25%

   (*CF* + *C*) > *FC* + 1............ 36   10%

   (*CF* + *C*) > *FC* + 2............ 41   11%

   SumC' = .88   (*SD* = 1.20)   *SumV* = .34   (*SD* = .75)   *SumY* = .73   (*SD* = 1.02)

   Afr = .51 (*SD* = .21)   (*Afr* < .40 = 106, 29%; *Afr* < .50 = 89, 25%)

   S = 2.39 (*SD* = 2.34)   (*S* > 2 = 137, 38%)

   Blends:R = 3.61:23.34

   CP = .03 (*SD* = .18)

Interpersonal

   COP = 1.08 (*SD* = 1.25)   (*COP* = 0 = 149, 41%; *COP* > 2 = 48, 13%)

   AG = .38 (*SD* = .80)   (*AG* = 0 = 270, 75%; *AG* > 2 = 12, 3%)

   Food = .48 (*SD* = .79)

   Isolate/R = .20 (SD = .15)

   H:(H)+Hd+(Hd) = 2.43 : 2.96

   (H)+(Hd):(A)+(Ad) = 1.60 : .71

   H+A:Hd+Ad = 11.27:3.55

   Sum T = .39 (*SD* = .59)   (*T* = 0 = 195, 54%; *T* > 1 = 52, 14%)

   GHR = 3.06 (*SD* = 2.03)

   PHR = 3.17 (*SD* = 3.18)   *GHR* > *PHR* = 168, 47%

Self-perception

$3r+(2)/R$ = .30 $(SD = .12$) $(3r+(2)/R < .33 = 146, 41\%\ 3r+(2)/R > .44 = 107, 30\%)$

$Fr + rF$ = .61 $(SD = 1.18)$ $(Fr + rF > 0 = 118, 33\%)$

FD = .70 $(SD = .96)$

$An+Xy$ = 1.38

MOR = .88 $(SD = 1.20)$ $(MOR > 2 = 41, 11\%)$

Ideation

a:p = 6.87: 3.04 $(p > a+1 = 51, 14\%)$

Ma:Mp = 2.38: 1.25 $(Mp > Ma = 94, 26\%)$

M = 3.60 $(SD = 2.92)$ $(M-$ = .88, $SD = 1.37$; M none = .02, $SD = .14)$

FM = 3.50 $(SD = 2.68$) m = 1.73 $(SD = 1.66)$

$2AB+Art+Ay$ = 2.10 $2AB+Art+Ay > 5 = 16, 4\%$
$(SD = 2.80)$

$Sum6$ = 4.13 $(SD = 3.97)$ $WSum6$ = 14.10 $(SD = 15.50)$

$Level\ 2\ Sp\ Sc$ = .85 $(SD = 1.45)$ $(Level\ 2\ Special\ Scores > 0 = 144, 40\%)$

Mediation

$Populars$ = 5.02 $(SD = 1.81)$ $(P < 4 = 74, 21\%; P > 7 = 31, 9\%)$

$XA\%$ = .74 $(SD = .12)$

$WDA\%$ = .77 $(SD = .12)$

$X+\%$ = .52 $(SD = .13)$

$X-\%$ = .25 $(SD = .12)$

$Xu\%$ = .22 $(SD = .10)$

$S-$ = .17 $(SD = .22)$

$XA\% > .89$	26	7%
$XA\% < .70$	131	36%
$WDA\% < .85$	105	29%
$WDA\% < .75$	140	39%
$X+\% < .55$	211	59%
$Xu\% > .20$	189	53%
$X-\% > .20$	113	31%
$X-\% > .30$	111	31%

Processing

Zf = 12.44 $(SD = 5.34)$

Zd = –2.59 $(SD = 4.97)$ $(Zd > +3.0 = 46, 13\%; Zd < –3.0 = 150, 42\%)$

W:D:Dd = 9.77:10.31:3.22 $(Dd > 3 = 115, 32\%)$

W:M = 9.77: 3.60

$DQ+$ = 5.83 $(SD = 4.10)$

DQv = 1.64 $(SD = 1.90)$ $(DQv > 2 = 105, 29\%)$

Constellations

PTI = 5	9	3%	$DEPI$ = 7	6	2%	CDI = 5	47	13%	$SCZI$ = 6	13	4%
PTI = 4	21	6%	$DEPI$ = 6	28	8%	CDI = 4	107	30%	$SCZI$ = 5	23	6%
PTI = 3	50	14%	$DEPI$ = 5	60	17%				$SCZI$ = 4	52	14%

S-Constellation Positive...... 2   1%

HVI Positive......................97   27%

OBS Positive........................2   1%

TABLE 21–3

Female Child Custody Litigant Sample (*N* = 368) Group Mean and Frequencies for Select Ratios, Percentages, and Derivations

R = 22.23 (*SD* = 8.45)	*L* = 1.02 (*SD* = 1.19)

EB: 3.77: .3.02   *EA* = 6.79 (*SD* = 3.63)

    eb = 4.73: 2.58   *es* = 8.66 (*SD* = 5.36) (*FM+m < Sum Shading*......... 125   34%)

    D Score = –0.55 (*SD* = 1.54)   *AdjD* = –0.08 (*SD* = 1.19)

EB style

    Introversive......................... 21   6%

    Pervasive Introversive...... 101   27%

    Ambient........................... 179   49%

    Extratensive........................ 15   4%

    Pervasive Extratensive....... 52   14%

    Avoidant........................... 132   36%

EA–es differences:D scores

    D score > 0......................... 49   13%

    D score = 0....................... 184   50%

    D score < 0....................... 135   37%

    D score < –1....................... 63   17%

    AdjD score > 0.................. 76   21%

    AdjD score = 0................ 206   56%

    AdjD score < 0.................. 86   23%

    AdjD score < –1................ 28   8%

Affect

    FC:CF + C = 1.87 : 1.93   (*Pure C > 0* = 74, 20%; *Pure C > 1* = 23, 6%)

    Pure C = .36 (*SD* = .71)

    FC > (CF + C) + 1............. 89   24%

    (CF + C) > FC + 1............. 42   11%

    (CF + C) > FC + 2............. 53   14%

    SumC' = .94   (*SD* = 1.11)   *SumV* = .28   (*SD* = .59)   *SumY* = .87   (*SD* = 1.25)

    Afr = .52 (*SD* = .22)   (*Afr < .40* = 109, 30%)

    S = 2.12 (*SD* = 2.02)   (*S > 2* = 125, 34%)

    Blends:R = 3.82 : 22.23

    CP = .03 (*SD* = .19)

Interpersonal

    COP = 1.29 (*SD* = 1.41)   (*COP* = 0 = 129, 35%; *COP > 2* = 65, 18%)

    AG = .28 (*SD* = .63)   (*AG* = 0 = 293, 80%; *AG > 2* = 5, 1%)

    Food = .38 (*SD* = .66)

    Isolate/R = .17 (*SD* = .13)

    H:(H)+Hd+(Hd) = 2.68 : 2.93   (*H* = 0 = 34, 9%; *H < 2* = 76, 21%)

    (H)+(Hd):(A)+(Ad) = 1.57 : .55

    H+A:Hd+Ad = 11.22:3.35

    Sum T = .49 (*SD* = .68)   (*T* = 0 = 178, 48%; *T > 1* = 82, 22%)

    GHR = 3.25 (*SD* = 1.98)

    PHR = 3.21 (*SD* = 2.76)   *GHR > PHR* = 175, 48%

Self-perception

$3r+(2)/R = .31$ $(SD = .13$) $(3r+(2)/R < .33 = 156, 42\%$ $3r+(2)/R > .44 = 115, 31\%)$

$Fr + rF = .48$ $(SD = .92)$ $(Fr + rF > 0 = 108, 29\%)$

$FD = .52$ $(SD = .88)$

$An+Xy = 1.71$

$MOR = .80$ $(SD = 1.38)$ $(MOR > 2 = 28, 8\%)$

Ideation

$a{:}p = 6.80{:} 2.75$ $(p > a+1 = 43, 12\%)$

$Ma{:}Mp = 2.59{:} 1.21$ $(Mp > Ma = 75, 20\%)$

$M = 3.77$ $(SD = 2.51)$ $(M\text{-} = .93, SD = 1.37; M none = .03, SD = .29)$

$FM = 3.11$ $(SD = 2.31$) $m = 1.62$ $(SD = 1.64)$

$2AB+Art+Ay = 2.27$ $(SD = 2.80)$ $2AB+Art+Ay > 5 = 12, 3\%$

$Sum6 = 4.51$ $(SD = 4.15)$ $WSum6 = 15.79$ $(SD = 17.79)$

$Level\ 2\ Sp\ Sc = .90$ $(SD = 1.63)$ $(Level\ 2\ Special\ Scores > 0 = 147, 40\%)$

Mediation

$Populars = 4.85$ $(SD = 1.75)$ $(P < 4 = 77, 21\%; P > 7 = 25, 7\%)$

$XA\% = .72$ $(SD = .13)$

$WDA\% = .76$ $(SD = .13)$

$X + \% = .51$ $(SD = .13)$

$X - \% = .26$ $(SD = .13)$

$Xu\% = .21$ $(SD = .10)$

$S\text{-} = .16$ $(SD = .21)$

$XA\% > .89$	29	8%
$XA\% < .70$	146	40%
$WDA\% < .85$	103	28%
$WDA\% < .75$	158	43%
$X + \% < .55$	223	61%
$Xu\% > .20$	186	51%
$X\text{-} \% > .20$	118	32%
$X - \% > .30$	127	35%

Processing

$Zf = 12.07$ $(SD = 4.95)$

$Zd = -1.55$ $(SD = 5.12$ $(Zd > +3.0 = 59, 16\%; Zd < -3.0 = 129, 35\%)$

$W{:}D{:}Dd = 9.70{:}9.46{:}3.07$ $(Dd > 3 = 117, 32\%)$

$W{:}M = 9.70{:} 3.77$

$DQ+ = 5.82$ $(SD = 3.62)$

$DQv = 1.45$ $(SD = 1.79)$ $(DQv > 2 = 97, 26\%)$

Constellations

$PTI = 5$	13	4%	$DEPI = 7$	8	2%	$CDI = 5$	26	7%	$SCZI = 6$	20	5%
$PTI = 4$	27	7%	$DEPI = 6$	34	9%	$CDI = 4$	94	26%	$SCZI = 5$	25	7%
$PTI = 3$	57	15%	$DEPI = 5$	62	17%				$SCZI = 4$	68	18%

S-Constellation Positive 3 1%

HVI Positive 84 23%

OBS Positive 0 0%

Traits and dynamics must be examined in relationship to the ex-spouse to understand fully how the conflict has developed and how specific interventions can be crafted.

Summary

Our group of child custody litigants' personality functioning, as reflected in their Rorschach protocols, is in many ways consistent with the clinical description of this population. They show marked deficits in managing interpersonal conflict; problematic ability to modulate, control,and tolerate their own affective experience; and difficulties engaging collaboratively in problem solving. Their emotional constriction may be a function of the difficulties that they have in processing complex affective states and leads to a defensive and constricted posture. Additionally, deficits in coping are primarily the result of their inability to engage with others emotionally and the difficulties these litigants have in processing complex feelings associated with the divorce.

The problem-solving deficits evidenced by this group seem to help explain why these parents are unable to keep their custody disputes outside the courtroom. Only 10% of our sample has an adaptive problem-solving style. Defensiveness, self-focus, a lack of capacity for empathy, and a distortion of others' motives characterize the thinking of the custody sample. Their distorted perceptions of the other parent, when added to their cognitive rigidity, result in a poor capacity to compromise or consider the other's perspective, leading to an ineffective resolution of custody issues and a lack of ability to engage cooperatively for the sake of their children. Self-perception in this group is also problematic. Parents either defend against a sense of inadequacy or they are self-absorbed and self-serving, unable in either case to take responsibility for their actions and projecting blame onto the other to protect their somewhat fragile sense of self. Because they are unable to reflect on their behavior and feel they must protect themselves against attack, change in treatment is often slow. Most importantly, therapists who help these families must understand the pull toward taking a side and aligning with the negative perception of the other parent, rather than constructively working on how to manage the relationship for the sake of the children.

Profound issues of trust color the views of these litigants, who have great difficulty experiencing their own losses and instead project their feelings outward. Additionally, the affectively charged boundary problems lead some of this group to try to align others with their views, including their own children. The distortions in reality testing and disturbances in thinking seem to reflect the deficits in managing affective responses that predominate the thought process of child custody litigants. These trends in the data can be compared to individual cases to elucidate areas of conflict and to develop treatment recommendations.

DIRECTIONS FOR FUTURE RORSCHACH RESEARCH

There is no doubt that the examination of Rorschach variables as it relates to child custody is a complex task. In keeping with Gacono and Meloy's (1994) groundbreaking work with antisocial and psychopathic populations and their recommendation for specific forensic Rorschach data sets, this chapter represents an important beginning in the process of understanding Rorschach base rates for the child custody population. Although this chapter marks the first published data set, any advance in research brings with it new questions and areas of exploration. The following are four areas that are important for the development of the forensic use of the Rorschach in child custody evaluations.

First, the most recent study of alienated children (Johnston, Walters, & Olesen, 2005) illustrates the ways in which the interaction of multiple variables must be utilized to understand how these cases develop. Not surprisingly, these children show deficits in perception, information processing, and psychological resources, impaired coping styles, and problems in appropriate expression and modulation of affect. Personality factors of parents are another influence that accounts for the outcome for these children. When evaluating families in the midst of a custody dispute, one must consider the dynamic interplay of parents' personality functioning and the child's psychological vulnerabilities. To this end, utilizing the Rorschach to examine pairs of parent protocols, and considering variables that in combination may lead to conflict, will be valuable (see Finn, 2002; Handler, 1997). As an example, the depressed and constricted victim of psychological abuse may be unable to negotiate with the seemingly calm, although narcissistic, spouse and it is through viewing the Rorschach of these kinds of couples in pairs that the data makes more sense. Additionally, comparing Rorschach protocols of parents who undergo child custody evaluations to those who do not may shed some light on the characteristics that distinguish the small percentage of couples who cannot resolve disputes about custody from those who can.

Second, Ganellen (chap. 5, this vol.) clearly points out that examining defensiveness and response style is critical in psycholegal evaluations. It has been an area of research with the MMPI–2 and child custody litigants (Bathurst et al., 1997; Bagby et al., 1999; Posthuma & Harper, 1998; Medhoff, 1999; Strong et al., 1999) and has been looked at in other forensic groups (Bannatyne, Gacono, & Greene, 1999). Examining response style and how it affects variables of the structural summary (Meyer & Viglione, 2006) will be important in determining the expected long-term consequences from a given Rorschach protocol for a parent involved in litigation around custody.

In particular, it will be helpful to evaluate constricted protocols (high *Lambda*, low *R*) to determine if this is a function of an avoidant coping style or defensiveness. The relationship between *Lambda* and the number of responses (*R*), and their impact on the variables in the structural summary, continues to be an area of research that may prove to be quite fruitful for the interpretation of protocols from child custody litigants. When response style was first considered an important variable in interpreting protocols, Exner (1991) discussed the effect of high *Lambda* protocols on a number of variables from the Structural Summary. More recently, Meyer and Viglione (2006) demonstrated ways in which examining high and low *R* protocols with high and low *Lambda* affected structural summary variables. Response engagement (Meyer, 1992) and complexity (Viglione & Meyer, 1998) are important variables that must be considered in interpreting the values in the structural summary and this is particularly true in forensic populations.

Further, in the case of *Avoidant* styles, it may help to determine interventions that may be useful in resolving custody issues. In the alternative, for defensive parents, it will be helpful to evaluate the degree to which this style is specific to the forensic case or more long-standing character issues, which will make them less capable of gaining from the input of others. Comparing constricted versus nonconstricted Rorschach protocols to other case characteristics and the ultimate outcome of the case will require long-term follow-up with these families.

Third, Johnston and Campbell (1988) described the narcissistic vulnerability of high conflict custody parents ranging from mild (45%), to moderate (36%), to severe (18%) and further noted the impact of narcissistic style on dispute resolution and on the post-divorce adjustment of children. Development of Rorschach data sets based on degree of narcissistic vulnerability may also be a useful direction in providing a more nuanced view of these parents. It may be valuable to determine if our group of litigants with *Reflection* responses in their protocols also has the paranoid core that has been observed clinically in this population.

Finally, as our sample is only from California, it will be useful to obtain protocols from other geographical areas to determine if there are regional differences or if our data is applicable to other parts of the country. Research by Schaffer et al. (1999) showed significant differences from Exner's published nonpatient norms. Their use of a sample only from California was discussed as one of the possible variables to account for these differences and, by extension, raises the question about the representativeness of our current sample.

ACKNOWLEDGMENT

The authors would like to thank Roger Greene for his assistance in analyzing this data set.

REFERENCES

Ackerman, M. J., & Ackerman, M. C. (1997). Custody evaluation practices: A survey of experienced professionals (revisited). *Professional Psychology: Research and Practice, 28*, 137–145.

Archer, R.A., & Krishnamuthry, R. (1993). A review of MMPI and Rorschach interrelationships in adult samples. *Journal of Personality Assessment, 61*, 277–293.

Bagby, R. M., Nicholson, R. A., Buis, T., Radovanovic, H., & Fidler, B. J. (1999). Defensive responding on the MMPI–2 in family custody and access evaluations. *Psychological Assessment, 11*, 24–48.

Bannatyne, L. A., Gacono, C. B., & Greene, R.(1999). Differential patterns of responding among three groups of chronic, psychotic, forensic outpatients. *Journal of Clinical Psychology, 55*(12), 1553–1565.

Bathurst, K., Gottfried, A. W., & Gottfried, A. W. (1997). Normative data for the MMPI–2 in child custody litigants. *Psychological Assessment, 9*(3), 205–211.

Blais, M. A., Hilsenroth, M. J., Castelbury, F., Fowler, J. C., & Baity, M. R. (2001). Predicting *DSM–IV* Cluster B personality disorder criteria from MMPI–2 and Rorschach data: A test of incremental validity. *Journal of Personality Assessment, 76*(1), 150–168.

Bonieskie, L. M. (2000). An examination of personality characteristics of child custody litigants on the Rorschach. *Dissertation Abstracts International, 61*(6-B), 3271.

Bow, J. N., & Quinnell, F. A. (2001). Psychologists' current practices and procedures in child custody evaluations: Five years after American Psychological Association Guidelines. *Professional Psychology: Research and Practice, 32*, 261–268.

Caldwell, A. (2005). How can the MMPI–2 help child custody examiners? *Journal of Child Custody,* 2(1/2) 83–117.

Ellis, E. (2000). *Divorce wars: Interventions with families in conflict.* Washington, DC: American Psychological Association.

Erard, R. E. (2005). What the Rorschach can contribute to child custody and parenting time evaluations. *Journal of Child Custody,* 2(1/2), 119–142.

Erdberg, P., & Shaffer, T. W. (1999, July) *Tables for the International symposium on Rorschach nonpatient data: Findings from around the world I, II, III.* Paper presented at the IRS '99 16th Congress, Amsterdam.

Exner, J. E. (1991). *Alumni Newsletter.* Asheville, NC: Rorschach Workshops.

Exner, J. E., & Erdberg, P. (2005). *The Rorschach: A Comprehensive System: Vol. 2. Advanced interpretation* (3rd ed.). New York: Wiley.

Exner, J. E., Weiner, I. B., & Par Staff. (1995). *The Rorschach interpretative assistance program: Version 3.* Lutz, FL: Psychological Assessment Resources, Inc.

Finn, S. E. (2002, September). *The consensus Rorschach as brief therapy for couples.* Paper presented at the 17th International Congress of Rorschach and Projective Methods, Rome, Italy.

Gacono, C. B., & Meloy, J. R. (1994). *The Rorschach assessment of aggressive and psychopathic personalities.* Hillsdale, NJ: Lawrence Erlbaum Associates.

Gacono, C. B., Meloy, J. R., & Heaven, T. R. (1990). A Rorschach investigation of narcissism and hysteria in antisocial personality disorder. *Journal of Personality Assessment, 55,* 270–279.

Ganellen, R. J. (1996). *Integrating Rorschach and MMPI–2 in personality assessment.* Hillsdale, NJ: Lawrence Erlbaum Associates.

Glick, P. C. (1988). The role of divorce in the changing family structure: Trends and variations. In S. A. Wolchik & P. Karoly (Eds.), *Children of divorce: Empirical perspectives on adjustment* (pp. 3–33). New York: Gardner Press.

Graham, J. R. (2000). *MMPI–2: Assessing personality and psychopathology* (3rd ed.). New York: Oxford University Press.

Handler, L. (1997). He says, she says, they say: The consensus Rorschach. In J. R. Meloy, M. W. Acklin, C. B. Gacono, J. F. Murray, & C. A. Peterson (Eds.), *Contemporary Rorschach interpretation* (pp. 499–533). Mahwah, NJ: Lawrence Erlbaum Associates.

Hoppe, C., & Kenney, L. (1994, August). *A Rorshach study of the psychological characteristics of parents engaged in child custody/visitation disputes.* Paper presented at the 102nd annual convention of the American Psychological Association, Los Angeles, CA.

Janson, H., & Olsson, U. (2001). A measure of agreement for internal or nominal multivariate observations. *Educational and Psychological Measurement, 61,* 227–289.

Janson, H., & Olsson, U. (2004). A measure of agreement for interval or nomimal multivariate observations by different sets of judges. *Educational and Psychological Measurement, 64,* 62–70.

Johnston, J. R. & Campbell, L.E.G. (1988). *Impasses of divorce.* New York: Wiley.

Johnston, J. R. Campbell, L.E.G., & Tall, M. C. (1985). Impasses to the resolution of custody and visitation disputes. *American Journal of Orthopsychiatry, 55,* 112–119.

Johnston, J. R., & Roseby, V. (1997). *In the name of the child: A developmental approach to understanding and helping children of conflicted and violent divorce.* New York: The Free Press.

Johnston, J. R., Walters, M. G., & Olesen, N. W. (2005). The psychological functioning of alienated children in custody disputing families: An exploratory study. *American Journal of Forensic Psychology, 23*(3), 39–64.

Lee, M. (1996, January). *Using the Rorschach in child custody evaluations.* Paper presented at the second Child Custody Symposium of the Association of Family and Conciliation Courts, Clearwater, FL.

Medhoff, D. (1999) MMPI–2 validity scales in child custody evaluations: Clinical versus statistical significance. *Behavioral Sciences and the Law, 17,* 409–411.

Meloy, J. R., & Singer, J. (1991). A psychoanalytic view of the Rorschach comprehensive system "special scores." *Journal of Personality Assessment, 56*(2), 202–217.

Meyer, G. J. (1992). The Rorschach's factor structure: A contemporary investigation and historical review. *Journal of Personality Assessment, 59,* 117–136.

Meyer, G. J., & Viglione, D. J. (2006, March). *The influence of* R, Form %, R-Engagement, *and* Complexity *on interpretative benchmarks for the Comprehensive System variables.* Paper presented at Society of Personality Assessment Annual Meeting, San Diego, CA.

Posthuma, A. B., & Harper, J. F. (1998). Comparison of MMPI–2 responses of child custody and personal injury litigants. *Professional Psychology: Research and Practice, 29*(5), 437–443.

Shaffer, T. W., Erdberg, P., & Haroian, J. (1999). Current nonpatient data for the Rorschach, WAIS–R, and MMPI–2. *Journal of Personality Assessment, 73*(2), 305–316.

Singer, J. (2001, March). *The Rorschach and personality characteristics of child custody litigants.* Paper presented at the Society for Personality Assessment Annual Meeting, San Antonio, TX.

Strong, D. R., Greene, R. L., Hoppe, C., Johnston, T., & Olesen, N. (1999). Taxometric analysis of impression management and self-deception on the MMPI–2 in child-custody litigation. *Journal of Personality Assessment, 73*(1), 1–18.

Vigloine, D. J., & Meyer, G. J. (1998). *Complexity Index scoring principles.* Unpublished document.

Viglione, D. J., Meyer, G. J., & Exner, J. E. (2001). Superiority of *Form%* over *Lambda* for research on the Rorschach Comprehensive System. *Journal of Personality Assessment, 76*(1), 68–75.

Wallerstein, J. S., & Kelly, J. B. (1980). *Surviving the break-up: How children and parents cope with divorce.* New York: Basic Books.

Weiner, I. B. (1999). What the Rorschach can do for you: Incremental validity in clinical applications. *Assessment, 6,* 327–338.

Weiner, I. B. (2003). *Principles of Rorschach interpretation* (2nd ed.). Mahwah, NJ: Lawrence Erlbaum Associates.

SPECIAL TOPICS

22

BATTERED WOMAN SYNDROME: ASSESSMENT-BASED EXPERT TESTIMONY

Nancy Kaser-Boyd
Geffen School of Medicine, UCLA

Experts say that about one quarter of women in relationships will be physically abused during the course of a relationship (Eigenberg, 2001). Domestic violence is a common cause of marital failure (Levinger, 1966) and is raised frequently in divorce actions (Pagelow, 1992). Many women with chronic pain are battered women (Kaser-Boyd, 2004; Walker, 1994). Some women charged with child neglect or child abuse are battered women (Cammaert, 1988; Kaser-Boyd, 2004; Walker, 1994). Sometimes women who commit crimes are battered women who are acting at the direction of their violent partner, perhaps under duress. Clinicians who have not specialized in evaluating battered women may discover a need for a method to evaluate Battered Woman Syndrome in the course of answering other questions for the courts. This chapter illustrates the use of psychological tests, with special emphasis on the Rorschach, to evaluate battered women, determine whether there is Battered Woman Syndrome and its severity, and how to rule out malingering. This chapter is written especially for the practitioner who employs a battery of psychological tests, is skilled in the use of each test, and might use the Rorschach to add information that is not available from other sources. This chapter is written with two goals in mind: to explain and describe the experience of the battered woman and the effects of that experience and to illustrate how to capture and measure that experience using the Rorschach. Elsewhere, I have discussed the history and social context of battering, provided an overview of the assessment process, discussed severity, described the typical batterer, and suggested questions for providing testimony about Battered Woman Syndrome (Kaser-Boyd, 2004).

Battered Woman Syndrome as an area of expert testimony has a history of about 25 years. The term *Battered Woman Syndrome* was coined by Walker (1979) when she first described the now well-known patterns of domestic violence and its effects on the women who lived with this violence. Numerous clinical and research studies further delineated the effects of battering (Blackman, 1990; Browne, 1987; Douglas, 1987; M. A. Dutton, 1992; Hilberman & Munson, 1978; Rollstin & Kern, 1998). In the 1980s, a parallel process was occurring for other kinds of trauma (Burgess & Holmstrom, 1974;

Horowitz, Wilner, & Kaltreider, 1980; Keane, Malloy, & Fairbank, 1984; Terr, 1979; van der Kolk, 1987; Wilson & Walker, 1990) and others began to publish and speak about Posttraumatic Stress Disorder, first in soldiers with combat trauma and survivors of war, and then with other kinds of interpersonal violence. By the early 1990s, it became apparent that the psychological effects of battering were not greatly different than the effects of repeated trauma of other types. The experience of high levels of fear, helplessness, and physical and emotional threat were highly similar across many types of interpersonal and naturally caused trauma (i.e., flood, earthquake). Battered Woman Syndrome was categorized as a subtype of Posttraumatic Stress Disorder. The importance of this to assessment psychologists is that research on psychological tests on trauma populations has generalizability to battered women, with some cautions.

Some have taken exception to using the diagnostic category of Posttraumatic Stress Disorder for battered women, feeling that it pathologizes a normal reaction to extreme fear (M. A. Dutton, 1996). Because of this concern, the terminology in professional journals has changed over time and Battered Woman Syndrome is also often called "the effects of battering," whereas Domestic Violence is called "Intimate Partner Violence." Many states have codified the term *Battered Woman Syndrome* into law, making it unwise in the respective jurisdictions, to abandon this term.

There is also some controversy about referring to a battered woman or survivor of intimate partner violence as a "victim." In reality, the "victim" can be a man; however, national demographics indicate the overwhelming majority of victims of serious intimate partner violence are women. The phrase "survivor of intimate partner violence" is probably better than victim, although it is cumbersome. With all of this in mind, I use the term *battered person* and, because the word "victim" appears in many places surrounding domestic violence (e.g., as in the District Attorney's Victims' Assistance Program, or the journal *Victimology*), I do not avoid the word "victim."

Battered Woman Syndrome (BWS) is used in legal proceedings in a variety of ways. To begin with, in a criminal case, the prosecution may use BWS testimony to explain behavior of a complaining witness that otherwise may seem perplexing or cause her credibility to be questioned. In this type of testimony, it is often the case that there is no examination of the battered person. The testimony is *academic* in that it reviews research and clinical literature about the patterns seen in domestic violence and the effects of such violence on the victim. The thrust of this kind of testimony is to dispel myths or misconceptions about battered women and to explain behavior that may cause the jury to see the complaining victim as inconsistent or unreliable. For example, such academic testimony may be used to explain a delay in reporting or the recantation of an earlier report. The expert witness can explain why a given woman might have returned to her battering partner on previous occasions or why she did not take effective steps to protect herself (e.g., leaving or filing a restraining order). The witness might be asked a series of hypothetical questions that mirror the evidence of the case. In reality, this kind of testimony does not require skill in psychological assessment, although the expert witness needs to have some understanding about false accusations and malingering. If the expert manages to evaluate the complaining victim, the court will hear testimony about battered women in general, and about this battered woman in particular, with respect to how she resembles a typical battered woman. The expert is generally not allowed to testify that she found the woman *credible*, because this is the province of the jury, but by testifying that, for example, battered women recant, the woman's credibility is restored indirectly.

Battered Woman Syndrome may also be relevant in family court. Expertise in domestic violence can be especially important in making decisions about visitation and custody, because batterers may be especially volatile during a divorce and may pose a real threat to children or their estranged spouse. In fact, the period of separation is the most dangerous time for battered women and their children, because women are vulnerable to being killed while trying to leave. BWS is also highly relevant because battered women may look like they have a major mental disorder, which may preclude the woman being granted custody, when in fact they are exhibiting the effects of battering, which will likely resolve in time.

The most common use of expert testimony about Battered Woman Syndrome is probably in criminal court, where there are a number of applications. Table 22–1 summarizes these and their possible outcomes. Some may be appropriate during the guilt phase of a trial and some are appropriate only for sentencing.

Testimony about battering and its effect is most typically admissible to support a claim of self-defense, but in some states there are two forms of self-defense: perfect self-defense and imperfect self-defense. In *perfect self-defense,* there must be both a subjective and objective degree of threat to safety. A defendant must prove that she *honestly and reasonably* believed that she was in imminent or immediate danger of unlawful bodily harm, her use of force was necessary to save her life or prevent serious bodily injury, and the force used was not excessive in relation to the threatened force. She must also prove that she did not initiate the violence (Hempel, 2004). The legal meaning of "honestly" is

TABLE 22–1
Legal Relevance of Battered Woman's Syndrome

Court	Legal Argument
Criminal court	
Murder charges	Self-defense
	Imperfect self-defense
	Heat of passion
	Accidental, while protecting self
	Unconsciousness
Criminal court	
Other criminal charges (e.g., bank robbery, tax evasion possession or sale of drugs)	Duress
Spousal assault	Self-defense
	Accidental, while protecting self
At sentencing	Mitigation
Dependency court	Unable to protect

usually taken to denote the subjective perception, whereas "reasonably" refers to what a juror or person other than the defendant might think. In many cases involving past trauma, the survivor is hypervigilant to danger and she might honestly perceive imminent danger when even reasonable people, considering her circumstances, cannot do so. In such cases, California and some other states have the concept of *imperfect self-defense.* Here the woman need only show that she honestly (but not reasonably) believed that she was in imminent danger of bodily harm, and her use of force was necessary to save her life or prevent serious bodily injury (Hempel, 2004). As might be expected, a successful imperfect self-defense leads to a different penalty (voluntary manslaughter), whereas perfect self-defense results in an acquittal.

Until the case of *People v. Humphreys* (1996), Battered Woman Syndrome testimony seemed, at best, to lead to voluntary manslaughter. In many cases, however, it seems clear that a battered woman honestly and reasonably believed her life was in imminent danger. In *Humphrey,*[1] the California Appeals Court's language paved the way for testimony that addresses the reasonableness of the battered woman's belief. The court said, "Although the ultimate test of reasonableness is objective, in determining whether a reasonable person in the defendant's position would have believed in the need to defend, the jury must consider all of the relevant circumstances in which the defendant found herself" (p. 1083).

In cases where the battered woman is charged with assault, attempted murder, or murder, the expert should also consider the possibility that the crime was accidental. The most typical example is where the battered woman picks up a weapon (usually a gun, but it could be a knife or even a car) to assist her in backing away, or signaling the batterer to back away, and the situation goes very awry (i.e., in a panic to leave, the gun goes off or she hits her spouse with the car). In these cases, the mental state is not demonstrably different than when she deliberately shoots the weapon or uses a knife, except there is no evidence that she intentionally shot the weapon or used a car to run over her partner. Even in the less severe instance, unfortunately, it is often the battered woman who is charged with spousal assault (e.g., the battered woman throws a glass at the batterer to get him to back off, the glass shatters and he is cut). Determining whether she has Battered Woman Syndrome, and its severity, is equally relevant.

A battered woman may also be so terrified during an incident of domestic violence that she enters a dissociative state. Battered women frequently describe dissociative experiences in situations of extreme fear. Research indicates the dissociative reaction and its phenomenology is biologically mediated (see later for a description of the biology of fear). In a dissociative state, a battered woman's behavior is reactive and automatic, not mediated by higher cognitive functions like planning and reasoning. The core aspect of dissociation is a lack of conscious connection in a person's thoughts, memories, feelings, actions, or sense of identity. In the legal context, a dissociative state may qualify for the legal definition of *unconsciousness*, which can lead to an acquittal.

Battered women may kill or assault in *the heat of passion.* Battered women live in very provocative situations. The batterer typically feels that he can do and say whatever he pleases. Although the overwhelming majority of battered women say they are afraid to

---

[1]*People v. Humphrey* (1996) 13 Cal 4th 1073.

express anger toward their partner because of the long-term, high level of anxiety, there may be times when the woman is unable to control her emotions. Her emotional eruption may come at times that will be normally provocative for nearly any person, such as upon discovering that the batterer has molested their daughter or has had an affair. In such cases, the prosecution argument might be that the motive for the crime (e.g., murder or attempted murder) was simple anger, but understanding Battered Woman Syndrome can help the trier of fact more accurately understand her mental state and establish the appropriate level of culpability.

Additionally, Battered Woman Syndrome may be important in understanding a battered woman's behavior in other crimes. Battered women may be charged, in state and federal courts with bank robbery, drug smuggling, tax evasion, and a variety of other crimes. A battered woman may be capable of carrying out such crimes on her own, but in some cases there is a psychopathic and violent man planning the crimes and coercing the woman to participate. In some of these cases, the woman realistically fears she will be killed or seriously injured if she does not comply. In these cases, the legal defense of *duress* might be applicable. There are other cases that do not approach the level necessary for duress, but the effects of battering, including the mental effects of coercive control, can explain why she did not resist or go to authorities. Coercive control is of special concern in light of D. Dutton's (2002) research indicating that 40% of batterers are psychopathic. Fear, short of the legal standard for duress, will be most relevant to issues raised in sentencing (e.g., mitigation).

Early attempts to present evidence of the effects of battering were often blocked by judicial rulings about admissibility. Often there was a first stage before expert testimony, called a *Kelly–Frye* hearing, where the judge heard testimony about the scientific credibility of the research on Battered Woman Syndrome and decided whether testimony would truly help the trier of fact. Expert testimony on battering and its effects are now admissible to support a self-defense claim, at least to some degree, in every state and the District of Columbia (Parrish, 1996). Judges can still rule on whether this evidence is relevant, and they can limit the scope of testimony. In many cases, limiting instructions are more likely when the woman does not testify. Judges are cautious lest the battered woman's account slip in the back door, without an opportunity for the prosecution to cross-examine her. Experts are allowed to base their opinion on hearsay, but the judge may give a "limiting instruction," indicating that the jury can hear the material as the basis for the expert's opinion but not as fact.

Expert testimony on Battered Woman Syndrome will receive the most careful scrutiny when the case surrounds a killing. It is in such cases that a battery of psychological tests may be particularly useful to illustrate the effects of battering and to rule out malingering.

THE BATTERING EXPERIENCE

Battering exists on a spectrum, from mild to severe, and it can be psychological, physical, or sexual. Almost every relationship with domestic violence also includes a high level of psychological abuse. At the lower end, there is name calling (e.g, "stupid bitch," "whore," "fat pig"); the battered women say these names felt more damaging than hits and punches because they made them feel worthless. At the higher end, however, are threats to harm, such as "If you leave me, I will find you and hurt you" or "I will kill your parents." It is obvious that the effect will vary based on the type of abuse—from feelings of worthlessness to terror. Sexual abuse in the battering relationship also exists on a spectrum: from unwanted or too frequent sex; to forced, painful acts; to acts that are degrading or cause the woman to violate her own moral standards (e.g., to be forced into a *ménage a trois*). Physical abuse also can range from mild to moderate acts of physical aggression (pushing, slapping, hair pulling) to extraordinarily threatening and frightening acts of violence (threatened with guns, thrown out of a moving car, choked to unconsciousness).

Because battering exists on a continuum of severity, in evaluations of battered women it is important to understand the level of severity of violence experienced. This is crucial to understanding the effects of the battering in the case at hand. More severe violence is closely tied to more severe psychological effects (APA, 2000, p. 466; Browne, 1987). Elsewhere (Kaser-Boyd, 2004), I have suggested the use of a formal rating scale called the Spousal Assault Violent Acts Scale, which can be used as a starting point for a clinical interview that follows up on the number of incidents of particular forms of violence and the woman's subjective perception of the incident (e.g., Did she think she would die?, Did she feel immobilized?, etc.) This is a crucial point in discussing severity: In the field of trauma, and in victimology, it is the victim's *perception* of the event that causes the psychological effects. If the battered person perceives significant threat, then she is more likely to have the level of fear that creates a trauma disorder.

The issue of severity is closely tied to our ideas (and misconceptions) of the nature of Battered Woman Syndrome. A simplistic view of a battered woman might be of someone who is rather dependent, with low self-esteem, rather passive and self-effacing. Some authors talk about "learned helplessness," again referring to a passive, resigned state. In reality, however, women seen in the legal context usually have suffered more serious levels of psychological and physical violence. Living in a violent and threatening relationship creates strong emotions (e.g., fear or intense ambivalence) and dramatic methods of coping (denial, emotional numbing, avoidance, substance abuse). The powerful experience of fear cannot be overlooked. Many battered women conduct their daily lives unable to predict when the violence will suddenly erupt, or knowing that a battering will occur if some particular event happens (e.g., a neighbor comes by to say hello). This means that a battered woman will have a high level of constant anticipatory anxiety or dread, punctuated by moments or hours of extreme fear or terror. Chronic anxiety may interfere with sleep and concentration, impair the ability to work, and have numerous health effects associated with any chronically stressful environment in which safety is in serious question.

The peaks of fear or terror, on the other hand, bring the full biological response to threat (LeDoux, 1996). The brain responds in a very definite way to threat (see Fear, 2003). At times of high threat, the brain signals an alarm that releases cortisol, which in turn causes the release of norepenephrine (known more commonly as adrenalin). Fear/threat messages go directly to the more "primitive" part of the brain, where a reaction can be immediate (run, fight, hide), as opposed to rational or deliberative (i.e., responses that are more of a secondary, rational reaction to threat and take place in the frontal cortex). A massive influx of cortisol is associated with a decrease in the brain's serotonin level, which is implicated in a number of psychiatric/psychological disorders. The secondary neurochemical effects may be responsible for some of the observed effects of battering (e.g., depression, poor emotional control, impaired sleep).

Human beings who have lived through very threatening events have a highly consistent clinical picture. First, they become sensitized to danger and to their own vulnerability. This is described even in individuals who suffered a traumatic event years ago (e.g., Holocaust survivors, combat veterans, rape trauma survivors, and others). Individuals with these experiences say they can no longer entertain the belief that the world is safe or that they will be unharmed. This phenomenological experience of threat has been codified into our diagnostic manual (*DSM–IV–TR*, APA, 2000) under Posttraumatic Stress Disorder. Symptoms of the effects of extreme threat/fear or trauma include a heightened sense of danger, biological and psychological hyperarousal and hypervigilance, re-experiencing or flooding with the intense memories of the trauma, or with the feeling associated with the threat (e.g., fear, vulnerability, profound sadness, despair, loss, or anger). These intense emotions alternate with efforts to back away from horrific memories and terror-filled emotion. In diagnostic terms, this is a cluster of avoidance symptoms and includes denial, emotional numbing, avoiding reminders, dissociation, or self-medicating with drugs or alcohol.

When the traumatic or profoundly threatening events are interpersonal, and prolonged, a set of features that *DSM–IV* calls "associated descriptive features" are observed. These include impaired affect modulation; self-destructive and impulsive behavior; dissociative symptoms; somatic complaints; feelings of ineffectiveness, shame, despair, or hopelessness; feeling permanently damaged; a loss of previously sustained beliefs; hostility; social withdrawal; feeling constantly threatened; impaired relationships with others; or a change from the individual's previous personality characteristics. Herman (1992) refers to this as Complex Posttraumatic Stress Disorder or Disorders of Extreme Stress, Not Otherwise Specified (DESNOS). There is now considerable acceptance of a set of complex effects that come from prolonged interpersonal trauma (van der Kolk, Roth, Pelcovitz, Sunday, & Spinazzola, 2005).

There are some experiences that deserve special emphasis with battered woman, in part because they are crucial to assessing Battered Woman Syndrome. One is the feeling of entrapment. Herman (1992) likens this to trauma while under captivity. Battered women frequently feel that they cannot get away from their batterer. Rhodes and McKenzie (1998) examined the research on the reasons battered women stay in battering relationships. In the more severe cases of domestic violence, battered women say they were very fearful of leaving (Kaser-Boyd, 2004); many say they feel entrapped, because of the variety of dire consequences threatened by the batterer (threats to kill her, kill himself, or kill other loved ones). A second common feeling is that of devaluation. Battered women feel damaged, worthless, and sometimes shameful. The experience of physical injury and violent sexual assault often, in addition, results in feeling fragmented, with permeable body boundaries. The accomplished Rorschacher can hypothesize, at this point, what Rorschach scores might be found in battered women.

THE BIPHASIC NATURE OF TRAUMA DISORDERS

Van der Kolk (1987) noted that the florid intrusive symptoms of trauma alternate with defensive avoidance. Our *DSM–IV* manual summarizes the criteria for Posttraumatic Stress Disorder as if the symptom clusters occur in tandem, but in reality there is a time sequence to trauma symptoms that makes sense when we think about the human capacity to cope and adapt. When patients are seen soon after a trauma (e.g., from immediately after to many months after), trauma memories are still fresh and coping or defense mechanisms have not congealed. The patient likely is actively experiencing intrusive recollections and nightmares, and the emotions of fear, anger, despair, and so on that accompany interpersonal trauma. They are likely hypervigilant and hyperaroused (sleeping poorly, monitoring the batterer's moods, checking on the children, etc.).

As time goes on, most trauma survivors try hard to push these painful memories and feelings out of their awareness. Some say, rather simply, "I just tried not to think about it." For others, the avoidance is more akin to repression, or an involuntary suppression of the painful memories (for a discussion of the neurobiology of fear, see Schachter, 1996). During this stage, the patient is likely still hypervigilant, perhaps still experiencing poor sleep and a startle response, but seems "flat" or detached. In the Defensive Avoidance stage of PTSD, the survivor appears to be emotionally constricted. In the process of avoiding the painful feelings from the trauma, it is as if all feeling is to be avoided lest the survivor again feel intensely vulnerable. There are more literary ways to describe this state (unable to experience joy, detached) or clinical descriptions (schizoid, depressed). Overt trauma symptoms (e.g., intrusive recollections, intense emotions) can be elicited during stages of defensive avoidance, by "triggers, " which can bring back the trauma memories and feelings in their full intensity. The avoidant stage of PTSD can continue for quite some time, perhaps assuming what appears like the new "personality" of the survivor.

This discussion should make obvious that psychological test results will vary depending on the state at the time of testing. The same is true of any psychological disorder with a fluctuating course (e.g., Bipolar Disorder). This is a critical point when one is testing a woman and the referral question is "Does this woman have Battered Woman Syndrome?" Take a commonly used psychological test, the Minnesota Multiphasic Personality Inventory (MMPI). In the easy case, a battered woman is psychologically tested with the MMPI–2 and the results resemble the results of Kahn, Welch, and Zillmer (1993) or Rosewater and Walker (1985)—elevated *F*, and elevated Clinical scales 2, 4, 6, 7, 8. The woman is still flooded with symptoms from the battering. Suppose, however, that the MMPI is completely unelevated, and the Validity scales *L* and *K* are elevated? This is an expected MMPI profile for a survivor in the stage of defensive avoidance. This is intuitively obvious to the assessment psychologist, because elevated Validity scales are a hallmark of the employment of psychological defenses. Clinical experience with hundreds of battered women supports this finding with the MMPI, and with the Millon Clinical Multiaxial Inventory (MCMI) as well, where the survivor who has had some time to recover, seems quite defensive and there are no real elevations on clinical scales. Indeed,

M. A. Dutton (1992), in her study of the MMPIs of battered women, found five distinct profiles, including one with no clinical elevations.

THE RORSCHACH AND TRAUMA

Emotional constriction may well be the most common long-term expression of PTSD, and the diagnosis is likely to be missed when the survivor is in the stage of emotional constriction. Van der Kolk and Ducey (1989) note that in some PTSD survivors, overt signs of continuing preoccupation with the trauma are absent in the clinical interview, but will be tapped by the Rorschach. The Rorschach has been suggested as the ideal tool to "trigger" trauma memories and feelings, a process that may be similar to traumatic reliving in nightmares (van der Kolk & Ducey, 1989). The abstract images, coupled with vibrant colors (especially red), seem to call out images of harm and danger in individuals with trauma experiences. The Rorschach may provide essential information not tapped by self-report measures (Levin & Reis, 1997). The Rorschach's structural data and content are useful indices to current symptoms and psychological processes (Armstrong & Kaser-Boyd, 2003). The Rorschach provides important data about perceptual accuracy, coping resources, stress tolerance, modulation of affect, and hypervigilience, to name some of the indices that are useful in the measurement of trauma (Kaser-Boyd, 1993).

There is a growing literature, in children and adults, on the Rorschach and trauma. This chapter focuses on adults, but see Armstrong and Kaser-Boyd (2004) for a review of studies with children that illustrate the early appearance of disturbances in perception and affect that result from trauma. van der Kolk and Ducey (1984, 1989) introduced the idea of the "co-arcted" Rorschach protocol, which is a type of protocol that was seen in survivors in the avoidant stage of the disorder. Examining 14 records of Vietnam combat veterans, they collected 10 "flooded" protocols and 4 "co-arcted" protocols, and discussed the latter as evidence of psychic numbing. They also noted an unusually elevated number of *Inanimate Movement* responses (m), which they took to reflect a perception of threatening forces beyond one's control. The flooded records were characterized by extensive use of color and seemingly uncensored percepts of traumatic war events, including numerous blood and anatomy responses. Souffrant (1987) used the Rorschach with 60 combat veterans with and without overt symptoms of PTSD, and found that m and the ratio $FC:CF + C$ (particularly unstructured color responses) differentiated the two groups. Hartman et al. (1990) collected Rorschachs on 41 inpatient Vietnam combat veterans with PTSD and found both high *Lambda* and low *Lambda* records, and a tendency toward severe perceptual distortion and ineffective coping strategies. Swanson, Blount, and Bruno (1990) studied 50 Vietnam combat veterans with PTSD and noted low affective ratios, which they linked to the tendency to avoid emotionally laden situations. Their sample, like Hartman's, had impaired reality testing, and like Souffrant's, had elevated m and unmodulated affect.

Several Rorschach studies focused on civilian disasters. Modlin (1967) collected 40 records from postaccident patients and discussed emotional constriction. The records were described as simple, literal, unimaginative, stoic, and conventional, with limited and constricted capacity for emotional expression. Cerney (1990) used the Rorschach to study 48 inpatients who had suffered traumatic loss. Some had suffered the traumatic loss of a loved one and others had been abused or had witnessed serious violence. She noted two types of protocols: either constricted protocols, absent color and with minimal content of a markedly aggressive nature; or color-dominated responses, with numerous primitive and aggressive percepts. Levin (1990, 1993) collected 27 Rorschachs from a heterogeneous sample of adults with PTSD. Her subjects had suffered a variety of traumatic events, including rape, violent assault, bombings, fires, and other major accidents. Her subjects attempted to avoid affectively provocative stimuli (low *Affective ratios*), but had elevations in scores measuring unmodulated affect. They had positive *Hypervigilance Indices* and a number of concrete trauma-related percepts. As with the Vietnam samples, reality testing was impaired. Levin emphasized the presence of *Inanimate Movement* (*m*) in her sample, citing Schachtel's (1966) interpretation of the inanimate movement response as the "attitude of the impotent spectator."

Women with sexual abuse histories have received some attention in Rorschach research. Saunders (1991) studied 33 women with histories of childhood sexual abuse and found them to produce more color-dominated responses, disturbances in thought processes, and primary process breakthroughs connected with sexual and aggressive content. Samples of sexually abused girls have almost identical findings. Zivney, Nash, and Hulsey (1988) examined the Rorschach records of 80 girls, divided into two groups— those molested before age 9 and those molested after age 9. Those molested early had the most disturbed cognition. Leifer, Shapiro, Martone, and Kassem (1991) replicated this finding. Zivney et al. (1988) found elevations of *m*, *Y*, and *Morbids*. Leifer et al. found more sexual responses and more scores associated with penetration of body boundaries. Franchi and Andronikof-Sanglade (1993) collected Rorschachs from 17 genitally circumcised Moslem women residing in France. Although none spoke directly about their circumcisions in interviews, their Rorschach records frequently mentioned the size, presence, or absence of the clitoris (e.g, "Everything has been taken away." or "That is the same female sex organ as before, only the clitoris is bigger." These records had high *Lambda* and low *F + %*. Also, the subject's cognitive functioning was characterized by a preponderance of magical thinking, and a number of defensive strategies aimed at distancing reality. Fifty-one percent of the group had a positive *PTI*.

Armstrong (1994) used the Rorschach with 119 patients with dissociative identity disorder, who had histories of severe childhood abuse. This sample was described as having low *Lambda*, a large number of *Blends*, atypical reality testing, and the presence of concrete trauma-related percepts, defined as a combination of special scores *Morbid* and *Aggressive* and *Blood*, *Sex*, and *Anatomy* contents. These findings formed the basis of her Trauma Content scale. The Trauma Content Index consists of the sum of the Exner Contents of *Sex*, *Blood*, *Anatomy*, *Morbids*, and *Aggressive*, divided by the total number of responses. A *TC/R* of .3 and above was hypothesized to suggest traumatic intrusions.

The Rorschach study most pertinent to battered women (Kaser-Boyd, 1993) studied 28 battered women who killed their battering spouses. The protocols displayed cognitive constriction, a lack of internal resources for problem solving, an ambitensive and passive problem-solving style, intense and poorly modulated affect, poor scanning of the stimulus field, and unconventional reality testing. At the time of the study, I was still learning about the nature of Posttraumatic Stress Disorder, particularly about the biphasic response to trauma, and the predominance of emotional constriction in individuals who struggle against traumatic images. In the sample, I noted that this group of battered women differed from the normative sample on *Lambda* ($M = 1.03$, compared to Exner mean of .59), and that almost half of the sample had *Lambda* greater than .85, or were obviously quite emotionally constricted when they were given the Rorschach. Having subsequently tested hundreds of battered women, it seems clear that many of the records discussed in Kaser-Boyd (1993) represent battered women in the constricted or avoidant phase of PTSD. When the sample was divided between high *Lambda* and low *Lambda* records, there were clear differences. Women with low *Lambdas* generated profiles that looked virtually psychotic. These records are often infused with morbid and aggressive images (i.e., bruised or bleeding bodies or body parts, threatening animals or malevolent creatures) and images of entrapment. They had a high number of *Inanimate Movement* responses (*m*). These seem to communicate the phenomenological experience of being battered. Consider the Rorschach responses of Marie R, who had been battered and, more importantly, she had been subjected to forced, painful sex (rape and sodomy):

Card II

A broken chest, somebody busted 'em in the chest, broken, bleeding. I: It's like this is your chest here, and they hit you here in the heart, the heart exploded from the top because they hit you there, and then part of your lungs or kidneys or whatever would be down here. It would be like an x-ray of the chest where somebody just punched it and there's blood spots just where it's bruised. (Bruised?) The color. (Exploded?) The burst of the fingers, but the splatter going out from it. The splatter effect there, you know how when you hit a water balloon, how it just splatters?

Card III

Two ovaries here, the hip bones, and this could possibly be the womb for a baby or something and they got hit in the stomach and busted it up. I: Two bloodstains coming down. Looks like they coulda been pinned against the wall and whoever had 'em there just put their hand up and then the blood was running down the wall, all the extra blood was, off their hands.

Card IV

A weird critter coming after somebody or something, going to attack 'em. It's got a little tail for a stinger. It's got the two feelers on the back side, and on his arms, and the there's biters on the front. I: Fear, run, hide. (tears) These he could sting ya with, his legs, and it's like he throws his front layer of skin, flappies or whatever, kinda like the uh, what are those big fish on the bottom of the ocean? The round ones that flop around, like a big pancake with a little tail? Do you know what I'm talking about? Like a Manta Ray. This is kinda like that, and they throw their skin back and that's what actually sticks to ya, where they can cling on ... tear ya apart. And once he gets ya in this part here, he just wraps around ya and engulfs ya and your whole body's just paralyzed and you just, you're gone.

Or, consider the Rorschach responses of Cathy W, who also reported physical and sexual violence at the hands of her husband:

Card II

That's blood. It's my blood and his blood. It's when he's kicking me, throwing kicks. I don't want to look at that one anymore. He's on the right, here, because he's always right. He has to be right! Blood. I've been bloody before, from a kick, or throwing a dish on the floor. He would throw them on the ground and they would slash my leg. I stopped cooking with glass.

Card X

That's our whole family in disarray. Splattered (beginning to cry). It's just everything gone mad. He and I are holding hands, here, and there is blood all over us, on both of us. Here are the kids, together but apart from us. They are away from all the blood and the hurt. There are bugs around us. They snap and they bite, and the flowers are torn apart from the vines. The colors, they were beautiful but now they are pulled apart from the pain. The children have their backs toward us so they don't have to see.

These are highly unusual, idiosyncratic responses. The average person (and the average patient!) could not conceive of responses this laden with injury and despair. A battered woman in the flooded stage of PTSD may have elevations on the Thought Disorder Index, as well as indices measuring depression and suicidality. The *Hypervigilance Index* is often elevated, illustrating their compulsive scanning of the environment for cues of danger. Table 22–2 summarizes typical findings in battered women with high *Lambda* and low *Lambda*.

The content of Rorschach responses often is a window into the examinee's experience of the world. The Exner (1993, 2003) Comprehensive System, following the lead of older Rorschach scoring systems, did not include a category for threatening percepts, or for fear, although there is a special score for *Aggressive* content (*AG*) and one for *Morbid* content (*MOR*) that captures the fear of harm or sense of disintegration. Ephraim and Kaser-Boyd (2003) have proposed the Preoccupation with Danger Index, which includes four content categories: fear, threat, harm, and violent confrontation.[2] The scoring categories were derived from clinical work with survivors of severe domestic violence and of torture/state violence. To date, the *Danger Index* (*DI*) has been formally studied with two groups of trauma survivors: refugee seekers who had been victims of political torture, and battered women referred for pretrial evaluation. Both groups were significantly higher on the *DI* than a group of normal volunteers. The mean number of danger contents was 5.55 for battered women and 6.33 for refugees. The mean number of danger contents for the comparison group was 1.25. Armstrong's Trauma Content Index has not been studied specifically with battered women, but in clinical samples (Kaser-Boyd, 1993; Kaser-Boyd, 2004) it is often found to be positive

---

[2]Fear: A living or imaginary being is portrayed as endangered or fearful. *Threat*: A living or imaginary being, or force, is portrayed as endangering, scary, threatening, destructive, or malevolent. *Violent confrontation*: Portrayal of a fight, clash, combat, or war. *Harm*: Portrayal of destruction, or failure to protect boundaries; includes also barrier responses that emphasize the need to protect/shelter the body-self against danger.

TABLE 22–2

Expected Rorschach Scores in Battered Woman's Syndrome

Clusters	High Lambda (Lambda > .85)	Low Lambda (Lambda < .85)
Cognitive clusters	High *Pure F*	*M–*
	Low *M*	*X + % < .60*
		F + % < .60
		Special scores
Affective cluster	Low *Afr*	*S > 1*
	Low *C* and *CF*	*Y > 2*
		C and *Pure C > 2*
Stress v. controls		*m > 1*
	D > 0	*D > –1*
	EA > es	*EA < es*
Self and other	*COP*	*MOR > 2*
	Fr > 0	*AG > 1*
Indices	*CDI*	*PTI*
	HVI	*DEPI*

when the woman is in a flooded stage of PTSD. Bornstein's Oral Dependency Scale (1999) may have some utility in studying battered women, because many have results on other tests that suggest dependency, but to date this scale has not been tested on battered women.

In addition to its capacity to tap images of trauma and measure hypervigilance and preoccupation with danger, the Rorschach may be a difficult test to malinger (see Ganellen, chap. 5, this vol., for a more extensive coverage of malingering on the Rorschach). Although self-report inventories can seem like symptom checklists, the Rorschach is an ambiguous task. The average defendant does not know what the forensic psychologist is looking for, and does not have access to journals or professional books that would provide a cookbook for a trauma Rorschach protocol. As with other studies of malingering (see Ganellen, chap. 5, this vol., about the Dramatic Content scale), an intuitive approach to faking a trauma disorder might involve delivering numerous "blood and guts" responses, but these would also need to be accompanied by some of the Rorschach scores associated with trauma, such as Armstrong's Trauma Context Index (Armstrong & Loewenstein, 1991).

A far more common strategy is to dampen down and give a short, defensive Rorschach, with a low response level or a high *Lambda*. Woods et al. (2003) cites one Rorschach malingering study (Frueh & Kinder, 1994) as evidence that PTSD can be malingered. Woods et al. notes that the malingerers actually had more indicators of PTSD than the veterans. A quick look at the methodology of this study reveals that these veterans were years away from their trauma experience. The study authors did not acknowledge the important difference between high *Lambda* and low *Lambda* records—protocol means, in fact, indicated that most of the sample was in the constricted or avoidant phase of the disorder. Thus, it is not surprising that they could not be differentiated from controls.

The Rorschach is but one part of a comprehensive forensic assessment battery that includes a thorough review of the Discovery (original police reports, investigation interviews, photographs, audio or videotapes, autopsy photographs, etc.), a forensic interview, collateral interviews, and psychological testing with other instruments. In a typical evaluation, I might structure the test battery with the Minnesota Multiphasic Personality Inventory (MMPI–2), the Millon Clinical Multiaxial Inventory (MCMI–III), the Rorschach (RIM), the Trauma Symptoms Inventory (TSI), and if I suspect dissociative symptoms, the Dissociative Experiences Scale (DES).

CASE EXAMPLE

Wendy W. was arrested after she hit her estranged partner with a baseball bat. She had hidden in his closet for many hours, seemingly waiting for him to fall asleep so she could sneak out undetected, but he woke up and she hit him. Wendy was a pretty 42-year-old Anglo woman who worked as a fashion designer. The relationship had been brief but intense, and Wendy reported a variety of instances of psychological and sexual abuse. She had one previous relationship that was abusive, and her father was a dominant man who lost control on one occasion and beat her severely. She had also survived a horrifying rape when she was much younger. She was an outgoing, creative, fun-loving woman who was rejection-sensitive and had a history of becoming distraught when love relationships ended. She had converted to a new religion in order to satisfy her partner, and she had been the sole support of their household until shortly before the arrest, when she lost her job and the boyfriend moved on to greener pastures. The prosecution theory was that she snuck into his apartment to kill him, out of anger that he left her. She said she entered his apartment to try to talk to him, but grew frightened before he realized she was there, and hid in a closet.

In the weeks prior to the crime, she had grown increasingly distraught. She said she was unable to get to sleep without a self-hypnosis ritual that involved visualizing cutting her wrists and watching the blood drain out. She was keeping an elaborate journal about her prayers to God. Although she was also in therapy, the therapist seemed undertrained and inexperienced in treating individuals with her history of trauma. He suggested she call her physician and get a prescription for Xanax, which she did.

Wendy was evaluated within the first 3 months of her arrest. She was tested with a battery of psychological tests, including the MMPI–2, the MCMI–III, and the Rorschach. Somewhat unusual for the criminal courts, private funding was available for an extended forensic assessment, and she did not disclose the sadistic sexual abuse she had endured until she had been seen for 6 months.

The MMPI–2 was remarkable for its extreme elevation on Scale 3 ($T = 94$). At this level, dissociative symptoms were a clear possibility. Patients with this elevation have been described as having hysterical psychotic episodes and transitory psychotic spells (for a clear description of Hysterical Psychosis, see van der Hart, Witztum, & Friedman, 1993). Her next highest elevation was on Scale 2 ($T = 88$), reflecting her despair, feelings of worthlessness, and guilt. Surprisingly, scales in the "psychotic" end of the profile were not elevated, but her preoccupation with God and with trancelike states is characteristic of a hysterical psychosis. The MCMI had Axis I elevations on Major Depression and Dysthymia, and Axis II elevations on Avoidant, Dependant, and Self-Defeating. This is a classic profile for battered women (Kaser-Boyd, 2004).

It was the Rorschach that best illustrated her profound despair and her unique perceptions of reality. The content of her responses told the story of her abuse and subsequent rejection, her sense of damage and fragmentation, and her complicated mix of painful emotions. For example, on Card II, she said:

> It looks like a ballet dancer. … These are her feet. She's on her toes and this is her torso. I don't know why the body would be open in the middle. Maybe some sort of emblem hanging on a chain. (Open in the middle?) Maybe her body is not present, just the pieces she wears, almost as if on a hanger. I see it both ways, as a costume with a medallion, and as a woman ripped apart with her heart torn out, and blood all over her clothes. I see it both ways, but it scares me this other way, so I said clothing on a hanger.

Or, on Card III, she said,

> It looks like two people holding on to something and it looks like their hearts have been torn out of their bodies, but they are connected … just like they are trying to pull away … almost like they are attached and can't get away, pulling and pulling, too tightly connected … and an explosion blew them apart, but their hearts are still connected … and I keep wanting to say that this is matter, like their minds have been hurt too, because it also looks like blood behind their heads.

In the forensic use of the Rorschach, the formal scores are the first focus for interpretive hypotheses, because it is from the scores that the individual's deviation from "normal" can be ascertained. Wendy's formal scores were clearly remarkable (see column 1 of Table 22–3). For example, $MOR = 9$, where the mean for nonpatient adults was .70 (Exner & Erdberg, 2005, Table 22–1). This underscored her profound sense of vulnerability and damage. Her protocol showed the presence of intense, painful affects—anger ($S = 7$), anxiety and helplessness ($Y = 5$), and painful introspection ($V = 2$). Her thinking was overly complex and imbued with emotion (*Blends* = 13), she was pathologically self-involved, probably in response to vulnerability, and there was much distortion surrounding her perception of others ($M- = 9$, and a clear indication of thought disorder ($PTI = 6$). Her two *Sex* contents were clearly above the mean (.19 for nonpatient adults, Exner & Erdberg, 2005, Table 22–1), as were her 3 *An + Xray*, and 3 *Blood* contents (i.e., her Trauma Content Index was positive). Wendy clearly evidenced a profound disturbance of both thought and affect, and she had a number of scores associated with trauma.

Wendy was re-tested with the Rorschach after lengthy psychotherapy (during which she was tried and acquitted}. The therapy was insight-oriented, focusing on gaining insight about her choices, and improving her judgment, her self-image, and most importantly, her sense of safety. Table 22–3 illustrates the changes in her Rorschach record as her defenses reorganized, and her fear and vulnerability began to recede. Her thinking became less complex. Although still infused with emotion, the distortion around human interaction decreased considerably ($M-$ was 9 after arrest and 3 after therapy), and she was able to see the potential for positive human relationships ($COP = 3$). Her intense, painful introspection and overwhelming anxiety and anger had abated (drops in S, Y, and V). PTI was still high, reflecting her rather idiosyncratic way of viewing the world, but she was significantly less self-involved and less fragmented. Although her protocol at Time 2 shows clear improvements, in many respects it still reflects PTSD. Her therapy continued

TABLE 22–3

Wendy W. Repeated Measures

	Time 1 After Arrest	Time 2 After Therapy
Cognitive clusters	Blends = 13	Blends = 11
	Zd = +13.5	Zd = +11
	X + % = .21	X + % = .27
	X – % = .58	X – % = .36
	M– = 9	M– = 3
	WSum6 = 13	WSum6 = 11
Affective cluster	S = 7	S = 2
	V = 2	V = 0
	Y = 5	Y = 2
	FC:CF = 1:6	FC:CF = 0:4
Stress v. controls	m = 3	m = 6
	EA:es = 18.5:16	EA:es = 12:7
	Y = 5	Y = 2
Self/other	Fr = 1	Fr = 0
	COP = 0	COP = 3
	AG = 3	AG = 1
	MOR = 9	MOR = 1
Indices	CDI = 2	CDI = 0
	HVI = 0	HVI = 0
	PTI = 6	PTI = 5
	DEPI = 7	DEPI = 3
Contents	Sx = 2	Sx = 1
	An + Xray = 3	An + Xray = 3
	Hd = 5	Hd = 1
	Bl = 3	Bl = 0

and now, at 5 years post-arrest, she has remained emotionally stable, is working at a creative job and earning a living, and she has formed a stable relationship with a man.

RORSCHACH TESTIMONY IN BATTERED WOMAN SYNDROME

The examples from battered women's Rorschach protocols presented earlier are dramatic and have the considerable potential of adding "flesh to the bones" of the data from the MMPI, the MCMI, and even to the Rorschach formal scores, but should the expert witness with this type of material rely on individual, dramatic, and illustrative Rorschach responses or on the structural data? It should not be a decision about one or the other. The ideal approach is testimony that begins with the formal scores (e.g., with Wendy, her *Morbids*, her *Vista*, her *m + Y*, her *PTI*—all potent data about the degree of her emotional disarray) and gives several illustrations with Rorschach content.

In a jury trial, the expert is well advised to keep her discussion of formal Rorschach scores very simple. In the celebrated trial of Sirhan Sirhan, for the murder of Robert Kennedy (see Kaiser, 1970), a reporter for the *Los Angeles Times* wrote about the impact of Rorschach testimony on jurors:

> For more than a month, they have listened to such psychiatric verbal shorthand as C-prime response, small animal movement, inanimate movement, large human response, pure form response, large M and small FM, Large F and little C and TH column. It is debatable how efficiently the jurors have been able to translate such arbitrary terms into their meaningful emotional equivalents, but the mere effort has exacted a toll that was apparent Monday as they listened to still more of the same, with faces that ranged a gamut of expression from boredom to stupefaction.

To minimize "stupefaction" for the trier of fact, it is advisable to simplify Rorschach testimony by picking several key variables or indices that best capture the relevant mental state, compare them to the normative sample, and tie them to findings from other tests. The value of presenting rich clinical description along with scoring variables cannot be underestimated. Indeed, the research of Krauss and Sales (2001) indicated empirically that testimony rich in clinical example was more persuasive to juries than actuarially based scientific testimony.

With the same principle in mind, the expert should try to keep testimony about psychometric issues like reliability and validity as simple as possible, because a series of cross-examination questions and answers about these technical topics is hard for the average juror to follow. The ideal approach for the expert witness, here, is to prepare for a blistering critical cross-examination on reliability, validity, and utility, as if sitting for the oral examination for the American Board of Assessment Psychology, but also prepare to talk about the Rorschach's validity in very simple, common sense terms (Gacono, Evans, & Viglione, 2002). In my experience, cross-examination questions about the Rorschach are usually quite general, perhaps because it is also hard for the average attorney to plow through all of the technical discussions that have been published in the last several years about the Rorschach (as well as understand psychometric issues). The questions attempting to undermine Rorschach testimony are therefore more along the lines of "Isn't it true, Doctor, that the Rorschach is a highly controversial test?" The chapter in this text by Weiner is excellent preparation for this type of questioning. In addition, I usually prepare to defend the validity of the particular scores on which I'm relying. For example, I do remind myself about the research literature on *m* or on *MOR*.

Initially, there was considerable anxiety about the publication of *What's Wrong With the Rorschach* (Woods, Nezwarski, Lilienfeld, & Garb, 2003). Although this book received considerable interest from journalists, and provides a number of incendiary quotes that can be used in cross-examination, a book that begins with the lead author's own Rorschach and his unabashed acceptance of the positive Exner interpretative statements and rejection of negative interpretations is a testament to bias. Others (e.g, Meloy, 2005) have cited the authors' inaccuracies in quoting their own work (e.g, serious errors in reporting work on *Reflections*), as well as more general flaws, including the failure to cite literature that supports the Rorschach. The recent White Paper published by the Society for Personality Assessment (2005) succinctly summarizes the scientific support for the Rorschach, and lists over 75 references.

CONCLUSIONS

The Rorschach has much to offer a comprehensive assessment of Battered Woman Syndrome. It is extremely sensitive to trauma disorders, and its abstract nature seems to serve as a trigger for traumatic images. There are many other Rorschach scores that have emerged as clear markers for battered woman, as this chapter illustrates. In using the Rorschach for this clinical population, it is crucial to remember that mean Rorschach scores for battered women cannot reflect the individual variation of the unique person, with her own trauma experience. It is especially important to remember that trauma disorders have a biphasic presentation, and a perfectly bland Rorschach with a high *Lambda* may be a trauma protocol. As with any other psychological test, the Rorschach should be used in combination with other pieces of assessment data.

Newer indices (e.g., the Danger Index and the Oral Dependency Scale) have clear applicability to battered women and deserve further research. To date, battered women's Rorschach protocols have been found to closely resemble trauma protocols from other trauma populations. The future will likely add new Rorschach data from groups of battered women and trauma survivors.

REFERENCES

American Psychiatric Association. (2000). *Diagnostic and statistical manual of mental disorders* (4th ed., text rev.). Washington, DC: Author.

Armstrong, J. G. (1994). Reflections on multiple personality disorder as a developmentally complex adaptation. *Psychoanalytic Study of the Child, 49*, 340–364.

Armstrong, J. G., & Kaser-Boyd, N. (2003). Projective assessment of psychological trauma. In M. Hilsenroth & D. Segal (Eds.), *Objective and projective assessment of personality and psychopathology: Vol. 2. Comprehensive handbook of psychological assessment* (pp. 500–512). New York: Wiley.

Armstrong, J. G., & Loewenstein, R. J. (1990). Characteristics of patients with multiple personality and dissociative disorders on psychological testing. *Journal of Nervous and Mental Disease, 178*, 445–454.

Blackman, J. (1990). Emerging images of severely battered women and the criminal justice system. *Behavioral Sciences and the Law, 8*, 121–130.

Bornstein, R. F. (1999). Criterion validity of objective and projective dependency tests: A meta-analytic assessment of behavioral prediction. *Psychological Assessment, 11*, 48–57.

Browne, A. (1987). *When battered women kill.* New York: The Free Press.

Burgess, A. W., & Holmstrom, L. L. (1974). Rape trauma syndrome. *American Journal of Psychiatry, 131*, 981–986.

Cammaert, L. A. (1988). Non-offending mothers: A new conceptualization. In L. E. A. Walker (Ed.), *Handbook on sexual abuse of children* (pp. 309–325). New York: Springer.

Cerney, M. (1990). The Rorschach and traumatic loss: Can the presence of traumatic loss be detected from the Rorschach? *Journal of Personality Assessment, 55*(3–4), 781–789.

Douglas, M. A. (1987). The battered woman syndrome. In D. J. Sonkin (Ed.), *Domestic violence on trial* (pp. 39–54). New York: Springer.

Dutton, D. (2002). *The abusive personality: Violence and control in intimate relationships.* New York: Guilford.

Dutton, M. A. (1996). Validity of "battered woman syndrome" in criminal cases involving battered women. In M. Gordon (Ed.), *The validity and use of evidence concerning battery and its effects in criminal trials: Report responding to Section 40507 of the violence against women act* (p. 17020). Washington, DC: U.S. Department of Justice.

Dutton, M. A. (1992) Understanding women's responses to domestic violence: A redefinition of battered woman syndrome. *Hofstra Law Review, 21*(4), 1191–1242.

Eigenberg, H. M. (2001). *Woman battering in the United States: Till death do us part.* Prospect Heights, IL: Waveland Press.

Ephraim, D., & Kaser-Boyd, N. (2003, March). *A Rorschach index to assess preoccupation with danger.* Paper presented at the annual meeting of the Society for Personality Assessment, San Francisco, CA.

Exner, J. E. (1993). *The Rorschach: A comprehensive system. Vol. 1: Basic foundations* (3rd ed.). New York: Wiley.

Exner, J. E. (2003). *The Rorschach: A comprehensive system* (4th ed.). New York: Wiley.

Exner, J., & Erdberg, P. (2005). *The Rorschach: A Comprehensive System: Vol. 2. Advanced interpretation* (3rd ed.). Hoboken, NJ: Wiley.

Fear: The brain plus emotions. (2003, March). *Discover Magazine*, 33–39.

Franchi, V., & Andronikof-Sanglade, A. (1993). Methodological and epistemological issues raised by the use of the Rorschach Comprehensive System in cross-cultural research. *Rorschachiana, 18*, 118–133.

Frueh, B. C., & Kinder, B. N. (1994). The susceptibility of the Rorschach inkblot test in malingering of combat-related PTSD. *Journal of Personality Assessment, 62*(2), 280–198.

Gacono, C., Evans, F. B., & Viglione, D. (2002). The Rorschach in forensic practice. *Journal of Forensic Psychology Practice, 2*(3), 33–54.

Hartman, W., Clark, M., Morgan, M., Dunn V., Fine, A., Perry, G., & Winsch, D. (1990). Rorschach structure of a hospitalized sample of Vietnam veterans with PTSD. *Journal of Personality Assessment, 54*(1–2), 149–159.

Hempel, C. L. (2004). Battered women who strike back: Using expert testimony on battering and its effects in homicide trials. In B. J. Cling (Ed.), *Sexualized violence against women and children* (pp. 71–97). New York: Guilford.

Herman, J. L. (1992). Complex post traumatic stress disorder: A syndrome in survivors of prolonged and repeated trauma. *Journal of Traumatic Stress, 5*(3), 377–389.

Hilberman, E., & Munson, K. (1978). Sixty battered women. *Victimology, 2*(3 & 4), 460–471.

Horowitz, M., Wilner, N., & Kaltreider, N. (1980). Signs and symptoms of post-traumatic stress disorder. *Archives of General Psychiatry, 37*, 85–92.

Kahn, F. I., Welch, T. L., & Zillmer, E. A. (1993). MMPI–2 profiles of battered women in transition. *Journal of Personality Assessment, 60*(1), 100–111.

Kaiser, R. B. (1970). *R.F.K. must die!: A history of the Robert Kennedy assassination and its aftermath.* New York: Dutton.

Kaser-Boyd, N. (1993). Rorschachs of women who commit homicide. *Journal of Personality Assessment, 60*(3), 458–470.

Kaser-Boyd, N. (2004). Battered Woman Syndrome: Clinical features, evaluation, and expert testimony. In B. J. Cling (Ed.), *Sexualized violence against women and children.* New York: Guilford.

Keane, T. M., Malloy, P. F., & Fairbank, J. A. (1984). Empirical development of an MMPI subscale for the assessment of combat-related posttraumatic stress disorder. *Journal of Consulting and Clinical Psychology, 52*, 888–891.

Krauss, D. A., & Sales, B. D. (2001, June). The effects of clinical and scientific expert testimony on juror decision making in capital sentencing. *Psychology, Public Policy, and Law, 7*(2), 267–310.

LeDoux, J. (1996). *The emotional brain: The mysterious underpinnings of emotional life.* New York: Simon & Schuster.

Leifer, M., Shapiro, J. P., Martone, M. W., & Kassem, L. (1991). Rorschach assessment of psychological functioning in sexually abused girls. *Journal of Personality Assessment, 56*, 14–28.

Levin, P., & Reis, B. (1997). Use of the Rorschach in assessing trauma. In J. P. Wilson & T. M. Keane (Eds.), *Assessing psychological trauma and PTSD* (pp. 529–543). New York: Guilford.

Levin, P. (1990). A normative study of the Rorschach and post-traumatic stress disorder. *Dissertation Abstracts International, 51*, 08-B, 4057.

Levin, P. (1993). Assessing PTSD with the Rorschach projective technique, In J. Wilson & B. Raphael (Eds.), *International handbook of traumatic stress syndromes.* New York: Plenum Press.

Levinger, G. (1966). Sources of marital dissatisfaction among applicants for divorce. *American Journal of Ortnopsychiatry, 89*, 804–806.

Meloy, J. R. (2005). Some reflections on *What's wrong with the Rorschach? Journal of Personality Assessment, 85*, 344–346.

Modlin, H. (1967). A post accident anxiety syndrome: Psychosocial aspects. *American Journal of Psychiatry, 123*(8), 1008–1012

Pagelow, M. D. (1992). Adult victims of domestic violence. *Journal of Interpersonal Violence, 7*(1), 87–120.

Parrish, J. (1996). Trend analysis: Expert testimony on battering and its effects in criminal cases. *Wisconsin Women's Law Journal*, 11, 75, 78, 83–87, 99–100, 112–115, 117–118, 121–123, 127, 131.

People v. Humphrey. (1996). 13 Cal 4th 1073.

Rollstin, A. O., & Kern, J. M. (1998). Correlates of battered woman's psychological distress: Severity of abuse and duration of the postabuse period. *Psychological Reports, 82*(2), 387–394.

Rhodes, N. R., & McKenzie, E. B. (1998). Why do battered women stay?: Three decades of research. *Aggression and Violent Behavior, 3*, 391–406.

Rosewater, L. B., & Walker, L. E. A. (Eds.). (1985). *Handbook of feminist therapy: Women's issues in psychotherapy.* New York: Springer.

Saunders, E. (1991). Rorschach indicators of chronic childhood sexual abuse in female borderline inpatients. *Bulletin of the Menninger Clinic, 55*, 48–70.

Schachtel, E. (1966). *Experimental foundations of Rorschach's test.* New York: Basic Books.

Schacter, D. L. (1996). *Searching for memory: The brain, the mind, and the past.* New York: Basic Books.

Society for Personality Assessment. (2005). Status of the Rorschach in clinical and forensic practice: An official statement by the Board of Trustees of the Society for Personality Assessment. *Journal of Personality Assessment, 85*(2), 219–237.

Souffrant, E. (1987). The use of the Rorschach in the assessment of post traumatic stress disorder among Vietnam combat veterans (Doctoral dissertation, Temple University, 1987). *Dissertation Abstracts International, 48,* 04B.

Swanson, G., Blount, J., & Bruni, R. (1990). Comprehensive system Rorschach data on Vietnam combat veterans. *Journal of Personality Assessment, 54*(1–2), 160–169.

Van der Hart, O., Witztum, E., & Friedman, B. (1993). From hysterical psychosis to reactive dissociative psychosis. *Journal of Traumatic Stress, 6*(1), 43–63.

van der Kolk, B. A. (1987). *Psychological trauma.* Washington, DC: American Psychiatric Press.

van der Kolk, B. A., & Ducey, C. (1984). Clinical implications of the Rorschach in posttraumatic stress disorder. In B. A. van der Kolk (Ed.), *Posttraumatic stress disorder: Psychological and biological sequelae* (pp. 30–42). Washington, DC: American Psychiatric Press.

van der Kolk, B. A., & Ducey, C. (1989). The psychological processing of traumatic experience: Rorschach patterns in post traumatic stress disorder. *Journal of Traumatic Stress, 2*(3), 259–274.

van der Kolk, B. A., Roth, S., Pelcovitz, D., Sunday, S., & Spinazzola, J. (2005). Disorders of extreme stress: The empirical foundation of a complex adaptation to trauma. *Journal of Traumatic Stress, 18*(5), 389–399.

Walker, L. E. A. (1979). *The battered woman.* New York: Harper & Row.

Walker, L. E. A. (1994). *Abused women and survivor therapy: A practical guide for the psychotherapist.* Washington, DC: American Psychological Association.

Wilson, J. P., & Walker, A. J. (1990). Toward an MMPI trauma profile. *Journal of Traumatic Stress, 3*(1), 151–168.

Wood, J. M., Nezworski, M. T., Lilienfeld, S. O., & Garb, H. N. (2003). *What's wrong with the Rorschach?* San Francisco: Jossey-Bass.

Zivney, O. A., Nash, M. R., & Hulsey, T. L. (1988). Sexual abuse in early versus late childhood: Differing patterns of pathology as revealed on the Rorschach. *Psychotherapy—Theory, Research, and Practice, 25,* 99–106.

23

THE RORSCHACH AND IMMIGRATION EVALUATIONS

F. Barton Evans
Private Practice, Bozeman, MT

The use of forensic psychological experts in immigration matters is a developing and evolving area of practice (Evans, 2000; Frumkind & Friedland, 1995), which has increasingly provided attorneys with valuable and, at times, essential evidence in representing their clients before the U.S. Citizenship and Immigration Service (USCIS) and the Immigration Court (IC).[1] Yet, psychological assessments adequate in clinical settings or forensic reports based solely on clinical treatment frequently fail to address the more stringent standards of objectivity and neutrality required for psychological assessment in the legal setting (see Weiner & Hess, 2006; Melton, Petrila, Poythress, & Slobogin, 1998) and the particularities of IC (Frumkind & Friedland, 1995).

The requirement for factual information obtained in an objective way in forensic assessment makes the use of psychological testing with its empirical methods a natural fit with the requirements of the court. Few instruments have the broad international usage (Ritzler, 2001; Viglione, 1999; Viglione & Hilsenroth, 2001; Viglione & Meyer, chap. 2, this vol.), complete with international norms (Erdberg, 2005; Erdberg & Schaffer, 1999), as the Rorschach Comprehensive System (CS) (Exner, 2003).[2] The purpose of this chapter is to provide an overview of areas where forensic psychological assessment and expert testimony may be useful in immigration practice and to discuss the value of the Rorschach in such evaluations within each area. Whereas this chapter discusses the special value of the Rorschach in forensic evaluation in immigration issues, it must be emphasized that all forensic psychological assessment must be conducted using a multimethod approach (see Erdberg, chap. 27, this vol.).

---

[1]Immigration Court also includes the Board of Immigration Appeals (BIA), which are administratively under the purview of the Department of Homeland Security.

[2]Throughout this chapter, all references to the Rorschach are to the CS (Exner, 2003), the only Rorschach with sufficient empirical validity to be admissible in court (Gacono, Evans, & Viglione, 2002 and chap. 1, this vol.; McCann, Evans, chap. 3, this vol.).

AREAS OF PRACTICE OF FORENSIC PSYCHOLOGY IN IC

Because the practice of immigration law addresses a broad and diverse set of legal issues, the following areas are most pertinent for the application of psychological expertise (Evans, 2000), including:

1. The assessment of torture and rape for asylum and Convention Against Torture (CAT) claims.
2. The assessment of physical, sexual, and psychological abuse and extreme mental cruelty in claims for permanent residence of a battered spouse or children of a U.S. citizen under Subtitle G—Protections for Battered Immigrant Women and Children of *The Violence Against Women Act of 1998* (VAWA).
3. The assessment of extreme hardship in suspension of deportation proceedings.
4. The assessment of recidivism and dangerousness for exceptions to mandatory deportation for aggravated felony and for parole from indefinite suspension.

The kinds of evidence provided by psychological experts vary according to area, reflecting different information probative to the court. Additionally, as a general rule, each kind of case will call for different kinds of psychological expertise and therefore different experts. The following sections outline the kinds of information and expertise that are valuable in immigration cases and the role of the Rorschach in these areas of immigration law.

In addition to professional and scientific knowledge, it is essential that the forensic psychologists have a working understanding of the legal issues relevant to each IC area. Gathering, weighing, and presenting psychological assessment information for the court is significantly different from standard clinical protocols. As a result, there are fundamental differences between the forensic examiner and the mental health clinician (Greenberg & Shuman, 1997). The most important difference between these roles is that the forensic examiner must take an objective, neutral stance in the evaluation, although, in the case of the assessment of torture and psychological trauma, neutrality must be understood in a broader context (Evans, 2005).

ASYLUM AND CONVENTION AGAINST TORTURE

Perhaps the best known use of psychological and psychiatric evaluation on immigrations matters involves asylum and CAT claims (see Evans, 2000; Jacobs, Evans, & Patsilides, 2001a, b). Individuals seeking political asylum often arrive in the United States with little more than the clothes on their back, lacking the documentation to support their claims. A claim of asylum has two grounds, both of which must be met. Asylum seekers must have a well-founded fear of persecution, either fear of future persecution or the experience of past persecution of such severity that it would be inhumane to return to their country of origin. Next, persecution must be on account of one or more of the five qualifying grounds: race, religion, nationality, membership in a particular social group, or political opinion. Often these individuals claim torture and rape to be a part of their persecution, although there are other grounds for asylum (e.g., fear of female genital mutilation because of membership in a group unprotected by their government; see *Matter of Kasinga*, 1996; Kassindja & Miller, 1998). For an extensive coverage of the legal issues involved in asylum law, see Anker (1998).

Sadly, the widespread use of torture and rape as instruments of persecution and repression is well documented (Dross, 2000). At the same time, immigration attorneys, USCIS asylum officers and attorneys, and IC judges are left with a bewildering array of stories and behaviors from asylum seekers that are difficult to interpret and to substantiate. In addition, immigration judges (IJ) are confronted with torturous stories of human cruelty. Additionally, because the burden of proof is on the asylum seekers, they are faced with sharing horrific, incomprehensible, and degrading experiences in an adversarial setting (Dignam, 1992). Forensic psychologists, psychiatrists, and social workers with expertise in psychological trauma can provide expert opinions about the impact and severity of torture and rape (and therefore the credibility of claim), as well as the psychological consequences of deportation.

The use of forensic psychological assessment of asylum/CAT claims for the immigration courts rests on two overlaying general principles: an in-depth knowledge of the psychological impact of torture and rape and a clear understanding of the way in which such information is germane within the legal context (see Committee on the Ethical Guidelines for Forensic Psychologists, 1991; Frumkind & Friedland, 1995; Hess & Weiner, 1999; Melton et al., 1998; Shapiro, 1984). As Evans (2000) identified, in-depth psychological knowledge required in asylum/CAT claims encompasses psychological expertise in three distinct areas:

1. Knowledge of the literature on the impact and psychological sequelae of torture, rape, and other forms of interpersonal violence, including the impact of severe trauma in general (see Herman, 1992; Pelcovitz et al., 1997; Putnam, 1989; van der Kolk, McFarlane, & Weisaeth, 1996) and addressing such issues as impaired memory (Herlihy, Scragg, & Turner, 2002).

2. Familiarity with the psychological assessment of psychological trauma beyond what can be gathered in a clinical interview (see Evans, 2000; Garb, 1998). Such assessment includes understanding the various empirically derived psychological assessment instruments as well as structured and semistructured interviews (e.g., see Briere, 1995; Butcher, 1998; Butcher, Williams, Graham, Tellegen, & Kaemmer, 1989; Foa, Riggs, Dancu, & Rothbaum, 1993).

3. Knowledge of how both the psychology of trauma and the assessment of trauma operate in the context of cross-cultural issues (Frumkind & Friedland, 1995), including increased sensitivity toward the respondent undergoing the evaluation (Stark, 1996). Far too often in forensic psychology, the terms *objective* and *neutral* have been interpreted as disbelieving and remote (Evans, 2005), which is anathema to women and men struggling to describe overwhelming torture experiences (Mollica, Wyshak, & Lavelle 1987; Mollica et al., 1992). The examiner's stance of benevolent neutrality (see Evans, 2005; Weigert, 1970) allows the asylum seekers to share their story as they choose to represent it.

ASSESSMENT OF TORTURE AND RAPE AND THE RORSCHACH

The first caveat for psychological testing of torture victims is that the assessor must be mindful that the test-taking situation, and even the choice of psychological instrument, may evoke overwhelming memories and feelings of the torture situation (Pope & Garcia-Peltoniemi, 1991). Nowhere is this concern more relevant than with the use of the Rorschach. In their exploratory study using the Rorschach with Vietnam war veterans, van der Kolk and Ducey (1984, 1989) noted two distinct patterns of response—traumatic flooded presentations and traumatic avoidant presentations—reflecting biphasic response to trauma, in which intrusion and emotional flooding alternate with avoidance and psychic numbing (van der Kolk, 1994). Given its capacity to evoke powerful reactions, the Rorschach should be approached with caution.

My assessment experience of approximately 100 torture victims leads me to note a striking phenomenon. Instead of one or the other of the elements of the biphasic response dominating the experience of the torture victim, I found that the horrific and relentless intrusive experiences of the torture, regardless of whether the victim is awake or asleep, overwhelm pervasive and extreme attempts at avoidance and numbing. This pattern indicates that victims can literally get no relief, no matter how much effort they put forth. This futile effort to seek relief through avoidance and dissociation is at the essence of the torture experience. Torture methods are frequently so sophisticated that, unlike many traumatic experiences, there is no way to escape or mitigate the pain and the "terrible knowledge" (Jay, 1991) accompanying it. Victims carry this appalling legacy with them and are tortured over and over again.

This experiential pattern of torture victims has important implications for the use of the Rorschach in such assessments. As Jacobs et al. (2001a, b) stated, the use of the Rorschach with torture victims should be considered with extreme caution. These individuals risk becoming overwhelmed emotionally by the evocative images in the test. For example, think about Card II and imagine how a tortured person can integrate the darkness and color with its powerful pull for images of blood, damage, and despair. Once victims experience Card II, they may shut down or wretchedly re-experience terrifying events. The experience may be simply too much—especially, for example, for those whose torture was relatively recent; for those who were tortured when they were young; for those where rape, sexual humiliation, and torture were used frequently and in concert; or for those where the types and variety of torture methods were especially atrocious.

Despite these cautions using the Rorschach with victims of torture and extreme violence, in other circumstances it remains a valuable assessment method. Ephraim (2002) points out the notable strengths of the Rorschach in trauma assessment and how it can be used well to assess cognitive disturbances associated with intrusive recollections, differentiating avoidant and numbing defense patterns, changes in identity and relatedness, and problems with self-regulation and dissociation in cases of concurrent early trauma. Ephraim presents seven vignettes in his article, four of women who were raped, threatened, and harassed by police and other governmental groups and three of older men who had been imprisoned and tortured. The women did not appear to be victims of systematic torture, but were victims of state violence. In these cases, Rorschach might be productively used to assess such individuals (except perhaps the 16 year old) as part of their asylum application because of the powerful way it can both illustrate the inner world of their traumatic experiences and support their claim, or alternatively, be indicative of malingering or deception. It is unclear when the three men, all in their mid- to late 30s, were tortured, or how frequently or how severely. The Rorschach might also be considered with these individuals as well, especially if their torture was not recent and if their avoidant/numbing symptoms were prominent and made it difficult to assess their experience through interview and more focused trauma-specific assessment methods.

Also, in his study of Mexican homosexuals, both those in Mexico and those illegally in the United States, Tori (1989) used the Rorschach. For members of scapegoated and persecuted groups, the test can be used to elucidate dysphoric mood, distorted perceptions, and significant difficulties coping with an increasingly dangerous social environment as they may legitimately be seeking asylum.

In summary, the Rorschach should be used with caution in the forensic assessment of asylum seekers, especially when political torture and rape is at issue before the court. It has the potential for overwhelming fragile defenses and subjecting the asylum seeker to the devastating, and likely unnecessary reviving, of terrifying emotions. The Rorschach is perhaps most usefully considered when it is unclear whether the individual was sophisticatedly malingering symptoms of trauma or being deceptive about a torture experience. Additionally, the Rorschach can be valuable in revealing more temporally distant traumatic experiences of asylum seekers, long since buried by the avoidant/numbing symptoms of PTSD. Lastly, the Rorschach can be of great value in demonstrating the profound underlying terror and anguish brought on by systematic government scapegoating and persecution of particular groups.

DOMESTIC ABUSE AND VAWA

A related area of psychological expertise relevant to immigration attorneys is the psychological assessment of domestic abuse, including spousal abuse and child abuse. Considerable professional and scientific literature has emerged in recent years, which has well described the psychology of women (e.g., Dutton, 1992; Walker, 1979, 1984, 1994) and men (e.g., Bergman & Brismar, 1992; Smith & Loring, 1994) subjected to physical, sexual, and psychological abuse in their intimate relationships. Additionally, D. G. Dutton (1995, 1998) has developed valuable profiles of men who batter, which can be used to provide validation of women's descriptions of their reportedly abusive husbands. Immigration attorneys may find themselves in need of documenting spousal or child abuse as part of their clients' petition for permanent residency under Subtitle G—Protections for Battered Immigrant Women and Children of the Violence Against Women Act of 1998 (VAWA). It is important to note that the abused spouse definition under this section of VAWA covers men as well as women.

Immigrant spouses and children of abusive U.S. citizens find themselves in a desperate situation when they are under the virtual control and enslavement of the abusive spouse. In such situations, the abusive citizens will not support their immigrant spouse's or child's applications for permanent residency and often threaten to have their family members deported if these individuals do not tolerate the abuse and comply with their wishes. In extreme cases, battered women and men report that they feel entrapped and afraid of leaving because of a variety of severe threats (Kaser-Boyd, 2004); for example, the abuser may talk about defaming these individuals' reputations in their home country to further enforce the threats of divorce and deportation. An in-depth forensic psychological assessment can be crucial evidence in establishing the reported physical, sexual, or psychological abuse or extreme mental cruelty, as well as the credibility of the respondent. In addition, in suspension of deportation proceedings, psychological evidence of extreme hardship (see later) to the abused respondent also can be useful based on other relevant factors such as mental disorder and the need for treatment, medical problems, longevity in the United States, family ties to other U.S. citizens and permanent residents, and cross-cultural factors (e.g., cultural reactions to divorce in the abused spouse's home country).

ASSESSMENT OF DOMESTIC ABUSE AND THE RORSCHACH

Specific psychological instruments have been developed that can be highly useful in objectively documenting the types and degree of interpersonal violence of men toward women and vice versa (see Abusive Observation Behavior Checklist, Dutton, 1992; Conflict Tactics Scales, Strauss, 1979).[3] Although substantial, these instruments do little to bring alive the inner experience of battered immigrant women and men. These individuals feel devalued, damaged, worthless, and ashamed. Physical injury and sexual assault can further lead them to experience the loss of bodily integrity (Kaser-Boyd, chap. 22, this vol.). The Rorschach can greatly assist in making known the inner reality of the battered spouse and help corroborate claims of abuse (Kaser-Boyd, 1993).

Kaser-Boyd (1993) studied the Rorschachs of women who killed their battering spouses. Consistent with the biphasic response of trauma victims (van der Kolk, 1994) and the Rorschach in the early van der Kolk and Ducey studies (1984, 1989), she found these women's Rorschach records divided between high *Lambda* and low *Lambda* styles, suggesting the former group in the constricted or avoidant phase and the latter group in the flooded and intrusive phase. As would be expected, high *Lambda*, constricted or avoidant phase women showed Rorschach indicators of cognitive constriction, low internal resources for problem solving, ambitent and passive problem-solving styles, poorly modulated affect, poor scanning for details in the environment, and eccentric reality testing. Women with low *Lambda*, flooded records produced profiles that indicated anxiety ridden feelings of helplessness (*m*), were permeated thematically with morbid and aggressive images and images of entrapment, showing clear signs of "traumatic psychosis" (see Kaser-Boyd & Evans, chap. 13, this vol.). These Rorschach images dramatically communicate the phenomenological experience of being battered.

---

[3]Although the abuse of immigrant children is included under VAWA, this chapter focuses on the more frequent assessment of abused immigrant adults.

Additionally, intermittent dissociation and dissociative disorders are regularly found among severely battered women (Coons, Cole, Pellow, & Milstein, 1990). The Rorschach has proven to be an excellent assessment instrument of dissociative disorders (Armstrong, 2002; Brand, Armstrong, & Loewenstein, 2006; Scroppo, Weinberger, Drob, & Eagle, 1998), especially Armstrong's Trauma Content Index (Armstrong, 1991; Armstrong & Lowenstein, 1990). In particular, Brand et al. (2006) reported on a large Rorschach sample of 100 psychiatric in-patients who were severely dissociated and found clear signs of traumatic avoidance and traumatic intrusion in this population (for a detailed discussion see Kaser-Boyd & Evans, chap. 13, this vol.).

As mentioned earlier, the Rorschach can also be useful in assessing malingering and deception in trauma-based evaluations. Evans (2004) reported a case of a battered Pakistani woman seeking a hardship waiver. Whereas other psychological testing and interview data were equivocal, the Rorschach showed clear evidence of profound psychological disturbance consistent with her description of very severe childhood physical abuse and spousal battering. Sadly, this woman became severely dissociated during the administration of the Rorschach and experienced a period of increased severe depression afterward. In such circumstances, the benefits of receiving the extreme hardship waiver due to past domestic abuse outweighed the cost, although at the price of severe distress during the evaluation.

EXTREME HARDSHIP WAIVER

The concept of the hardship waiver essentially allows the immigration judge the discretion to suspend removal of an individual who otherwise would be deported for a violation of immigration law because of the privation it would cause to qualifying spouse, children, or parents. Hake (1994) points out that the term *hardship* in immigration law carries with it a qualifier that can vary from exceptional to extreme to extremely unusual, although the criteria for hardship are not well defined and the terms essentially interchangeable. Hake and Banks (2005) noted six major areas for extreme hardship to the spouse or child of the individual in deportation proceeding: medical hardships, psychological hardships, career or educational disruptions, very serious financial hardships, sociocultural hardships upon relocation to the home, and significant risk of physical harm due to political or sectarian violence.

The most obvious area of extreme psychological hardship involves a qualifying family member's mental disorder (e.g., depression or schizophrenia) and the impact of deportation on the individual's condition, especially if appropriate treatment would not be available in the destination country. The formal assessment of malingering and deception (see Rogers, 1997) can also help the court with issues involving credibility of a claim of extreme psychological hardship (Evans, 2000; Frumkind & Friedland, 1995).

Another application of forensic psychology to extreme hardship waivers is the "family impact statement," which establishes the impact of loss through deportation of a parent, child, or spouse on the family. Although there is no research on the impact of deportation on children, there is ample psychological literature that can illustrate the psychological impact of loss of a parent. For example, the literature strongly indicates the short-term and long-term deleterious impact of the loss of a parent on children through death (e.g., Kaffman & Elizur, 1984; Lehman, Lang, Wortman, & Sorenson, 1989), divorce (e.g., Amato & Keith, 1991; Wallerstein & Kelly, 1980; Wolchik & Karoly, 1988), and all forms of parental absence (Amato & Keith, 1991). The assessment of children facing loss of a parent through deportation can establish depression, anxiety, or other mental disorders, or special psychosocial factors that could be exacerbated by the loss. Further considerations could include the psychological impact of removing the child to a different culture with a different language and—a critical factor often overlooked—the psychological impact of the extreme loss of financial resources on children's development (see Brooks-Gunn & Duncan, 1997).

Similarly, psychological assessment can also evaluate the U.S. citizen spouse or elderly parent for mental disorder, either caused or exacerbated by loss (see Carnelley, Wortman, & Kessler, 1999; Maciejewski, Prigerson, & Mazure, 2001), for the impact of loss on health (see Martikainen & Valkonen, 1996), and for vulnerability to suicide after profound and sudden loss (see de Vries, Davis, Wortman, & Lehman, 1997; Li, 1995). Finally, consistent with Horowitz's (1993) research on stress response syndromes, social disruption of the family arising from the deportation of a spouse or parent can also trigger powerful stress responses. More specifically, as Lin (1986) has noted, the social disruption experienced by refugees commonly results in powerful emotional and behavioral manifestations of distress, including depression, anxiety, dissociation, and even reactive psychosis. The loss of a family member to deportation can activate a similar process.

EXTREME HARDSHIP WAIVERS AND THE RORSCHACH

Unlike the assessment of psychological trauma underlying its use in asylum and VAWA evaluations, the Rorschach serves a more general role in psychological testing in extreme psychological hardship evaluations. It is especially useful in evaluating several areas specific to the kinds of distress experienced by families anticipating the loss of a family member through deportation. First, the Rorschach can be used to substantiate and support underlying processes in mental disorders. As Hake (1994) has noted, the presence of a preexisting or coincident mental disorder is an important factor to consider for granting a waiver of extreme hardship. Whereas the Rorschach is not designed to diagnose *DSM–IV* (American Psychiatric Association, 1994) mental disorders (Exner, 2003), it can be highly useful in providing a fine-grained assessment of factors underlying mental disorder and its nexus to the psycholegal issue before the immigration court.

Second, when a wife or husband faces the sudden and irrevocable loss of a spouse (see Hays, Kasl, & Jacobs, 1994a), especially when there has been a past history of dysphoria (see Hays, Kasl, & Jacobs, 1994b), the Rorshach can also provide documentation of situational, although often severe, emotional distress underlying the common reactions of depression (e.g., *D/AdjD*; *DEPI*) and helplessness (e.g., *m* and *FY*). Moreover, as both Horowitz (1993) and Lin (1986) noted, acute reactive psychosis is also a known stress response to the social disruption experienced by family members in response to the dislocation of a spouse and parent through deportation. The Rorschach is uniquely suited to assess both the cognitive decompensation (e.g., *PTI*, including *WSUM6*) and intense emotional distress in acute reactive psychosis or its prodromal phase.

Third, the Rorschach can also be highly useful in gauging vulnerability and resiliency necessary to assess the psycholegal question of "extreme hardship beyond the normal stress of separation due to deportation." The presumption in the immigration court is that individuals must show that the hardship due to the deportation of their spouse is extreme. The following case example is illustrative.

Mrs. S was a 34-year-old married woman with a 4-year-old son, whose husband was placed in removal proceedings because of an aggravated felony committed 15 years prior. Despite a childhood background of poverty, abuse, and neglect, she was a very competent midlevel manager for a telecommunications company and was a successful athlete in college. Also, despite her seeming strengths, Mrs. S claimed that the loss of her husband would be devastating to her. A psychological evaluation was conducted to assess her claim of extreme psychological hardship. The results of her PAI were of marginal validity due to a defensive response style in which she denied psychological problems. Her Rorschach was interpretatively useful and documented her vulnerability to severe depression characterized by low self-esteem and a lack of emotional and interpersonal resources with which to handle stress. She currently experienced exceptionally high levels of situational stress, as well as a chronic vulnerability to becoming upset, anxious, and disorganized. Mrs. S was highly susceptible to decompensation under stress, as demonstrated by her difficulty in thinking logically and coherently. She was withdrawn and isolated interpersonally and her social skills were limited, except in clearly structured situations. In summary, consistent with her history of tragic loss and emotional neglect, the psychological assessment revealed that Mrs. S was an emotionally vulnerable individual with high susceptibility to depression. It was clear that she had developed a very positive relationship with her husband, which provided considerable stability in her life despite her background. Based in part on the psychological assessment of extreme hardship to his wife, Mr. S was granted a waiver of deportation and a recent follow-up with their attorney indicated that Mrs. S continues to function adequately, although with previously mentioned limitations.

This case illustrates how powerfully the Rorschach can bring alive the inner experience of individuals whose character defenses all but shut out inner suffering in their daily lives and on objective testing. As Hake and Banks (2005, p. 417) state, "Exceptional cases may require a report from a forensic psychologist. In the rare cases, where there is no apparent outward hardship, but there is in fact very serious and unusual inward hardship." In such circumstances, the Rorschach may provide critical information for fully documenting a claim of extreme psychological hardship.

ASSESSMENT OF PAROLE AND RECIDIVISM

Another role for forensic psychologists involves expert evaluation and testimony on immigration court issues involving the parole of individuals in indefinite detention and in suspension of mandatory deportation following an aggravated felony (for a more extensive coverage of this aspect of criminal immigration law, see Kesselbrenner & Rosenthal,

1984, with updates through 2006). Indefinite detention in the immigration context occurs when a foreign national who is a legal permanent resident or is in the United States illegally commits a deportable criminal offense, but cannot be returned to the country of origin for a variety of reasons, such as Convention Against Torture or the unwillingness for a foreign country to receive deportees. In such instances, the immigrant is placed in indefinite detention, literally an open-ended imprisonment until conditions in the country of origin allow for deportation to occur. Parole from indefinite detention involves two primary areas in which expert opinion may be useful. The first involves parole for "emergent reasons" of aliens who are detained after arrival in the United States without proper documentation. Such emergent reasons include serious medical conditions (e.g., severe mental disorder). Appropriate psychological assessment can help establish the presence and credibility of a mental disorder. As Frumkind and Friedland (1995) point out, the psychologist expert can also consider the psychological impact of detention and imprisonment (see Haney & Zimbardo, 1998; Zimbardo, 1973). This assessment, combined with an assessment of potential dangerousness (see Monahan & Steadman, 1994; Webster, Douglas, Eaves, & Hart, 1997), can help establish whether or not continued confinement is in the best interest of the public. The use of such expert forensic mental health assessment and testimony was important in establishing the deleterious effects of incarceration in the landmark female genital mutilation case of Fauziya Kassindja (Kassindja & Miller, 1998).

An additional area for psychological expertise involves parole from indefinite detention of undeportable aliens who are incarcerated for aggravated felonies. The use of Rorschach, along with powerful psychological tools such as the Hare Psychopathy Checklist–Revised (Gacono, Loving, Evans, & Jumes, 2002; Hare, 1993, 2003), the Violence Risk Assessment Guide (Harris, Rice, & Cormier,1993), and the HCL–20 (Webster et al., 1997), can provide attorneys with valuable information regarding violent recidivism and the potential danger to the public of parole of an incarcerated alien. As described by Rosenberg and Evans (2003),[4] the same methodology is used as crucial evidence in petitioning the USCIS for exceptions to mandatory deportation for aggravated felony, especially concerning the rehabilitation and future recidivism risk.[5]

THE RORSCHACH IN ASSESSMENT OF PAROLE AND RECIDIVISM

To date, the most extensive research on the forensic use of the Rorschach has been the work of Gacono and his colleagues on antisocial and psychopathic personalities in criminal settings (see Gacono & Meloy, 1994; Gacono, Gacono, & Evans, chap. 16, this vol.). Recently, this literature has been applied to forensic assessment of criminal matters in immigration court (Evans, 2000; Rosenberg & Evans, 2003), which in conjunction with

---

[4]This article contains a detailed legal analysis when recidivism and dangerousness may be at issue, such as those involving release from detention and various forms of relief from removal based on a conviction.

[5]There are two prongs in the determination of a waiver of removal of an aggravated felon (i.e., a person convicted of a felony carrying a sentence of greater than one year). The first prong is whether or not the individual has been rehabilitated, including future risk of danger to the community and recidivism. The second prong involves extreme hardship to a qualifying U.S. citizen or legal permanent resident spouse, child, or parent.

the PCL–R (Hare, 2003) and risk assessment/recidivism risk assessment tools such as the Level of Service Inventory–Revised (LSI–R) (Andrews & Bonta, 1995) can assist in determinations of parole from indefinite detention and of waivers of deportation. Because risk/recidivism assessment tools have important limitations (see Zamble & Quinsey, 1997, for the problem static, "tombstone" markers), the Rorschach allows for a thorough assessment of dynamic variables when assessing risk. Additionally, substantial forensic Rorschach reference group data (Gacono, Gacono, & Evans, chap. 16, this vol.) allow for further empirical comparisons regarding the degree to which a particular individual is similar or dissimilar to known criminal populations. Such data is especially useful in assisting immigration judges, because the presence of recidivistic criminals in immigration court has a much lower base rate than in federal and state criminal courts.

The following case example is illustrative of how the Rorschach provided important information in assisting a judge's determination of the rehabilitation and future recidivism risk of a 30-year-old legal permanent resident male placed in deportation proceedings for an aggravated felony committed 9 years earlier after recent parole from USCIS detention.

Mr. W came to the United States from a Caribbean country at age 12 with his family. Within several years, he became involved with other adolescent antisocial peers and the predatory adults who supplied illegal drugs. He reported that his participation led to 14 arrests, both as a juvenile and as an adult, until he was convicted for possession with intent to distribute marijuana at age 18. He had no legal or behavioral difficulties before coming to the United States and was never involved in stealing from others, vandalizing property, cruelty toward animals, or fire setting, nor was he enuretic after toilet training. After his last arrest, Mr. W determined to leave his life in the drug culture, which he did by no longer associating with past street friends and by getting training and a job as an auto-mechanic. Shortly afterward, he met his current wife and had a daughter with her. He became increasingly involved in raising his daughter and stepson, becoming the more nurturing of the two parents, and was noted for his reliability at work.

A psychological evaluation was conducted to assess his claim of rehabilitation. His PCL–R score, while elevated due to his past arrests, was significantly lower than the average incarcerated felon and his PAI was valid and showed situational anxiety, but otherwise indicated no psychopathology. The results of Mr. W's Rorschach indicated fewer psychological resources for coping with the demands of everyday living, although he used an avoidant style and overly simplistic way of looking at the world to maintain a stable psychological equilibrium. He showed good reality testing and sound judgment, indicating an ability to recognize and act on conventional expectations and modes of behavior and to engage in adaptive interpersonal behaviors. Most importantly, the results did not suggest that Mr. W had the aggressiveness, chronic excitement seeking and poor impulse control, externalization of responsibility, lack of remorse, and callous disregard for others found in chronic criminal offenders.

Mr. W was granted a waiver of deportation by the immigration judge, in substantial part due to the results of his evaluation of rehabilitation and the finding of extreme psychological hardship to his wife, who had a long history of depression, and to his children with whom he was deeply bonded. A recent follow-up with his attorney indicated that he continues to do well at work and at home, including fathering another child with whom he is also very close.

This case illustrates how the Rorschach can provide important psychodynamic information in assessing recidivism risk in criminal immigration issues. As Rosenberg and Evans (2003) stated, such evaluations can help provide "Another Chance," or what Maruna (2001, p. 26) calls *desistence* (i.e., "the long-term abstinence from crime by individuals who had previously engaged in a persistent pattern of criminal offending" or the process of "making good"). Indeed, in such circumstances, the Rorschach may provide critical information for fully documenting a claim of rehabilitation and recidivism risk. Such evaluations afford families and individuals relief from often overly harsh criminal immigration laws when immigrants have successfully been rehabilitated.

CONCLUSIONS

In closing, the application of the principles of forensic psychology to immigration court is an exciting and expanding area. Productive alliances can be forged between immigration attorneys, the immigration court, and psychologist experts. This chapter has been an initial attempt to explicate where and how the Rorschach may be used in immigration court and USCIS administrative proceedings to provide relevant, and often critical, information. The psycholegal issues in immigration court are diverse and complex, but also highly rewarding for the forensic examiner who is willing to both understand the legal issues involved and their nexus to psychological assessment. This chapter has attempted to highlight how the Rorschach can be used in such evaluations in the context of relevant legal issues. It is my view that the Rorschach can be very helpful when used appropriately in forensic evaluation in immigration court.

ACKNOWLEDGMENT

I wish to express my gratitude to Judy Maris for her support and invaluable editing help.

REFERENCES

Amato, P. R., & Keith, B. (1991). Parental divorce and the well-being of children: A meta-analysis. *Psychological Bulletin, 110,* 26–46.

American Psychiatric Association. (1994). *Diagnostic and statistical manual of mental disorders* (4th ed.). Washington, DC: American Psychiatric Press.

Andrews, D. A., & Bonta, J. (1995). *The Level of Service Inventory–Revised manual.* North Tonawanda, NY: Multi-Health Systems.

Anker, D. (1998). *Law of asylum in the United States* (3rd ed.). Cambridge, MA: Refugee Law Center.

Armstrong, J. G. (1991). The psychological organization of multiple personality disordered patients as revealed in psychological testing. *Psychiatric Clinics of North America, 14,* 533–546.

Armstrong, J. G. (2002). Deciphering the broken narrative of trauma: Signs of traumatic dissociation on the Rorschach. In A. Andronikof (Ed.), *Rorschachiana XXV: Yearbook of the International Rorschach Society* (pp. 11–27). Ashland, OH: Hogrefe & Huber.

Armstrong, J. G., & Loewenstein, R. J. (1990). Characteristics of patients with multiple personality and dissociative disorders on psychological testing. *Journal of Nervous and Mental Disease, 178,* 445–454.

Bergman, B. K., & Brismar, B. G. (1992). Do not forget the battered male!: A comparative study of family and non-family violence victims. *Scandinavian Journal of Social Medicine, 20*, 179–183.

Brand, B. L., Armstrong, J. G., & Loewenstein, R. J. (2006). Psychological assessment of patients with dissociative identity disorder. *Psychiatric Clinics of North America, 29*, 145–168.

Briere, J. (1995). *Trauma Symptom Inventory*. Odessa, FL: Psychological Assessment Resources.

Brooks-Gunn, J., & Duncan, G. J. (1997). The effects of poverty on children. *Future of Children, 7*, 55–71.

Butcher, J. (Ed.). (1998). *International adaptations of the MMPI–2*. Minneapolis: University of Minnesota.

Butcher, J., Williams, C., Graham, J., Tellegen, A., & Kaemmer, B. (1989) *MMPI–2: Manual for administration and scoring*. Minneapolis: University of Minnesota.

Carnelley, K. B., Wortman, C. B., & Kessler, R. C. (1999). The impact of widowhood on depression: Findings from a prospective survey. *Psychological Medicine, 29*, 1111–1123.

Committee on the Ethical Guidelines for Forensic Psychologists. (1991). Specialty guidelines for forensic psychologists. *Law and Human Behavior, 1*, 655–665.

Coons, P. M., Cole, C., Pellow, T. A., & Milstein, V. (1990). Symptoms of posttraumatic stress and dissociation in women victims of abuse. In R. P. Kluft (Ed.), *Incest-related syndromes of adult psychopathology* (pp. 205–225). Washington, DC: American Psychiatric Association.

de Vries, B., Davis, C. G., Wortman, C. B., & Lehman, D. R. (1997). Long-term psychological and somatic consequences of later life parental bereavement. *Omega: Journal of Death & Dying, 35*, 97–117.

Dignam, Q. (1992). The burden and the proof: Torture and testimony in the determination of refugee status in Australia. *International Journal of Refugee Law, 4*, 343–363.

Dross, P. (2000). Survivors of politically motivated torture: A large, growing, and invisible population of crime victims. *Office of Victims of Crime Report*. Washington, DC: Office of Justice Programs, U.S. Department of Justice.

Dutton, D. G. (1998). The *abusive personality*. New York: Guilford.

Dutton, D. G. (1995). The *batterer: A psychological profile*. New York: Basic Books.

Dutton, M. A. (1992). *Empowering and healing the battered woman*. New York: Springer.

Ephraim, D. (2002). Rorschach trauma assessment of survivors of torture and state violence. In A. Andronikof (Ed.), *Rorschachiana XXV: Yearbook of the International Rorschach Society* (pp. 58–76). Ashland, OH: Hogrefe & Huber.

Erdberg, P. (2005, July). *Intercoder agreement as a measure of ambiguity of coding guidelines* Paper presented at the 18th International Congress of Rorschach and Projective Methods, Barcelona.

Erdberg, P., & Schaffer, T. W. (1999, July). *International symposium on Rorschach nonpatient data: Findings from around the world*. Paper presented at the International Congress of Rorschach and Projective Methods, Amsterdam, The Netherlands.

Evans, F. B. (2000). Forensic psychology and immigration court: An introduction. In R. Auerbach (Ed.), *Handbook of immigration and nationality law: Vol. 2. Advanced topics* (pp. 446–458). Washington, DC: American Immigration Lawyers Association.

Evans, F. B. (2004). Family violence, immigration law, and the Rorschach. In A. Andronikof (Ed.), *Rorschachiana XXVI: Yearbook of the International Rorschach Society* (pp. 147–157). Ashland, OH: Hogrefe & Huber.

Evans, F. B., III. (2005). Trauma, torture, and transformation in the forensic assessor. *Journal of Personality Assessment, 84*, 25–28.

Exner, J. (2003) *The Rorschach: A Comprehensive System: Basic foundations* (4th ed.). New York: Wiley.

Foa, E. B., Riggs, D., Dancu, C., & Rothbaum, B. (1993). Reliability and validity of a brief instrument for assessing post-traumatic stress disorder. *Journal of Traumatic Stress, 6*, 459–473.

Frumkind, I. B., & Friedland, J. (1995). Forensic evaluations in immigration cases: Evolving issues. *Behavioral Sciences and the Law, 13*, 477–489.

Gacono, C. B., Evans, F. B., III, & Viglione, D. J. (2002). The Rorschach in forensic practice. *Journal of Forensic Psychology Practice, 2*, 33–54.

Gacono, C. B., Loving, J. L., Evans, F. B., III, & Jumes, M. T. (2002). The Psychopathy Checklist–revised: PCL–R testimony and forensic practice. *Journal of Forensic Psychology Practice, 2*, 11–32.

Gacono, C., & Meloy, R. (1994). *The Rorschach assessment of aggressive and psychopathic personalities*. Hillsdale, New Jersey: Lawrence Erlbaum Associates.

Garb, H. N. (1998) *Studying the clinician: Judgment research and psychological assessment*. Washington, DC: American Psychological Association.

Greenberg, S. A., & Shuman, D. W. (1997). Irreconcilable conflict between therapeutic and forensic roles. *Professional Psychology: Research & Practice, 28*, 50–57.

Hake, B. A. (1994). Hardship waivers for J–1 physicians. *Immigration Briefings, 94*(2), 1–71.

Hake B. A., & Banks, D. L. (2005). The Hake Hardship Scale: A quantitative system for assessment of hardship in immigration cases based on a statistical analysis of AAO decisions. *Bender's Immigration Bulletin, 10*, 403–420.

Haney, C., & Zimbardo, P. (1998). The past and future of U.S. prison policy: Twenty-five years after the Stanford Prison Experiment. *American Psychologist, 53*, 709–727.

Hare, R. D. (1993) *Without conscience: The disturbing world of the psychopaths among us*. New York: Guilford.

Hare, R. D. (2003). *Hare Psychopathy Checklist–Revised* (2nd ed.). North Tonawanda, NY: Multi-Health Systems.

Harris, G. T. Rice, M. E., & Cormier, C. A. (1993). Violent recidivism of mentally disordered offenders: The development of a statistical prediction instrument. *Criminal Justice and Behavior, 20*, 315–335.

Hays, J. C., Kasl, S. V., & Jacobs, S. C. (1994a). The course of psychological distress following threatened and actual conjugal bereavement. *Psychological Medicine, 24*, 917–927.

Hays, J. C., Kasl, S. V., & Jacobs, S. C. (1994b). Past personal history of dysphoria, social support, and psychological distress following conjugal bereavement. *Journal of the American Geriatrics Society, 42*, 712–718.

Herlihy, J., Scragg, P., & Turner, S. (2002). Discrepancies in autobiographical memories—Implications for the assessment of asylum seekers: Repeated interviews study. *British Medical Journal, 324*(7333), 324–327.

Herman, J. (1992). *Trauma and recovery*. New York: Basic Books.

Hess, A., & Weiner, I. (1999). *The handbook of forensic psychology* (2nd ed.). New York: Wiley.

Horowitz, M. J. (1993). Stress-response syndromes: A review of posttraumatic stress and adjustment disorders . In J. P. Wilson & B. Raphael (Eds.), *International handbook of traumatic stress syndromes* (pp. 49–60). New York: Plenum.

Jacobs, U., Evans, F. B., & Patsilides, B. (2001a). Forensic psychology and documentation of torture. Part I. *Torture, 11*(3), 85–89.

Jacobs, U., Evans, F. B., & Patsilides, B. (2001b). Forensic psychology and documentation of torture. Part II. *Torture, 11*(4), 100–102.

Jay, J. (1991, November/December). Terrible knowledge. *Family Therapy Networker*, 18–29.

Kaffman, M., & Elizur, E. (1984). Children's bereavement reactions following death of the father. *International Journal of Family Therapy, 6*, 259–283.

Kaser-Boyd, N. (1993). Rorschachs of women who commit homicide. *Journal of Personality Assessment, 60*, 458–470.

Kaser-Boyd, N. (2004). Battered Woman Syndrome: Clinical features, evaluation, and expert testimony . In B. J. Cling (Ed.), *Sexualized violence against women and children: A psychology and law perspective* (pp. 41–70). New York: Guilford.

Kassindja, F., & Miller, L. M. (1998). *Do they hear you when you cry*. New York: Delta.

Kesselbrenner, D., & Rosenthal, L. D. (1984). *Immigration law and crimes*. New York: Clark Boardman Callaghan/Thomson West.

Lehman, D. R., Lang, E. L., Wortman, C. B., & Sorenson, S. B. (1989). Long-term effects of sudden bereavement: Marital and parent/child relationships and children's reactions. *Journal of Family Psychology, 2*, 344–367.

Li, G. (1995). The interaction effect of bereavement and sex on the risk of suicide in the elderly: An historical cohort study. *Social Science & Medicine, 40*, 825–828.

Lin, K. (1986). Psychopathology and social disruption in refugees . In C. L. Williams & J. Westermeyer (Eds.), *Refugee mental health in resettlement countries* (pp. 61–73). Washington, DC: Hemisphere.

Maciejewski, P. K., Prigerson, H. G., & Mazure, C. M. (2001). Sex differences in event-related risk for major depression. *Psychological Medicine, 31*, 593–604.

Martikainen, P., & Valkonen, T. (1996). Mortality after the death of a spouse: Rates and causes of death in a large Finnish cohort. *American Journal of Public Health, 86*, 1087–1093.

Maruna, S. (2001). *Making good: How ex-convicts reform and rebuild their lives.* Washington, DC: American Psychological Association.

Matter of Kasinga, 21 I & N Dec. 357 (BIA 1996).

Melton, G., Petrila, J., Poythress, N., & Slobogin, C. (1998). *Psychological evaluations for the court* (2nd ed.). New York: Guilford.

Mollica, R. F., Caspi-Yavin, Y., Bollini, P., Truong, T., Tor, S., & Lavelle, J. (1992). The Harvard Trauma Questionnaire. Validating a cross-cultural instrument for measuring torture, trauma, and posttraumatic stress disorder in Indochinese refugees. *Journal of Nervous and Mental Disease, 180*, 111–116.

Mollica, R. F., Wyshak, G., & Lavelle, J. (1987). The psychosocial impact of war trauma and torture among Southeast Asian refugees. *American Journal of Psychiatry, 144*, 1567–1572.

Monahan, J., & Steadman, H. J. (Eds.). (1994). *Violence and mental disorder: Developments in risk assessment.* Chicago: University of Chicago Press.

Pelcovitz, D., van der Kolk, B. A., Roth, S. H., Mandel, F. S., Kaplan, S., & Resick, P. A. (1997). Development of a criteria set and a structured interview for disorders of extreme stress (SIDES). *Journal of Traumatic Stress, 10*(1), 3–16.

Pope, K. S., & Garcia-Peltoniemi, R. E. (1991). Responding to victims of torture: Clinical issues, professional responsibilities, and useful resources. *Professional Psychology: Research and Practice, 22*, 269–276.

Putnam, F. W. (1989). *Diagnosis and treatment of multiple personality disorder.* New York: Guilford.

Ritzler, B. A. (2001). Multicultural usage of the Rorschach. In L. A. Suzuki, J. G. Ponterotto, P. J. Meller (Eds.), *Handbook of multicultural assessment: Clinical, psychological, and educational applications* (2nd ed., pp. 237–252). San Francisco: Jossey-Bass.

Rogers, R. (Ed.). (1997). *Clinical assessment of malingering and deception* (2nd ed.). New York: Guilford.

Rosenberg, L. D., & Evans, F. B (2003). Another chance: Forensic psychological assessment of recidivism and dangerousness in immigration adjudications. *Bender's Immigration Bulletin, 8*(9), 768–779.

Scroppo, J. C., Weinberger, J. L., Drob, S. L., & Eagle, P. (1998). Identifying dissociative identity disorder: A self-report and projective study. *Journal of Abnormal Psychology, 107*, 272–284.

Shapiro, D. L. (1984). *Psychological evaluation and expert testimony: A practical guide to forensic work.* New York: Van Nostrand Reinhold.

Smith, R., & Loring, M. T. (1994). The trauma of emotionally abused men. *Journal of Psychology, 31*(3/4), 1–4.

Stark, A. E. B. (1996). Posttraumatic stress disorder in refugee women: How to address PTSD in women who apply for political asylum under grounds of gender-specific persecution. *Georgetown Immigration Law Journal, 11*(3), 167–197.

Straus, M. (1979). Measuring intrafamily conflict and violence: The Conflict Tactics Scales. *Journal of Marriage and the Family, 41*, 75–88.

Tori, C. D. (1989). Homosexuality and illegal residency status in relation to substance abuse and personality traits among Mexican nationals. *Journal of Clinical Psychology, 45*, 814–821.

Wallerstein, J. S., & Kelly, J. B. (1980). *Surviving the breakup: How children and parents cope with divorce.* New York: Basic Books.

Walker, L. E. (1979). *The battered woman.* New York: Harper & Row.

Walker, L. E. (1984). *Battered woman syndrome*. New York: Springer.

Walker, L. E. (1994). *Abused women and survivor therapy*. Washington, DC: American Psychological Association.

Webster, D. D., Douglas, K. S., Eaves, D., & Hart, S. D. (1997). *HCR–20: Assessing risk for violence* (2nd ed.). Burnaby, BC: Mental Health, Law, and Policy Institute, Simon Fraser University.

Weiner, I. B., & Hess, A. K. (Eds.). (2006). *The handbook of forensic psychology* (3rd ed.). Hoboken, NJ: Wiley.

Weigert, E. (1970). *The courage to love*. New Haven, CT: Yale University Press.

Wolchik, S. A., & Karoly, P. (1988). *Children of divorce: Empirical perspectives on adjustment*. New York: Gardner Press.

van der Kolk, B. A. (1994). The body keeps score: Memory and the evolving psychobiology of posttraumatic stress. *Harvard Review of Psychiatry, 1,* 235–265.

van der Kolk, B. A., & Ducey, C. (1984). Clinical implications of the Rorschach in post-traumatic stress disorder. In B. A. van der Kolk (Ed.), *Post-traumatic stress disorder: Psychological and biological sequelae* (pp. 29–42). Washington, DC: American Psychiatric Press

van der Kolk, B. A., & Ducey, C. (1989). The psychological processing of traumatic experience: Rorschach patterns in PTSD. *Journal of Traumatic Stress, 2,* 259–263.

van der Kolk, B., McFarlane, A., & Weisaeth, L. (Eds.). (1996). *Traumatic stress*. New York: Guilford.

Viglione, D. J. (1999). A review of recent research addressing the utility of the Rorschach. *Psychological Assessment, 11*(3), 251–265.

Viglione, D. J., & Hilsenroth, M. J. (2001). The Rorschach: Facts, fictions, and future. *Psychological Assessment, 13*(4), 452–471.

The Violence Against Women Act (VAWA), Title IV of the Violent Crime Control and Law Enforcement Act of 1994 (P.L. 103–322). Subtitle G—Protections for Battered Immigrant Women.

Zamble, E., & Quinsey, V. (1997). *The criminal recidivism process*. Cambridge, England: Cambridge University Press.

Zimbardo, P. G. (1973). The psychological power and pathology of imprisonment. *Catalog of Selected Documents in Psychology, 3,* 45.

24

THE USE OF THE RORSCHACH IN PROFESSIONAL FITNESS TO PRACTICE EVALUATIONS

Scott C. Stacy

Peter Graham

Acumen Assessments, Inc., Lawrence, KS

George I. Athey, Jr.

Heritage Mental Health Clinic, Topeka, KS

The use of the Rorschach Inkblot Method (RIM) for measuring personality functioning has a very rich history. The RIM has been employed within psychiatric hospital settings (Athey, 1974, 1986; Frieswyk & Colson, 1980; Kleiger, 1999; Klopfer, Ainsworth, Klopfer, & Holt, 1954; Rapaport, 1950, 1951; Rapaport, Gill, & Schafer, 1945), intensive outpatient assessments (Shevrin & Shectman, 1973), team evaluations of physicians having licensure and legal issues related to mental health status (Graham & Stacy, 2004; Katsavdakis, Gabbard, & Athey, 2004; Stacy & Graham, 2006), and forensic contexts (Gacono & Meloy, 1994; Gacono, Evans, & Viglione, 2002; Meloy, 1991; Meloy, Hansen, & Weiner, 1997; McCann, 1998; Piotrowski, 1996; Weiner, Exner, & Sciara, 1996; Weiner, 1977, 1995, 1996, 1998, chap.6, this vol.). Within a battery of psychological tests, clinical data, and collateral information, the RIM has been useful in clarifying an examinee's perception, problem solving, affect/emotion regulation, thought organization, and reality testing.

This chapter outlines procedures for conducting fitness to practice evaluations of licensed professionals. It illustrates how the RIM provides important information that cannot be acquired by self-report inventories or collateral information alone. This assessment data is integral to making determinations about a licensee's functional status and capacities, rehabilitative potential, risk for recidivism, and suitability for treatment/education. Finally, it presents structural summary data from four groups of licensees (professional sexual misconduct, PSM; chemical dependency, CD; psychiatric, Psych; and disruptive behavior, DB) referred for fitness to practice evaluations.

PROFESSIONAL FITNESS TO PRACTICE EVALUATIONS

Referrals for professional fitness to practice evaluations come from several sources, ranging from self-referral and referral by colleagues to licensure boards, offices of professional conduct, departments of health, hospital boards and executive committees, professional practices, the office of the chief disciplinary council, and professional health/assistance programs. Referrals are made for the same general reasons as "fitness-for-duty" evaluations with law enforcement personnel and personnel engaged in other high-risk occupations (Gormally, chap.15, this vol.; Weiss, Weiss, & Gacono, chap. 25, this vol.). These referrals are initiated whenever "there is reasonable cause to suspect that the [licensee] may pose a significant risk of harm to self or others in the workplace" and/or "when there is reasonable cause to suspect that the [licensee] may have a psychological, psychiatric, or substance use disorder, or psychological/psychiatric symptoms that significantly interfere with his or her ability to perform the essential functions of the position" (Borum, Super, & Rand, 2003, p. 140).

When the referral comes from a licensing or regulatory body, the evaluation takes place in an administrative law context. Even when the referral is from another source, it may be reviewed within an administrative law context. This underscores the need to treat all materials as potentially discoverable. It is not uncommon for evaluation results, particularly those involving sexual misconduct, to end up in administrative, civil, or criminal court settings—sometimes 2 to 3 years after the evaluation was initiated. Additionally, a member of the evaluation team may be required to provide expert testimony. With this in mind, evaluators must carefully structure the evaluation process and any reports following forensic guidelines (including the use of informed consent; Ewing, 2003; Goldstein, 2003; Packer & Borum, 2003). State regulations and professional ethical principles define acceptable ethical and legal behaviors of licensed professionals. Forensic examiners must have a clear understanding of the relevant regulations that apply their fitness to practice.

Legal determinations regarding guilt/innocence and culpability are related to, but different than, fitness to practice determinations. Guilt or innocence bear on whether or not a statute was violated. Culpability involves levels of blameworthiness with regard to statutory violation. Affirmative defenses related to state of mind and context (e.g., insanity, duress, provocation, and mental/emotional disturbance) can impact determinations of blameworthiness, guilt, and discipline/punishment (Goldstein, Morse, & Shapiro, 2003). Psychiatric/psychological fitness determinations are also related to questions of state of mind and context, but do not necessarily require that a statute or regulation be violated. Functional, ethical, and legal problems can each give rise to questions about fitness. The evaluator offers expert testimony regarding fitness, whereas regulatory bodies make findings of fact related to guilt and culpability.

Various professional associations (American Psychological Association, 2006; Anfang, Faulkner, Fromson, & Gendel, 2005) and regulatory boards (Federation of State Medical Boards, 2006) have developed guidelines for fitness to practice evaluations and for subsequent rehabilitation. These guidelines define impairment, professional assistance programs, roles and functions of licensing boards, and disciplinary and rehabilitative processes. They also outline the qualifications and role of the forensic evaluator(s) (as distinct from a therapeutic or clinical role), limits in confidentiality, necessary historical and collateral information, and components of the psychiatric and psychological examination. These guidelines require that the evaluation includes only information relevant to the referral question and makes explicit the rationale for all conclusions. In addition to being conversant with the relevant literature, examiners should be familiar with the basic functions and psychological capacities necessary for a licensee to successfully perform their professional duties.

The general goals of the evaluation are fourfold:

1. Identify the nature and severity of any psychiatric, psychological, medical, cognitive, or character impairment or disorder.
2. Identify any aggravating and mitigating circumstances that may have predisposed the licensee to impairment or behavioral problems.
3. Establish an explanatory hypothesis.
4. Estimate the risk for recidivism, including recommendations for treatment, monitoring, and/or supervision methods that will decrease the likelihood of future inappropriate behavior.

For example, is the licensee suffering from a mental or cognitive disorder that would impair their ability to function in a clinical role? A family medicine physician might be able to function adequately with a Wechsler Adult Intelligence Scale (WAIS–III) Block Design score of 8 (Wechsler, 1997). However, a vascular surgeon with this score would likely need further neuropsychological testing and possibly a historical review of their technical competency. An internist who has engaged in sexual misconduct with a markedly elevated *WSum6* score secondary to numerous *FABCOM*s and *ALOG*s and evidence of affect dysregulation ($m = 4$; $FC:CF + C = 3:7$; $Blends:R = 22:34$) would more than likely be deemed unsuitable to practice in the immediate future (given convergence with other data), because these indices signal serious problems with maintaining conceptual boundaries, logical thinking, and affect regulation. A related determination involves the evaluation of "character." Johnson and Campbell (2002) argue for the relevance of both character and fitness requirements in evaluating professionals. They define the essential characteristics of fitness as involving personality adjustment, psychological health, and of character as involving integrity, prudence, and caring.

Utilizing the assessment data, the team establishes an explanatory hypothesis that helps clarify why and how behaviors are encroaching into the licensee's professional life. These findings directly inform treatment and possibly the nature of disciplinary action. The evaluation will come to conclusions along a continuum of fitness determinations:

1. The licensee is capable of practicing without treatment/educational interventions or restrictions.
2. The licensee is capable of practicing as long as appropriate treatment/monitoring/supervision requirements are in place.
3. The professional undergoing the evaluation is fit to practice with concurrent treatment/monitoring/supervision requirements and restrictions (e.g., may not treat females).

4. The licensee is incapable of practicing until successfully completing primary treat-ment/rehabilitation followed by some combination of monitoring/supervision and/or restrictions.

5. The examinee is unfit to practice based on compelling evidence clearly outlined in the report (e.g., organic brain-based disorder, high predatory inclination, chronic and per-vasive mental disorder, etc.).

INFORMED CONSENT AND ALLIANCE IN THE EVALUATION PROCESS

Establishing an alliance is intrinsically difficult when conducting a fitness to practice evaluation. Often beginning within a legal context, the risk of iatrogenic paranoid as-sumptions about the evaluation is heightened. At the outset, it is critical to acknowledge the externally prompted nature of the evaluation. However, at the same time, the evalua-tor must clearly indicate the nonbiased nature of the process and the steps undertaken to ensure this process (e.g., multidisciplinary team, neutral position of team, etc.). Informed consent is used to document the licensee's understanding of the evaluation as a forensic rather than a clinical process (Greenberg & Shuman, 1997). The licensee's failure to ac-knowledge consent by signature and failure to sign appropriate authorizations to release information to the referral source would constitute reasons for suspension of the evalua-tion process.

When obtaining informed consent, delineation of potential benefits and risks should be stated. One potential benefit would be that the licensee's case might be understood dif-ferently than is represented by the concerns of the referral source. Another potential ben-efit might be that the licensee's difficulties that have been outside their awareness might be remedied so as to facilitate a plan to return to work. Potential risks are that the li-censee's capability to practice could be limited, restricted, or revoked. Unlike most fo-rensic evaluations, these assessments serve multiple functions. Whereas they address the issue of fitness to practice, they also serve as a potential entry to the treatment and reha-bilitation process. Therefore, it is common practice to provide assessment feedback to the examinee.

THE FITNESS TO PRACTICE EVALUATION

Evaluation procedures are chosen based on the presenting complaint. For example, in the case of professional sexual misconduct, a procedure aimed at ruling out predation or severe character pathology will be important. When a history of strange or bizarre be-havior is noted, organic disorder or psychosis will be important to rule out. Consistent with a convergent data model (see also Gacono et al., 2002; Gacono, Evans, & Viglione, chap. 1, this vol.), the examiner will strategically select assessment methods. Each as-sessment process should be individualized to address the question(s) under consider-ation and may include medical screening, substance abuse screening, a review of collateral information, psychosocial/developmental history, sexual history, and psy-chological testing.

Medical Screening

Medical problems can manifest in behaviors that appear to be psychological in origin. For example, the disinhibition, lack of insight, and defensiveness that may occur with early onset dementia could be misunderstood as a severe personality disorder or bipolar illness. Metabolic disease can manifest in various mood-related problems. Various medications (i.e., tamoxifen for the treatment of cancer) can cause significant mood and cognitive difficulties. A complete medical examination with appropriate laboratory studies can be helpful to rule out a physical cause for the problem(s) under investigation.

Substance Abuse Screening

Substance abuse screening is a routine component of the fitness to practice evaluation, even absent a substantiated history of substance abuse/dependence. We recommend using a multipanel drug screen that includes testing for a wide variety of illegal and prescription drugs of abuse and alcohol metabolites (ethylglucuronide, or EtG). If heavy substance use is suspected in the past (e.g., within the past 3 months), a hair test enables the evaluator to investigate this possibility.

Collateral Information

An examination of collateral information is recommended in any forensic evaluation. Prior psychological evaluations, information from colleagues, patient statements, regulatory agency investigations, advocacy organizations, family members, and formal complaints are the most frequent sources of collateral information. The licensee should also be encouraged to bring collateral information that they believe will be pertinent to the evaluation process.

Psychosocial/Developmental History

A thorough developmental history helps to identify any psychodynamic linkages between formative object relations, paradigms/role-relationship models/schemas, and the licensee's present experiences and behaviors. Additionally, licensees who are overachievers and who may also have a brain-based (e.g., ADHD) or pervasive developmental disorder can exhibit behaviors in adulthood similar to personality disorder symptomatology. For example, Asperger's Disorder and the associated lack of sufficient filters for social judgment are the result of a congenital incapacity to empathize and mentalize emotional experiences. This can result in behaviors that may be perceived as belligerent, narcissistic, and antisocial. When considering this diagnosis, it is important to carefully evaluate peer relationship history and history of involvement in unusual and narrowly focused activities. Similarly, childhood trauma and its resulting impact on affect and thought regulation (Allen, 1995, 2001) can manifest in adults in the form of traumatic reenactments leading to various kinds of ethical problems, such as disruptive behavior or professional sexual misconduct.

Comprehensive Sexual History

In cases where sexual misconduct is an issue, a thorough sexual history can aid in ruling out the presence of compulsive sexual behavior or paraphilic interests or practices. An Abel Assessment for Sexual Interest (Abel Screening, Inc., 1995) provides additional information concerning sexual interest. The inclusion of the licensee's sexual information and history can be problematic when the licensee's history of affairs or particular sexual interests are not directly linked to the referral question(s). When including a licensee's sexual history, the evaluators should clearly articulate the relevance of this information. The evaluation team can exclude from the final report sensitive information that is not critically linked to the referral questions, conclusions, or recommendations.

Psychological Testing

Consistent with a convergent data model of evaluation (see also Gacono et al., 2002; Gacono et al., chap. 1, this vol.), the examiner will want to strategically select a battery of psychological and cognitive tests and screening measures meant to address the various personality, diagnostic, historical, behavioral, and functional factors that may be contributing to the presenting problem. The combination of psychological tests and clinical interviews provide the data necessary to rule out deception and malingering, cognitive/neuropsychological deficits, latent or frank psychosis, affect/mood instability, bipolar spectrum disorder, depression, impulse control, anxiety, paraphilic, and thought disorders. Within the context of analyzing this data, functional capacities and historical risk factors will need to be taken into consideration. When appropriate and available, actuarial risk assessment instruments that evaluate historical, clinical, dispositional, and contextual variables in a systematic and empirically valid manner are recommended.

Polygraph Examination

This form of structured interviewing can be very helpful when the licensee is contesting the validity of the allegations. It may also be helpful when the licensee believes that he is the victim of a sham peer review process (cases of disruptive behavior or other alleged untoward behaviors). When employing the polygraph, the questions asked need to be focused on past behavior and not intent. This method is useful for the licensee to be forthcoming and to rule out the possibility of deception by those leveling allegations.

Multidisciplinary Team Model

Making a determination regarding a licensee's fitness to practice in isolation (e.g., one examiner) is potentially fraught with complications. Countertransference dynamics in fitness to practice evaluations are ubiquitous. Employing a multidisciplinary team model where all members present clinical data, review collateral information, explore personal and professional biases, challenge each other's conceptualizations, and arrive at a consensus protects the accuracy, reliability, and validity of the process. The team can include a psychiatrist, psychologist, social worker, and an internist or well-trained general medical practitioner (e.g., family medicine physician), as well as other specialists as needed.

Communicating the Results

Unlike most forensic evaluations, typically, the primary clinician identified within the team structure will provide both the licensee and referral source verbal feedback. Then the primary clinician will generate a written report that:

1. Employs a convergent data methodology aimed at resolving prominent discontinuities.
2. Assigns weight to the various types of disturbance indicated by the results of psychological tests, history, and observed behaviors.
3. Establishes an explanatory hypothesis that allows consumers of the report to understand the etiological factors that predisposed the licensee to engage in the problematic behaviors.

The final report will also include a *DSM–IV–TR* diagnosis, if applicable, a statement regarding the licensee's risk for recidivism and rehabilitative potential, a medical/psycholegal statement regarding the licensee's fitness to practice, and recommendations for treatment, monitoring, and supervision, if indicated.

THE UTILITY OF THE RORSCHACH IN FITNESS TO PRACTICE EVALUATIONS

The RIM literature related to the evaluation of physicians and other professional groups is limited. Sion, Akatli, and Kemalof (1954) report a high proportion of anxiety responses in studying practicing physicians ($N = 100$). In their study of practicing and nonpracticing physicians, Miller and Salomon (1962) found a high number of *Whole* responses (*W%*), few *Human Movement* responses (*M*), relatively numerous *Color-Dominated Form* responses (*CF*), and some *White Space* responses (*S*). Interestingly, this Rorschach pattern, where aspirations (*W*) outstrip real-world abilities (*M*), has been linked to grandiosity (Gacono & Meloy, 1994; Weiner, 1966) and poor self-appraisal skills.

Typically, when a licensee is faced with a fitness to practice evaluation, their attitude is that the "problem" is external rather than inside.[1] More often than not, they are not able to acknowledge their distress. In this regard, examiners tend to be working with individuals whose inappropriate behaviors or distress is either denied or outside of their awareness. Because the RIM has no cues to social desirability and image maintenance, the manner in which the examinee relates during the administration of the Rorschach (and the entire assessment process) is often revealing. For example, rigid and highly form-dominated protocols (low *Afr*, high *F*, low *Color*, high *C'*, and low *W* responses) suggest

---

[1]It should be noted that, occasionally, licensees come to the attention of regulatory agencies and of others in positions of authority secondary to sham peer review processes or patently false allegations. However, this is a rare occurrence.

that treatment is going to be structured around a fact-driven, educational process with efforts to increase affect tolerance. Those protocols that are "loose" and affect-laden with disruptions in logic (high *CShad Blends*, *CF* + *C* > *FC*, high *Afr*, and/or elevated *WSum6*) will need rehabilitation that is highly educational but also designed toward increasing self-regulation skills. In either case, helping the licensee to understand how RIM findings provide a model for their real-world psychological and interpersonal functioning develops a bridge between evaluation and treatment. A final caveat is that protocols that suggest severe impairment, and consequently the likelihood of never returning to practice, must have ample corroborating information to support such findings.

The following ratios, percentages, and derivations represent four subgroups of licensee data: Professional sexual misconduct (*PSM*, *N* = 70), chemical dependency/abuse (*CD*, *N* = 37), psychiatric difficulties (*Psych*, *N* = 55), and disruptive behavior (e.g., anger management problems; *DB*, *N* = 78) that typically present for fitness to practice evaluations. Approximately 95% of these individuals came from the evaluation of physicians. The remaining 5% were psychologists, dentists, or attorneys. Ninety-six percent of these individuals were male.[2]

This is a prospective study based on data gathered over a period of approximately 7 years. We consider our data to be preliminary. All examiners were licensed psychologists with extensive experience in RIM administration, scoring, and interpretation (Comprehensive System, Exner, 1991, 1993). An interrater reliability study was conducted on 10 randomly sampled protocols. The percent agreement is as follows: *Location* = 96.03%, *Developmental Quality* = 95.15%, *Determinants* = 85.46%, *Form Quality* = 89.42%, *Pair(s)* = 91.0, *Content(s)* = 85.46%, *Popular* = 87.0%, *Z score* = 94.83%, *Special Scores* = 89.0%.

Core Characteristics, Stress Tolerance

There are common patterns shared by all of our groups. From the standpoint of validity, licensees exhibit a willingness to engage in the testing process (*R Mean*: *PSM* = 21.8; *CD* = 24.62; *Psych* = 28.02; *DB* = 23.65) with little evidence of defensiveness (*Lambda*: *PSM* = .37; *CD* = .54; *Psych* = .60; *DB* = .53). This contrasts with self-report inventories that typically exhibit moderately high levels of defensiveness in these groups. Most of our subjects were ambient, a finding consistent with the real-world difficulties these individuals have in managing stressful situations. Unable to rely on a predictable problem-solving strategy when experiencing stress, these licensees tend to act out or make poor decisions. Essentially, they "psychologically decompensate" in areas where they are most vulnerable (e.g., stress regulation, thinking and processing emotionally charged information, and managing self and other relationships). Another way of describing this vulnerability is that licensees function adequately when performing non-emotional, medical tasks but demonstrate potentially serious problems in the interpersonal aspects of their job.

---

[2]The authors are interested in exploring gender differences. However, doing so in this chapter is beyond the scope of this early endeavor.

TABLE 24-1
Group Means and Frequencies for Selected Ratios, Percentages, and Derivations for Impaired Licensees

	PSM (N = 70)			CD (N = 37)			Psych (N = 55)			DB (N = 78)		
	Mean	*SD*	*f*	*Mean*	*SD*	*f*	*Mean*	*SD*	*f*	*Mean*	*SD*	*f*
Introversive	n/a	n/a	32.85	n/a	n/a	32.43	n/a	n/a	30.90	n/a	n/a	23.07
Extratensive	n/a	n/a	18.57	n/a	n/a	29.72	n/a	n/a	32.72	n/a	n/a	24.35
Ambient	n/a	n/a	48.57	n/a	n/a	37.83	n/a	n/a	36.36	n/a	n/a	52.56
R =	21.80	7.80	70.00	24.62	11.36	37.00	28.02	13.12	55.00	23.65	11.65	78.00
Lamba =	0.37	0.35	65.00	0.54	0.56	37.00	0.60	0.64	55.00	0.53	0.48	75.00
EB =	4.21 : 3.79	n/a	n/a	3.76 : 3.07	n/a	n/a	4.11 : 3.71	n/a	n/a	3.46 : 3.31	n/a	n/a
EA =	8.01	4.55	70.00	6.82	3.03	37.00	7.83	3.07	55.00	6.78	3.48	78.00
eb =	6.24 : 8.79	n/a	n/a	6.92 : 9.93	n/a	n/a	6.84 : 9.58	n/a	n/a	6.21 : 7.37	n/a	n/a
es =	15.03	7.27	70.00	16.65	8.28	37.00	16.42	8.46	55.00	13.58	6.75	78.00
D =	-2.37	2.18	70.00	-3.35	2.80	37.00	-2.93	2.57	55.00	-2.22	2.02	78.00
Adj es =	8.75	n/a	n/a	8.44	n/a	n/a	8.85	n/a	n/a	7.64	n/a	n/a
AdjD =	-0.74	1.37	70.00	-1.62	1.73	37.00	-1.02	1.39	55.00	-0.86	1.38	78.00
FM =	4.03	2.19	69.00	4.57	2.50	36.00	4.51	2.88	53.00	4.04	2.78	74.00
SumC' =	2.87	2.05	62.00	3.11	2.26	33.00	2.91	2.29	45.00	2.41	2.00	63.00
SumT =	1.03	0.91	47.00	1.57	1.79	24.00	1.38	1.52	36.00	1.06	1.22	47.00
T > 1	n/a	n/a	28.57	n/a	n/a	32.43	n/a	n/a	43.63	n/a	n/a	24.35
m =	2.21	2.00	60.00	2.35	2.24	28.00	2.33	2.00	42.00	2.17	2.23	62.00
SumV =	0.86	1.50	34.00	1.19	1.45	21.00	0.84	1.22	24.00	0.68	1.03	34.00
Sum Y =	4.03	3.04	67.00	3.86	3.23	36.00	4.45	3.81	50.00	3.22	2.73	66.00
Affect												
FC:CF+C =	3.81 : 1.76	n/a	n/a	3.59 : 1.22	n/a	n/a	3.93 : 1.65	n/a	r/a	3.59 : 1.45	n/a	n/a
Pure C =	0.26	0.55	14.00	0.11	0.31	4.00	0.20	0.58	7.00	0.14	0.52	8.00
SumC:WsumC =	2.87 : 3.79	n/a	n/a	3.11 : 3.07	n/a	n/a	2.91 : 3.72	n/a	n/a	2.41 : 3.31	n/a	n/a
Afr =	0.57	0.22	70.00	0.48	0.18	37.00	0.57	0.21	55.00	0.54	0.17	78.00
S =	2.74	2.14	63.00	3.05	2.96	31.00	3.36	2.97	50.00	2.79	2.41	69.00
Blends:R =	0.36	0.19	70.00	0.35	0.18	37.00	0.30	0.19	52.00	0.29	0.19	75.00
CP =	0.03	n/a	n/a	0.05	n/a	n/a	0.01	n/a	n/a	0.03	n/a	n/a

(continued)

TABLE 24–1 (continued)

	PSM (N = 70)			CD (N = 37)			Psych (N = 55)			DB (N = 78)		
	Mean	SD	f	Mean	SD	f	Mean	SD	f	Mean	SD	f
Ideation												
a:p =	6.97 : 3.49	n/a	n/a	7.59 : 3.08	n/a	n/a	6.93 : 4.11	n/a	n/a	6.54 : 3.15	n/a	n/a
Ma:Mp =	2.81 : 1.37	n/a	n/a	2.76 : 1.00	n/a	n/a	2.58 : 1.56	n/a	n/a	2.40 : 1.09	n/a	n/a
2AB+ (Art+Ay) =	3.06	3.05	70.00	1.84	1.68	37.00	2.55	2.22	55.00	2.35	2.04	78.00
MOR =	1.47	1.83	42.00	0.76	1.57	12.00	1.42	1.68	38.00	1.19	1.41	47.00
Sum6 =	3.96	3.63	65.00	4.00	3.47	32.00	4.91	5.35	50.00	2.69	3.16	63.00
WSum6 =	13.09	14.89	65.00	13.49	13.50	32.00	16.02	19.31	50.00	8.09	10.78	63.00
M- =	0.44	0.84	20.00	0.49	0.86	11.00	0.67	1.11	21.00	0.45	1.33	16.00
M none =	0.00	n/a	n/a	0.00	n/a	n/a	0.00	n/a	n/a	0.00	n/a	n/a
Mediation												
XA% =	0.87	0.09	70.00	0.84	0.10	37.00	0.82	0.11	55.00	0.87	0.08	78.00
WDA% =	0.88	0.09	70.00	0.85	0.10	37.00	0.85	0.10	55.00	0.88	0.08	78.00
X-% =	0.13	0.09	67.00	0.16	0.10	34.00	0.17	0.11	52.00	0.13	0.08	72.00
S- =	0.66	1.09	29.00	0.84	1.26	17.00	0.96	1.39	24.00	0.73	0.11	78.00
P =	4.50	1.90	69.00	4.00	1.74	37.00	4.31	2.51	52.00	4.60	1.62	78.00
X+% =	0.60	0.12	70.00	0.56	0.12	37.00	0.53	0.14	55.00	0.57	0.13	78.00
Xu% =	0.27	0.12	69.00	0.27	0.13	37.00	0.29	0.11	55.00	0.30	0.11	78.00
Processing												
Zf =	14.06	5.13	70.00	14.54	7.61	37.00	15.93	7.13	55.00	14.19	5.93	78.00
W:D:Dd =	11.3:9.0:1.4	n/a	n/a	11.22:10.7:2.7	n/a	n/a	12.3:12.1:3.6	n/a	n/a	11.5:9.6:2.5	n/a	n/a
W:M =	11.3 : 4.2	n/a	n/a	11.2 : 3.7	n/a	n/a	12.3 : 4.1	n/a	n/a	11.5 : 3.5	n/a	n/a
Zd =	3.02	5.64	70.00	3.05	5.09	37.00	2.91	5.37	55.00	2.72	5.53	78.00
PSV =	0.21	1.00	7.00	0.43	0.95	10.00	0.36	1.02	9.00	0.17	0.59	8.00
DQ+ =	6.93	3.69	69.00	7.51	4.73	35.00	7.45	3.44	54.00	6.44	3.66	78.00
DQv =	0.36	0.94	13.00	0.38	1.00	7.00	0.51	1.32	13.00	0.58	4.42	18.00
Self-Perception												
3r+(2)/R =	0.42	0.17	70.00	0.41	0.17	37.00	0.41	0.18	55.00	0.42	0.18	78.00
Fr+rF =	0.77	1.12	32.00	0.73	1.03	15.00	0.80	1.24	21.00	0.99	1.43	36.00
Fr+rF > 1	n/a	n/a	17.14	n/a	n/a	21.62	n/a	n/a	20.00	n/a	n/a	30.76

SumV =	0.86	1.15	34.00	1.19	1.45	21.00	0.84	1.22	24.00	0.68	1.03	34.00
FD =	1.23	1.28	50.00	1.68	1.73	26.00	1.20	1.38	31.00	1.13	1.32	42.00
An+Xy =	2.07	n/a	n/a	2.36	n/a	n/a	1.74	n/a	n/a	1.63	n/a	n/a
MOR =	1.47	n/a	n/a	0.76	1.57	12.00	1.42	1.68	38.00	1.19	1.41	47.00
H:(H)+Hd+(Hd) =	2.84 : 2.98	n/a	n/a	2.73 : 2.92	n/a	n/a	2.93 : 4.17	n/a	n/a	2.54 : 2.63	n/a	n/a
Interpersonal												
COP	0.83	1.24	35.00	0.73	1.06	15.00	1.11	1.42	30.00	0.74	0.97	38.00
AG	0.66	1.03	26.00	0.65	1.12	12.00	0.95	1.53	22.00	0.53	0.89	26.00
GHR:PHR	3.54 : 2.96	n/a	n/a	3.04 : 3.27	n/a	n/a	3.49 : 4.05	n/a	n/a	3.40 : 2.46	n/a	n/a
a:p	6.97 : 3.49	n/a	n/a	7.59 : 3.08	n/a	n/a	6.93 : 4.11	n/a	n/a	6.54 : 3.15	n/a	n/a
Food	0.44	0.94	19.00	0.38	0.85	8.00	0.45	0.87	16.00	0.53	0.89	26.00
SumT	1.03	0.91	47.00	1.57	1.79	24.00	1.38	1.52	36.00	1.06	1.22	47.00
H Content	6.46	4.00	70.00	5.92	3.35	35.00	7.09	4.65	54.00	5.50	3.95	77.00
Pure H	2.84	2.07	65.00	2.37	1.91	32.00	2.93	1.92	50.00	2.54	2.00	73.00
PER	0.83	1.24	28.00	0.70	1.11	17.00	0.89	1.42	22.00	0.82	1.36	33.00
Isol. Index	0.15	0.11	61.00	0.15	0.12	32.00	0.17	0.16	0.49	0.16	0.11	70.00
Pairs (2)	6.61	3.98	69.00	7.41	4.45	37.00	8.76	6.96	54.00	6.72	4.88	76.00
Special Scores												
DV	0.64	0.93	30.00	0.76	0.94	17.00	0.98	1.45	25.00	0.59	0.87	31.00
INCOM	0.79	0.95	37.00	0.43	0.75	12.00	0.62	0.82	25.00	0.46	0.80	24.00
DR	0.71	1.23	24.00	1.00	1.45	15.00	1.22	1.95	27.00	0.69	1.19	29.00
FABCOM	0.57	0.80	30.00	0.62	0.85	17.00	0.65	0.88	24.00	0.33	0.55	23.00
DV2	0.06	0.23	4.00	0.00	0.00	0.00	0.11	0.45	4.00	0.03	0.16	2.00
INCOM2	0.31	0.95	12.00	0.24	0.59	6.00	0.25	0.79	8.00	0.15	0.56	7.00
DR2	0.26	0.82	8.00	0.30	0.83	5.00	0.24	0.66	9.00	0.09	0.33	6.00
FABCOM2	0.21	0.58	10.00	0.19	0.56	4.00	0.27	0.77	8.00	0.09	0.29	7.00
ALOG	0.39	0.91	15.00	0.46	0.79	12.00	0.49	0.95	16.00	0.23	0.99	8.00
CONTAM	0.01	0.12	1.00	0.00	0.00	0.00	0.07	0.32	3.00	0.03	0.16	2.00
AB	0.46	0.94	16.00	0.05	0.23	2.00	0.18	0.47	8.00	0.12	0.39	7.00
PSV	0.21	1.00	7.00	0.43	0.95	10.00	0.36	1.02	9.00	0.17	0.59	8.00

Internal emotional and ideational pressures are extreme in all groups (*es: PSM* = 15.03, *CD* = 16.65, *Psych* = 16.42, *DB* = 13.58). Even the lowest *es* mean score among groups is nearly two standard deviations above the nonpatient adult mean. There is evidence of significant environmental and internal stressors impinging on coping capacities (*D:PSM* = –2.37; *CD* = –3.35; *Psych* = –2.93; *DB* = –2.22). Inconsistent with their public image, this population is far from calm and unflappable. Instead, they are "anxious, tense, nervous, and irritable ... with limited tolerance for frustration and resulting proclivity for impulsiveness ... [with] susceptibility to unwelcome, unpleasant, and episodic losses of self-control" (Weiner, 1998, p. 145). Consistent with behavioral descriptions, these individuals manifest what Weiner describes as incapacitation, high levels of stress, vulnerability to losses of self-control that lead to embarrassment and agitation, and distress that is clearly noticeable to others.

Even when high levels of situational stress (*m, Y: PSM* = 2.21, 4.03; *CD* = 2.35, 3.86; *Psych* = 2.33, 4.45; *DB* = 2.17, 3.22) are controlled, these individuals exhibit lingering internal emotional and ideational pressures, dysphoria, and painful self-reflection (*C', V: PSM* = 2.87, .87; *CD* = 3.11, 1.19; *Psych* = 2.91, .84; *DB* = 2.41, .68). This is consistent with a chronic stress disorder (Weiner, 1998). Although licensees are understandably feeling powerless, chronic levels of anxiety are defensively partitioned off by narcissistic and obsessive-compulsive defenses (e.g., idealization, devaluation, externalization, displacement, isolation of affect, reaction formation, undoing, etc., and increased *Y, V,* and *m* with elevated *2AB + Art + Ay*), and/or by the use of substances or compulsive/impulsive behaviors. All groups except for the *CD* group show a high level of intellectual abstraction that keeps them distant from actual, empathic engagement with themselves and others. After completing treatment, however, the authors have noticed that most licensees appear better equipped to take advantage of their potential for thoughtful self-reflection (*FD: PSM* = 1.23; *CD* = 1.68; *Psych* = 1.20; *DB* = 1.13). It is interesting to note that physicians, in general, are initiated into a culture of overextension and disregard for their own well-being. So, it makes sense that the RIM would reveal what many of us have observed.

Affect

All groups evidence high levels of negativism and oppositional tendencies (*S : PSM* = 2.74, *CD* = 3.05, *Psych* = 3.36, *DB* = 2.79). Elevated *C', V,* and *m* increase their vulnerability to periods of dysphoria, anhedonia, and resentment. This emotional set provides the template for acting-out that is mediated by poor judgment. A slightly higher than normal *Blends:R* ratio (*PSM* = .36, *CD* = .35, *Psych* = .30, *DB* = .29) suggests a moderately increased level of affective complexity. This level of complexity within the context of other vulnerabilities suggests higher levels of emotional confusion than compared to nonpatient adult norms. It is understandable why these individuals employ defensive efforts to wall off emotionally charged experiences.

Thinking and Processing

The level of cognitive distortions, arbitrary and circumstantial reasoning, and confusion is typically high across all groups (*WSum6: PSM* = 13.09; *CD* = 13.49; *Psych* = 16.02; *DB*

= 8.09). It is very important to determine the nature and etiology of the licensee's ideational difficulties when signs of thought disturbance emerge in the structural summary. In this population, these difficulties ($WSum6$ = 13–20) usually stem from a mood disorder or the byproducts of engrained personality functioning and associated ego deficits and defenses. In cases where there is a developmental history of trauma, the astute examiner will scrutinize the protocol content, data, and sequence of scores to observe whether or not affect-based symbolic representations of trauma intrude into the perceptions of the licensee (see Kleiger, 1999, for details). Spoiled responses within a protocol[3] or $FABCOM2s$[4] that seem to pop out from nowhere can be explored during feedback to see if peculiar themes embedded in the licensee's responses mirror trauma-based affect states that may be influencing current interpersonal modes of relating. Examinees exhibiting these kinds of difficulties along with elevations of *Diffuse Shading* (*Y*), *Inanimate Movement* (*m*), and *Unmodulated Affect* (*CF* + *C* > *FC*) provide further evidence for the possibility of trauma having an impact on functioning (Kleiger, 1999). These types of difficulties are not uncommon occurrences amongst *PSM*, *DB*, and *Psych* populations.

All examinees show a mild predisposition to individualistic and unconventional perspectives (*Xu%: PSM* = .27, 4.5; *CD* = .27, 4.0; *Psych* = .29, 4.31; *DB* = .30, 4.60). These professionals strive and aspire to succeed more than the average population, whereas their ideational coping resources are at the same level as the nonpatient adult population (*W:M: PSM* = 11.31:4.21; *CD* = 11.22:3.76; *Psych* = 12.33:4.11; *DB* = 11.50:3.46). However, their higher level of striving is compromised by inefficient attempts to integrate information (*Zf, Zd: PSM* = 14.06, 3.02; *CD* = 14.54, 3.05; *Psych* = 15.93, 2.91; *DB* = 14.19, 2.72). Overall, these groups are high achievers who are overextending themselves by exceeding their psychological resources.

Self and Other Perception

Although all groups exhibit a relatively normal anticipation for intimacy (*T: PSM* = 1.03, *CD* = 1.57, *Psych* = 1.38, *DB* = 1.06), their ability to productively channel needs for emotional relatedness appears to be inhibited by a paucity of interest in others, as well as the expectation of interpersonal disappointment (*COP: PSM* = .83, *CD* = .73, *Psych* = 1.11, *DB* = .74). Their ability to experience people as whole objects with both reality-based positive and negative attributes is low (*H:[H] + Hd + [Hd]: PSM* = 2.84:2.98, *CD* = 2.73:2.92, *Psych* = 2.93:4.17, *DB* = 2.54:2.63). This appears to translate into others or objects (i.e., substance or compulsive behaviors) being used as narcissistic extensions of the self (*Fr + rf: PSM* = .77, *CD* = .73, *Psych* = .80, *DB* = .99). In this state of mind, needs for affirmation/mirroring may compromise decision-making judgment. Perhaps, in part due to their narcissistic predisposition, licensees within these groups also struggle with a fairly profound sense of isolation and painful/critical self-reflection (*V:PSM* = .86, *CD* = 1.19, *Psych* = .84, *DB* = .68).

---

[3]Card II: "This is a brightly colored butterfly ... [Inquiry] ... it's been smashed by something that's not on this card."

[4]Card IV: "This is a large man with John Deere tractor tread feet ... [Inquiry] ... His hair is being blown by the wind. ... the head's up here and is insecty ... makes it look like it's coming at me."

Typically, a high level of $An + Xy$ responses reflects a sense of vulnerability. The authors have noted that some physicians with these elevations ($An + Xy = PSM = 2.07$, $CD = 2.36$, $Psych = 1.74$, $DB = 1.63$) appear to be trying to invoke a sense of familiarity while engaging in a perceptual task that can feel ambiguous. In this regard, they may be trying to regulate anxiety. However, elevated An and Xy responses may also reflect a grandiose display of knowledge in an effort to invoke a sense of superiority (elevated Fr, as noted earlier). In this population, An and Xy responses can mean different things. For example, after exhibiting poor *Form Quality* or an illogical *Special Score*, an *Anatomy* and/or an *X-ray* percept may represent an adaptive effort to rejoin the task at hand by focusing on a familiar nonemotional perception. However, when feeling intimidated (e.g., negative transference), it is not uncommon for narcissistic licensees to defensively utilize omnipotence to regain a felt sense of superiority (Cooper, Perry, & Arnow, 1988; Gacono, Meloy, & Heaven, 1990). For example, "This here is a poorly executed laminotomy/microdiscectomy where the otomy has not been properly closed." "That's spelled L-A-M-I-N ... ." What makes it look like that? "It's clearly right there." In this kind of situation, the licensee is unwittingly demonstrating the projective identification phenomena that result in the alienation of people in the workplace. Whereas all of the *PSM*, *CD*, *Psych*, and *DB* groups share common characteristics, they also produce Rorschach patterns consistent with their presenting problems.

GROUP DIFFERENCES

Professional Sexual Misconduct (PSM)

Members of this group (predominantly physicians) have engaged in sexual contact with at least one patient. The mean age is 50 years old ($SD = 14.25$). As a result of thinking problems, self-esteem issues, and stress management and interpersonal/social deficits, these licensees exhibit significant problems maintaining appropriate boundaries. There is a striking link between this subgroup's unethical behaviors and their internal boundaries between representations. The distinction between their professional functioning (diagnosis and the provision of treatment) and friends, romantic partners, sexual acquaintances, and so on, becomes blurred ($INCOM = .79$; $INCOM2 = .31$; $FABCOM = .57$; $FABCOM2 = .21$). What might explain this vulnerability is their tendency to fluidity in thinking ($ALOG = .39$). Adding to this problem are emotions that derail their ability to stay on task ($DR = .71$; $DR2 = .26$). PSM individuals evidence a type of reasoning that Kleiger (1999) refers to as "coincidental thinking," where conclusions are based on circumstantial factors (p. 229). For example, the licensee feels attraction toward a patient but loses sight of the patient's status (e.g., feelings and perceptions derail professional process). Sometimes, this role transformation can occur when the patient is perceived by the licensee to be exhibiting flirtatious behavior, which can stimulate unmet needs ($T = 1.03$, $T > 1 = 29.57\%$). They may interpret this as meaning that the patient is interested in them and fail to consider that the patient's behavior may be a general personality characteristic. Deviations in expected amounts of conventionality ($P = 4.50$; $Xu\% = .27$; $X-\% = .13$) foster cognitive distortions (e.g., "I'm like a country doctor. I'm friends with all my patients."), which impair the licensee's ability to maintain professional boundaries. In light of Kleiger's conceptualization of thought disorder existing on a continuum, this group typically struggles more with "misorganization" than frank "disorganization" (p. 205). For example, in response to Card I, a licensee who had engaged in sexual misconduct remarked: "This is a woman with her wings outstretched and ready to fly."

The RIM also suggests a predisposition toward self-centeredness/narcissistic vulnerability ($Fr + rf = .77$; $Fr + rf > 1 = 17.14\%$) and dysphoria ($C' = 2.87$, $V = .86$, $m = 2.21$) that is not well managed ($W:M = 11.31:4.21$) ($D = -2.37$, $AdjD = -.74$). Although these individuals have the capability to engage in adaptive self-reflection ($FD = 1.23$; $EA = 8.01$), this ability appears to be derailed by painful introspection ($V = .86$), the sense of feeling damaged ($MOR = 1.47$), emotional distancing ($2AB + [Art + Ay] = 3.06$), emotional constriction (C'), and feelings of helplessness ($Y = 4.03$). More often than not, the PSM examinee is more hypersensitive than thick-skinned and oblivious. These problems set the interpersonal stage for the licensee to unleash his or her unmet needs for comforting contact toward an idealizing but narrowly perceived patient ($H:[H] + Hd + [Hd] = 2.84:2.98$; $COP = .83$; $Sx = .77$) in the hopes that such a relationship will restore self-esteem and psychological equilibrium with little perceived risk of rejection. Because of these difficulties, the professional/fiduciary relationship is vulnerable to being unwittingly transformed and distorted leading to various forms of interpersonal professional boundary problems.

In the absence of data to support psychopathy, predatory inclination, or a paraphilic disorder, most licensees who engage in PSM are what many have termed "love sick"—where the licensee's needs eclipse the ability to reflect on a situation with some objectivity. The following response to Card X captures the overly symbolic, derailed, sadomasochistic psychodynamics of a male licensee who "fell in love" with a female patient after experiencing many years of marital problems, depression, and family disruption. In addition to this, he also has a history of catastrophic event trauma that occurred in late adolescence:

> Kind of reminds me of my wife's and my relationship. Me and my perception being the color in the relationship. With my wife in somewhat of a passive-aggressive mode in this top position here. And then this colored part representing more the life/relationship part. I wanted to bring emotions into the relationship. When you flip it around with me on top with the color representing her going places, doing things, and buying things and I am up here as the governor going ... we're not going any further until we can break some real ground.

Chemical Dependency (CD)

The mean age of this group is 47 years old ($SD = 9.35$). Individuals who struggle with chemical dependency/abuse have problems regulating their internal emotional ($D = -3.35$; $V = 1.19$; $S = 3.05$; $Y = 3.86$; $V = 1.19$) and ideational experiences ($m = 2.35$; $WSum6 = 13.49$, $M- = .49$). Of all the groups, the CD examinees manifest the highest level of chronic ideational and emotional pressure from internal and external sources ($es = 16.65$; $AdjD = -1.62$). Substance abuse can be understood as a maladaptive way to compensate for coping deficits that, at the same time, exacerbates the licensee's difficulties. The data in this section appears to psychometrically explicate and validate the disease paradigm of substance abuse and dependency.

The CD population exhibits a high level of needs for closeness ($T = 1.57$, $T > 1 = 32.43\%$). At the same time, they have problems engaging in adaptive social interactions where those needs might be appropriately met ($COP = .73$). The loneliness and emotional deprivation they feel translates into using substances and/or superficial ties to others in the service of gratifying self-centered needs ($Fr + rf = .73$, $Fr + rf > 1 = 21.62\%$). This would be consistent with self-reports of feeling cradled, energized, and empowered by opioids, omnipotent after using cocaine, and feeling less inhibited by the effects of alcohol.

The combination of oppositional attitude and negativistic avoidance ($S = 3.05$) in this population potentiates acting-out behaviors mediated by impaired thought processes ($WSum6 = 13.49$; $S- = .84$; $Xu\% = .27$; $X-\% = .16$). The CD examinee has difficulty accurately assessing the impact of substance abuse on their lives. They have difficulty recognizing the association between resentment and ill-advised action. This cluster of illogical thinking, oppositionality, and idiosyncratic perceptions of the world may reflect what is referred to in the field of addictionology as "denial." Diverting opioid use to get "high" or avoid symptoms of withdrawal speaks to how the CD group's decision making is driven by a high degree of arbitrary, concrete, and emotionally derailed reasoning ($ALOG = .46$; $INCOM = .24$; $DR2 = .30$).

Like the other groups, licensees with CD problems tend to "bite off more that they can chew" ($Zf = 14.54$; $Zd = 3.05$; $W:M = 11.22:3.76$), and not recognize the negative impact of their substance use on daily living. With this in mind, it is not uncommon to see the emergence of an exacerbation of substance-related problems emerge in middle age when internal resources begin to decline both naturally and as a result of trying to maintain a "youth-driven" practice.

Psychiatric Disorders (Psych)

The mean age of the psychiatric group is 46 years old ($SD = 10.19$). The central presenting symptoms in this group include mood disorders (depression, bipolar disorder), anxiety disorders (especially anxiety associated with relationship-based trauma in early development), and personality disorders (both internalizing, self-defeating and externalizing, dysregulated types). There are indications of significant situational and longstanding psychological vulnerability in this group ($D = -2.93$, $AdjD = -1.02$).

The Psych group exhibits a strong need for comforting contact ($T = 1.38$, $T > 1 = 43.63\%$, $Pairs = 8.76$, $Food = 0.45$). However, it appears as though dysphoric depressive constraint of emotional response ($C' = 2.91$), negativism ($S = 3.36$), painful internal reflection ($V = 0.84$), and feelings of helplessness ($Y = 4.45$) interfere with their being able to realize comfort in adaptive, nondistorted interpersonal relationships ($H = 2.93$, $PHR = 4.05$, $COP = 1.11$, $X-\% = 0.17$, $Xu\% = 0.25$; $S- = 0.96$). Licensees in this group are difficult to get along with in a professional environment. They are preoccupied with themselves and their own needs ($Fr + rF = 0.80$, $Fr + rf > 1 = 20\%$) and have a strong inclination to experience themselves as "right," even when exhibiting incorrect assumptions ($ALOG = .49$). Their bravado is really a sham ($V = .84$, $MOR = 1.42$) and others realize this when they act in a manner that is arbitrary and even odd. These licensees are often labeled as troublemakers or "weird" when, in fact, they are suffering from an undiagnosed or poorly managed psychiatric disorder. However, this is often not directly confronted by others (particularly subordinates) because technically they are more often than not very bright and sometimes very accomplished.

The difficulties mentioned previously are not unexpected given that a large number of individuals in this group suffer from a bipolar illness and/or history of severe early relationship-based trauma and resulting personality problems ($INCOM2$, $FABCOM2$, and DR scores are at levels 12.5, 9.0, and 24.0 times greater than the nonpatient population, respectively).

The internal state of these licensees is mired in depressive isolation and vulnerability to emotionally based distortions in their sense of self and others. The technical aspect of their professional life is one arena where they can maintain some sense of constancy in their self-definition—often becoming the sole basis for their identity and self-worth. Nonetheless, their interactions with others convey the fact that something is wrong. Oftentimes, this is not attended to until the licensee's personal and professional functioning precipitously collapses.

Disruptive Behavior (DB)

Members of this group (Mean age = 48, $SD = 8.89$; almost entirely physicians) have engaged in angry and explosive outbursts, physical aggression toward coworkers, intimidation, harassment, yelling, and other disruptions. Their disruptive behavior poses either a direct or an indirect threat to patient safety. Disruptive behavior results from an interaction of social skills deficits, logical distortions about coworkers' intentions and organizational conditions, personal overextension, and overstimulation from environmental stressors. These individuals have considerable technical skill but show significant deficits in navigating the interpersonal aspects of their work environment. Low interest in or low anticipation of cooperative engagement in interactions with others ($COP = .74$; $Pairs = 6.72$) and self-centeredness ($Fr + rF = .99$, $Fr + rF > 1 = 30.76\%$) interferes with collaborative teamwork. Further, their ability to incorporate the positive and negative attributes of others is low ($H:[H] + Hd + [Hd] = 2.54 : 2.63$). This lack of realistic engagement with others results in nonempathic disregard for the experiences and rationales of others. This group copes by thinking about how things "should" be as opposed to how they realistically could be or need to be (Akhtar, 1996). They use concrete, unrealistic, and "loose" thinking that has a strained logic to it in order to justify their responses ($X-\% = .13$; $Xu\% = .30$; $S-\% = .73$; $P = 4.60$; $WSum6 = 8.09$; $INCOM2 = .15$; $ALOG = .23$; $Level\ 2\ Special\ Scores = .36$).

These individuals expect too much from themselves ($W:M = 11.5:3.46$; $Zd = 2.72$) and do not understand why those around them do not share in their perception of priorities and sources of stress and strain. This group's substantial internal emotional and ideational pressures ($m = 2.17$) and unprocessed dysphoric feelings of helplessness ($Y = 3.22$) disrupt a coherent stream of associations and behaviors ($DR = .69$). This results in behaviors that are abrasive and alienating. As one disruptive surgeon once exclaimed to the rest of the team after explosively venting on his coworkers, "all right, you guys need to calm down now." They remain unaware that they have a deficit with regard to being able to muster sufficient adaptive capacities to alter their chronically stressful conditions ($EA = 6.78$; $es = 13.58$; $D = -2.22$; $AdjD = -.86$). As a result, they do not make changes in their life and work situation or rally empathy for themselves and others to be able to work their way out of tough situations through cooperation and collaboration.

Interestingly, this population perceived fewer *Aggressive* responses ($AG = .53$) than that of the nonpatient adult population ($AG = 1.11$). This finding suggests that those functional variables that are less face obvious and less open to manipulation by conscious defensiveness are more pertinent to the evaluation of disruptiveness than obvious and more easily manipulated response contents (e.g., manifestly aggressive themes), or as hypothesized by Gacono and Meloy (1994), represent the egodystonic nature of aggression to these individuals. An exploration of other aggressive imagery (Gacono, Gacono, Meloy, & Baity, 2005) may be very useful in understanding the behavior of this group.

CONCLUSIONS

Conducting a fitness to practice evaluation is a complex endeavor. This type of highly specialized evaluation requires knowledge about forensic/legal issues; the capacity to integrate multiple theoretical perspectives with psychological test data and behavioral observations; a clear understanding of the multiple professional functions, practice settings, and ethical guidelines associated with the licensee's type of practice; and a firm understanding of how all of these components are translated into determinations about the issue of "fitness."

Our RIM data is preliminary and our sample sizes are rather small. However, although there are similarities in Rorschach indices among our four subgroups, their difficulties and vulnerabilities manifest in diverse ways. These differences, in turn, impact rehabilitative potential and the form of treatment. For example, the origins and treatment of thought organization problems and impulsivity are quite different for licensees who are disruptive and have a history of posttraumatic stress versus those with a bipolar illness. Although both may require similar medication(s), the goals of treatment regarding insight and behavioral change will differ. Disruptive physicians with posttraumatic stress will need to lower their vulnerability to thematic triggers. Disruptive physicians with a bipolar illness must adapt to an illness that compromises their thinking and requires adherence to proper medication management and an enhanced self-care regimen. The RIM plays a unique and vital role in separating out these personality nuances.

Future RIM research might include larger samples and data on licensees (particularly physicians) who have never been mandated to undergo a fitness to practice evaluation and who have no history of unethical, criminal, violent, or impaired conduct. Compiling a nonpatient sample of physician RIM data will help to identify common vulnerabilities in this population. At the same time, such a sample could also help to identify indices that specifically differentiate adaptive from maladaptive patterns of responding to the predictable stressors of professional life.

To the best of our knowledge, this chapter represents a first effort to systematically study the implementation of the RIM in fitness to practice evaluations. The data elicited by the RIM offers forensic examiners a standardized sample of licensees' psychological functioning that is not accessible from self-report or collateral information alone and therefore integral to the fitness to practice evaluation.

ACKNOWLEDGMENT

The views in this chapter are solely the authors', and may or may not reflect the views of any of the authors' past, current, or future affiliations.

REFERENCES

Abel Screening, Inc. (1995). Abel Assessment for Sexual Interest. Atlanta: Abel Screening, Inc.

Akhtar, S. (1996). "Someday ..." and "if only ..." fantasies: Pathological optimism and inordinate nostalgia as related forms of idealization. *Journal of the American Psychoanalytic Association, 44*(3), 723–753.

Allen, J. G. (1995). *Coping with trauma: A guide to self-understanding.* Washington, DC: American Psychiatric Press.

Allen, J. G. (2001). *Traumatic relationships and serious mental disorders.* Chichester, England: Wiley.

American Psychological Association. (2006). *Advancing colleague assistance in professional psychology.* Monograph available electronically at http://www.apa.org/practice/acca_monograph.Html

Anfang, S. A., Faulkner, L. R., Fromson, J. A., & Gendel, M. H. (2005). The American Psychiatric Association's resource document on guidelines for psychiatric fitness-for-duty evaluations of physicians. *Journal of the American Academy of Psychiatry and Law, 33*(1), 85–88.

Athey, G. (1974). Schizophrenic thought organization, object relations and the Rorschach test. *Bulletin of the Menninger Clinic, 38*, 406–429.

Athey, G. (1986). Rorschach thought organization and transference enactment in the patient-examiner relationship. In M. Kissen (Ed.), *Assessing object relations phenomena* (pp. 19–50). Madison, CT: International University Press.

Borum, R., Super, J., & Rand, M. (2003). Forensic assessment for high-risk occupations. In A. Goldstein (Ed.), *Handbook of psychology: Vol. 11. Forensic psychology* (pp. 133–147). New York: Wiley.

Cooper, S., Perry, C., & Arnow, D. (1988). An empirical approach to the study of defense mechanisms: Reliability and preliminary validity of the Rorschach Defense scales. *Journal of Personality Assessment, 52*(2), 187–203.

Ewing, C. P. (2003). Expert testimony: Law and practice. In A. Goldstein & I. B. Weiner (Eds.), *Handbook of psychology: Vol. 11. Forensic psychology* (pp. 55–68). New York: Wiley.

Exner, J. (1991). *The Rorschach: A Comprehensive System: Vol. 2. Interpretation* (2nd ed.). New York: Wiley.

Exner, J. (1993). *The Rorschach: A Comprehensive System: Vol. 1. Basic foundations* (3rd ed.). New York: Wiley.

Federation of State Medical Boards. (2006). *Addressing sexual boundaries: Guidelines for state medical boards.* Policy Monograph.

Frieswyk, S., & Colson, D. (1980). Prognostic considerations in the hospital treatment of borderline states: The perspective of object relations theory and Rorschach. In J. Kwawer, H. Lerner, P. Lerner,

& A. Sugarman (Eds.), *Borderline phenomena and the Rorschach test* (pp. 229–255). Madison: International University Press.

Gacono, C. B., Evans, F. B., & Viglione, D. (2002). The Rorschach in forensic practice. *Journal of Forensic Psychology Practice, 2*(3), 33–53.

Gacono, C. B., Gacono, L. A., Meloy, J. R., & Baity, M. (2005). Rorschach Extended Aggression scores. *Rorschachiana, 27*, 164–190.

Gacono, C. B., & Meloy, R. (1994). *The Rorschach assessment of aggressive and psychopathic personalities.* Hillsdale, NJ: Lawrence Erlbaum Associates.

Gacono, C. B., Meloy, J. R., & Heaven, T. (1990). A Rorschach investigation of narcissism and hysteria in antisocial personality. *Journal of Personality Assessment, 55*(1–2), 270–279

Goldstein, A. M. (2003). Overview of forensic psychology. In A. M. Goldstein (Ed.), *Handbook of psychology: Vol. 11. Forensic psychology* (pp. 3–20). Hoboken, NJ: Wiley.

Goldstein, A. M., Morse, S. J., & Shapiro, D. L. (2003). Evaluation of criminal responsibility. In A. M. Goldstein (Ed.), *Handbook of psychology: Vol. 11. Forensic psychology* (pp. 381–406). Hoboken, NJ: Wiley.

Graham, P., & Stacy, S. (2004, April). *The difficulties of assessment.* Paper presented at the Federation of Physician Health Programs Southeast and Western Conferences. Albuquerque, NM.

Greenburg, S., & Shuman, D. (1997). Irreconcilable conflict between therapeutic and forensic roles. *Professional: Psychology: Research and Practice, 23*(1), 50–57.

Johnson, W. B., & Campbell, C. D. (2002). Character and fitness requirements for professional psychologists: Are there any? *Professional Psychology: Research and Practice, 33*(1), 46–53.

Katsavdakis, K., Gabbard, G., & Athey, G. (2004). Profile of impaired health professionals. *Bulletin of the Menninger Clinic, 68*(1), 60–72.

Kleiger, J. (1999). *Disordered thinking and the Rorschach: Theory, research, and differential diagnosis.* Hillsdale, NJ: Analytic Press.

Klopfer, B., Ainsworth, M. D., Klopfer, G., & Holt, R. (1954). *Developments in the Rorschach technique: Vol. 1. Techniques and theory.* New York: World Book.

McCann, J. (1998). Defending the Rorschach in court: An analysis of admissibility using legal and professional standards. *Journal of Personality Assessment, 70*(1), 125–144.

Meloy, R. (1991, Fall/Winter). Rorschach testimony. *Journal of Psychiatry and the Law*, 221–235.

Meloy, R., Hansen, T., & Weiner, I. B. (1997). Authority of the Rorschach: Legal citations during the past 50 years. *Journal of Personality Assessment, 69*, 53–62.

Miller, L., & Salomon, F. (1962). Test de Rorschach de medicines praticiens [Rorschach tests of medical experts]. *Bulletin de la Societe du Rorschach at des Methodes Projectives de Langue Francaise, 13/14*, 20–27.

Packer, I. K., & Borum, R. (2003). Forensic training and practice. In A. Goldstein & I. B. Weiner (Eds.), *The handbook of psychology* (Vol. 11, pp. 21–32). New York: Wiley.

Piotrowski, C. (1996). The Rorschach in contemporary forensic psychology. *Psychological Reports, 78*(2), 458.

Rapaport, D. (1950). The theoretical implications of diagnostic testing procedures. *Congres International de Psychiatric, 2*, 241–271.

Rapaport, D. (1951). States of consciousness: A psychopathological and psychodynamic view. In M. Gill (Ed.), *The collected papers of David Rapaport* (pp. 385–404). New York: Basic Books.

Rapaport, D., Gill, M., & Schafer, R. (1945). *Diagnostic psychological testing* (rev. ed.; R. Holt, Ed.). New York: International University Press.

Shevrin, H., & Shectman, F. (1973). The diagnostic process in psychiatric evaluations. *Bulletin of the Menninger Clinic, 37*(5), 451–494.

Sion, M., Akatli, S., & Kemalof, S. (1954). De certaines reponses d'anxietie dans les protocols de Rorschach des medicines [Certain answers of anxiety in the Rorschach protocols of physicians]. *Beiheft zur Schweizerischen Zeitschrift fur Psychologie und ihre Anwendungen, 25*, 155–173.

Stacy, S., & Graham, P. (2006, January). *Professional sexual misconduct: Where we have been, where we are, and where we are going.* Paper presented at Sexual Boundary Violations: A National Conference for Regulatory Boards, Federation of State Medical Boards National Conference. Dallas, TX.

Wechsler, D. (1997). *Wechsler Adult Intelligence Scale—III.* San Antonio, TX: The Psychological Corporation.

Weiner, I. B. (1966). *Psychodiagnosis of schizophrenia.* New York: Wiley.

Weiner, I. B. (1977). *Approaches to Rorschach validation.* In M. A. Rickers-Ovsiankina (Ed.), *Rorschach psychology* (2nd ed., pp. 575–608).

Weiner, I. B. (1995). Methodological considerations in Rorschach research. *Psychological Assessment, 7,* 330–337.

Weiner, I. B. (1996). Some observations on the validity of the Rorschach Inkblot Method. *Psychological Assessment, 8,* 206–213.

Weiner, I. B. (1998). *Principles of Rorschach interpretation.* Mahwah, NJ: Lawrence Erlbaum Associates.

Weiner, I. B., Exner, J., & Sciara, A. (1996). Is the Rorschach welcome in the courtroom? *Journal of Personality Assessment, 72*(2), 422–424.

25

THE USE OF THE RORSCHACH IN POLICE PSYCHOLOGY: SOME PRELIMINARY THOUGHTS

Peter A. Weiss

Interfaith Medical Center, Brooklyn, NY

William U. Weiss

University of Evansville, Indiana

Carl B. Gacono

Private Practice, Austin, TX

Police psychology involves the application of psychological knowledge and research to the field of law enforcement. Much of the police psychologist's responsibilities include evaluation and treatment, program development, and conducting research.[1] The movement toward community policing (President's Commission on Law Enforcement, 1973) and the Civil Rights Act of 1964, which created penalties for civil rights violations by police departments (Rostow & Davis, 2004), have increased interest in police psychology. These issues have encouraged police departments to consider psychological factors in selecting and evaluating police officers. The need to ensure the emotional health of both candidates and seasoned officers is now well recognized.

Psychological assessment has long been essential to police psychology. Assessment has been utilized in pre-employment screening, fitness for duty referrals, and treatment planning. When testing is needed, police psychologists have mostly relied on self-report measures, such as the Minnesota Multiphasic Personality Inventory–2 (MMPI–2), the California Psychological Inventory (CPI), Personality Assessment Inventory (PAI), and Inwald Personality Inventory (IPI) (Rostow & Davis, 2004; Weiss, 2002; Weiss, Johnson, Serafino, & Serafino, 2001).

---

[1]Several professional organizations represent and recognize the police psychologist. The American Psychological Association includes Police Psychology as a subdivision of Division 18, Psychologists in Public Service. The Society for Police and Criminal Psychology offers a Diplomate in Police Psychology. The International Association of Chiefs of Police has a Police Psychological Services Section whose members resolve to promote the implementation of effective police psychological services.

Although it is less frequently used, there are some compelling reasons why the Rorschach Inkblot Method (RIM) may be useful to police psychologists (Weiss, 2002; Zacker, 1997). The test's ability to bypass volitional controls may be especially useful in pre-employment screening evaluations where the applicant is frequently invested in presenting themselves in a good light (Gacono, Evans, & Viglione, 2002). The RIM is more resistant to malingering than self-report inventories and can provide accurate information about personality with resistant clients (Ganellen, chap. 5, this vol.). Additionally, the RIM has the ability to elucidate personality traits in ways that differ from the other instruments (Gacono & Evans, preface, this vol.; Weiss, 2002; Zacker, 1997). This chapter discusses three areas—pre-employment screening, fitness for duty evaluations, and treatment planning—where the RIM could be useful in augmenting the traditional assessment battery.

EMPLOYMENT SCREENING OF POLICE OFFICERS

Applicants to police departments complete an extensive pre-employment process. In addition to filing a formal application, they participate in interviews with police administrators, extensive background checks, drug testing, strength and fitness tests, and literacy tests. The exact procedures vary among police departments. Individuals with serious problems (e.g., criminal records, inappropriate behavior during the job interview, and/or substance abuse problems) are eliminated from employment consideration prior to a formal psychological evaluation. The Americans With Disabilities Act mandates that medical and psychological evaluations be conducted after all other factors are considered (Flanagan, 1995).

The psychological evaluation occurs after these initial screening procedures, so examinees are, generally, emotionally stable (Weiss, Davis, Rostow, & Kinsman, 2003). The psychological evaluation ensures that the candidates do not exhibit psychopathology or personality characteristics that would interfere with their job performance. The psychologist conducting the pre-employment evaluation must be very familiar with the roles and stresses involved in police work.

Although the vast majority of city, county, and state governments require a pre-employment psychological evaluation (Weiss, Zehner, Davis, Rostow, & Decoster-Martin, 2005), guidelines for these evaluations vary greatly. Some jurisdictions mandate specific procedures, including the use of specific psychological tests, such as the Minnesota Multiphasic Personality Inventory–2 (MMPI–2). Other jurisdictions simply specify that all applicants have a "psychological evaluation"and leave the procedures to the discretion of the police psychologist. Similar to any forensic evaluation, the examiner must be aware of the laws or regulations that govern this work (Melton, Petrila, Poythress, & Slobogin, 1997; Shapiro, 1984).

The psychological evaluation involves an in-depth clinical interview and, nearly always, one or more psychological assessment instruments. As the agency, rather than the applicant, is the client, informed consent specifies the relationship of the examiner to the applicant, and allows for information to be released to the personnel office. It is essential that the psychologist review the applicant's file, which contains all of the aforementioned information from the application process, prior to conducting the psychological evaluation. The clinical interview is a comprehensive one and consists of a mental status examination, and an assessment of other areas of psychosocial functioning.

Self-report personality inventories such as the MMPI–2 and the PAI are most frequently administered (Weiss, 2002; Weiss et al., 2001), because relationships to future job performance have been demonstrated (Graham, 2005). Officer candidates with significant psychopathology on the MMPI do not perform well as police officers. Studies with the original MMPI found high scores on the *Ma* and *Pd* scales were correlated with excessive aggression, eventual termination, and poor supervisory ratings in several of these studies (Bartol, 1991; Hargrave, Hiatt, & Gaffney, 1988; Shusman, Inwald, & Knatz, 1987). A comparison of MMPI and MMPI–2 profiles of officer applicants found similar profiles (Hargrave, Hiatt, Ogard, & Carr, 1994). Studies with the MMPI–2 have confirmed and extended the earlier MMPI findings. They have found elevated *Pd*, *Ma*, *Hs*, *Hy*, and *Pa* scale scores to significantly correlate with termination and poor ratings by supervisors (Brewster & Stoloff, 1999; Weiss, Serafino, Serafino, Willson, & Knoll, 1998).

Findings related to response style can also be useful in forming opinions about an applicant's employability. In particular, high scores ($T > 65$) on the *L* scale of the MMPI–2 have been shown to discriminate between successful officers and those who exhibit problem behaviors, such as corruption, insubordination, and misinterpretations of the law or procedure (Boes, Chandler, & Timm, 1997; Weiss et al., 2003). Candidates with elevated *L* scale scores were more likely to be terminated (Weiss et al., 2003). Weiss et al. (2003) recommend using a raw score of 8 (T-score = 70) as a cutoff for both males and females on the *L* scale. Elevated Negative Impression PAI scale scores have been shown to predict subsequent performance problems, including conduct mistakes, inappropriate use of a weapon, neglect of duty, suspension, and reprimands by supervisors (Weiss, Rostow, Davis, & Decoster-Martin, 2004).

Other self-report instruments such as the California Psychological Inventory (CPI) and the Inwald Personality Inventory (IPI) have been useful in identifying characteristics of successful and unsuccessful police officers (Hogan & Kurtines, 1975; Inwald & Shusman, 1984; Mufson & Mufson, 1998; Shusman et al., 1987). Officers who had higher police academy grades and class standing, as well as fewer disciplinary actions after 3 years of employment, scored higher on the CPI Capacity for Status and Achievement via Independence scales, and lower on the Tolerance and Psychological Mindedness scales than unsuccessful officers (Hogan & Kurtines, 1975). IPI findings have suggested that poor performance ratings and termination correlate with elevated scores on the Driving Violations and Lack of Assertiveness scales and low scores on the Type A and Rigid Type scales (Mufson & Mufson, 1998).

Typically, most candidates who complete the psychological evaluation are hired. Candidates who fail can appeal this finding. They may request review or obtain a second evaluation from a different psychologist. Most police departments have guidelines for such an appeal. It should be noted that the psychologist conducting pre-employment evaluations is usually a consultant. Consequently, the referring department is not required to follow the psychologist's recommendations, although most do.

Despite extensive screening procedures, performance problems that are psychologically related continue to receive attention (Davis, Rostow, Pinkston, Combs, & Dixon, 2004). As a result, police psychologists continually seek to refine their methods for officer selection. As noted by Scrivner (1994):

> [Screening measures are] limited almost exclusively to psychological tests and pre-employment clinical interviews. New screening technologies could enable psychologists to examine such areas as a candidate's decision making and problem-solving abilities and quality of interaction with others. These dimensions are important for resolving situations without using excessive force and are particularly relevant to hiring officers who will work in community policing. (p. 2)

The RIM may be one such method.

THE RORSCHACH IN PRE-EMPLOYMENT SCREENING

Several studies support the RIM's potential for screening police officer candidates (Weiss, 2002; Zacker, 1997). Prior to the Comprehensive System (Exner, 2003), researchers have utilized Rorschach variables to aid in predicting job satisfaction, as well as to identify characteristics of successful officers (Kates, 1950; Matarazzo, Allen, Saslow, & Wiens, 1964). Using the Klopfer scoring system to study job satisfaction and interest in police officers, Kates (1950) found that officers who showed a high level of interest in their job gave more *M* than *Color* responses and had higher *M Form Quality* than those who had less interest in their job. Officers who reported high job satisfaction gave fewer *Color* and *Popular* responses than those who reported lower levels of job satisfaction. Officers who were motivated to increase their job level gave more *Color* than *M* responses. Whereas these findings were not interpreted according to the Comprehensive System, the increased *Color* could have been related to the emotional experience of dissatisfaction, and consequently, the stimulus for one to increase (change) their job level. Increased *M* could have related to an *Introversive* style and greater tolerance for job frustrations. Unfortunately, whereas this study (Kates, 1950) provides interesting information about police personality characteristics, it does not address job performance.

A requirement for using the RIM in police selection is that it be admissible, because unsuccessful job candidates occasionally challenge the findings. The applicant may claim that an error was made in the evaluation or that it was conducted incorrectly. Other reasons for contested hiring include accommodation requests under the Americans With Disabilities Act, accusations of gender or ethnic bias on the part of the psychologist, or the validity of the psychological tests (Hibler & Kurke, 1995). In this regard, the current version of the Comprehensive System for scoring and interpretation (Exner, 2003) has been shown to be both reliable and valid, and recent investigators have shown that the Comprehensive System meets the Daubert standards (McCann, 1998; Gacono et al., 2002; Gacono, Evans, & Viglione, chap. 1, this vol.; Viglione & Meyer, chap. 2, this vol.; McCann, Evans, chap. 3, this vol.).

The Rorschach possesses several features that may make it desirable in the selection process. First, it has the ability to provide valid information about personality functioning even in situations where the examinees are motivated to present themselves in a good light. Second, the Rorschach Comprehensive System has been extensively researched in areas that bear a direct relationship to the personality characteristics that are routinely assessed as part of the pre-employment psychological evaluation. In this regard, the RIM is no different than other personality measures. The majority measure dimensional aspects of personality that are important to forming forensic questions (e.g., employability). The measures do not directly answer the question of employability or job performance. But, traits measured by self-report measures, such as the RIM, are useful in forming opinions. It is the role of the evaluator to integrate the information to form a forensic opinion. For example, Capacity for Control and Stress Tolerance (which includes the *EA, es, D,* and *AdjD* variables), Interpersonal Perception and Behavior (which includes the *CDI, COP, AG,* and *PER* variables), and the Mediation (including the *XA%, WDA%,* and $X - \%$ variables) and Ideation clusters (variables such as the *PTI, WSum6, M–,* and *EB)* appear particularly important as stress tolerance, interpersonal functioning, and reality testing are all critical to the high stress levels inherent in police work. Finally, the RIM provides unique information about individuals with personality disorders.

Impression Management

The Rorschach is more resistant to the effects of positive impression management than are self-report inventories like the MMPI–2 (Ganellen, 1994, chap. 5, this vol.). Whereas individuals may be able to successfully deny psychopathology on self-report personality inventories, many individuals with these defensive profiles produce valid Rorschachs (Ganellen, 1994). Police psychologists recognize the defensive posture of most job applicants including their approach to the MMPI–2 (Graham, 2005; Kornfeld, 1995). Graham (2005) summarizes findings of personnel selection studies by stating that MMPI–2 findings are frequently moderately to significantly defensive. This increases the incremental value of the RIM. Indeed, Zacker (1997) found in a study of 53 applicants to suburban police departments that the RIM provided information that was incremental to the data provided by two self-report measures (IPI & MMPI–2; Zacker, 1997). In particular, the RIM provided useful information in the areas of coping deficits and reality testing.

Personality Characteristics

Three main clusters of Comprehensive System (CS; Exner, 2003) appear to be directly relevant to police work. Capacity for Control and Stress Tolerance is important because policing is a high stress profession (Weiss, 2002). *EA* is a direct measure of an individual's psychological resources (Exner, 2003). Police work may require average or even above-average resources. Police applicants with above-average *es* scores may have difficulties due to high levels of psychological stress (Exner, 2003). Additionally, the *D* and *AdjD* scores may identify those individuals who become disorganized and impulsive when placed in stressful situations (Exner, 2003) with individuals with low scores ($D < 0$) being particularly vulnerable.

Performing effectively as a law enforcement officer requires considerable interpersonal skill. Officers must interact successfully with a large number of individuals with differing personality characteristics. Although the Interpersonal cluster contains several variables (e.g., *AG, COP, GHR:PHR*, and *PER*) worth investigating, perhaps the *Coping Deficit Index (CDI)* is the most relevant. Zacker (1997) found that police officer applicants who show no evidence of psychopathology on the MMPI–2 or other self-report inventories sometimes exhibit a positive *CDI*. Individuals with positive scores on this variable typically have a long history of interpersonal problems (Exner, 2003). They are often regarded by others as inept in interpersonal relationships and have limited social skills (Exner, 2003). Because of the nature of police work, this finding could be associated with poor officer performance.

Making clear, efficient decisions, often in ambiguous or difficult situations, is essential to police work. The *Perceptual Thinking Index (PTI)* directly assesses thinking processes. Elements of the *PTI* include variables, such as the *WSum6* and *M*–, which assess distorted and peculiar thinking. Whereas individuals with the kind of thinking difficulties suggested by a positive *PTI* are frequently screened out in the initial stages of the hiring process, this information may serve as a guide for further questioning. The *EB* (*Erlebnistypus*) may also be useful as individuals with an *Ambitent* style may have problems with the difficult decisions, particularly those that occur under stress (Weiss, 2002). The Mediation cluster (*XA%, WDA%*) can identify individuals with impaired reality testing. Such individuals have difficulty accurately interpreting everyday events, which may lead to their having difficulties with police work.

Another notable aspect of the RIM is its ability to elucidate levels of personality organization (Meloy, Acklin, Gacono, Murray, & Peterson, 1997). Although the Rorschach does not provide specific diagnostic information, it is useful in assessing Axis II personality issues. Zacker (1997) observed that the Rorschach may be more useful at identifying individuals with problematic personality characteristics than the MMPI–2, which emphasizes Axis I-type symptoms. Combining the two approaches adds incrementally to the psychologist assessment yield. Certainly, information about personality organization is useful to police selection, because individuals with personality disorders have severe and chronic psychological problems that could interfere with their work performance. One of the groups Scrivner (1994) identified as "violence-prone officers" consisted of officers with personality disorders. They were described as having pervasive and enduring personality traits that are manifested in antisocial, narcissistic, paranoid, or abusive tendencies.

In summary, the RIM appears to have considerable potential as an assessment measure in pre-employment screening. When used in combination with a clinical interview, self-report measures, and history, the RIM may be of considerable benefit. However, research is needed to validate the Rorschach use for police selection.

FITNESS FOR DUTY

The fitness for duty evaluation (FFDE) is another area where traditional psychological tests are administered. FFDEs are conducted when an officer's inappropriate conduct appears to relate to psychological problems. The FFDE is defined as "a specialized mental health examination designed to inform the law enforcement executive responsible for the officer's supervision of issues of mental impairment that may impact upon the ability of the officer to perform his duty in a safe and effective manner" (Rostow & Davis, 2004, p. 62).

Among the most common FFDE referrals are suspected psychopathology, excessive force issues, substance abuse, repeated poor judgment, domestic violence, sexual misconduct, and work-related posttraumatic stress disorder (Rybicki & Nutter, 2002; Stone, 1995). The FFDE referral is initiated by a supervisor. The goal of the evaluation is to provide recommendations regarding disciplinary action or treatment. Whereas guidelines for FFDEs may vary, a set of general guidelines drafted by the International Association for Chiefs of Police may be found at their Web site at http://www.iacp.org. These 22 guidelines are not legally binding, although most departments have based their procedures on them.

At the beginning of a fitness for duty evaluation, the psychologist will obtain consent identifying the purpose of the evaluation and limits of confidentiality. If the officer refuses to give informed consent, then the FFDE procedure is terminated and the department is informed of the officer's refusal. In this initial stage, officers occasionally attempt to circumvent the FFDE and either directly refuse to participate or come with recording devices, attorneys, or union representatives. This problem is usually minimized by consulting the formal departmental policies on FFDEs. For example, some departments have officers sign documents when they are hired to explain and establish the departmental procedure for requesting psychological or medical examinations.

As part of the FFDE, the police psychologist typically reviews the officer's records, including collateral information, and conducts a detailed clinical interview. This interview is focused on the behavior of concern, but will also include a detailed mental status examination. Following the interview, the examinee completes a battery of tests. These might include the Shipley Institute of Living Scale, the MMPI–2, the Millon Clinical Multiaxial Inventory–III (MCMI), and the PAI (Rostow & Davis, 2004) or, depending on the referral question, the 16PF, CPI, Inwald Personality Inventory, and NEO–PI. In some cases, the RIM has been used (Rybicki & Nutter, 2002). Neuropsychological tests may be included as needed. The psychologist will then prepare a written report and submit it to the referring department.

Typically, an FFDE provides the following recommendations to the referring department:

1. The officer is unfit and is unlikely to become fit in the foreseeable future.
2. The officer is unfit but with treatment is likely to become fit in the foreseeable future.
3. The officer shows no mental health problems.
4. Malingering or an invalid presentation. (Rostow & Davis, 2004).

The Americans With Disabilities Act, which requires employers to assist unfit employees by helping to provide them with treatment and therapy (Stone, 1995) is an important consideration in formulating treatment recommendations. Rostow and Davis's (2004) recommendation, that the officer is unfit and is unlikely to become fit in the foreseeable future, is made only when further treatment is deemed not to be helpful. This might occur with a traumatic brain injury or a psychotic break. With the recommendation that the officer is unfit but is likely to become fit in the foreseeable future, the officer is referred for appropriate treatment. The fitness for duty evaluator may review progress but should not be involved in treatment, because this may constitutes a conflict of interest (Greenburg & Shuman, 1997).

The recommendation that the officer "shows no mental health problems," is made when the officer is referred because of conflicts and/or behaviors that are not found to be related to psychological factors. For example, an officer's behavior might reflect corrupt practices or inappropriate racial attitudes rather than psychopathology. Dispositions in such cases would be disciplinary. The officer referred for a FFDE may provide a "fake-good" presentation or circumvent the evaluation by malingering. If this is the case, then it is the responsibility of the FFDE evaluator to report this and make the recommendation that the presentation was invalid.

The FFDE report is a forensic rather than a clinical evaluation. The client in the FFDE is the referring police department rather than the officer. Whereas the psychologist can make certain recommendations for the officer, the final disposition rests with the referring department.

THE RORSCHACH IN FITNESS FOR DUTY EVALUATIONS

The RIM has been used at times for fitness for duty evaluations in police psychology (Rybicki & Nutter, 2002). Admissibility in court is a significant issue with FFDEs. There is always the possibility of a legal challenge, especially in a case where the psychologist doing the FFDE decides on recommendation 1, that is, that the officer is unfit and is unlikely to become fit in the foreseeable future.

Typically, police officers who exhibit characteristics during the clinical interview and psychological testing that are indicative of severe psychopathology will usually be classified as "unfit and unlikely to become fit in the foreseeable future." On the RIM, this would typically manifest itself in results indicative of severe thinking problems. A positive *PTI* is characteristic of individuals with bizarre thinking and poor reality testing. Such individuals often are diagnosed with psychotic disorders such as schizophrenia or schizoaffective disorder. Combined with a history of problematic and erratic behavior, as well as support from a well-conducted clinical interview, these data would provide support for this recommendation.

Another FFDE finding is when an officer is clearly unfit but may become fit for duty in the future. This category is associated with many psychological disorders; the most frequent being depression, personality disorders, posttraumatic stress disorder, and substance abuse. Such disorders often become evident due to the stressful nature of police work (Skolnick, 2000). Whereas the police psychologist must use the RIM in the context of an entire evaluation, various findings can aid in making such a determination.

Depressed individuals may present with a positive *Depression Index* (*DEPI*) on the Rorschach (Exner, 2003). Such individuals often experience severe psychological distress, depression, and a variety of behavioral problems related to depression and anxiety.

Such a finding would indicate that an officer should be referred for treatment focusing on that officer's affective problems.

Uncovering personality disorders in a FFDE is more problematic, because there is no single "borderline" or "personality disordered" RIM profile (Murray, 1997; Peterson, 1997). Some indicators of personality disorders, however, may include reflection responses, mild thought disorder (*Sum6* and *WSum6*), and disturbances on the Mediation variables (*XA%*, *WDA%*, *X–%*). However, RIM findings of borderline personality organization need thorough support from collateral sources. Officers found to have personality disorders that impact their work performance may be referred for treatment.

Posttraumatic stress disorder (PTSD) represents an important issue for police psychologists because of its frequency, as well as its seriousness (Rostow & Davis, 2004). Stone (1995) reported that nearly 4% of all fitness for duty evaluations he conducted involved confirmed PTSD, although this figure may be an underestimate, because a larger portion of those he assessed were classified as having "suspected psychopathology." Beginning with van der Kolk and Ducey (1984, 1989), the RIM has been used to assess psychological trauma in combat situations, often similar to situations experienced by many inner-city police officers. Sloan, Arsenault, and Hilsenroth (2002) found numerous variables sensitive to psychological trauma in combat situations, which may prove valuable in assessing police trauma. Hallett's (2002) dissertation on the impact of vicarious traumatization in law enforcement professionals found the Rorschach especially useful in assessing trauma exposure, the tendency for police personnel with histories of child abuse to work in units with high exposure to trauma, and the vulnerability of officers with trauma history to dissociative and anxiety disorders. Additionally, typical symptoms of PTSD, such as depression and anxiety, may be revealed by the RIM. Individuals whose overall presentation is similar to PTSD based on the history, clinical interview, and test data should be referred for psychological/psychiatric treatment as a result of the FFDE.

Substance abuse problems also figure prominently in FFDEs (Rostow & Davis, 2004). Although the RIM is not an instrument that directly measures substance abuse problems, it has value in the clinical assessment of individuals helping to identify what personality vulnerabilities underlie the problematic behavior (Exner & Erdberg, 2005). This, in turn, directs treatment planning.

The third finding, that there is no obvious psychological problem, indicates that performance problems are not due to psychological factors. If, in addition to other data, RIM variables are generally within the normal range (see Exner, 2003; Exner & Erdberg, 2005), this finding should be made. It should be noted that this finding does not mean that the officer has no performance problems; it merely means that they are not due to psychological factors.

Typically, an invalid or malingering presentation (Rostow & Davis, 2004) will involve either an excessively defensive stance in which an individual denies any and all psychological difficulties, or one in which an individual attempts to malinger mental illness in order to obtain a more sympathetic recommendation. In such cases, the RIM may be particularly useful. Excessive defensiveness will result in a denial of psychological difficulties in clinical interviews and on self-report inventories. Self-report data may reveal high scores on fake-good validity scales, such as the *L* and *K* on the MMPI–2 (Exner

& Erdberg, 2005; Graham, 2005). Some individuals with fake-good self-report profiles, however, will produce RIMs indicative of psychopathology in the same evaluation (Ganellen, 1994; Gacono et al., 2002).

For example, a malingering profile on the MMPI–2 is characterized by extreme elevations on the clinical scales and an F scale well above 100. If this profile is found in conjunction with a relatively normal Rorschach protocol, or with one that has serious inconsistencies (Exner & Erdberg, 2005), then the clinician may have added information supporting a case for malingering.

TREATMENT PLANNING

The usefulness of the Rorschach in the treatment planning has been well documented (Exner, 2003; Maruish, 2004, Mortimer & Smith, 1983; Weiner, 2004; Gacono, Jumes, & Gray, chap. 11, this vol.). Police officers will typically be referred for treatment for a variety of problems, including posttraumatic stress disorder, depression, alcohol and substance abuse, and antisocial behavior.

Police officers can be self-referred, referred by the department, or more frequently, they are encouraged to attend treatment by family members. Unusual stresses, as well as the unusual hours of separation from family members, contribute to police officers having one of the highest rates of divorce and family problems (Rostow & Davis, 2004). Officers typically exhibit extreme authoritarian behaviors as an adaptive response to police work (Skolnick, 2000), which are not adaptive in family and social relationships. Family problems may be exacerbated by the authoritarian behavior resulting from stress, anxiety, and isolation (Fromm, 1941). When self-referred or referred by family, the usual therapist–client confidentiality applies. When officers are referred for treatment by their departments (FFDE evaluation), a specific treatment provider and access to the officer's medical records should be requested (Rostow & Davis, 2004).

Whereas a comprehensive discussion of the use of the RIM for treatment planning is beyond the scope of this chapter, useful descriptions can be found elsewhere (Exner, 2003, Exner & Erdberg, 2005; Gacono, 1998; Gacono et al., chap. 1, this vol.; Jumes, Oropeza, Gray, & Gacono, 2002; Maruish, 2004; Mortimer & Smith, 1983; Weiner, 2004). This section focuses on several specific issues that suggest the RIM may be useful for treatment planning with police officers.

Treating police officers requires an understanding of the police culture. The general attitude of most officers toward psychological treatment is one of mistrust. Although the existence of a unique "police personality" is controversial (Twersky-Glasner, 2005), some characteristics must be acknowledged. The so-called blue wall of silence is one of these; this is essentially the belief that "Cops don't tell on cops" (Skolnick, 2000), to which might be added the notion that "Cops don't want to tell on themselves." Police officers often do not present to treatment with "psychological problems" because having psychological problems is considered a sign of weakness (Rostow & Davis, 2004). Instead, officers may present vague, nonspecific behavioral complaints, for example, "My marriage just isn't going well." This stance may cause a defensive response set on self-report assessment measures. The RIM would be helpful in treatment planning because of its value in obtaining personality information in the presence of resistance.

Traditional assessment measures, such as the MMPI–2, generally deal with symptom-related issues. For purposes of treatment planning, information about personality organization is also desirable. Several RIM variables provide information that might guide treatment (Weiner, 2004). The Cluster Analysis approach to interpretation (Exner, 2003; Exner & Erdberg, 2005) identifies and prioritizes key areas of clinical concern. This approach emphasizes particular aspects of psychological functioning based on certain key variables. For example, if an individual shows a positive score on the *Depression Index* (*DEPI*), then the search routine suggests interpreting variables and issues related to affect before exploring others. It would be likely in this case that affect is the most important clinical issue for that individual and would provide the most important information (Exner, 2003; Exner & Erdberg, 2005).

Additionally, the RIM may be useful in identifying impediments to treatment (Weiner, 2004). For example, the *a:p* ratio measures the ability of an individual to consider other perspectives and to be cognitively flexible. Individuals with an *a:p* ratios above 2:1 tend to be inflexible and to cling to their existing ideas. An individual's ability to engage in introspective behavior (presence of *FD*), might be a positive prognostic sign. The presence of one *Texture* (*T*) response might also be a positive indication, as *T*-less individuals tend to be more interpersonally distant and more difficult to engage in psychotherapy. Also, individuals with lower *D* scores might be more motivated to change due to their current levels of stress.

RIM variables can also alert the treating psychologist to nature of resistances to therapy (trait vs. state). For example, an officer may be experiencing distress (a low *D* score), exhibit cognitive flexibility (normal *a:p* ratio), have an ability to connect with others (the presence of *T*), and be introspective (presence of *FD*), but not want to engage in treatment because of the social norms associated with police culture. This kind of officer would provide less of a challenge than a person with fewer personality resources. An officer whose resistance is more character based, as indicated by a *D* score of 0 or greater, an *a:p* ratio greater than 2:1, no *T* responses, or no *FD* responses, would pose a different set of issues for treatment.

From a structural perspective, the RIM also has indices that are useful in clinical assessment of common psychological problems. The *Depression Index* (*DEPI*) is particularly well suited for assessing the depressive, frustrating feelings (*FC'*, *C'F*, *C'*, *S*). The Interpersonal cluster (including variables such as the *CDI, Reflections, T, COP, AG, PER,* and *GHR:PHR*) would be particularly useful in understanding treatment issues, as police frequently present for treatment with marital, family, or other interpersonal difficulty. Indices such as the *CDI, Reflection* responses, and *T* responses could be used to help identify the causes of interpersonal and family problems, and then provide a focus for structural or strategic family therapy, or individual therapy focusing on interpersonal issues. For example, an officer with a positive *CDI* might be helped by emphasizing more adaptive communications skills, whereas one with Reflections, might require careful attention in therapy to avoid narcissistic injuries from the therapist and/or family members, which might result in premature termination of therapy.

Officers with unusual levels of T (either 0 or ≥ 2) would benefit from individual and family interventions oriented toward awareness of family needs for interpersonal contact, closeness, and appropriate boundaries.

Other variables in the Interpersonal cluster also appear to have potential here. The *GHR:PHR* ratio, which measures how adaptive an individual's interpersonal functioning is, can be helpful in understanding the cause of interpersonal problems. Variables that relate to expectations and personal style in relationships with others (*COP, AG, PER*) can also be useful. For example, individuals with more *AG* responses in comparison to *COP* tend to anticipate aggressive interactions with others as being commonplace. Individuals with large numbers of *PER* responses tend to be rather authoritarian in their dealings with others.

Obviously, the treatment approach taken by the psychologist as a result of such an evaluation will depend on the client's individual personality characteristics. A sample evaluation of a police officer who presented to treatment with serious psychological problems can be found in Peterson (1997). This individual exhibited interpersonal, stress, and affective problems, which in the context of the overall evaluation showed a borderline personality organization. Peterson asserts that the goal for the therapist in such a case is more effective integration of the individual's personality. However, not all individuals require the same kind of treatment approach.

CONCLUSIONS

Much validation research is needed, but the RIM has considerable potential for use in police psychology. Areas such as police selection (Weiss, 2002; Zacker, 1997), FFDE evaluations (Rybicki & Nutter, 2002), and treatment planning (Peterson, 1997) are appropriate for including the RIM. At present, the RIM is a useful method of personality assessment that is supported by much research (Exner, 2003). Further research in the area of police psychology would serve to increase its popularity and usefulness.

Whereas many research applications exist, perhaps the most important would be to determine if there are Rorschach predictors of police misconduct. Episodes of inappropriate aggression and violence are of particular concern to police departments. Improved methods of identifying individuals at risk for violence would improve police/community relations and protect the department from legal actions.

One obstacle to the RIMs use has been concerns about admissibility. However, it is clear that the Rorschach Comprehensive System is admissible (McCann, Evans, chap. 3, this vol.). Another obstacle to its wider acceptance is its "purported" labor intensive nature, and thus, "cost." Cost, in this sense, usually refers to an unwanted increase in a departmental budget. However, as noted by Hughes, Gacono, and Owen (in press):

Although novice examiners typically take longer to administer and score the RIM than advanced examiners, unlike many self-report measures, it is the skill level of the examiner rather than anything inherent in the test that determines administration and scoring time (Gacono et al., 1997). On average it takes an experienced examiner about an hour and a half to administer and score a Rorschach including the in-putting of raw data through scoring software (e.g., ROR-SCAN, Rorschach Interpretive Assistant Program).

The cost benefits of administering the RIM must be put in a context. As described by Hughes, Gacono, and Owen (2007):

> [The] psychologist must, however, carefully weigh the importance of RIM data (including information regarding the person's attitudes and behaviors while completing the test) when deciding on this cost–benefit issue. With experience, the RIM can be administered in an efficient manner. As part of a multi-method assessment strategy the value of the Rorschach is considerable. While a single method of data collection (e.g., behavioral rating scales) may indeed be less time/cost intensive at the outset, it may also lead to a narrow and limited understanding of the individual (Meyer et al., 2001), for which subsequent, expanded and costly data collections may be required (Meyer et al., 2001). Performance based measures, such as the RIM, add incrementally to self-report data (Gacono et al., 2002). Stricker and Gold (1999) stress the value of both nomothetic (normative) and idiographic (thematic) approaches to personality assessment and they suggest that RIM information is more useful for understanding automatic processes (unconscious), longitudinal, and structural dimensions of functioning. Clearly, a thoughtful and comprehensive assessment can better serve the student and reduce assessment costs. (Mattlar, 2004)

The true cost of adding the RIM to the assessment battery, however, must be balanced against the costs of failure to do so. The costs are many when an experienced police officer is lost, "burned out," or has instances of police misconduct, or when the recruit resigns within the first year of police work because of job-related "stress."

Whereas the use of the RIM in police psychology is in its early stages, psychologists have previously advocated and recommended its use (Weiss, 2002; Zacker, 1997). We hope this chapter may encourage police psychologists to continue using the RIM and studying its efficacy. The vast potential of the RIM use in police psychology is yet to be determined.

REFERENCES

Bartol, C. R. (1991). Predictive validation of the MMPI for small-town police officers who fail. *Professional Psychology: Research and Practice, 22*, 127–132.

Boes, J. O., Chandler, C. J., & Timm, H. W. (1997). *Police integrity: Use of personality measures to identify corruption-prone officers.* Monterey, CA: Defense Personnel Security Research Center.

Brewster, J., & Stoloff, M. L. (1999). Using the good cop/bad cop profile with the MMPI–2. *Journal of Police and Criminal Psychology, 14*(2), 29–34.

Davis, R. D., Rostow, C. D., Pinkston, J. B., Combs, D. R., & Dixon, D. R. (2004). A re-examination of the MMPI–2 aggressiveness and immaturity indices in law enforcement screening. *Journal of Police and Criminal Psychology, 19*(1), 17–26.

Exner, J. E., Jr. (2003). *The Rorschach: A Comprehensive System: Vol. I. Basic foundations and principles of interpretation* (4th ed.). New York: Wiley.

Exner, J. E., Jr., & Erdberg, P. (2005). *The Rorschach: A Comprehensive System: Vol. 2. Advanced interpretation* (3rd ed.). New York: Wiley.

Flanagan, C. L. (1995). Legal issues regarding police psychology. In M. I. Kurke & E. M. Scrivner (Eds.), *Police psychology into the 21st century* (pp. 93–107). Hillsdale, NJ: Lawrence Erlbaum Associates.

Fromm, E. (1941). *Escape from freedom.* New York: Henry Holt.

Gacono, C. B. (1998). The use of the Psychopathy Checklist–Revised (PCL–R) and Rorschach in treatment planning with antisocial personality disordered patients. *International Journal of Offender Therapy and Comparative Criminology, 4*(1), 49–64.

Gacono, C. B., Decato, C. M., Brabender, V., & Goertzel, T. G. (1997). Vitamin C or *Pure C*. The Rorschach of Linus Pauling. In J. R. Meloy, M. W. Acklin, C. B. Gacono, J. F. Murray, & C. A. Peterson (Eds.), *Contemporary Rorschach interpretation* (pp. 421–451). Mahwah, NJ: Lawrence Erlbaum Associates.

Gacono, C. B., Evans, F. B., & Viglione, D. J. (2002). The Rorschach in forensic practice. *Journal of Forensic Psychology Practice, 2*(3), 33–53.

Ganellen, R. J. (1994). Attempting to conceal psychological disturbance: MMPI defensive sets and the Rorschach. *Journal of Personality Assessment, 63,* 423–437.

Graham, J. R. (2005). *MMPI–2: Assessing personality and psychopathology* (4th ed.). New York: Oxford University Press.

Greenburg, S., & Shuman, D. (1997). Irreconcilable conflict between therapeutic and forensic roles. *Professional Psychology: Research and Practice, 23*(1), 50–57.

Hallett, S. J. (1996). Trauma and coping in homicide and child sexual abuse detectives. *Dissertation Abstracts International: Section B: The Sciences and Engineering,.57*(3), 2152B.

Hargrave, G. E., Hiatt, D., & Gaffney, T. W. (1988). $F + 4 + 9 + Cn$: An MMPI measure of aggression in law enforcement officers and applicants. *Journal of Police Science and Administration, 16,* 268–273.

Hargrave, G. E., Hiatt, D., Ogard, E. M., & Karr, C. (1994). Comparison of the MMPI and MMPI–2 for a sample of peace officers. *Psychological Assessment, 6,* 27–32.

Hibler, N. S., & Kurke, M. I. (1995). Ensuring personal reliability through selection and training. In M. I. Kurke & E. M. Scrivner (Eds.), *Police psychology into the 21st century* (pp. 57–91). Hillsdale, NJ: Lawrence Erlbaum Associates.

Hogan, R., & Kurtines, W. (1975). Personological correlates of police effectiveness. *Journal of Psychology, 91,* 289–295.

Hughes, T., Gacono, C. B., & Owen, P. F. (2007). Current Status of Rorschach Assessment: Implications for the School Psychologist. Psychology in the Schools, 44(8), 281–291.

Inwald, R. E., & Shusman, E. J. (1984). The IPI and MMPI as predictors of academy performance for police recruits. *Journal of Police Science and Administration, 12*(1), 1–11.

Jumes, M. T., Oropeza, P. P., Gray, B. T., & Gacono, C. B. (2002). Use of the Rorschach in forensic settings for treatment planning and monitoring. *International Journal of Offender Therapy and Comparative Criminology, 46*(3), 294–307.

Kates, S. L. (1950). Rorschach responses, Strong blank scales, and job satisfaction among policemen. *Journal of Applied Psychology, 34,* 249–254.

Kornfeld, A. D. (1995). Police officer candidate MMPI–2 performance: Gender, ethnic, and normative factors. *Journal of Clinical Psychology, 51,* 536–540.

Maruish, M. E. (2004). *The use of psychological testing for treatment planning and outcome assessment* (3rd ed.). Mahwah, NJ: Lawrence Erlbaum Associates.

McCann, J. T. (1998). Defending the Rorschach in court: An analysis of admissibility using legal and professional standards. *Journal of Personality Assessment, 70,* 125–144.

Matarazzo, J. D., Allen, B. V., Saslow, G., & Wiens, A. N. (1964). Characteristics of successful policemen and firemen applicants. *Journal of Applied Psychology, 48,* 123–133.

Mattlar, C. (2004). The Rorschach comprehensive system is reliable, valid and cost-effective. *Rorschachiana, 26,* 158–186.

Meloy, J. R., Acklin, M. W., Gacono, C. B., Murray, J. F., & Peterson, C. A. (Eds.). (1997). *Contemporary Rorschach interpretation*. Mahwah, NJ: Lawrence Erlbaum Associates.

Melton, G., Petrila, J., Poythress, N., & Slobogin, C. (1997). *Psychological evaluations for the courts: A handbook for mental health professionals and lawyers* (2nd ed.). New York: Guilford.

Meyer, G. J., Finn, S. E., Eyde, L., Kay, G. G., Moreland, K. L., Dies, R. R., Eisman, E. J., Kubiszyn, T. W., & Reed, G. M. (2001). Psychological testing and psychological assessment: A review of evidence and issues. *American Psychologist, 56,* 128–165.

Mortimer, R., & Smith, W. (1983). The use of the psychological test report in setting the focus of psychotherapy. *Journal of Personality Assessment, 47*(2), 134–138.

Mufson, D., & Mufson, M. A. (1998). Predicting police officer performance using the Inwald Personality Inventory: An illustration. *Professional Psychology: Research and Practice, 29*(1), 59–62.

Murray, J. F. (1997). The Rorschach search for the borderline holy grail: An examination of personality structure, personality style, and situation. In J. R. Meloy, M. W. Acklin, C. B. Gacono, J. F. Murray, & C. A. Peterson (Eds.), *Contemporary Rorschach interpretation* (pp. 123–138). Mahwah, NJ: Lawrence Erlbaum Associates.

Peterson, C. A. (1997). A borderline policeman: AKA, a cop with no *COP*. In J. R. Meloy, M. W. Acklin, C. B. Gacono, J. F. Murray, & C. A. Peterson (Eds.), *Contemporary Rorschach interpretation* (pp. 157–176). Mahwah, NJ: Lawrence Erlbaum Associates.

President's Commission on Law Enforcement and Administration of Justice. (1973). *Task force report: The police.* Washington, DC: Government Printing Office.

Rostow, C. D., & Davis, R. D. (2004). *A handbook for psychological fitness-for-duty evaluations in law enforcement.* Binghamton, NY: Haworth.

Rybicki, D. J., & Nutter, R. A. (2002). Employment-related psychological evaluations: Risk management concerns and current practices. *Journal of Police and Criminal Psychology, 17*(2), 18–31.

Scrivner, E. M. (1994). *Controlling police use of excessive force: The role of the police psychologist.* Rockville, MD: National Criminal Justice Reference Service.

Shapiro, D. (1984). *Psychological evaluation and expert testimony: A practical guide to forensic work.* New York: Van Nostrand Reinhold.

Shusman, E. J., Inwald, R. E., & Knatz, H. F. (1987). A cross validation study of police recruit performance as predicted by the IPI and MMPI. *Journal of Police Science and Administration, 15,* 162–169.

Skolnick, J. H. (2000). Code blue. *The American Prospect, 11*(10), 49–53.

Sloan, P., Arsenault, L., & Hilsenroth, M. J. (2002). Use of the Rorschach in the assessment of war-related stress in military personnel. *Rorschachiana: Yearbook of the International Rorschach Society, 25,* 86–122.

Stone, A. V. (1995). Law enforcement psychological fitness for duty: Clinical issues. In M. I. Kurke & E. M. Scrivner (Eds.), *Police psychology into the 21st century* (pp. 109–131). Hillsdale, NJ: Lawrence Erlbaum Associates.

Stricker, G., & Gold, J. R. (1999). The Rorschach: Toward a nomothetically based, idiographically applicable, configurational model. *Psychological Assessment, 11,* 240–250.

Twersky-Glasner, A. (2005). Police personality: What is it and why are they like that? *Journal of Police and Criminal Psychology, 20*(1), 56–67.

Van der Kolk, B. A., & Ducey, C. P. Clinical implications of the Rorschach in post-traumatic stress disorder. In B. A. van der Kolk (Ed.), *Post-traumatic stress disorder: Psychological and biological sequelae* (pp. 29–42). Washington: American Psychiatric Press.

van der Kolk, B., & Ducey, C. P. (1989). The psychological processing of traumatic experience: Rorschach patterns in PTSD. *Journal of Traumatic Stress, 2,* 259–274.

Weiner, I. B. (2004). Rorschach inkblot method. In M. E. Maruish (Ed.), *The use of psychological testing for treatment planning and outcome assessment* (3rd ed., 1123–1156). Mahwah, NJ: Lawrence Erlbaum Associates.

Weiss, P. A. (2002). Potential uses of the Rorschach in the selection of police officers. *Journal of Police and Criminal Psychology, 17*(2), 63–70.

Weiss, W. U., Davis, R., Rostow, C., & Kinsman, S. (2003). The MMPI–2 L scale as a tool in police selection. *Journal of Police and Criminal Psychology, 18*(1), 57–60.

Weiss, W. U., Johnson, J., Serafino, G., & Serafino, A. (2001). A three-year follow-up of the performance of a class of state police academy graduates using the MMPI–2. *Journal of Police and Criminal Psychology, 16*(1), 51–55.

Weiss, W. U., Rostow, C., Davis, R., & DeCoster-Martin, E. (2004). The Personality Assessment Inventory as a selection device for law enforcement personnel. *Journal of Police and Criminal Psychology, 19*(2), 23–29.

Weiss, W. U., Serafino, G., Serafino, A., Willson, W., & Knoll, S. (1998). Use of the MMPI–2 to predict the employment continuation and performance ratings of recently hired police officers. *Journal of Police and Criminal Psychology, 13*, 40–44.

Weiss, W. U., Zehner, S. N., Davis, R. D., Rostow, C., & Decoster-Martin, E. (2005). Problematic police performance and the Personality Assessment Inventory. *Journal of Police and Criminal Psychology, 20*(1), 16–21.

Zacker, J. (1997). Rorschach responses of police applicants. *Psychological Reports, 80*, 523–528.

26

THE RORSCHACH ASSESSMENT OF AGGRESSION: THE RORSCHACH EXTENDED AGGRESSION SCORES

Carl B. Gacono

Private Practice, Austin, TX

Lynne A. Gacono

Austin State Hospital, Austin, TX

J. Reid Meloy

University of California, San Diego

Matthew R. Baity

Massachusetts General Hospital, Boston, MA

The *Extended Aggression* scores were developed to quantify the aggressive Rorschach imagery produced by violent Antisocial Personality Disordered (ASPD; American Psychiatric Association, 1980) offenders. Despite their histories of real-world violence, these subjects produced few *Aggressive Movement* (*AG*; Exner, 1993) responses. Why didn't violent children, adolescents, and adults produce more *AG* responses? Considering their expression of uncensored pleasurable affect when relating their aggressive acts during interviews, conscious censoring (Exner, 1993; Meloy, 1988) did not adequately explain the paucity of *AG* responses among *sentenced* adults. Why would they describe their violent acts with pride and bravado during an interview and subsequently censor *AG* on the Rorschach? Conscious censoring among the Conduct Disorder (CD) children and adolescents, who frequently produced sexual content, seemed an equally unlikely explanation (Gacono, 1997).

Earlier Rorschach research (Holt & Havel, 1960; Rapaport, Gill, & Schafer, 1946, 1968; Schafer, 1954) provided clues to understanding the discrepancies between Rorschach production and the interview/historical data. Direct or implicit aggressive content was thought to imply tensions of aggressive impulse (Rapaport et al., 1946, 1968). Initial findings (Gacono, 1988; 1990; Heaven, 1988) suggested that the paucity of symbolized aggression, represented by *AG* movement, might be due in part to the ego-syntonic nature of aggression in ASPD and psychopathic subjects.[1] The clinical logic was that *AG* symbolized tensions of ego-dystonic aggression when produced by nonviolent patients. In the absence of binding the aggressive impulse, the habitually violent individual would, instead, act it out, thus vitiating the need to symbolize it. Table 26–1 offers some support for this hypothesis: Exner's (1995) character disordered sample produced lower *AG* frequencies than his adult nonpatients; violent children and adolescents produce lower *AG* frequencies than child and adolescent nonpatients; and the majority of the forensic subjects with known histories of violence produce less *AG* than nonpatients and the Gacono and Meloy clinical samples without histories of violence (Gacono, 1997; Gacono & Meloy, 1994).[2]

Despite the paucity of *AG* responses in ASPD records, other aggression imagery was not absent. Rather, the presence of other potentially scorable aggressive imagery (see Gacono, 1988, 1990, 1997) allowed for the development (Gacono, 1988) and refinement (Gacono & Meloy, 1994; Meloy & Gacono, 1992) of five additional scoring categories: *Aggressive Content (AgC), Aggressive Past (AgPast), Aggressive Potential (AgPot), Aggressive Vulnerability (AgV),* and *Sadomasochism (SM)* (see Gacono, Gacono, Meloy, & Baity, 2005).

Since their introduction (Gacono, 1988), the *Extended Aggression* scores have received considerable clinical interest and empirical study. As noted in the Rorschach Workshops' *Alumni Newsletter* (2000) concerning the work of the Rorschach Research Council, "Another project on which there has been good progress is the special score for *Aggressive Content* (AgC). Council has reviewed the criteria and guidelines for its applications and has evaluated the literature concerning it . ... A more precise interpretation of AgC responses will probably hinge on findings for other variables" (p. 13). Additionally, the ROR-SCAN Version 6 Rorschach Interpretive Scoring System (Caracena, 2002) now includes *AgC, AgPast, AgPot,* and *SM.* What began as an attempt to expand the scoring of Rorschach aggressive imagery in CD and ASPD subjects, has evolved into a larger study of aggression on the Rorschach. This appendix evaluates and summarizes the reliability and validity of the *Extended Aggression* scores and discusses their clinical meanings.

INTERRATER RELIABILITY

A search of PsycINFO between 1989 and 2003 using the key words Rorschach and aggressive, aggression, *AgC, AgPot, AgPast,* sadomasochism, sado-masochism, Gacono or Meloy, revealed that, since their introduction (Gacono, 1988), there have been eight published articles (Baity & Hilsenroth, 1999, 2002; Gacono, 1990; Gacono et al., 1992; Kamphui, Kugeares, & Finn, 2000; Meloy & Gacono, 1992; Mihura & Nathan-Montano,

---

[1]The psychopath's ego-syntonic relationship to aggression is exemplified by a psychopath who while intoxicated wandered through a section of town looking for an individual he planned to murder. Instead he killed a 15-year-old male stranger. His comment after killing the boy was, "I was going to kill someone anyway."

[2]The higher rates of *AG* among the sexual homicide perpetrators (compared to other forensic samples) might appear to be antithetical to this hypothesis; however, increased rates of *AG* (compared to other forensic samples) are theoretically consistent with their ambivalent relationship to aggression. Increased *AG* has been consistently predicted and found for this particularly disturbed group of individuals despite their histories of both affective and predatory real-world violence.

TABLE 26–1

Frequency of Aggressive Movement Responses (AG)

Exner (1995) Subjects				Gacono & Meloy Subjects			
Group	*N*	*Mean (SD)*	*%*	*Group*	*N*	*Mean (SD)*	*%*
Children				*Conduct-Disordered*			
Age 5	90	1.23 (.67)	91%	Ages 5–12[b]	72	.60 (1.04)	32%
Age 6	80	30 (.56)	25%				
Age 7	120	1.20 (.40)	100%				
Age 8	120	.93 (.58)	80%				
Age 9	140	1.37 (.78)	91%				
Age 10	120	1.57 (.62)	100%				
Age 11	135	1.42 (.57)	100%				
Age 12	120	1.08 (.66)	82%				
Adolescents				*Conduct-Disordered*			
Age 13	110	1.18 (.91)	77%	Ages 13–17[b]	179	.53 (.84)	35%
Age 14	105	1.30 (.92)	85%	Males[c]	79	.65 (.96)	38%
Age 15	140	1.14 (.91)	74%	Females[c]	21	.33 (.66)	24%
Age 16	140	1.20 (.99)	76%				
Adults				*Adult Antisocial (ASPD)*			
Nonpatient Adults	700	1.18 (1.18)	67%	Males[b]	108	.50 (.85)	54%
Schizophrenic	320	1.26 (1.85)	50%	Females[b]	69	.62 (.84)	45%
Character Disordered	180	.41 (.67)	31%	Schizophrenic[b]	100	.75 (1.17)	40%
				Female Psychopaths[e]	28	.57 (.92)	39%
				Male Psychopaths[b]	30	.50 (.82)	43%
				Sexual Homicide[b]	38	.82 (.90)	58%
				Adult Outpatient			
				Forensic/Paranoid Schizophrenic[d]	90	.54 (.96)	36%
				Forensic/Bipolar[d]	40	.68 (1.09)	38%
				Forensic/Undiff Schizophrenic[d]	38	.74 (1.13)	37%
				Forensic/ Schizoeffective[d]	59	.64 (.89)	44%
				Narcissistic[a]	18	.78 (1.21)	50%
				Borderline[a]	18	1.39 (1.33)	72%
				Borderline Female[b]	32	1.60 (2.2)	69%

Note. % = is the percentage of subjects that produced at least one aggressive movement response.

[a]Gacono, Meloy, & Berg (1992). [b]Gacono & Meloy samples. [c]Gacono & Meloy (1994). [d]Gacono, & Gacono samples (data analyzed by Dr. Exner at Rorschach Workshops). [e]Cunliffe & Gacono (2005).

2001; Mihura, Nathan-Montano, & Alperin, 2003) and approximately 12 dissertations (several additional dissertations were discovered through additional searches) that have included the *Extended Aggression* scores. When interrater agreement was reported, it has been good (i.e., > .75; Fleiss, 1981).

Table 26–2 summarizes the interrater reliability of the *Extended Aggression* scores from seven published studies (Baity & Hilsenroth, 1999; Baity & Hilsenroth, 2002; Kamphuis, Kugeares, & Finn, 2000; Huprich, Gacono, Schneider, & Bridges, 2004; Meloy & Gacono, 1992; Mihura & Nathan-Montano, 2001; Mihura et al., 2003), six dissertations (Cohan, 1998; Darcangelo, 1997; Levy, 1998; Margolis, 1992; Neubauer, 2001; White, 1999), and one book chapter (Ephriam, Occupati, Riquelme, & Gonzales, 1993; Riquelme, Occupati, & Gonzales, 1991). Percent agreement means ranged from 86% (*AgPot*) to 99.5% (*SM*). One low percent agreement finding, 50% for *AgPot* (White, 1999), lowered the mean scores. The combined mean for kappa coefficients and intraclass correlation coefficients (ICCs) ranged from .84 (*AgPast*) to .96 (*SM*).

VALIDITY RESEARCH

Not surprisingly, because these are the most frequently produced scores, *AgC*, *AgPast*, and/or *AgPot* have been studied in the majority of studies. Only three studies investigated *SM* and no studies investigated *AgV*. The following sections describe the validity research, primarily from published studies, for each of the *Extended Aggression* scores. Dissertation studies are used mostly to highlight methodological limitations. For readers unfamiliar with the *Extended Aggression* scores, each section begins with a brief description of how the variable is coded along with sample responses.

Aggressive Content (AgC)

AgC is coded for content popularly perceived as predatory, dangerous, malevolent, injurious, or harmful (Gacono, 1988; Meloy & Gacono, 1992). Consider two examples: Card VI: "It's a gun." Card IX: "It's a demon with claws" (this second percept would only receive one *AgC* score; "A dragon attacking a demon" would receive two *AgC*s). *Popular* responses are not coded as *AgC* unless embellished with aggressive imagery (i.e., Card V "a bat" [not *AgC*]; "A vampire bat" [score *AgC*]).[3] Gacono's surveys of mental health workers and college students provided guidelines for scoring *AgC* (Gacono & Meloy, 1994; Meloy & Gacono, 1992). In order to ascertain the robustness of the Gacono and Meloy (1994) *AgC* guidelines, Baity, McDaniel, and Hilsenroth (2000) surveyed an undergraduate student group utilizing the Gacono and Meloy aggressive objects, a sample of potentially aggressive objects not located in Gacono and Meloy's work (e.g., bear, bee, Bigfoot, etc.), and a list of neutral objects taken from practice scoring protocols in Exner's Comprehensive Sys-

---

[3]Some studies did not report excluding aggressive objects from *AgC* scoring that qualified as a *Popular* (e.g., a "tiger" to D1 on Card VIII). Many authors did not indicate that they had scored multiple occurrences of a single aggressive category within a response (i.e., if two different objects within a single response qualify for an *AgC*, score two *AgC*s; same for *AgPast*, *AgPot*, etc.).

TABLE 26–2

Inte-rater Agreement for the Rorschach Extended Aggression Scores

Study	N	AgC	AgPot	AgPast	SM	Sample Studied
Baity & Hilsenroth (1999)	25	99%	100%	99%	—	Cluster A, B, & C Personality Disorders
		.95[a]	1.0[a]	.79[a]	—	
Baity & Hilsenroth (2002)	20	.88[a]	—	—	—	Psychiatric reference groups from Exner's (1993) normative sample
Cohan (1998)	20	86%	83%	88%	—	Forensic outpatient sex offenders
Darcangelo (1997)	5	.97[b]	.92[b]	.95[b]	—	Male incarcerated rapists
Gacono et al. (1992)	30	95%	100%	96%	—	Cluster B/Personality Disorders
Huprich et al. (2004)	19	97%	99%	99%	99%	Psychopaths, Pedophiles, Sexual Homicide Perpetrators
		.90[a]	.83[a]	.89[a]	.91[a]	
Levy (1998)	14	93%	97%	98%	—	Physically abused children
Meloy & Gacono (1992)	30	95%	100%	96%	—	ASPD incarcerated males
Mihura & Nathan-Montano (2001)	50	.85[a]	.76[a]	.85[a]	—	Undergraduate college students
Mihura et al. (2003)	70	.89[a]	.88[a]	.94[a]	—	Undergraduate college students
Neubauer (2001)	20	95%	99.60%	97.70%	—	Nonpatient adults
		.80[a]	.66[a]	.65[a]	—	
Riquelme et al. (1991)/Ephriam et al. (1993)	40	—	97%	97%	—	Nonpatient adults (Venezuela)
White (1999)	33	73%	50%	86%	—	Forensic outpatients

Note. N = Number of protocols scored for interrater agreement. [a]Kappa coefficients (k). [b]Intraclass correlations (ICC).

tem Workbook (e.g., apple, butterfly, candle, etc.; Exner, 1995b). Most of Gacono and Meloy's aggressive objects fit the definition of *AgC* and could be further delineated by categories (weapons, animal/part animal, environmental danger, fictional creature) and aggressive adjectives (scary, frightening, evil, angry, or mean; Baity et al., 2000). This research reinforced using the original *AgC* tables as a scoring guide rather than an exhaustive list. The authors also demonstrated that *AgC* definitions remained consistent over time (a 1-month test–retest reliability check produced an $r = .99$).

AgC is the most frequently occurring *Extended Aggression* score in all studies. This variable was thought to represent identification with aggressive objects, and in certain cases, highly cathected object representations of weapons or violent acts (Gacono & Meloy, 1994). The relationship between *AgC* and aggressive identification, ideation, or preoccupation has been supported in several studies. In a sample of personality disordered outpatients, Baity and Hilsenroth (1999) found that *AgC* was the strongest predictor of both the total number of *DSM–IV* criteria for Antisocial Personality Disorder (ASPD) and scores on the MMPI–2 Antisocial Practices Scale (APS). The findings of Mihura and colleagues (Mihura & Nathan-Montano, 2001; Mihura et al., 2003) suggested that, in college samples, elevated *AgC* represented an ego-dystonic relationship to aggression that caused disorganization (feelings of less control) and defensive use of projection. Elevated *AgC* signals the need to explore the presence of aggressive figures and events in the client's past that may have contributed to an "identification with the aggressor" (Freud, 1936).

Baity and Hilsenroth (2002) also linked *AgC* to histories of real-world aggression. They found that more behavioral aggressiveness (based on an Aggression Chart Rating scale) was significantly correlated with a greater number of *AgC*, *AG*, and *Morbid* responses (*MOR*; Exner, 1993). Among these three responses, *AgC* was the only nonredundant, significant predictor of aggressiveness; specifically, *AG* and *MOR* did not account for significant variance beyond that provided by *AgC*. An $AG \geq 3$ cutoff was also effective in ruling out nonaggressive chart summaries (Specificity = .88 and Negative Predictive Power = .84), but demonstrated only a limited ability to identify cases with aggression (Sensitivity = .28 and Positive Predictive Power = .36; Baity & Hilsenroth, 2002). The ability to identify aggressive cases was greatly improved when either the *AgC* ≥ 3 or $AgC \geq 4$ cutoffs were used (Sensitivity = .72 and .61, respectively). In summary, the *AG* cutoff was more effective in excluding "nonaggressive" histories, whereas the *AgC* cutoffs were more effective for identifying "aggressive" histories. Most important from the Baity and Hilsenroth (2002) research was that increases in *AgC* scores were more strongly related to reports of highly aggressive behavior than current Comprehensive System variables (CS; Exner, 1993).

Darcangelo (1997) found that higher *AgC* and *AG* scores were associated with higher ratings of both general and sexual aggression for incarcerated male rapists. In female nonpatients without a criminal history, Neubauer (2001) found that *AgC* was related to self-reported contained anger, but not to self-reported physical aggression. He concluded that in his sample *AgC* "could be a means of sublimating aggressive energy" or indicate "one's current level of anger." In comparison, Mihura et al. (2003) investigated *AgC* in a college student sample and found that *AgC* correlated with the Personality Assessment Inventory (PAI; Morey, 1991) Physical Aggression subscale, Borderline Features scale, and its Affective Instability and Identity Problems subscales. Methodological differences between the Neubauer and Mihura et al. studies could account for the contrast in finding a significant relationship between *AgC* and self-reported physical aggression.

Aggressive Past (AgPast)

AgPast is coded for any response in which an aggressive act has occurred or the object has been the target of aggression (Gacono, 1988). Consider an example: Card X: "It's a cat that had its head cut off" (Gacono, 1988, p. 20). *AgPast* responses may represent masochistic tendencies (Meloy & Gacono, 1992) or internal representations related to victimization (Gacono & Meloy, 1994). By definition, all *AgPast* responses would also be scored as *MOR*; however, *Morbid* responses without aggressive connotations are not scored as *AgPast* (e.g., "It's a sad person."). Indeed, Baity and Hilsenroth (1999) found a strong relationship between *MOR* and *AgPast* scores in Axis II outpatient Personality Disorders. Of note, *Morbid* responses have been associated with aggression turned against the self (Hilsenroth, Hibbard, Nash, & Handler, 1993; Westen, 1990).

Several studies have reported findings that are consistent with Gacono and Meloy's (1994) conceptualization of *AgPast* as indicating self-damage, masochism, or an early traumatic experience of having been aggressed against. Baity and Hilsenroth (1999) found that combined with *Morbid* responses and Holt's (1977) primary process variable, *AgPast* loaded (.90) onto a factor labeled, "Aggression at Objects." Stepwise regression analysis with the aggression variables and selected scales of the MMPI–2 indicated that *AgPast* was the only significant predictor of scores on the Anger scale. Consistent with previous theories (Gacono & Meloy, 1994), they noted, "This suggests that the identification of the self as damaged or spoiled might arise from a history of being in an unstable environment potentially resulting in victimization. More severe aggressive environments might be expected to foster greater feelings of resentment and inner turmoil that may manifest on certain indices of anger" (Baity & Hilsenroth, 1999, p. 106).

Kamphuis et al. (2000) included *AgPast* in their study of three nondissociative outpatient groups: those with a history of sexual abuse, those with suspected but unconfirmed sexual abuse, and those with no sexual abuse. Although there was no significant mean difference among these groups, the *AgPast* score was significantly correlated with the intensity of violent or sadistic sexual abuse in the group with confirmed sexual abuse. Based on these findings, Kamphuis and colleagues suggested that "Those sexually abused clients with significant numbers of *AgPast* scores in their Rorschachs will have the greatest difficulties overcoming the negative effects of their abuse" (p. 220).

Two studies discovered relative elevations of *AgPast* in the Rorschach records of a male offender group where an early history of victimization would be expected (Huprich et al., 2004; White, 1999). Pedophiles were two times more likely to have at least one *AgPast* than those without the diagnosis (White, 1999). Huprich et al. (2004) found even higher elevations of *AgPast* in the records of sexual homicide perpetrators compared to nonviolent pedophiles.

Similar to Baity and Hilsenroth's (1999) findings, Neubauer (2001) found that *AgPast* was related to several self-report anger scales: contained anger, state anger, trait anger, and hostility in female college students. He concluded that the presence of *AgPast* suggested feelings of frustration, resentment, being mistreated, and/or suspiciousness. The Mihura et al. (2003) findings shed further light on *AgPast* in a college sample as they found that *AgPast* was most strongly associated with interpersonal submissiveness, the PAI Borderline Self-Harm and Negative Relationships subscales and, to a lesser degree, with the Physical Aggression subscale. In certain nonpatient samples, *AgPast* scores may signal a defensive strategy where internalization of one's anger and hostility results in passivity, and even impulsively self-destructive behavior.

Aggressive Potential (AgPot)

AgPot has been defined as any response in which an aggressive act is getting ready to occur. Usually the act is imminent (Gacono, 1988). Consider an example: Card X: "These two are going to give them a surprise. They are waiting to lop their heads off. They won't even know what hit them" (Gacono, 1988, pp. 20–21). *AgPot* was thought to relate to sadism (Meloy & Gacono, 1992) or an identification with predatory objects or a preoccupation with predation (Gacono & Meloy, 1994).

Early research suggested that *AgPot* may occur more frequently in Cluster B Personality Disorders (Gacono et al., 1992) than nonpatients (Margolis, 1992). Consistent with this observation, White (1999) found that female offenders with BPD were approximately 3½ times more likely to have at least one *AgPot* response than those not diagnosed with BPD. Other research has found *AgPot* related to problems modulating one's aggressive urges. For example, Huprich et al. (2004) found that *AgPot* scores were significantly higher for sexual homicide perpetrators than for both nonsexually offending psychopaths and nonviolent pedophiles. In a college sample, Mihura et al. (2003) found that *AgPot* was related to the PAI Aggression scale and its Physical Aggression subscale, the Borderline Self-Harm scale, and their PAI measure of suicidal ideation with impulsivity.

AgC, AgPast, and AgPot Combinations

Two studies by Mihura and colleagues combined *AgC* (aggressive identity) with *AgPot* (aggressive urges) using *Z scores* to see if this variable was more highly related to their external criteria than either variable in isolation. Indeed, protocols that contained elevations of both *AgPot* and *AgC*, versus either of these scores alone, were more highly associated with a PAI measure of outwardly expressed aggression (Mihura et al., 2003). Whereas elevated rates of *AgC* were associated with viewing a significant other as less controllable when the relationship felt threatened, elevated rates of both *AgC* and *AgPot* were associated with not only viewing the significant other as less controllable, but also as more controlling. Mihura et al. (2003) also combined *AgPot* (aggressive urges) and *AgPast* (victimization) using *Z scores*, and found that this combination was more highly associated with a PAI measure of inwardly expressed aggression than either of these scores in isolation.

Finally, Levy (1998) investigated gender differences for *AgC*, *AgPot*, and *AgPast* in children with severe and chronic physical abuse, hypothesizing that physically abused boys would show higher rates of externalized aggression on the Rorschach than physically abused girls. Consistent with expectations, the physically abused boys had higher levels of both *AgC* and *AgPot* than did physically abused girls, with no significant differences for *AgPast*.

Aggressive Vulnerability (AgV)

AgV is coded when the subject identifies a percept as vulnerable to attack, exploitation, or indicates that the object has taken steps to protect itself from predation. Take the following example: "It's a butterfly and here is where it needs to cover up so the predators can't attack it" (Gacono & Meloy, 1994, p. 277). Like *AgPast*, it suggests a passive relationship to aggressive impulses. Unlike *AgPast*, rather than suggesting a masochistic identification, it suggests a sensitivity or preoccupation with vulnerability or being exploited, injured, or victimized. There has been no published research on this variable since its introduction in Gacono and Meloy (1994).

Sadomasochism (SM)

SM is scored when a response contains devalued, aggressive, or morbid content accompanied by pleasurable affect expressed by the subject (Gacono, 1988; Meloy, 1988). Consider the following example: Card VII: "A lady dancing and she got her head blown off (laughs)." The pleasurable affect is usually expressed through smiling or laughing, but the examiner should be careful to not interpret anxious behavior as pleasurable affect. Because *SM* requires observation during test administration, it can generally be accurately scored from archival protocols only when the examiner recorded the patient's affective expressions; consequently, it has been the second least researched of the aggression scores.

Studies that investigated *SM*, however, produced findings consistent with the interpretation of *SM* as reflecting a sadistic orientation. Gacono (1988, 1990) first reported frequencies for *SM* in groups of psychopathic and nonpsychopathic ASPD offenders. In an expanded sample (*N* = 43), Meloy and Gacono (1992) found that *SM* differentiated between Hare Psychopathy Checklist–Revised (PCL–R; Hare, 1991) identified psychopathic ASPD (PCL–R $\geq$ 30) and nonpsychopathic ASPD offenders (P–ASPDs = 41%; NP–ASPDs = 14%). Huprich et al. (2004) found that sexual homicide perpetrators produced higher frequencies of *SM* than nonviolent pedophiles (none of the pedophiles met the criteria for ASPD or psychopathy; respective frequencies; 24% and 3%). In Darcangelo's (1997) adult rapist sample, *SM* was also significantly related to elevated PCL–R scores and ratings of sexual sadism. Neubauer (2001) found no occurrences (0%) of *SM* in a female adult nonforensic sample.

DISCUSSION

Gacono and Meloy (1994) wrote, "The various indices of aggressive responses to the Rorschach appear to be a rich source for understanding the structure and dynamics of an individual's intrapsychic aggression ..." (p. 278). Since that time, additional research has supported and refined, rather than refuted, the original interpretations for these variables. None of the extant research has discredited Gacono and Meloy's hypothesis that the paucity of the *AG* response in CD and ASPD populations may relate to the ego-syntonic nature of aggression in CD, ASPD, or psychopathic individuals.[4] This hypothesis does not exclude the possibility that any given patient may be consciously censoring *AG*. The impact of response style (Bannatyne, Gacono, & Greene, 1999) and the assessment context (forensic, research) must always be considered when evaluating an individual protocol (Gacono, Evans, & Viglione, 2002) for the presence or absence of aggressive imagery. However, the fact that a particular Rorschach response can be censored does not mean that it was censored. For the original Gacono (1988, 1990) ASPD samples and later Gacono and Meloy (1992, 1994) samples, consistent findings across age groups and discrepancies between interview and Rorschach administration suggest an ego-dystonic relationship to aggressive impulses that stimulates *AG* production.

The notion that *AgC* represents a preoccupation or an identification with aggressive objects has also been supported (Baity & Hilsenroth, 1999, 2002; Darcangelo, 1997; Mihura et al., 2003; White, 1999). *AgC* is produced frequently enough that when combined with *AG*, it has the potential to add incrementally to understanding both violent patients and nonpatients with no documented histories of violence. For example, with sexual homicide perpetrators (Gacono, Meloy, & Bridges, 2000; Meloy, Gacono, & Kenney, 1994) or rapists (Darcangelo, 1997) elevated *AG* (intensity of the ego-dystonic impulse) and increased *AgC* (aggressive identifications) in conjunction with other Rorschach identified sexual preoccupations, cognitive deficits, and personality vulnerabilities provide a window into the object relations, defenses, and impulses that drive the perpetrator's real-world sexual violence (Gacono, Meloy, & Bridges, 2000). In these sexually violent subjects, Rorschach identified impulses (*AG*) and identifications (*AgC*) await only a situational spark to ignite them. Whereas combined aggression coding more accurately captures the underlying psychodynamics of patients with histories of real-world aggression, like many other Rorschach variables, interpretations should be made while also considering the degree to which poor reality testing, cognitive slippage, and other drive derivatives infuse the record.

Correlations with severe aggression in sexual trauma (Kamphuis et al., 2000), self-reported self-destructive behaviors (Mihura et al., 2003), interpersonal submissiveness (Mihura & Nathan-Montano, 2001), and anger (Baity & Hilsenroth, 1999; Neubauer, 2001) support links between *AgPast* and a history of having been aggressed against, a masochistic identification, a passive orientation toward aggressive impulses, and/or ambivalence concerning expressing aggression (aggression turned inward). *AgPast* appears to reflect internalized object relations related to victimization with accompanying resentment and anger (aggression directed toward self). However, whereas *AgPast* may signal a propensity for self-harm in some patients, for patients who are characterologically predisposed to commit violence toward others (ASPD, psychopaths) it may also be a marker for their feelings of entitlement to retaliate.

---

[4]Whereas the *Extended Aggression* scores first appeared in Gacono (1988), this hypothesis first appeared in Meloy and Gacono (1992).

Research findings with *AgPot* are more limited, although the extant literature is consistent with the interpretation of *AgPot* as representing aggressive impulses. This is supported by *AgPot*'s more frequent occurrence in protocols of sexual homicide perpetrators (compared to nonviolent pedophiles; Huprich et al., 2004), offenders with a BPD diagnosis (White, 1999), and in college students with higher PAI scores on inwardly and outwardly directed aggressive impulses (Mihura et al., 2003). Because many studies report rather low base rates of *AgPot*, interpretations of *AgPot* may be more useful when considered in conjunction with other aggression variables. For example, Mihura and her colleagues suggest that when a protocol contains both *AgPot* and *AgC* (vs. either variable alone), aggressive urges are more likely (Mihura et al., 2003; Mihura & Nathan-Montano, 2001). Like its name, *Aggressive Potential* may represent a "potential" for acting on aggressive impulses; other variables in the protocol, such as *AgC* (toward others) or *AgPast* (toward self), may suggest the direction of the action. Given the low base rates for both *SM* (sadism) and *AgPot* (aggressive urges/potential), combining the two scores might be explored; however, the degree of conceptual overlap between these variables remains to be seen.

Although Gacono and Meloy (1994) have suggested that *AgPot* may represent sadism, *SM* is the Rorschach aggression score most obviously linked to sadism. Unfortunately, *SM* is one of the least studied of the aggression scores. This is likely due to the fact that it may be difficult to score using archival CS Rorschach data, because the pleasurable affect must be observed and recorded. Additionally, when it does occur, it does so infrequently. We don't want to, however, discount the extant research. The three studies that did include *SM* in investigating offender populations found that *SM* was related to psychopathy (Meloy & Gacono, 1992), higher PCL–R scores (Darcangelo, 1997), and/or sadism (Darcangelo, 1997; Huprich et al., 2004). Darcangelo (1997) found that *SM* was significantly related to ratings of sexual sadism expressed during rape as well as in other behaviors. These studies suggest that SM might be used as a type of behavioral coding that indicates a greater likelihood of sadistic behaviors in everyday life.

The senior author has also examined Rorschach responses for *SM* that can be coded in a manner that does not require examiner observation. Scoring verbalized projected sadism may be useful for identifying this worrisome trait. That is, when projecting sadism, rather than displaying pleasurable affect, the examinee attributes sadistic attitudes to the Rorschach percept or personalizes (often coded with a *PER*) the sadistic activity of the percept. An example of "sadistic attribution" includes a subject perceiving a human face and stating, "He's smiling like he's going to hit you." The percept, rather than the examinee, contains the pleasurable affect. An example of "personalized sadism" includes (Card III), "It's a fly. It's far out. I've been going to mental health counseling since 13 or 16. (Inquiry?) A fly, got big eyes. When I was little, I used to pull flies' eyes off" (Gacono & Meloy, 1994, p. 277). Researchers must consider that whereas empirical links between real-world behavior and the original *SM* coding have been demonstrated, there has been no research with this expanded coding. Also, this expanded coding may capture different aspects of a patient's relationship to sadism than the ego-syntonic relationship linked to the original coding. Quite likely, the manner in which the patient expresses their sadistic impulses (directly, projected, with anxiety, and so forth) on the Rorschach tells us something about their relationship to the impulse. The question that remains is not the importance of assessing the sadistic impulse, but the best empirical Rorschach measure with which to do it.

Trends in the research have also highlighted the need for interpreting these aggression scores within the context of the patient's personality organization and the presence or absence of real-world aggression in their history. Although still representing an identification, the presence of AgC aids in understanding the disruptive impact of aggressive impulses on certain college samples with little real-world histories of aggression (Mihura & Nathan-Montana, 2001; Neubauer, 2001). These findings support an ego-dystonic relationship to aggressive impulse (AG) and identifications (elevated AgC scores). Whereas AgC in these nonpatient samples coincides with feelings of less control and the need to modulate the impulse through projection, in forensic populations correlations with the number of ASPD criteria, scores on the Antisocial Practices Scale (MMPI–2), and institutional chart ratings of aggressive behavior, support an ego-syntonic relationship to the aggressive identification and aggressive preoccupations (Gacono & Meloy, 1994). The use of sequence analysis to study the presence of other variables in the record, such as *Diffuse Shading* (*FY, YF, Y*) and *Inanimate Movement* (*m*), may help further delineate the forensic patients' relationship to their aggressive impulses (Meloy & Gacono, 1992).

The unpublished dissertation studies help us to understand methodological problems when studying the Rorschach and aggression. Most frequently, studies have failed to incorporate a conceptually accurate basis for predicting group differences. A glaring example includes the use of chart reported offense histories, alone, as the independent measure for determining aggressive versus nonaggressive groups. This procedure is problematic for several reasons. First, it is not uncommon for violent offenders to have an absence of formal charges or convictions (arrestable offenses) in their records. Secondly, the impact of plea bargaining can result in convictions that are quite different from the actual charges. Finally, any particular offense category may capture a diverse array of motivations and behaviors. With the exception of an extreme behavior such as sexual homicide, with its very low base rate of occurrence, researchers must carefully consider the limitations of using "rap sheets" or patient records to quantify levels of aggression. Although these studies may provide useful descriptive data (relative frequency of the *Extended Aggression* scores within the given population), they do little to aid in understanding the utility of the scores in differentiating among levels of aggression. A related conceptual error in the offender Rorschach research is predicting that a Rorschach variable(s) will differentiate among two heterogeneous, but similar groups (e.g., hypothesizing differences between a group of ASPD offenders and a group of control offenders; the appropriate comparison is comparing PCL–R identified psychopaths with low PCL–R scorers; see Gacono, Loving, & Bodholdt, 2001). When interpreting a lack of "significant between group differences," one must first consider if there was a carefully considered and valid theoretical rationale for predicting differences and evaluate whether the proposed or established clinical meaning of the variables was accurately reflected in the study's hypothesis (Gacono & Meloy, 1994; also see Gacono et al., 2001). An evaluation of this latter point requires a sophisticated understanding of violent offenders and, also, how the Rorschach actually works.

High *Lambda* forensic samples represent another concern when evaluating frequencies or proportions of any Rorschach content-based item (see Cohan, 1998; White, 1999). Any comparison of content-based items means and frequencies with more normally distributed *Lambda* samples must be done with caution. Constricted protocols (high *Lambda*) are consistent with certain forensic patients' inadequacy and limited psychological resources (Bannatyne et al., 1999); however, the corresponding reduction in content-based items means and frequencies limit direct comparisons to nonconstricted samples. Whereas findings from constricted populations may represent a true estimate of the relative proportion of the given variable within the population studied, comparing between study means or frequencies is not possible. In this regard, the vast majority of well-designed studies in this area have produced findings consistent with the clinical meanings of the *Extended Aggression* scores, but issues related to Rorschach administration, scoring, and sample characteristics (*Lambda, R*) limit between study comparisons of descriptive data. Although an important consideration whenever Rorschach content-based items are studied, controlling for R may be especially important for AgC, because it occurs frequently enough that comparing AgC score proportions, means, or subjects who produce greater than or equal to 3 may be more useful than comparing frequencies of individuals who produce at least one. Regardless, *Lambda* and R must be considered when comparing mean scores or frequencies for the *Extended Aggression* scores across studies.[5] Considering descriptive data within the context of *Lambda* and R is especially crucial when comparing AgC mean scores between criminal and noncriminal samples.

Research done by summing the raw *Extended Aggression* scores assumes that each score has the same meaning or assesses the same criteria and/or that each type of variable contributes equally to measuring the criteria (e.g., one AgC is equal to one $AgPot$). Aggregated variables can be created by calculating Z scores per variable and summing the Z scores (see Mihura et al., 2003; Mihura & Nathan-Montano, 2001), but the aggregation of variables should always be based on a theoretical rationale, rather than just convenience to increase variable frequencies. Two final problems were apparent in several of the dissertations. First, inappropriate statistical procedures were used for comparing categorical data. Second, researchers failed to report interrater agreements for the *Extended Aggression* scores, level of aggression measure, diagnosis, and so forth.

---

[5]Compared to the mean R for nonpatient adults ($M = 22.32$; $SD = 4.40$; CS, Exner, 2001), the mean R for most criminal samples is lower ($M \approx 17$–19), whereas the mean R is *higher* for sex offender groups ($M \approx 26$–29). Additionally, most studies finding AgC significantly related to ratings of aggressive behavior and self-reported aggressive urges have controlled AgC for R. However, *Lambda* and R may be only two of several factors that account for differences in mean scores. Administration errors, qualities within the population studied (relationship to aggressive impulse), and so forth may also contribute to differences.

CONCLUSIONS

Research findings have been consistent with Gacono and Meloy's (1994) interpretations for the *Extended Aggression* scores. Whereas the integration of other assessment data, including Rorschach scores, provides the best picture of personality, these single Rorschach *Extended Aggression* scores each appear to capture unique aspects of aggressive drive derivatives: *AG* representing aggressive drive intensity (ego-dystonic or ego-syntonic dependent on the population studied), *AgC* symbolizing an aggressive identification (forensic samples) or preoccupation (forensic and college samples), *AgPot* indicating aggressive urges or a potential to translate aggression into action, *AgPast* suggesting a victimized object representation, and *SM* indicating sadism and a link to psychopathy (Holt, Meloy, & Strack, 1999).[6]

In addition to capturing unique aspects of the aggressive impulse, these variables expand the examiner's ability to code a variety of aggressive imagery not included in the Comprehensive System. The importance of increased scoring potential needs to be underscored. This was the senior author's sole intent when he observed the paucity of *AG* movement coupled with the presence of these scores; that was to be able to code the diverse Rorschach aggressive imagery produced in the forensic samples (see Table 26–1; Gacono, 1988, 1997). The forensic examiner always integrates data from multiple sources in formulating hypotheses and offering opinions (see the preface to this text). In this regard, the *Extended Aggression* scores are very useful idiographically; however, the sophisticated researcher always couches interpretation within a thorough understanding of the difference between aggressive preoccupations and identifications and violent action. Quite likely, no combination of Rorschach variables in isolation, and certainly not a single variable, will ever be successful in predicting violent behavior. Violence does not occur in a vacuum, but is best understood within a psycho-biological-situational context (Espinosa, 2001). To expect otherwise is naive and asks too much of the Rorschach. Like any Rorschach variable, the usefulness of the *Extended Aggression* scores occurs when they are viewed in conjunction with a patient's psychology, history, and situation.

Recent research with nonforensic populations also supports the need to examine *Extended Aggression* responses, particularly *AgC*, *AgPast*, and *AgPot*. The extant research suggests that there are individual differences for the production of Rorschach aggressive imagery, and that it can be qualitatively and quantitatively different depending on the person's legal and psychological history. As exemplified in Exner's *Rorschach Primer* (2000) and Rorschach computer software (e.g., Caracena, 2002), Rorschach technology is becoming more sophisticated. The days of generic interpretations of variables applied to everyone are over, and advanced algorithms individualizing interpretations of Rorschach findings are becoming the standard of practice. Although *AgV*, *AgPot*, and *SM* hold promise and should not be forgotten (due to their low frequencies of occurrence),

---

[6]Using the *Extended Aggression* scores, Huprich et al. (2004) found significant correlations in the proportionally predicted directions (which would not have occurred with *AG* alone) between aggression and oral dependency among nonsexually offending psychopaths, nonviolent pedophiles, and sexual homicide offenders.

this current research supports including the more frequently appearing *AgC* and *AgPast* in the Comprehensive System.

ACKNOWLEDGMENTS

The authors wish to thank Chris Piotrowski and Amy Mashberg for conducting literature searches and Joni Mihura and Donald Viglione for their comments and suggestions. The views expressed in this chapter are solely the authors' and may not reflect the views of any of the authors' past, present, or future affiliations. this chapter is a revised version of Gacono, Gacono, Meloy, & Baity, The Rorschach Extended Aggression Scores, from *Rorschachiana: Yearbook of the International Rorschach Society* (2005). It is reprinted with permission.

REFERENCES

American Psychiatric Association. (1980). *Diagnostic and statistical manual of mental disorders* (3rd ed.). Washington, DC: Author.

Baity, M. R., & Hilsenroth, M. J. (1999). Rorschach aggression variables: A study of reliability and validity. *Journal of Personality Assessment, 72,* 93–110.

Baity, M. R., & Hilsenroth, M. J. (2002). Rorschach Aggressive Content (*AgC*) variable: A study of criterion validity. *Journal of Personality Assessment, 78,* 275–287.

Baity, M. R., McDaniel, P. S., & Hilsenroth, M. J. (2000). Further exploration of the Rorschach Aggressive Content (*AgC*) variable. *Journal of Personality Assessment, 74,* 231–241.

Bannatyne, L. A., Gacono, C. B., & Greene, R. (1999). Differential patterns of responding among three groups of chronic psychotic forensic outpatients. *Journal of Clinical Psychology, 55,* 1553–1565.

Caracena, P. F. (2002). *ROR-SCAN version 6 Rorschach interpretive system.* Laredo, TX: ROR-SCAN.

Cohan, R. D. (1998). A comparison of sex offenders against minors and rapists of adults on selected Rorschach variables. *Dissertation Abstracts International, 59*(5), 2471B. (UMI No. 9834544)

Cohen, J. (1992). A power primer. *Psychological Bulletin, 112,* 155–159.

Darcangelo, S. M. (1997). Psychological and personality correlates of the Massachusetts Treatment Centre classification system for rapists (Doctoral dissertation, Simon Fraser University, Canada, 1997). *Dissertation Abstracts International, 58*(4), 2115B.

Ephriam, D., Occupati, R., Riquelme, J., & Gonzales, E. (1993). Gender, age and socioeconomic differences in Rorschach thematic content scales. *Rorschachiana, 18,* 68–81.

Espinosa, S. (2001). *The difference between aggressive and non-aggressive hospitalized adolescents in their projected aggression and developmental levels of object relations functioning* (Doctoral dissertation, Seton Hall U, College Education and Human Services). *Dissertation Abstracts International, 61*(12-B), 6703.

Exner, J. E. (1993). *The Rorschach: A Comprehensive System: Vol 1. Basic foundations* (2nd ed.). New York: Wiley.

Exner, J. E. (1995a). *Issues and methods in Rorschach research.* Hillsdale, NJ: Lawrence Erlbaum Publishers.

Exner, J. E. (1995b). *A Rorschach workbook for the Comprehensive System* (4th ed.). Asheville, NC: Rorschach Workshops.

Exner, J. E. (2000). *A primer for Rorschach interpretation.* Asheville, NC: Rorschach Workshops.

Exner, J. E. (2001). *A Rorschach workbook for the Comprehensive System* (5th ed.). Asheville, NC: Rorschach Workshops.

Fleiss, J. (1981). *Statistical methods for rates and proportions.* New York: Wiley.

Freud, A. (1936). *The ego and the mechanisms of defense.* New York: International Universities Press.

Gacono, C. B. (1988). *A Rorschach analysis of object relations and defensive structure and their relationship to narcissism and psychopathy in a group of antisocial offenders.* Unpublished doctoral dissertation, U. S. International University, San Diego.

Gacono, C. B. (1990). An empirical study of object relations and defensive operations in antisocial personality. *Journal of Personality Assessment, 54,* 589–600.

Gacono, C. B. (1997). Is the Rorschach Aggression Movement response enough? *British Journal of Projective Psychology, 42,* 5–10.

Gacono, C. B., Evans, B., & Viglione, D. (2002). The Rorschach in forensic practice. *Journal of Forensic Psychology Practice, 2*(3), 33–53.

Gacono, C. B., Gacono, L. A., Meloy, J. R., & Baity, M. (2005). The Rorschach Extended Aggression scores. *Rorschachiana, 27,* 164–190.

Gacono, C., Loving, J., & Bodholdt, R. (2001). The Rorschach and psychopathy: Toward a more accurate understanding of the research findings. *Journal of Personality Assessment, 77,* 16–38.

Gacono, C. B., & Meloy, J. R. (1994). *The Rorschach assessment of aggressive and psychopathic personality.* Hillsdale, NJ: Lawrence Erlbaum Associates.

Gacono, C. B., Meloy, J. R., & Berg, J. L. (1992). Object relations, defensive operations, and affective states in narcissistic, borderline, and antisocial personality. *Journal of Personality Assessment, 59,* 32–49.

Gacono, C. B., Meloy, J. R., & Bridges, M. R. (2000). A Rorschach comparison of psychopaths, sexual homicide perpetrators, and non-violent pedophiles: Where angels fear to tread. *Journal of Clinical Psychology, 56,* 757–777.

Hare, R. (1991). *Manual for the Revised Psychopathy Checklist.* Toronto: Mulit-Health Systems.

Heaven, T. R. (1988). *Relationship between Hare's Psychopathy Checklist and selected Exner Rorschach variables in an inmate population.* Unpublished doctoral dissertation, United States International University, San Diego.

Hilsenroth, M. J., Hibbard, S. R., Nash, M. R., & Handler, L. (1993). A Rorschach study of narcissism, defense, and aggression in borderline, narcissistic, and Cluster C personality disorders. *Journal of Personality Assessment, 60,* 346–361.

Holt, R. R. (1977). A method for assessing primary process manifestations and their controls in Rorschach responses. In M. A. Rickers-Ovsiankina (Ed.), *Rorschach psychology* (2nd ed., pp. 375–420). Huntington, NY: Krieger.

Holt, R. R., & Havel, J. (1960). A method for assessing primary and secondary process in the Rorschach. In M. A. Rickers-Ovsiankina (Ed.), *Rorschach psychology* (pp. 263–315). New York: Wiley.

Holt, S., Meloy, J. R., & Strack, S. (1999). Sadism and psychopathy in violent and sexually violent offenders. *Journal of the American Academy of Psychiatry Law, 27,* 23–32.

Huprich, S. K., Gacono, C. B., Schneider, R.B ., & Bridges, M. R. (2004). Rorschach oral dependency in psychopaths, sexual homicide perpetrators, and nonviolent pedophiles. *Behavioral Sciences & the Law, 22,* 345–356.

Kamphuis, J. H., Kugeares, S. L., & Finn, S. E. (2000). Rorschach correlates of sexual abuse: Trauma content and aggression indexes. *Journal of Personality Assessment, 75,* 212–224.

Levy, A. E. (1998). Gender differences among physically abused children on Rorschach indices of adaptive patterns. (Doctoral dissertation, California School of Professional Psychology at Alameda, 1997). *Dissertation Abstracts International, 58*(9), 5127B.

Margolis, J. D. (1992). Aggressive and borderline-level content on the Rorschach: An exploratory study of some proposed scoring criteria. (Doctoral dissertation, California School of Professional Psychology at Alameda, 1992). *Dissertation Abstracts International, 54,* 2805.

Meloy, J. R. (1988). *The psychopathic mind: Origins, dynamics, and treatment.* Northvale, NJ: Aronson.

Meloy, J. R. (2000). The nature and dynamics of sexual homicide: An integrative review. *Aggression and Violent Behavior, 5,* 1–22.

Meloy, J. R., & Gacono, C.B. (1992). The aggression response and the Rorschach. *Journal of Clinical Psychology, 48,*104–114.

Meloy, J. R., Gacono, C., & Kenney, L. (1994). A Rorschach investigation of sexual homicide. *Journal of Personality Assessment, 62,* 58–67.

Mihura, J. L., & Nathan-Montano, E. (2001). An interpersonal analysis of Rorschach aggression variables in a normal sample. *Psychological Reports, 89,* 617–623.

Mihura, J. L., Nathan-Montano, E., & Alperin, R. J. (2003). Rorschach measures of aggressive drive derivatives: A college student sample. *Journal of Personality Assessment, 80*(1), 41–49.

Morey, L. C. (1991). *Personality Assessment Inventory: Professional manual.* Odessa, FL: Psychological Assessment Resources, Inc.

Neubauer, L. M. (2001). The relationship between behavior ratings of aggression and an aggression coding system of the Rorschach in a non-patient female sample (Doctoral dissertation, California School of Professional Psychology at Fresno, 2001). *Dissertation Abstracts International, 61*(11), 6143B.

Rapaport, D., Gill, M. M., & Schafer, R. (1946). *Diagnostic psychological testing* (Vol. 1). Chicago: Year Book Publishers.

Rapaport, D., Gill, M. M., & Schafer, R. (1968). *Diagnostic psychological testing.* New York: International Universities Press.

Riquelme, J., Occupati, R., & Gonzales, E. (1991). *Rorschach: Estudio de contenidos. Datos normativos para de sujetos no pacientes di Caracas y su area metropolitana. Aportes al sistema comprensivo de Exner* [Rorschach: Study of the content. Normative data for nonpatient subjects from the greater Caracas area. According to Exner's Comprehensive System]. Unpublished raw data.

Rorschach Workshops. (2000). *2000 alumni newsletter.* Asheville, NC: Author.

Schafer, R. (1954). *Psychoanalytic interpretation in Rorschach testing.* New York: Grune & Stratton.

Shaffer, T. W., Erdberg, P., & Haroian, J. (1999). Current nonpatient data for the Rorschach, WAIS–R, and MMPI–2. *Journal of Personality Assessment, 73,* 305–316.

Westen, D. (1990). Towards a revised theory of borderline object relations: Contributions of empirical research. *International Journal of Psycho-Analysis, 71,* 661–693.

White, D. O. (1999). A concurrent validity study of the Rorschach extended aggression scoring categories. *Dissertation Abstracts International, 59*(9), 5152B. (UMI No. 9907543).

27

MULTIMETHOD ASSESSMENT AS A FORENSIC STANDARD

Philip Erdberg
Private Practice, Corte Madera, CA

> The evidence indicates that clinicians who use a single method to obtain patient information regularly draw faulty conclusions. (Meyer et al., 2001, p. 150)

The year was 1956. Personality assessment as we know it —barely 30 years old—was flourishing. The Rorschach arrived first. Its use in Europe during the 1920s and its introduction to the United States in the mid–1930s assured its historical primacy. But, by 1956, some upstarts were nipping at its heels.

Out in Minnesota in 1943, psychologist Starke Hathaway and psychiatrist J. Charnley McKinley took some items from the old Cornell Medical Inventory, some from psychiatric textbooks, some from their own clinical experience, and brought midwestern empiricism to personality assessment with the Minnesota Multiphasic Personality Inventory.

Even earlier, in 1935, Henry Murray and his colleague C. D. Morgan at the Harvard Psychological Clinic published an article, entitled "A Method for Investigating Phantasies: The Thematic Apperception Text," in the *Archives of Neurology and Psychiatry*, which launched the TAT.

So, by the mid–1950s, personality assessment was flourishing. There was, however, a small problem. None of the giants—Bruno Klopfer, Starke Hathaway, Henry Murray, to name a few—were talking to each other. But they were certainly talking about each other.

And that's how it came to be that Volume II of Klopfer's Rorschach series (1956), included a chapter by Edwin S. Shneidman that contained an extraordinary diagram (1956, p. 614). Paper-and-pencil self-report tests were represented as an airplane cruising over the landscape, able only, as Shneidman (1956, p. 613) delicately put it, to identify "conscious attitudes" and "those defensive psychic efforts amenable to conscious control." Shneidman represented picture-thematic tests as a kind of glass-bottom boat that could spot a few blurry shapes near the surface: maybe a preconscious motive, perhaps just some seaweed floating by. And then there was the Rorschach. Here was the intrapsychic submarine, able, as Shneidman wrote enthusiastically, "to go 'deeper' and get at the primary ways in which an individual perceptually organizes his world—ways of which the individual is mostly unaware or unconscious" (p. 613).

The diagram is perhaps the earliest example of the sort of monomethod bias that has characterized personality assessment—to its detriment—since its very beginning.

And even though Rapaport, Gill, and Schafer (1946) at the Menninger Foundation in Topeka stressed the necessity of a battery of tests, even though the developers of the different instruments supported the idea of synthesizing test findings, psychology training programs tended to identify themselves with one or another personality assessment instrument and did not emphasize an integrative approach.

It turns out that Rapaport and his colleagues were right, and this chapter reviews the accumulated evidence supporting the efficacy of multimethod assessment and suggesting that it should be a standard in forensic practice. But, it is important to note that the idea of integrating test findings continues to be a difficult one for psychologists to embrace. Archer and Krishnamurthy (1993) noted: "There will be many situations in which the results of the Rorschach and the MMPI are either somewhat inconsistent or clearly contradictory. In these situations, the test interpreter must make the clinical decision to emphasize certain aspects of test findings, while suppressing the results from other sources of test data. ... In determining which results to emphasize, we must consider the relative reliability and validity of the specific data sources" (p. 138).

It is the purpose of this chapter to suggest that suppressing contradictory findings from two or more reliable and valid tests is exactly the wrong thing to do.

Back in 1946, Meehl and Hathaway wrote that the best data set from which to predict a criterion involves multiple variables that are not highly correlated with each other. This is the idea of *incremental validity*: The accuracy and validity of judgments improves when additional sources of information are added, as compared to decisions based on only one source of information. Meyer and his colleagues (2001) looked at the question of whether different assessment methods provide incremental as opposed to redundant or inaccurate information, and concluded that "distinct assessment methods provide unique information ... at best, any single assessment method provides a partial or incomplete representation of the characteristics it intends to measure" (p. 145).

It is helpful to consider some examples from a variety of areas. Meyer (1996) gives an illustrative example from astrophysics. Astrophysicists use optical, infrared, and ultraviolet telescopes to identify gasses in distant parts of the universe. If only optical techniques were used, it would be impossible to tell hydrogen and helium apart, because they both look pale blue in the visible light spectrum. However, by bringing in infrared and ultraviolet telescopes, it becomes possible to identify hydrogen, because it has a characteristic pattern in the infrared part of the spectrum and no radiations at all in the ultraviolet spectrum. The infrared and ultraviolet pattern for helium is exactly the opposite of that for hydrogen. As Meyer (1996) explains, "Despite the fact that infrared and ultraviolet methods 'disagree,' astronomers do not consider one method to be less valid than the other. Rather, they recognize their strengths and limitations ... they also know each method is differentially sensitive to particular wavelengths of radiation ... they are able to use the 'disagreements' between optical, infrared, and ultraviolet readings to gain a more thorough understanding of the cosmological universe" (p. 560).

It is the same in psychological assessment. It is important to understand the differential usefulness of different tests, moving away from the idea that one technique is more valid than another. Each has its strengths and its limitations, and using multiple methods allows a more comprehensive description of the individual. It may be helpful to list some of the different "telescopes" forensic psychologists have available and briefly summarize the strengths and limitations of each:

1. Interviews do a good job of describing the important themes around which individuals have organized their life. Open-ended questions like, "In the best of possible worlds, how would you like to spend your time?" allow them to articulate what is most significant in their psychological organization. But interviews have their limitations. The skill of the interviewer is a significant variable; and it is often difficult to assess the extent to which impression management, the wish to present oneself in a particular way, influences what the person says.

2. Self-report measures like the MMPI–2 give individuals an opportunity to describe themselves and the problems they are experiencing. These instruments can cover a wide variety of topics in a systematic way. They are limited by the person's insightfulness and psychological mindedness, ability to make accurate judgments, ability to describe oneself accurately relative to other people, and motivation to communicate in an honest and straightforward manner.

But objectively accurate self-ratings are not what self-report measures can most importantly provide. We know that people do not rate themselves very accurately, if we compare their ratings with those of outside observers or external criteria. A meta-analysis done by Mabe and West (1982) surveyed 55 studies involving correlations between a person's self-ratings of ability and some external measure of that ability. These studies involved nonpatients and the average correlation for all the studies between self-ratings and some external criterion measure was .29. In areas in which there is very substantial feedback, like athletic skills, the correlations averaged .47. For more subjective, interpersonal areas, the correlations dropped dramatically. In 41 studies relating self-estimate of managerial ability with some external criterion variable such as ratings by coworkers, the average correlation was .04.

Meyer (1996) phrased it diplomatically when he concluded that "self-ratings cannot be viewed as veridical reflections of a consensual reality" (p. 569). But "consensual reality" is not the goal of self-report measures. What they provide is data about the individuals' self-understanding and the problems that they are experiencing. And that kind of data is one important building block in comprehensive psychological assessment.

3. Performance-based personality tests like the Rorschach and the Thematic Apperception Test allow us to observe how individuals handle moderately ambiguous perceptual-cognitive tasks, giving us information about their psychodynamics and stylistic approaches. The stimulus materials and the person's engagement with the task are among the variables that can limit the yield these instruments can provide.

4. Interviews with others who know the person well, observer rating scales, and review of school, job, and criminal history records bring in another important source of

information, the consensual realities that someone else's view of the person can provide. There is no doubt that the observer's relationship with the individual influences the observations and that different observers will likely generate contradictory findings. Again, far from being problematical, the integration of these contradictory findings can result in a more nuanced description of the individual. It is natural that different observers, in different settings, with different kinds of relationships with the person being evaluated, would have different perspectives. For example, teachers, parents, and clinicians come up with very different behavior ratings for children and adolescents on measures like the Achenbach Child Behavior Checklist (Achenbach, McConaughy, & Howell, 1987). The fact that teachers, parents, and clinicians do not agree with each other does not imply invalidity. Instead, it can lead to more fine-grained descriptions of the individual.

As Meyer (1997) noted, comprehensive assessment requires the psychologist to "recognize what type of information each method can reveal ... . When using different methods, the assessment clinician must work to create a sophisticated portrait of the patient that makes use of all the data—even when the methods are superficially discrepant, as it is just such disagreements that often provide a richer understanding of defensive structures and struggles to adapt" (p. 327).

Monomethod bias—suppressing contradictory information or differentially weighting data from one kind of test versus another—threatens the validity of personality assessment. Cook and Campbell (1979) have pointed out that any single operational definition of a construct and any single method to measure that construct must necessarily be incomplete. That brings us to another reason why it has been hard for psychologists to embrace the importance of test integration. Test developers have suggested, albeit inadvertently, and test users have perhaps been too willing to assume that their scales measure the length and breadth of a construct. It's understandable that this would happen. How frequently are psychologists in clinical or forensic situations asked "Is he depressed?" or "Is he schizophrenic?" And how comforting it is to have an MMPI–2 Depression scale or a Rorschach Schizophrenia Index. The problem is that, despite their names, no single scale measures all the elements that comprise a broad construct like depression or schizophrenia.

It was for that reason that, when Exner (2003) revised the Schizophrenia Index, he also renamed it. It is no longer the Schizophrenia Index but rather the Perceptual Thinking Index. It is an index that provides information about the person's reality testing and about the presence of faulty logic and cognitive slippage. These are two important elements of schizophrenic spectrum disorders, but they are not the whole story. As an example, some of the elements that the MMPI–2 Scale 8 can provide (e.g., bizarre sensory experiences and difficulties with planning) allow us to provide a picture that more extensively represents the full scope of schizophrenic pathology.

Another example of the incremental validity that multimethod assessment can furnish, this time about the construct of dependency, comes from the work of Robert Bornstein. Bornstein (1998) asked male and female college students to complete a self-report, the Interpersonal Dependency Inventory, and he also gave them the Rorschach. He found that self-report measures tap what McClelland and his colleagues (1989) would have called self-attributed motives, or features that the individuals acknowledge as characteristic of their day-to-day function. On the other hand, Bornstein found that performance-based measures like the Rorschach tap what McClelland would have called implicit motives. These are features that affect behavior automatically and without the individuals having much awareness that their behavior is influenced by these components. Bornstein's findings replicated previous research in suggesting that, although women typically obtain higher scores than men on objective dependency measures, there are no significant gender differences on projective measures of this construct. This multimethod, "two-telescope" approach allows a more refined understanding, because it turns out that the "wavelength signature patterns" of men and women are different for dependency.

Up to this point, this chapter has highlighted the importance of multimethod approaches in general, and the examples used have come from the research, group-data literature. It will now be helpful to turn to the individual case, which is the context in which forensic psychologists work.

Single-method approaches place individuals at risk. Meyer and his colleagues (2001, p. 150) put it succinctly: "A single clinician using a single method (e.g., interview) to obtain information from a patient will develop an incomplete or biased understanding of the patient. To the extent that such impressions guide diagnostic and treatment decisions, patients will be misunderstood, mischaracterized, misdiagnosed, and less than optimally treated."

Given the unambiguous research findings, it seems clear that multimethod personality assessment should represent the standard of practice in forensic work with individuals. Meyer and his colleagues (2001) put it well when they wrote:

> Just as optimal research recognizes that any method of measurement and any single operational definition of a construct are incomplete, optimal clinical assessment should recognize that the same constraints exist when measuring phenomena in the life of a single person. Furthermore, just as effective research recognizes how validity is maximized when variables are measured by multiple methods, particularly when the methods produce meaningful discrepancies, the quality of individual assessment can be enhanced by clinicians who integrate the data from multiple methods of assessment. (p. 150)

This multimethod approach, which takes advantage of the agreements, disagreements, and unique contributions of multiple data sources, does best by forensic clients. The complexity they bring requires multitrait, multimethod approaches. No cardiologist would assess a person's cardiovascular function with just an electrocardiogram, and the issues forensic psychologists assess are at least as complex. Even when the referral question involves what seems to be a single issue, an approach that brings in cognitive, neuropsychological, and personality components expands our ability to provide a comprehensive picture. Within personality assessment, a multimethod approach to specific constructs such as depression or impulsivity insures that we come closer to assessing the full range of the construct. There can be little argument that such an approach represents an important standard for forensic psychology practice.

REFERENCES

Achenbach, T. M., McConaughy, S. H., & Howell, C. T. (1987). Child/adolescent behavioral and emotional problems: Implications of cross-informant correlations for situational specificity. *Psychological Bulletin, 101*, 213–232.

Archer, R. P., & Krishnamurthy, R. (1993). A review of MMPI and Rorschach interrelationships in adult samples. *Journal of Personality Assessment, 61*(2), 277–293.

Bornstein, R. F. (1998). Implicit and self-attributed dependency strivings: Differential relationships to laboratory and field measures of help seeking. *Journal of Personality and Social Psychology, 75*(1), 778–787.

Cook, T. D., & Campbell, D. T. (1979). *Quasi-experimentation: Design and analysis issues for field settings.* Boston: Houghton Mifflin.

Exner, J. E. (2003). *The Rorschach: A Comprehensive System* (4th ed.). New York: Wiley.

Hathaway, S. R., & McKinley, J. C. (1943). *The Minnesota Multiphasic Personality Inventory.* Minneapolis, MN: University of Minnesota Press.

Klopfer, B. (1956). *Developments in the Rorschach technique: Vol. II. Fields of application.* Oxford, England: World Book Co.

Mabe, P. A., & West, S. G. (1982). Validity of self-evaluation of ability: A review and meta-analysis. *Journal of Applied Psychology, 67*, 434–452.

McClelland, D. C., Doestner, R., & Weinberger, J. (1989). How do self-attributed and implicit motives differ? *Psychological Review, 96*, 690–702.

Meehl, P. E., & Hathaway, S. R. (1946). The *K* factor as a suppressor variable in the MMPI. *Journal of Applied Psychology, 30*, 525–564.

Meyer, G. J. (1996). The Rorschach and MMPI: Toward a more scientifically differentiated understanding of cross-method assessment. *Journal of Personality Assessment, 67*(3), 558–578.

Meyer, G. J. (1997). On the integration of personality assessment methods: The Rorschach and MMPI. *Journal of Personality Assessment, 68*(2), 297–330.

Meyer, G. J., Finn, S. E., Eyde, L. D., Kay, G. G., Moreland, K., Dies, R. R., et al. (2001). Psychological testing and psychological assessment. *American Psychologist, 56*(2), 128–165.

Morgan, C. D., & Murray, H. A. (1935). A method for investigating phantasies: The Thematic Apperception Test. *Archives of Neurology and Psychiatry, 34*, 289–306.

Rapaport, D., Gill, M., & Schafer, R. (1946). *Diagnostic psychological testing: The theory, statistical evaluation, and diagnostic application of a battery of tests* (Vol. 2). Chicago: Year Book Publishers.

Shneidman, E. S. (1956). Some relationships between the Rorschach technique and other psychodiagnostic tests. In B. Klopfer (Ed.), *Developments in the Rorschach technique: Vol. II, Fields of application.* Oxford, England: World Book.

A

THREE COMMENTARIES
ON "WHAT'S WRONG WITH THE RORSCHACH?"

Appendix A contains three critiques of "What's Wrong With the Rorschach?" The first two (Gacono & Evans, 2004; Martin, 2003) were invited book reviews; the third (Meloy, 2005) was a commentary.

Martin, E. H. (2003). Scientific critique or confirmation bias?: An analysis of "What's wrong with the Rorschach" by Wood, Nezworski, Lilienfeld, & Garb. *The National Psychologist, 121*(5), 19. Reprinted with permission.

Scientific Critique or Confirmation Bias?
by Hale Martin, PhD

"What Is Wrong With the Rorschach?" by James M. Wood, M. Teresa Nezworski, Scott O. Lilienfeld, and Howard N. Garb purports to be a scientific critique of the Rorschach. However, my hope to find an unbiased critical review of the Rorschach was disappointed. I found the book replete with thinking errors that led me to question the conclusions, if not the motives of the authors. Moreover, the authors' understanding of psychological assessment in general and of the role of the Rorschach in assessment is inadequate for the task they attempt in this book. Unintentionally, the book presents a powerful argument for more, not less, training in graduate schools in the Rorschach and psychological assessment.

Perhaps the most prevalent thinking error in the book is selective abstraction. The authors focus almost exclusively on negative findings without adequately considering positive results. For example, they focus extensively on the fact that approximately 70 studies included in John Exner's volumes are not peer reviewed and published in professional journals. They accurately conclude that some of these studies appear to contain flaws or are too sketchy to be critiqued. While this seems to be a valid criticism of some of Exner's work, the authors pay little attention to the 1,793 studies on the Rorschach published in peer review professional journals between 1977 and 1997 (identified by Hiller, Rosenthal, Bornstein, Berry, & Brunell-Neuleib, 1999). The fact is that there are many good peer reviewed studies of the Rorschach that contribute to its validity that the authors ignore. Similarly they frequently magnify facts that support their beliefs and minimize facts that contradict their beliefs.

Selective abstraction is also evident in their attack on Comprehensive System norms. The authors extol the sample reported by Shaffer, Erdberg, and Haroian in 1999, which they present as evidence that the current Comprehensive System norms overpathologize. However, they ignore the obvious flaws in the Shaffer, Erdberg, and Haroian study, such as collecting approximately two thirds of their "normal" sample from volunteer blood bank donors in California, small sample size ($n = 123$), and using graduate students in training for the critical test administration.

The authors of this book justifiably rail against the error discovered in 1999 (by a person "favorably disposed to the Rorschach") that 221 protocols included in the Comprehensive System norms were duplicates. No one could argue that this error was not an egregious one, but the authors fail to mention that when the error was corrected, the norms actually did not change much. They also ignore the fact the Rorschach Workshops has been carefully collecting a new normative sample (at last check $n = 350$) that generally supports the Comprehensive System norms that have been in use.

Arbitrary inference and overgeneralization are other thinking errors found throughout the book. In chapter 1, Wood presents the case of Rose Martelli, in which a psychologist allegedly relied solely on indicators from a Rorschach in the face of "manifest" information to the contrary to negatively impact the outcome of a custody case. As is commonly known among well-trained psychologists, no one test and certainly no one indicator provides sufficient information from which to draw firm conclusions. It is the pattern of scores within tests, the pattern of tests within batteries, and test results in context with all the diverse information that can be gathered that are central to any conclusions that can be drawn in an assessment. This principle is profoundly important to competent assessors. However, Wood inaccurately concludes the injustice that ensued was the fault of the Rorschach, not the psychologist conducting the assessment. He further overgeneralizes this instance to imply that this is how the Rorschach is typically used, and furthermore, implies that these miscarriages of justice based on the Rorschach are common.

Erroneous personalization is also apparent in the book. In chapter 11 the authors assume that Finn's 2002 Presidential address to the Society of Personality Assessment focused on the authors' attacks on the Rorschach. The speech actually focused on assessment in a managed care environment and not the Rorschach or the authors of this book. This personalization is one of several in the book that lead to significant distortions. Furthermore, the authors commit many of the errors they caution against in chapter 11, including the use of testimonials and anecdotes to support claims and falling victims to their own confirmation bias, among others. The result of all these thinking errors is a distorted and inaccurate analysis of the Rorschach, ironically in the name of science.

In general, the authors write as if there is some conspiracy by those "favorably disposed to the Rorschach" to inflate the reliability and validity of the Rorschach. The evidence seems to indicate otherwise. It has been those "favorably disposed to the Rorschach" that have discovered and published the errors the authors report in this book and that have welcomed debate in "their" journals about weaknesses in the Comprehensive System.

Finally, the authors include advice to attorneys in chapter 12 on how to circumvent the APA ethics code to get access to raw test data for use in court. I find this disturbing in that

I believe there are reasons for ethical principals, in this instance to protect assessment data from misuse by those who do not have the expertise to understand it. It seems to me irresponsible if not unethical to encourage others to disregard this concern.

In summary, this book does nothing to lead in a responsible direction. It is important to be critical of any scientific endeavor in order to keep it honest, but this book seems less of a scientific critique than strenuous confirmation bias. The book's arguments lead me to value competent training in the Rorschach and psychological assessment, training the authors of this book obviously missed.

Gacono, C. B., & Evans, F. B. (2004). Entertaining reading but not science: Book review of "What's wrong with the Rorschach?" *International Journal of Offender Therapy and Comparative Criminology, 48*(2), 253–257.

Entertaining Reading But Not Science

By Carl B. Gacono, PhD, and F. Barton Evans, PhD

James M. Wood, M. Teresa Nezworski, Scott O. Lilienfeld, and Howard N. Garb in "What's Wrong With the Rorschach?" provide a collection and rehashing of their critiques. While their zeal for protecting the public is undeniable, several critical caveats are necessary in order to interpret the information presented in "What's Wrong With the Rorschach?" First, like interpreting Rorschach results, the experienced Rorschach practitioner (those thoroughly familiar with the administration, interpretation, relevant research, have conducted their own research—as labeled by Wood et al. (p. 80), Klopfer's "limited number"—those truly proficient with the test) will gain the most from this text. This level of sophistication is necessary to separate scientific fact from Wood et al's frequent forays into fiction. Secondly, when reading "case or clinical examples" or other testimonials offered in this text, it is essential for the reader to differentiate between inherent structural weaknesses in the Rorschach and poor clinical practice (understand how tests are actually used in clinical practice, i.e. the problem of using one source of information for generating hypotheses, which should never be used in isolation). This essential differentiation is conspicuously missing from Wood et al's text. Consequently, examples of poor or even unethical clinical practice are used to denounce weaknesses in the psychometrics of the Rorschach, leaving the critical reader perplexed about why such obvious distinctions are not noted.

Thirdly, and related to clinical and forensic practice, an understanding of how personality tests (not just the Rorschach) are used is necessary to assess the Wood et al critique. Specifically, it is well known among competent practitioners that personality tests, while relevant to forming clinical and forensic opinions, never answer the ultimate clinical (suicidality, diagnosis) or forensic questions (competency, insanity, and so forth) by themselves. As stated by Gacono, Loving and Bodholdt (2001), "Psychological testing is helpful in formulating diagnosis and assessing dimensional aspects of syndromes but is seldom used as the sole measure for making a diagnosis" (2001, p. 24). The competent assessment psychologist understands that psychological assessment and the role of individual methods within it entails the use of a comprehensive and carefully chosen battery of psychological tests, interviews, collateral information, etc. Yet, for example, the authors of "What's Wrong With the Rorschach" use the failure of the Rorschach test to predict the ultimate success of aviation cadets as an indication of the inadequacy of the test itself (p. 164). This standard would be an inappropriate use of any single personality test including the MMPI–2, MCMI–III, PAI, and so forth, leaving the reader deeply puzzled about why Wood et al would use such a device to indict the test.

The fourth, and perhaps the most important issue, is that this "Rorschach" book is written by individuals who are not Rorschach, or even assessment, experts. This lack of expertise, we believe, directly impacts how issues are presented and discussed. The result is that "What's Wrong With the Rorschach?" is replete with plausible sounding criticisms that are in reality "straw person" arguments. This rhetorical device falls into two main categories: (1) Criticisms targeted toward the Rorschach that are actually examples of poor clinical or forensic practice, and (2) Criticisms of the Rorschach based on an inaccurate understanding of how the instrument is used (i.e., using sign approaches to diagnose rather than for describing dimensional aspects of personality; see Gacono, Loving, & Bodholdt, 2001; Gacono, Evans, & Viglione, 2002). For example, the straw person rhetoric is no more evident than in the authors' discussion of computing percent agreement for determining interrater reliability (pp. 227–228). The authors provide a method for computing interrater reliability and then indicate why it is faulty. While their presentation sounds and is plausible, it is based on a disquietingly inaccurate portrayal of how percent agreement is computed for Rorschach variables, which is methodologically completely and unequivocally erroneous! From a scientific perspective, what is disturbing about this example is that, even when presented with information to the contrary,[1] the authors have stuck with their inaccurate beliefs and continue to use them as a basis for supporting their arguments. It is equally disturbing that this example is not an isolated incident, but part of a larger pattern of misconception and inaccurate information.

Finally, "What's Wrong With the Rorschach" contains much blatantly inaccurate information. For example, in the study cited on page 251–252, the authors state, "… the same researcher who administered the Rorschach to prisoners also rated their levels of psychopathy. As we explained in Chapter Two such a procedure is vulnerable to confirmation bias, because the researchers' ratings of psychopathy may be unconsciously influenced by the Rorschach responses." While the study may have had methodological issues, the fact that in every case the PCL–R and ASPD diagnosis were completed prior to the Rorschach makes the authors' statement related to the influence on Rorschach responses impossible. It's hard to believe that Rorschach scores could influence a diagnosis that had already been made! On page 266 and elsewhere the authors refer to "Rorschach indicators of psychopathy" that have been disproven. These "indicators" were only representative of one constellation of variable for one sub-type of psychopathy. They were never meant to diagnose psychopathy, which is not even a diagnosis. As stated by Gacono & Meloy (2002): "Although the PCL–R alone suffices to determine the

---

[1]On page 228 they note that "Exner proceeded to explain how he calculated 'percentage agreement' (% correct), yet the authors dismissed it (also see Gacono, Meloy, & Bridges, 2000).

presence or absence of psychopathy, assessment generally involves more than arriving at a simple diagnosis (Gacono et al., 2001). Other personality instruments ... add to our clinical understanding of the ASPD diagnosed or psychopathic individual. These instruments were not specifically designed to 'diagnose' psychopathy, and not surprisingly fail to do so (Gacono et al., 2001). ... It is recommended that several other tests be employed to further delineate the behavioral and intrapsychic characteristics (dimensional aspects) of antisocial and psychopathic subjects" (p. 364).

Another incomprehensible inaccuracy stated in "What's Wrong With the Rorschach" includes using the dominance of Rorschachers in both the Society of Personality Assessment (SPA) and the Journal of Personality Assessment (JPA) to cast doubt on, or even dismiss, any research that originates from this group. Although both SPA and JPA originated from interest in the Rorschach, the complete dominance of Rorschachers in JPA or SPA is simply not factual. For example, in reviewing the three volumes comprising number 79 of JPA (2002), of the 28 articles not included as special issues (Number 2—"multicultural assessment teaching methods and competence evaluations") 5 included the Rorschach (one was not even a research study, another was a joint MMPI–2/Rorschach article), 8 the MMPI–2, 2 the PAI, 1 the Millon, 1 the Hand test, 1 the TAT, and the rest other (NEO and so forth). A similar trend has been reflected in both workshops and presentations at the SPA mid winter meetings. Additionally, the most recent president of SPA is Steve Finn, Ph.D. an internationally known expert on the MMPI–2, not the Rorschach. This "selective abstraction" (Martin, 2003) severely detracts from any scientific merit that might be attributed to this text. Given the authors' claim of a higher level of scientific acumen than the average Rorschacher, such disregard for factual evidence, the core value of science, is deeply troubling. As such, we recommend that, in reading "What's Wrong With the Rorschach?," each and every study cited by the authors must be carefully scrutinized for selective abstraction and bias to see if it is portrayed accurately. Perhaps, the following statement from the authors' article on clinical assessment in a recent *Annual Review of Psychology* give us some understanding of where their true biases lie: "It is interesting to imagine a time when psychologists may replace their Rorschach cards with a DNA kit and a pocket scanner" (Wood et al., 2002, p. 535).

However, given these above caveats, the experienced Rorschacher will still find this book to be useful and informative. Its strength lies in tracing the evolution of the test which is correctly anchored in the context of the development of clinical psychology (Chapters 2–6). In offering a chronology of the Rorschach's evolution, the authors accurately present many of the early weaknesses of the test, for example, the discrepancies among the systems and discounting the use of normative data for anchoring interpretation by some early Rorschach systems. The authors also accurately confirm the complexity of the test when they list the levels of experience required to use the test (p. 80). In quoting Klopfer they also correctly identify the use of the instrument as one that identifies dimensional aspects of personality that can only be interpreted within a configural context. Specifically, simple sign approaches to interpretation largely fail to capture the usefulness of any personality test. Specifically, not only are some traits situationally influenced, traits such as the Rorschach variable that is associated with anger can manifest differently within a given individual.

In tracing the history of the instrument the authors rightly cite Hertz as a voice of reason and share both Beck's and her concerns related to the over reliance on the test and their combined "voice of reason" related to the appropriate use of the instrument. This is indeed a legitimate criticism of some Rorschach practice (overinterpretation; stretching the test beyond what it can do), but not of inherent qualities of the test. Ironically, the authors themselves fall prey to inflating the Rorschach's worth. They use example after example of what amounts to poor clinical practice where the Rorschach is extended beyond its capabilities. It appears that they are not aware of the test's limitations based on a deep understanding of the underlying validity research.

The authors of "What's Wrong With the Rorschach" are also correct that there is no personality test that is an "X-ray of the mind," an unfortunate phase attributed to it by some of the earlier, though importantly not current, advocates of the Rorschach. This observation does not detract from the insights gained in classroom presentations of blind analysis. Some classroom techniques used by master clinicians to teach and educate should never be confused with actual clinical practice, where competent practitioners use of a comprehensive battery of tests including clinical interviewing and the use of collateral information. It is important to note though that the authors' informative review of the Rorschach's history in the 1940s, 1950s, and early 1960s does a good job tracing the evolution of the instrument, they do not provide an adequate base for critiquing the psychometric strengths and weaknesses of the test since the Comprehensive System (7 of the 12 chapters are devoted to the years prior to the Comprehensive System).

In summary, while "What's Wrong With the Rorschach?" provides a useful summary of their previously stated papers necessary these days for essential task of preparing Rorschachers for addressing its authors' criticisms of the test, it presents a surprisingly unbalanced and unscientific critique of the instrument given the authors' cry for greater scientific rigor for the Rorschach. It might have been more useful and scientific for the authors to succinctly outline both the instruments strengths and weaknesses. In failing to do so, the authors weaken or even negate the fact that some of their criticisms have merit and deserve further study. Unfortunately, the manner in which their information is presented will leave the reader with the task of sorting out the intellectual wheat from the unscientific and biased chaff. Perhaps one of the great ironies of "What's Wrong With the Rorschach?" is that the authors are acutely aware of the power of confirmation bias. As Wood et al (2003) state, "It's no big secret that people tend to notice and remember information that's consistent with their prejudices (p. 159)" and when discussing confirmation basis, "despite their PhDs, psychologists aren't immune to the biases we've discussed (p. 161)." While whether or not the current status of Rorschach rests on shaky grounds is never truly illuminated in this text, it is clear that logic behind many of the author's criticisms appears to firmly rest on the shifting sands of their own biases.

REFERENCES

Gacono, C. B. (2002). Introduction to a special series: Forensic psychodiagnostic testing. *Journal of Forensic Psychology Practice, 2*(3), 1–10.

Gacono, C. B., Evans, B., & Viglione, D. (2002). The Rorschach in forensic practice. *Journal of Foren-sic Psychology Practice, 2*(3), 33–53.

Gacono, C. B., Loving, J., & Bodholdt, R. (2001). The Rorschach and psychopathy: Toward a more accurate understanding of the research findings. *Journal of Personality Assessment, 77*(1), 16–38.

Gacono, C. B., & Meloy, J. R. (2002). Assessing antisocial and psychopathic personalities. In J. Butcher (Ed.), *Foundations of clinical personality assessment* (2nd ed.). Oxford University Press.

Gacono, C. B., Meloy, J. R., & Bridges, M. (2000). A Rorschach comparison of psychopaths, sexual homicide perpetrators, and nonviolent pedophiles: Where angels fear to tread. *Journal of Clinical Psychology, 56*(6), 757–777.

Martin, H. (2003). Scientific critique or confirmation bias? *National Psychologist, 121*(5), 19.

Meloy, J. R. (2005). Some reflections on "What's wrong with the Rorschach?" *Journal of Personality Assessment, 85*(3), 44–46.

Meloy, J. R., Acklin, M., Gacono, C. B., Peterson, C., & Murray, J. (1997). *Contemporary Rorschach interpretation.* Mahwah, NJ: Lawrence Erlbaum Associates.

Wood, J. M., Garb, H. N., Lilienfeld, S. O., & Nezworski, M. T. (2002). Clinical assessment. *Annual Review of Psychology, 53*, 519–543.

Some Reflections on *What's Wrong With the Rorschach?*

By J. Reid Meloy, PhD, ABPP, Department of Psychiatry,
University of California, San Diego

I have followed the most recent controversies concerning the Rorschach with a myriad of feelings, such as curiosity, annoyance, delight, and occasional trepidation. One of the most recurrent emotions I have felt was admiration at the statistical knowledge of some of the participants in this academic debate, a level of understanding I would like to eventually achieve.

My decision to not engage in this debate has most recently dissolved with a professional experience that I wish to share; one that may shed some light on a limited aspect of the controversy. I was retained as a Rorschach expert in a forensic matter involving the civil commitment of a "sexually violent predator" in the State of Washington (*In Re the Detention of John Robinson,* Yakima County Superior Court No. 97–2–03149–3). I subsequently gave a deposition in the case. My role was quite circumscribed, relatively straightforward, and focused upon the strength and limitations of the use of the Rorschach to understand the personality and psychology of the subject. Neither prosecution nor defense were advancing the belief that the Rorschach was designed as a risk assessment instrument, or that the test could determine whether or not the subject was a sexually violent predator. No competent professional would make such a claim.

In my preparation for both deposition and testimony, I submerged myself in the scientific articles relevant to the current controversies surrounding the reliability, validity, and norms of the test. A summary of the findings and opinions of these authors are widely available and do not warrant repetition here, and are likely well known to members of the Society for Personality Assessment and other psychologists who follow the literature. It was also suggested by the retaining attorney that I be familiar with a book he vaguely referred to as "The Trouble With the Rorschach." My search for this book led me to *What's Wrong With the Rorschach?* by James Wood, Teresa Nezworski, Scott Lilienfeld, and Howard Garb (2003). I purchased it and began to read.

When I open a technical or professional book for the first time, I test it in two ways: I read to see if I will learn something new, and I read to see if the authors accurately convey knowledge I already possess. The first question posed no difficulty, since I immediately learned something about the personality and psychology of James Wood, the first author, through a "blind analysis" of his own Rorschach in the first chapter. The only trouble with this new knowledge—which actually seemed a bit too private and somewhat bizarre—was its veracity: how could Dr. Wood "who was recently given the test" (p. 2) by an unidentified person produce a valid protocol when he arguably knows the test in exquisite detail, including all the structural ratios and indices?

But I did learn some new facts concerning the Rorschach's history if I continued to cast aside the trivialization in Wood et al.'s choice of words, e.g., "with impeccable timing, Klopfer launched his sales efforts in a market that was just beginning to expand" (p. 52)—what psychological test is not dependent on marketing for its economic success? I was also a bit troubled by some factual errors, such as the statement that David Levy was an "American psychologist" (p. 49). He was actually a psychiatrist. I was also continuously reminded of the bold red title of the book whenever I set it down or picked it up: What's Wrong With the Rorschach? I found the title quite ironic given Wood et al.'s important reminder that we all be sensitive to confirmatory bias: "the door to subjectivity, bias, and the common human tendency to find what one is expecting" (p. 45). It was clear that their book title advocated a certain point of view, rather than setting forth a balanced look at the Rorschach. Could this be commercial advocacy in the guise of science? Could I expect to find what's *right* with the Rorschach in a book with such a title? I read on, more certain of a likely motive to devalue on the part of the authors, but uncertain of their reasons to do so.

As the book's material became more contemporary, I began my second test: could the authors accurately convey knowledge to me that I already possessed? My first surprise came on p. 244: "Exner's former student Don Viglione argued that the Rorschach was useful for predicting new crimes by murderers and rapists." I personally know Don Viglione. I could not imagine him saying this. My shock prompted me to search for the footnote on p. 369, which led me to the actual reference on p. 410. I then looked at the referenced article. Here is what Dr. Viglione (1999) actually wrote,

> Taken together, the evidence suggests that Rorschach aggressive content within simplistic records from forensic evaluations may be a specific but not a very sensitive indicator of the potential for behavioral dyscontrol.

> Such was the case in a very impressive longitudinal, predictive field study (Rose & Bitter, 1980). The Palo Alto Destructive Content Scale, a scale encompassing general aggression but emphasizing the notion of victim and attack, predicted with a large effect size (Cohen's $d = 1.7, p < .002$) reoffense after release from prison in a group of rapists and murderers. Certainly, any extra tool to predict reoffense might be very useful (p. 258).

I did not suspect deliberate exaggeration, but I found it. This tremor, however, did not prepare me for the emotional jolt I was to experience when I read Wood et al.'s narrative concerning the research Carl Gacono and I conducted on various samples of antisocial children, adolescents, and adults beginning in 1985, much of it captured in our book, *The Rorschach Assessment of Aggressive and Psychopathic Personalities* (Gacono & Meloy, 1994). Wood et al. critiqued our work by selecting "for example" the relation between reflection responses and psychopathy to illustrate "a pattern distressingly common for the Rorschach," a lack of replication studies (p. 251). They then stated that "ten replication studies examined the relationship between reflection responses and psychopathy. Nine of the ten found no significant relationship" (p. 251).

Now suspicious of the accuracy and motivation of Wood et al., I once again searched the footnotes cited and the references. Here is what I found:

a. Of the ten studies, eight were doctoral dissertations that had never been peer reviewed and published in a scientific journal.
b. Not having immediate access to most of these dissertations, I did know one quite well. I had served on the dissertation committee of Murphy-Peaslee (1995) whom Wood et al. cite as one of the studies which found no significant relationship between psychopathic and nonpsychopathic subjects and their reflection responses. Dr. Murphy-Peaslee had only female inmates in her study, and did not have sufficient subjects that were psychopathic (PCL–R $\geq$ 30) to make such a comparison.
c. Wood et al. do acknowledge in a footnote (fn 136) that one study did find a significant difference (Loving & Russell, 2000). They failed to mention, however, that this was the only study that was submitted for publication, withstood peer review, and was published.
d. The tenth study appeared in a book chapter (Young, Justice, Erdberg & Gacono, 2000). Again, Wood et al. cite this as a nonsignificant finding. Knowing the authors, the study, and the book, I was dubious once again. My suspicions were well founded. Young et al. (2000) did not find a significant difference in the reflection responses of their psychopathic and nonpsychopathic subjects—the *p* value was nearly significant at .07—but they did find that the psychopaths produced three times as many reflection responses as the nonpsychopaths. Wood et al. do not mention this.

They then write, "similar negative findings were reported for the other 'psychopathic' Rorschach indicators identified by Gacono and Meloy" (p. 251). We, in fact, have never advocated the position that we had identified the Rorschach indicators of psychopathy, or a psychopathic constellation of scores, and have strongly cautioned against this. The sign approach to the Rorschach is not something we endorse, although Wood et al. seem to, and by inference suggest that we do too. Concerning our work with the reflection response, we wrote in 1990,

The mean (reflection) score for the severe psychopaths exceeded both the Exner nonpatient adults and outpatient character disordered groups, and the mean egocentricity score for the moderate psychopaths fell below all groups. Although this trend is consistent with our predictions, we suggest a conservative interpretation of this finding. Previous findings have failed to correlate level of psychopathy with the egocentricity ratio or degree of narcissism within an antisocial sample. (Gacono, Meloy, & Heaven, 1990, p. 275)

We further wrote in 1994,

> When interpreted within the context of the entire protocol, analysis of reflections provides information concerning the self-focusing process, the nature of the libidinal drive, internalized object relations, and the defensive use of grandiosity and withdrawal. We emphasize the context of the entire protocol since reflections should never be interpreted in isolation from other structural data, determinants, content, form quality, or psychodynamic content analysis. (Gacono & Meloy, 1994, p. 252)

In a similar vein, no one would interpret the Bizarre Sensory Experiences (BSE) scale as an indicator of schizophrenia in isolation from the other numerous relevant scales on the MMPI–2. Wood et al. finish their attack on our work by writing, "in any case, it now seems clear that Gacono and Meloy's findings are not replicable and that decisions made in forensic settings should not be informed by results from the Comprehensive System" (p. 252). They damn with distortions of detail, false imputation, and the construction of a straw man (Reflections indicate psychopathy!) which they then impale (No they don't!) to generally condemn the use of the entire CS system in a forensic setting.

Wood et al. appear to be quite familiar with our work, at least evident by the 12 citations to it in their book. I would have expected them to mention the CS Rorschach data that we generated on over 400 antisocial individuals—conduct disordered children, conduct disordered adolescents, antisocial personality disordered adult males and females, psychopathic adult males, sexual homicide perpetrators, antisocial schizophrenic males, and pedophiles—to be an important contribution toward the establishment of forensic norms for the instrument, something they desperately want to see. Not a word of these samples is mentioned in their book.

My selection of brief passages and references to explore in this book was not random and was both personally and professionally motivated. I have not meant this to be a comprehensive book review (Gacono & Evans, 2004; Martin, 2003). What I found, however, was quite disturbing. This is a tricky and crafty book which unfortunately sullies the scientific credibility of its authors. We generally trust scientists to accurately portray the findings upon which they base their opinions and conclusions. Wood et al. (2003) have sacrificed this trust at the altar of commercialism and confirmatory bias. I urge those who use the Rorschach in forensic evaluations and know the research, however, to be familiar with this book. The devil dwells in the details.

REFERENCES

Gacono, C. B., & Evans, B. (2004). Entertaining reading but not science: Book review of "What's wrong with the Rorschach?" *International Journal of Offender Therapy and Comparative Criminology, 48*, 253–257.

Gacono, C. B., & Meloy, J. R. (1994). *The Rorschach assessment of aggressive and psychopathic personalities*. Hillsdale, NJ: Lawrence Erlbaum Associates.

Gacono, C. B., Meloy, J. R., & Heaven, T. (1990). A Rorschach investigation of narcissism and hysteria in antisocial personality. *Journal of Personality Assessment, 55*, 270–279.

Loving, J., & Russell, W. (2000). Selected Rorschach variables of psychopathic juvenile offenders. *Journal of Personality Assessment, 75*, 126–142.

Martin, E. H. (2003). Scientific critique or confirmation bias?: An analysis of "What's wrong with the Rorschach?" by Wood, Nezworski, Lilienfeld & Garb. *The National Psychologist, 121*, 9.

Murphy-Peaslee, D. (1995). An investigation of incarcerated females: Rorschach indices and Psychopathy Checklist scores. *Dissertation Abstracts International, 56*, 0531B.

Rose, D., & Bitter, E. J. (1980). The Palo Alto Destructive Content Scale as a predictor of physical assaultiveness in men. *Journal of Personality Assessment, 44*, 228–233.

Viglione, D. (1999). A review of recent research addressing the utility of the Rorschach. *Psychological Assessment, 11*, 251–265.

Wood, J., Nezworski, M. T., Lilienfeld, S., & Garb, H. (2003). *What's wrong with the Rorschach?* San Francisco: Jossey-Bass.

Young, M., Justice, J., Erdberg, P., & Gacono, C. (2000). The incarcerated psychopath in psychiatric treatment: Management or treatment. In C. B. Gacono (Ed.), *The clinical and forensic assessment of pychopathy: A practitioner's guide* (pp. 313–331). Mahwah, NJ: Lawrence Erlbaum Associates.

AUTHOR INDEX

Schaye, N., 197, 198, *208*
Schaye-Glos, R., 197, 198, *208*
Scheid, T. L., 302, *319*
Schill, T., 182, *193*
Schiller, E., 422, *444*
Schinka, J. A., 271, *275*
Schlaes, J., 261, *273*
Schlesinger, L., 183, *193*
Schneider, R. B., 186, *192,* 332, *358,* 546, 547, 549, 550, 551, 553, 556, *558*
Schopp, R. F., 160, *173*
Schretlen, D., 24, *48*
Schretlen, D. J., 97, 100, 107, 108, *119,* 271, *276*
Schuerger, J. M., 25, *52*
Schultz, I. R., 261, *273*
Schumm, J. A., 267, *276*
Schutz, B. M., 234, 237, 239, 240, 244, 247, 249, 250, *254*
Schwartz, N. S., 9, *19*
Schwartz-Watts, D., 158, *171*
Schwarzwald, J., 261, *277*
Sciara, A., 3, 8, *20,* 56, *72,* 75, *77,* 214, *230,* 505, *525*
Sciara, A. D., 30, 32, 33, 38, *49,* 382, *391*
Sciara, T., *155,* 169, *173*
Scott, C., 158, *171*
Scott, H., 380, *392*
Scragg, P., 491, *502*
Scrivner, E. M., 530, 532, *541*
Scroppo, J. C., 264, 265, *276,* 495, *503*
Seamons, D. T., 68, *71,* 107, 116, *119*
Seelen, J., 56, *71,* 75, *77,* 245, *253*
Sellers, A. H., 271, *273*
Serafino, A., 527, 529, *541, 542*
Serafino, G., 527, 529, *541, 542*
Serin, R. C., 179, *193,* 380, *391*
Set, M. C., 380, *391*
Sewell, K., 179, *193,* 362, *378*
Sewell, K. W., 89, 94, *119,* 147, 148, *155,* 325, *359*
Shaffer, T., *19,* 31, 34, *51*
Shaffer, T. W., 31, 32, 34, 37, *49, 52,* 454, 455, 462, *463, 464, 559*
Shalev, A. Y., 258, *276*
Shalit, B., 263, *276*
Shapiro, D., 212, *232,* 328, *359,* 362, *378,* 528, *541*
Shapiro, D. L., 491, *503,* 506, *524*
Shapiro, E., 247, *253*
Shapiro, J. P., 265, *275,* 476, *486*
Share, M. C., *274*
Sharpe, J. P., 182, *193*
Shavzin, A. R., 107, *117*
Shaw, E. C., 176, *191*
Shectman, F., 505, *524*
Shedler, J., 4, 12, 13, *19*
Shenton, M., 165, 166, *170, 171, 172, 173*
Shenton, M. E., 259, *274*
Sheppard, K., 213, *231,* 326, *357,* 361, *377,* 383, *392*

Sherman, E. M. S., 91, *119*
Sherry, D., 63, *71*
Shevrin, H., 505, *524*
Shipley, S. L., 362, *378*
Shneidman, E. S., 561, *566*
Shrout, P. E., 9, *19,* 26, *52*
Shuman, D., 214, *231,* 508, *524,* 534, *540*
Shuman, D. W., 124, *137,* 161, *172,* 302, 310, *319,* 490, *502*
Shusman, E. J., 529, *540, 541*
Sidhu, L. S., 98, 104, *119*
Silbaugh, D., 362, 368, *377*
Silver, E., xiv, *xix,* 175, 178, 180, *193,* 213, 214, 230, *232*
Silver, R. J., 25, *52*
Simeon, D., 258, *274*
Sinday, S., 267, *277*
Sines, L. K., 25, *52*
Singer, H. K., 247, *254*
Singer, J., 445, 455, *463, 464*
Sion, M., 511, *524*
Skeem, J. L., 144, 150, 151, 152, *155,* 176, *190*
Skolnick, J. H., 534, 536, *541*
Slick, D. J., 91, *119*
Sloan, P., 266, *276,* 535, *541*
Slobogin, C., 121, *137,* 141, 142, 144, 145, 146, *154,* 157, 158, 159, 161, 162, 163, *172,* 196, 207, *208,* 212, 213, *232,* 489, 491, *503,* 528, *540*
Smith, A., 226, *232,* 372, *378,* 383, 385, *393*
Smith, A. M., 7, *19,* 328, 329, 331, *359*
Smith, B. L., 25, *51*
Smith, M., 166, *170*
Smith, R., 493, *503*
Smith, S., 167, *173*
Smith, S. R., 247, *254*
Smith, S. S., 362, *378*
Smith, W., 211, *232,* 536, *541*
Smoke, N., 165, *172*
Snooks, H., 237, *253*
Snowden, R. J., 179, 181, *191*
Solbogin, C., 421, 443, *444*
Solomon, Z., 258, 261, *276, 277*
Solovay, M., 165, 166, *171, 172, 173*
Sonnega, A., 256, *275*
Sorenson, S. B., 496, *502*
Souffrant, E., 475, *487*
Southwick, S. M., 257, 259, 260, *273, 276, 277*
Speth, E., 213, *231,* 326, *357,* 361, *377,* 383, *392*
Spinazola, J., 260, 267, *273*
Spinazzola, J., 204, *209,* 267, *277,* 473, *487*
Spitzer, R., 409, *420*
Sprock, J., 47, *52,* 248, *253*
Stacy, S., 505, *524, 525*
Stark, A. E. B., 491, *503*
Stattin, H., 46, *50*

Subject Index

A

Abel Assessment for Sexual Interest, 510
Abstraction responses, 328
Abusive Observation Behavior Checklist, 494
Accidental crime, battered woman syndrome and, 469, 470
Accommodations, for disability, 306
Achenbach Child Behavior Checklist, 564
Actuarial data, 188–189
Actuarial prediction, clinical *vs.,* 176–177
Actuarial risk assessment instruments, xvi
ADA. *See* Americans with Disabilities Act
ADEA. *See* Age Discrimination in Employment Act
Adjective, Rorschach used as, 84–85
Adjudication, forensic treatment evaluation at time of, 212
Adjudicative competence, 147
Administration, of Rorschach, 6, 63–64
Admissibility
    fitness for duty evaluations and, 534
    of psychological testimony, xv, 57–60
    of Rorschach findings, 10, 62–68, 75, 164, 538
Adolescents, conduct disordered, 7, 336–340
Affect cluster, 203–204, 214
    alterations in regulation of, 205
    in ASPD females, 340–341, 342
    in ASPD males, 344–345, 346
    in ASPD schizophrenics, 348, 349
    in bipolar outpatients, 432, 438
    in child custody litigants, 245–246, 450, 452–453, 456, 458
    Complex Posttraumatic Stress Disorder, 267
    in conduct disordered adolescents, 337, 338
    in conduct disordered children, 333, 334
    in female psychopaths, 363, 365
    in fitness to practice evaluations, 513, 516
    in paranoid schizophrenics, 427, 428
    in schizoaffective outpatients, 434–435, 439
    in sexual homicide perpetrators, 351, 352
    in undifferentiated/disorganized schizophrenics, 431, 436
Affective disorder, 247
Affective disregulation, trauma and, 258

Affective Ratio, 246, 264
Affective violence, 175, 219
Age Discrimination in Employment Act (ADEA), 282
Aggravation, death penalty and, 197
Aggression
    in antisocial personality disorder, 329–330, 345
    in conduct disordered adolescents, 340
    in conduct disordered children, 336
    extended aggression scores, 184–185, 186, 543–557
    in forensic outpatients, 442
    gender differences in, 374
    mental illness and, 175
Aggressive Content (AgC), 184, 185, 330, 544
    in child custody evaluation, 246
    combinations with *AgPast* and *AgPot,* 550–551
    interrater agreement for, 547
    PTSD and, 478
    research findings on, 552, 554, 556
    sexually violent subjects and, 552
    validity of, 546–549
Aggressive Content Scales, 15
Aggressive Movement (AG), 184–185, 330, 543–544
    in child custody evaluations, 245–246, 454
    frequency of, 545
    treatment response and, 215
Aggressive Past (AgPast), 184, 185, 330, 544, 556
    combinations with *AgC* and *AgPot,* 550–551
    interrater agreement for, 547
    sexual trauma and, 552
    validity of, 549–550
Aggressive Potential (AgPot), 184, 185, 330, 544, 553, 556
    combinations with *AgPast* and *AgC,* 550–551
    interrater agreement for, 547
    validity of, 550
Aggressive scores, 99, 101
Aggressive Vulnerability (AgV), 330, 544, 551
Albertsons, Inc. v. Kirkingburg, 304–305
Alcohol use, violence and, 175, 179
ALI. *See* American Law Institute
Alienated children, 461
Alliance, establishing in fitness to practice evaluations, 508